Clinical Skills
Documentation Guide for
Athletic Training

Second Edition

Clinical Skills Documentation Guide for
Athletic Training

Second Edition

HERB AMATO, DA, ATC
Associate Dean, Undergraduate Studies
James Madison University
Harrisonburg, Virginia

CHRISTY D. HAWKINS, MS, ATC
Director of Continuing and Professional Education
Thomas Nelson Community College
Hampton, Virginia

STEVEN L. COLE, MEd, ATC, CSCS
Assistant Athletic Director for Health Services
College of William and Mary
Williamsburg, Virginia

Delivering the best in health care information and education worldwide

www.slackbooks.com

ISBN 10: 1-55642-758-1
ISBN 13: 978-1-55642-758-9

The *Clinical Skills Documentation Guide for Athletic Training, Second Edition Instructor's Manual* is also available from SLACK Incorporated. Don't miss this important companion guide to the *Clinical Skills Documentation Guide for Athletic Training, Second Edition*. To obtain the instructor's manual, please visit http://www.efacultylounge.com

The procedures and practices described in this book should be implemented in a manner consistent with the professional standards set for the circumstances that apply in each specific situation. Every effort has been made to confirm the accuracy of the information presented and to correctly relate generally accepted practices. The authors, editor, and publisher cannot accept responsibility for errors or exclusions or for the outcome of the material presented herein. There is no expressed or implied warranty of this book or information imparted by it. Care has been taken to ensure that drug selection and dosages are in accordance with currently accepted/recommended practice. Due to continuing research, changes in government policy and regulations, and various effects of drug reactions and interactions, it is recommended that the reader carefully review all materials and literature provided for each drug, especially those that are new or not frequently used. Any review or mention of specific companies or products is not intended as an endorsement by the author or publisher.

SLACK Incorporated uses a review process to evaluate submitted material. Prior to publication, educators or clinicians provide important feedback on the content that we publish. We welcome feedback on this work.

Published by: SLACK Incorporated
                   6900 Grove Road
                   Thorofare, NJ 08086 USA
                   Telephone: 856-848-1000
                   Fax: 856-853-5991
                   www.slackbooks.com

Contact SLACK Incorporated for more information about other books in this field or about the availability of our books from distributors outside the United States.

Library of Congress Cataloging-in-Publication Data

Amato, Herb, 1956-
  Clinical skills documentation guide for athletic training / Herb Amato, Christy D. Hawkins, Steven L. Cole.-- 2nd ed.
     p. cm.
  Includes bibliographical references.
  ISBN-13: 978-1-55642-758-9 (softcover)
  ISBN-10: 1-55642-758-1 (softcover)
 1. Sports medicine. 2. Physical education and training. 3. Athletic trainers. I. Hawkins, Christy Venable, 1973- II. Cole, Steven L., 1954- III. Title.

RC1210.A434 2006
617.1'027--dc22

                              2006004602

Printed in the United States of America.

Last digit is print number: 10   9   8   7   6   5   4   3   2   1

Contents

Lower Quarter

Upper Quarter

Acknowledgments

Many thanks to our spouses, families, colleagues, and friends for their support in this endeavor. Special thanks to all the Certified Athletic Trainers who supervise Athletic Training Students.

We would also like to thank the following colleagues and students for their contributions with information gathering, reviewing, and editing. With their help, the second edition has been strengthened. They are: Jeff Konin, Steve Rathbone, Bridget McSorley, Jonathan "Andy" Carter, GM Pugh, Jason Hollar, Jessica Tanner, and Shannon Poplstein.

About the Authors

Herb Amato, DA, ATC was the Athletic Training Program Director for the past 18 years at James Madison University in Harrisonburg, Virginia. His current role at the University is an Associate Dean for Undergraduate Studies. He remains involved with Athletic Training Students in the classroom and with program/student assessment. He has been involved in the education of Athletic Training Students for 25 years at the university and high school levels. Herb has an extensive public speaking and consulting background and has published several articles in the areas of Athletic Training Education and clinical practice. He is also active in service at the community, university, and national levels.

Herb resides in Harrisonburg with his wife, Lori, and three daughters, Casey, Lyndy, and Jessy.

Christy D. Hawkins, MS, ATC is the Director of Continuing and Professional Education at Thomas Nelson Community College in Hampton, Virginia. In this position, she develops and implements educational programs for the local workforce. She also teaches health and physical education courses at the college. Since 1996, Christy has traveled to colleges and universities throughout the country as a workshop coordinator for Amato-Cole Educational Services (ACES Workshops). She has taught Athletic Training courses at the university level and has coordinated leisure classes for both children and adults. Christy received a Bachelor of Science degree from James Madison University and a Master of Science degree from the University of South Carolina. She is currently pursuing a second Master of Science degree focusing on adult education at Old Dominion University.

In her free time, Christy enjoys hiking and traveling, particularly to Alaska to visit her godchildren, Camille, Logan, and Elliot. She resides in Newport News with her husband, David, and three children from the animal kingdom, Jake, Autumn, and Timmie.

Steven L. Cole, MEd, ATC, CSCS is the Assistant Athletic Director for Health Services at the College of William and Mary, Williamsburg, Virginia. He oversees a staff of seven Certified Athletic Trainers and coordinates a regional network of health care specialists to provide athletic health care for nearly 600 student-athletes annually. In addition to his local role with the college, he coordinates an on-site sports medicine program for Busch Entertainment Corporation in Williamsburg, aimed at educating entertainers in the early recognition and self-management of common injuries. Steve is one of the cofounders of the ACES Preparatory Workshops for Athletic Training Students who are eligible to sit for the Board of Certification exam.

Steve has served as a consultant to various athletic programs, medical practices, and industrial corporations. He is the sports medicine consultant to Tidewater Physical Therapy Inc, a group of outpatient physical therapy clinics serving the Tidewater area of Virginia. He has extensive public speaking and consulting experience, from local to international, and has published several articles relevant to athletic health care and the administration of health care programs. Steve is a member of the Virginia High School League Sports Medicine Advisory Committee, the Legislative Committee for the Virginia Athletic Trainers' Association, and the Athletic Training Liaison to the Colonial Athletic Association.

A competitive triathlete, Steve resides in Williamsburg with his wife, Lonna, and two daughters, Sydney and Jahnessa.

Introduction

The purpose of this book is to provide the Athletic Training Student and Athletic Training Educator with a reference that focuses on clinical skills. This guidebook was written with both audiences in mind. The Athletic Training Student working toward Board of Certification (BOC) as an entry-level professional will find this book useful as both a learning tool and a study guide. As a learning tool, students may take notes on the individual skill sheets while listening to the instructor or reading from a reference text. As the student learns these practical skills in the classroom or clinical environment, this book can be used as a guide for practicing, with the final goal being mastery. As the student reviews skills acquired throughout the clinical experience in preparation for cognitive skills, clinical decision-making, and the practical skills application integration of the BOC certification exam, he or she can use this book as a study guide and evaluation tool. References and supplies needed are listed on each skill sheet. These tips allow the student to focus on the task at hand, rather than wasting time figuring out what is needed or where to find additional information.

The Athletic Training Educator or Approved Clinical Instructor (ACI) in an Athletic Training Education Program will also find this guide useful both in documenting student mastery of individual psychomotor skills and in helping students prepare for the interactive portion of the BOC exam. Since an ACI is responsible for formal instruction and evaluation of clinical proficiencies, this book is designed to serve as a documentation tool for the initial step of Learning-Over-Time. The building blocks of clinical proficiency are the individual skills. An example of a clinical proficiency may be the evaluation of the injured knee of a 17-year-old soccer player. There are numerous psychomotor skills needed in order to successfully evaluate that soccer player's knee.

In verifying student readiness to take the certification exam, the BOC no longer requires the logging of clinical hours. Instead, the BOC requires all candidates to graduate from an accredited undergraduate or entry-level master Athletic Training Education Program. Formal documentation of students' learning of specific clinical proficiencies over time is required as part of the accreditation process. Thus, the ACI must document when a skill/proficiency is taught, practiced, tested, and retested to verify student learning. The concept of Learning-Over-Time views clinical proficiency as the "big picture"; however, each of the proficiencies has many subsets or psychomotor skills. This guidebook is designed with documentation requirements in mind. It provides a suitable format for recording individual skills that may be used as part of a student's portfolio to record the mastery of proficiencies.

Additionally, this book is formatted to record a student's progress in mastering psychomotor skills; therefore, it provides a history of that student's clinical strengths and weaknesses. The ACI can then review that history to prepare a study plan with the student. With the knowledge of the student's clinical strengths and weaknesses, the educator is better prepared to assist the student in exam preparation and entry into the Athletic Training Profession.

SECTION ONE

I

INTRODUCTION

Chapter 1

OVERVIEW OF THE BOARD OF CERTIFICATION EXAMINATION

In 1969, the National Athletic Trainers' Association (NATA) developed an examination to certify entry-level professionals. A function of any certification examination is to demonstrate to the public that an individual is qualified to perform specific duties without causing harm. The first certification exam included two sections: a written portion and an oral/practical portion. While the written portion of the exam strived to test the candidate's basic knowledge of Athletic Training domains, the oral/practical portion of the examination sought to test the clinical skills of the candidate.

The candidate was asked to complete skills in four categories (taping/wrapping, evaluation, rehabilitation, and emergency management) within a given time frame. Examples included asking the candidate to explain and demonstrate his or her ability to tape an ankle, evaluate a shoulder, construct a rehabilitation program for an MCL sprain, or manage an athlete suspected of heat illness. While the intent of the oral/practical portion of the exam was to evaluate the clinical skills of a candidate, there was much concern over the discrepancy between what was "explained" and what was "demonstrated."

Every 5 years, a *Role Delineation Study* is conducted as the initial step in updating the Board of Certification (BOC) exam. The first step in this process is for the BOC to appoint a committee of subject matter experts. Through their work, performance domains for the practice of Athletic Training are defined. These performance domains are further broken down into tasks, knowledge areas, and skill abilities expected of a professional working in the field of Athletic Training.

The *Role Delineation Study*, published in 1994, led to changes in the design of the certification exam. The domain and task areas shifted from the previous study, which led to a different configuration of the written exam. The oral/practical portion of the exam was eliminated, giving rise to the current "practical exam."

With the changes to the practical exam came an emphasis on the demonstration of *psychomotor skills*, rather than the explanation of a skill. Psychomotor skills are "physical activities associated with mental processes." In other words, candidates must apply their knowledge of Athletic Training skills by demonstrating those skills during the practical portion of the exam. The key term here is "demonstrate." Candidates are no longer asked to explain and demonstrate, and candidates' verbal explanations are no longer taken into account when scoring the practical exam.

The fifth edition of the BOC *Role Delineation Study* was published in 2004 with minimal changes to the Domain Areas. The domain areas are as follows:

1. Prevention
2. Clinical Evaluation and Diagnosis
3. Immediate Care
4. Treatment, Rehabilitation, and Reconditioning
5. Organization and Administration
6. Professional Responsibility

A goal of the BOC Role Delineation Study is to set the minimum standards for entry into the Athletic Training Profession. This document establishes the blueprint for the BOC examination and will impact all Athletic Training students taking the BOC exam after April 2006.

The BOC announced that the certification exam will transition to a Computer-Based Exam (CBE). The three sections of the current exam (Written, Practical, and Written Simulation) will be phased out and integrated into one exam delivered by computer testing. The format of the CBE will evaluate Athletic Training Students in areas pertaining to cognitive skills, clinical decision-making, and practical skill application.

It is important for exam candidates, Program Directors, classroom faculty, and clinical instructors to continually seek current guidelines of the format and requirements of the BOC exam. The best source for current information may be found by accessing the BOC website (www.bocatc. org). The following links are most helpful:

- http://www.bocatc.org/resources/EXREDESIGN
- http://www.bocate.org/becomeatc/CANDIDATE (Candidate's Handbook)
- http://www.bocatc.org/becomeatc/SELF

Knowledge of the current format prevents surprises during the exam and helps lower stress levels on what is already a very stressful day.

How to Use This Book

Clinical Skill Assessments

Skill assessments comprise the majority of this book. They are organized into general categories. For the most part, skill assessments are specific outcomes or psychomotor skills listed as part of the Athletic Training Clinical Proficiencies within the *NATA Athletic Educational Competencies* (1999). The majority of the individual psychomotor skills contained herein are deemed necessary or useful for the successful performance of Athletic Training clinical proficiencies. These skills are used in the day-to-day duties of Athletic Training Students (ATS) as they progress toward mastering clinical proficiencies.

To gain the most from this practical exam guide, Athletic Training Students, and the Approved Clinical Instructor (ACI) should review the following instructions on how to use the skill assessments (Figure 2-1). Each skill assessment is divided into five sections:

A. Introduction of the specific psychomotor skill

B. Score sheet of the specific tasks that comprise the skill

C. Evaluation box

D. Scale of skill mastery

E. Information and supplies needed to demonstrate the skill

The individual components of each section will be further dissected and explained so that both the ATS and the ACI can gain maximum benefits from this guide.

Introduction of a Specific Psychomotor Skill

The introduction of a specific psychomotor skill is the first part of each skill assessment. This section focuses on the ATS's initial exposure to the skill. It also provides spaces to record peer review of the skill and the dates of practice opportunities prior to testing.

The middle of the top portion of the page, Figure 2-1 identifies the skill assessment classification by the place and unit in the study guide. Thus, in Figure 2-1A, the title of the unit and the number of the test within that unit are indicated. *Sensory Testing* is the title of the unit, therefore SST-L-Test 1 identifies this skill assessment as being the first test for the lower extremity.

The remaining components of this section allow the student and the ACI to record exposure to and practice sessions of the skill. The spaces marked *Peer Review* should be initialed and dated by a peer who observes the skill being performed. The number of peer reviews may be increased or decreased depending on the difficulty of the skill and the amount of practice the instructor requires prior to testing. It should also be made clear that peer reviews are not part of the formal documentation for Learning Over Time. Peer reviews should serve as learning tools.

Skill Acquisition refers to the student's initial exposure to the skill. Thus, this space should be completed with the class number (eg, AT 206) and the date the skill was introduced. The space marked *Practice Opportunities* allows for documentation of the structured opportunities by the student to practice the skill under the supervision of an instructor.

The Score Sheet for the Specific Tasks That Comprise a Skill

The score sheet for the specific tasks that comprise a skill (Figure 2-1B) opens with an explanation of the skill the student is being asked to perform. Following the ini-

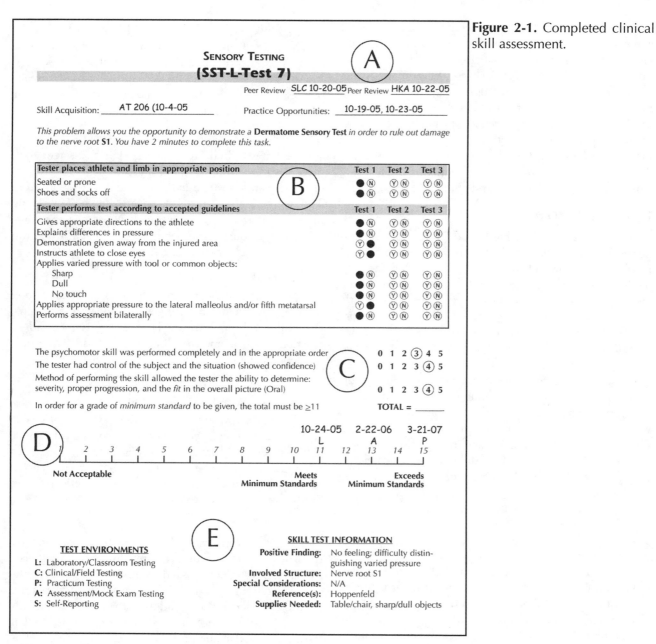

Figure 2-1. Completed clinical skill assessment.

tial statement of the skill, each individual task that contributes to that skill is listed. Blank circles, labeled *Y* or *N* (for yes and no), are provided next to each component of the skill. A response of *yes* indicates that the component of the skill was performed correctly. A negative response indicates that the component of the skill was either performed incorrectly or not at all. Note that the skill assessments in this section of the text are not weighted.

The correct responses for each *yes* or *no* section are objective; however, unless the instructor weights each response, the final score is somewhat subjective. The tester may choose to use different colored markers and/or use the corresponding letters of the method for testing (*L, C,*

P, A, or S) in order to document which circle was checked at a specific interval. The observed responses should be the same, whether they are checked by a peer or by a clinical instructor. However, the level set for mastery is subjective and should be determined by the ACI. For a student preparing for entry into the Athletic Training profession, the goal for mastery should be 100%. The student should strive to have as many *yes* boxes checked as possible.

This section (Figure 2-1B) may be used during the instruction, practice, or testing of a skill. During instruction, the student may use this score sheet, along with note-taking from class and review of other recommended references, to learn the skill. Each score sheet was developed using one or more references. However, total agreement between references does not occur in all cases, and for the purposes of this book, when disagreements occurred between the references, a decision was made based on the author's knowledge. Very few score sheets have 100% agreement of multiple sources. It is important to understand that all references do not say the same thing. This fact may be frustrating to a young professional. However, when disagreements between references occur, discussion of these differences can enhance the learning experience between students and clinical instructors.

EVALUATION BOX

The evaluation box (Figure 2-1C) begins to incorporate the individual psychomotor skills into the larger picture of the clinical proficiency. The higher the subjective score given, the greater the understanding of the overall skill. The first line of the evaluation box is directly related to the number of *yes* and *no* checks on the score sheet. The second line indicates the tester's confidence level in performing the skill. The third line is determined by verbal communication between the evaluator and the Athletic Training Student. This communication occurs in a series of questions to determine whether the student understands the purpose of the skill being tested and where it fits into a clinical proficiency. The minimum standard score of 11 or higher is arbitrary; however, it does represent 73% of the total possible points. This section can play a beginning role in documenting the Learning Over Time concept.

SCALE OF SKILL MASTERY

This section is designed to monitor the dates and methods used by the ACI when evaluation occurs. Figure 2-1D indicates that a student was tested three times over a 17-month period. In this example, the first testing situation was in a laboratory environment on 10-24-05. The placement of the *L* indicates that the score from the evaluation box meets minimum standards and was administered in a laboratory or classroom environment. The second test of the same skill occurred the following semester during program assessment. The placement of the A has moved closer to exceeding minimum standards. The final test date (3-21-07) indicates that the student was tested a year later in a practicum class and scored very well, based on the placement of the "P."

The letters *L*, *C*, *P*, *A*, and *S* are used to indicate the environment in which the skill assessment took place. While the following information indicates the authors' definitions for using these environmental indicators, these indicators may be adjusted to fit the testing methods used in individual Athletic Training Education Programs.

L: Laboratory or Classroom Testing

The letter *L* indicates that the skill assessment took place during a structured laboratory or classroom setting. These testing sessions may include formal lab tests, breakout sessions where testing occurs, or written exams that include practical testing.

C: Clinical/Field Testing

The letter *C* indicates that the skill assessment took place in the Athletic Training room, clinical setting, or on the athletic field and was performed by an ACI. This method of testing is based around the "teachable moment." Practice occurs during down-time in the clinical setting or during the observation of a skill when the student is actually performing it.

P: Practicum Testing

The letter *P* indicates that the skill assessment took place during scheduled testing at least one semester after the skill has been learned. This testing is included in practicum courses and the clinical packet associated with a practicum course.

A: Assessment/Mock Exam Testing

The letter *A* indicates that skill the assessment took place during assessment testing. This type of testing evaluates the same skill sets year after year. Program assessment gives students a baseline of strengths and weaknesses relative to their own performance in the previous year, to peers in the same class, and to previous Athletic Training Students in the same program.

S: Self-Reporting

The letter *S* indicates that the skill assessment took place when the student evaluated him- or herself. For example, if a student is asked whether he or she is confident in performing a specific skill and the answer is no, additional practice time is allotted to that student. This means of testing is not used as a replacement for formal testing or for documenting Learning Over Time but is helpful in finding weaknesses of the curriculum and of the individual student.

ADDITIONAL INFORMATION

Finally, valuable information (Figure 2-1E) to assist the student and ACI in finding additional reading material on the skill assessment can be found on the bottom right corner of the page. This area includes the following information: positive finding or purpose of the skill, the structures being assessed, special considerations unique to the skill assessment, the primary reference book(s) used in developing the score sheet, and any supplies needed for the student to perform the skill.

SECTION TWO

II

PRACTICAL SKILL ASSESSMENTS

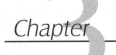

Chapter 3

AMBULATION ASSISTS/ MISCELLANEOUS

AMBULATION ASSISTS/MISCELLANEOUS
(AA-Test 1)

Peer Review_____   Peer Review _____

Skill Acquisition: _____   Practice Opportunities: _____

This problem allows you the opportunity to demonstrate **crutch fitting** *for an athlete. You have 4 minutes to complete this task.*

Tester places athlete and limb in appropriate position	Test 1	Test 2	Test 3
Standing with good posture	Ⓨ Ⓝ	Ⓨ Ⓝ	Ⓨ Ⓝ
Feet shoulder width apart	Ⓨ Ⓝ	Ⓨ Ⓝ	Ⓨ Ⓝ
Wearing low-heeled/flat shoes	Ⓨ Ⓝ	Ⓨ Ⓝ	Ⓨ Ⓝ
Tester measures athlete for ambulation device	**Test 1**	**Test 2**	**Test 3**
Places crutch slightly in front of the involved limb (2 to 4 inches)	Ⓨ Ⓝ	Ⓨ Ⓝ	Ⓨ Ⓝ
Places crutch slightly to the side of the involved limb (4 to 6 inches)	Ⓨ Ⓝ	Ⓨ Ⓝ	Ⓨ Ⓝ
Places axillary pad approximately 1 to 1.5 inches below axilla	Ⓨ Ⓝ	Ⓨ Ⓝ	Ⓨ Ⓝ
Places elbow in approximately 30 degrees flexion	Ⓨ Ⓝ	Ⓨ Ⓝ	Ⓨ Ⓝ
Tester checks ambulatory device for safety	**Test 1**	**Test 2**	**Test 3**
Tightens all fasteners	Ⓨ Ⓝ	Ⓨ Ⓝ	Ⓨ Ⓝ
Verifies axilla and hand grips are well-padded	Ⓨ Ⓝ	Ⓨ Ⓝ	Ⓨ Ⓝ
Verifies that rubberized tips are not damaged	Ⓨ Ⓝ	Ⓨ Ⓝ	Ⓨ Ⓝ
Instructs athlete to bear weight on hands, not axilla	Ⓨ Ⓝ	Ⓨ Ⓝ	Ⓨ Ⓝ

The psychomotor skill was performed completely and in the appropriate order   **0 1 2 3 4 5**

The tester had control of the subject and the situation (showed confidence)   **0 1 2 3 4 5**

Method of performing the skill allowed the tester the ability to determine:
severity, proper progression, and the *fit* in the overall picture (Oral)   **0 1 2 3 4 5**

In order for a grade of *minimum standard* to be given, the total must be ≥11   **TOTAL = _____**

1	2	3	4	5	6	7	8	9	10	11	12	13	14	15

Not Acceptable   **Meets**   **Exceeds**
                          Minimum Standards   **Minimum Standards**

TEST ENVIRONMENTS

L: Laboratory/Classroom Testing
C: Clinical/Field Testing
P: Practicum Testing
A: Assessment/Mock Exam Testing
S: Self-Reporting

SKILL TEST INFORMATION

Positive Finding:	N/A
Involved Structure:	N/A
Special Considerations:	Hand grips should be at the level of the greater trochanter
Reference(s):	Anderson et al; Houglum; Prentice (2003)
Supplies Needed:	Crutches of various sizes

AMBULATION ASSISTS/MISCELLANEOUS
(AA-Test 2)

Peer Review_____   Peer Review _____

Skill Acquisition: _____   Practice Opportunities: _____

This problem allows you the opportunity to instruct an athlete in the **nonweightbearing—tripod** *method of crutch walking. You have 4 minutes to complete this task*

Tester places athlete and limb in appropriate position	Test 1	Test 2	Test 3
Standing with good posture	Y N	Y N	Y N
Feet shoulder width apart	Y N	Y N	Y N
Wearing low-heeled/flat shoes	Y N	Y N	Y N
Tester verifies correct fit of ambulation device	**Test 1**	**Test 2**	**Test 3**
Places crutch slightly in front of the involved limb (2 to 4 inches)	Y N	Y N	Y N
Places crutch slightly to the side of the involved limb (4 to 6 inches)	Y N	Y N	Y N
Places axillary pad approximately 1 to 1.5 inches below axilla	Y N	Y N	Y N
Places elbow in approximately 30 degrees flexion	Y N	Y N	Y N
Tester instructs athlete in walking with ambulatory device	**Test 1**	**Test 2**	**Test 3**
Weight evenly distributed on crutches	Y N	Y N	Y N
Instructs athlete not put weight on axilla	Y N	Y N	Y N
Involved limb is off the floor (flexed position)	Y N	Y N	Y N
Athlete moves both crutches forward (6 to 8 inches)	Y N	Y N	Y N
Athlete swings the noninjured limb forward (swing-to) or (swing-through)	Y N	Y N	Y N
Repeat the above two steps	Y N	Y N	Y N

The psychomotor skill was performed completely and in the appropriate order   **0 1 2 3 4 5**

The tester had control of the subject and the situation (showed confidence)   **0 1 2 3 4 5**

Method of performing the skill allowed the tester the ability to determine:
severity, proper progression, and the *fit* in the overall picture (Oral)   **0 1 2 3 4 5**

In order for a grade of *minimum standard* to be given, the total must be ≥11   **TOTAL = _____**

```
1    2    3    4    5    6    7    8    9    10   11   12   13   14   15
|    |    |    |    |    |    |    |    |    |    |    |    |    |    |
```

Not Acceptable   **Meets**   **Exceeds**
                                    Minimum Standards   **Minimum Standards**

TEST ENVIRONMENTS

L: Laboratory/Classroom Testing
C: Clinical/Field Testing
P: Practicum Testing
A: Assessment/Mock Exam Testing
S: Self-Reporting

SKILL TEST INFORMATION

Positive Finding: N/A
Involved Structure: N/A
Special Considerations: N/A
Reference(s): Anderson et al
Supplies Needed: Crutches of various sizes

AMBULATION ASSISTS/MISCELLANEOUS
(AA-Test 3)

Peer Review_____   Peer Review _____

Skill Acquisition: _____   Practice Opportunities: _____

This problem allows you the opportunity to instruct an athlete in the **nonweightbearing—ascending and descending stairs (without a handrail)** *method of crutch walking. You have 4 minutes to complete this task.*

Tester places athlete and limb in appropriate position	Test 1	Test 2	Test 3
Standing with good posture	Ⓨ Ⓝ	Ⓨ Ⓝ	Ⓨ Ⓝ
Feet shoulder width apart	Ⓨ Ⓝ	Ⓨ Ⓝ	Ⓨ Ⓝ
Wearing low-heeled/flat shoes	Ⓨ Ⓝ	Ⓨ Ⓝ	Ⓨ Ⓝ
Tester verifies correct fit of ambulation device	**Test 1**	**Test 2**	**Test 3**
Places crutch slightly in front of the involved limb (2 to 4 inches)	Ⓨ Ⓝ	Ⓨ Ⓝ	Ⓨ Ⓝ
Places crutch slightly to the side of the involved limb (4 to 6 inches)	Ⓨ Ⓝ	Ⓨ Ⓝ	Ⓨ Ⓝ
Places axillary pad approximately 1 to 1.5 inches below axilla	Ⓨ Ⓝ	Ⓨ Ⓝ	Ⓨ Ⓝ
Places elbow in approximately 30 degrees flexion	Ⓨ Ⓝ	Ⓨ Ⓝ	Ⓨ Ⓝ
Tester instructs athlete in ascending stairs	**Test 1**	**Test 2**	**Test 3**
Weight evenly distributed on crutches	Ⓨ Ⓝ	Ⓨ Ⓝ	Ⓨ Ⓝ
Athlete steps up with uninjured leg	Ⓨ Ⓝ	Ⓨ Ⓝ	Ⓨ Ⓝ
Athlete follows with injured leg and crutches	Ⓨ Ⓝ	Ⓨ Ⓝ	Ⓨ Ⓝ
Tester instructs athlete in descending stairs	Ⓨ Ⓝ	Ⓨ Ⓝ	Ⓨ Ⓝ
Weight evenly distributed on crutches	Ⓨ Ⓝ	Ⓨ Ⓝ	Ⓨ Ⓝ
Athlete steps down with injured leg and crutches	Ⓨ Ⓝ	Ⓨ Ⓝ	Ⓨ Ⓝ
Athlete follows with uninjured leg	Ⓨ Ⓝ	Ⓨ Ⓝ	Ⓨ Ⓝ

The psychomotor skill was performed completely and in the appropriate order   0 1 2 3 4 5

The tester had control of the subject and the situation (showed confidence)   0 1 2 3 4 5

Method of performing the skill allowed the tester the ability to determine:
severity, proper progression, and the *fit* in the overall picture (Oral)   0 1 2 3 4 5

In order for a grade of *minimum standard* to be given, the total must be ≥11   TOTAL = _____

```
 1    2    3    4    5    6    7    8    9   10   11   12   13   14   15
 |____|____|____|____|____|____|____|____|____|____|____|____|____|____|
```

Not Acceptable   **Meets**   **Exceeds**
                            Minimum Standards   **Minimum Standards**

TEST ENVIRONMENTS

L: Laboratory/Classroom Testing
C: Clinical/Field Testing
P: Practicum Testing
A: Assessment/Mock Exam Testing
S: Self-Reporting

SKILL TEST INFORMATION

Positive Finding: N/A
Involved Structure: N/A
Special Considerations: If available, may use handrail (see references)
Reference(s):   Anderson et al; Houglum; Prentice (2003)
Supplies Needed: Crutches of various sizes

AMBULATION ASSISTS/MISCELLANEOUS
(AA-Test 4)

Peer Review_____   Peer Review _____

Skill Acquisition: _____   Practice Opportunities: _____

This problem allows you the opportunity to demonstrate **cane fitting** *for an athlete. This should include instruction on walking with a cane. You have 2 minutes to complete this task.*

Tester places athlete and limb in appropriate position	Test 1	Test 2	Test 3
Standing with good posture	Ⓨ Ⓝ	Ⓨ Ⓝ	Ⓨ Ⓝ
Feet shoulder width apart	Ⓨ Ⓝ	Ⓨ Ⓝ	Ⓨ Ⓝ
Wearing low-heeled/flat shoes	Ⓨ Ⓝ	Ⓨ Ⓝ	Ⓨ Ⓝ
Tester measures athlete for ambulation device	**Test 1**	**Test 2**	**Test 3**
Measure from greater trochanter of femur to the floor	Ⓨ Ⓝ	Ⓨ Ⓝ	Ⓨ Ⓝ
Adjust cane to the measured length	Ⓨ Ⓝ	Ⓨ Ⓝ	Ⓨ Ⓝ
Tester instructs athlete in walking with ambulatory device	**Test 1**	**Test 2**	**Test 3**
Cane is placed on uninjured side	Ⓨ Ⓝ	Ⓨ Ⓝ	Ⓨ Ⓝ
Athlete steps forward with cane and injured leg	Ⓨ Ⓝ	Ⓨ Ⓝ	Ⓨ Ⓝ
Athlete follows with uninjured leg	Ⓨ Ⓝ	Ⓨ Ⓝ	Ⓨ Ⓝ

The psychomotor skill was performed completely and in the appropriate order   0 1 2 3 4 5

The tester had control of the subject and the situation (showed confidence)   0 1 2 3 4 5

Method of performing the skill allowed the tester the ability to determine:
severity, proper progression, and the *fit* in the overall picture (Oral)   0 1 2 3 4 5

In order for a grade of *minimum standard* to be given, the total must be ≥11   TOTAL = _____

```
  1     2     3     4     5     6     7     8     9     10    11    12    13    14    15
  |     |     |     |     |     |     |     |     |     |     |     |     |     |     |
```

Not Acceptable   **Meets**   **Exceeds**
                              Minimum Standards   **Minimum Standards**

TEST ENVIRONMENTS

L: Laboratory/Classroom Testing
C: Clinical/Field Testing
P: Practicum Testing
A: Assessment/Mock Exam Testing
S: Self-Reporting

SKILL TEST INFORMATION

Positive Finding:	N/A
Involved Structure:	N/A
Special Considerations:	Instruct not to lean heavily on the cane (same instructions for the use of one crutch)
Reference(s):	Anderson et al; Houglum; Prentice (2003)
Supplies Needed:	Canes of various sizes, measuring device

AMBULATION ASSISTS/MISCELLANEOUS
(AA-Test 5)

Peer Review_____   Peer Review _____

Skill Acquisition: _____   Practice Opportunities: _____

*This problem allows you the opportunity to instruct an athlete in the **four-point gait method** of crutch walking. You have 4 minutes to complete this task.*

Tester places athlete and limb in appropriate position	Test 1	Test 2	Test 3
Standing with good posture	Ⓨ Ⓝ	Ⓨ Ⓝ	Ⓨ Ⓝ
Feet shoulder width apart	Ⓨ Ⓝ	Ⓨ Ⓝ	Ⓨ Ⓝ
Wearing low-heeled/flat shoes	Ⓨ Ⓝ	Ⓨ Ⓝ	Ⓨ Ⓝ
Tester verifies correct fit of ambulation device	**Test 1**	**Test 2**	**Test 3**
Places crutch slightly in front of the involved limb (2 to 4 inches)	Ⓨ Ⓝ	Ⓨ Ⓝ	Ⓨ Ⓝ
Places crutch slightly to the side of the involved limb (4 to 6 inches)	Ⓨ Ⓝ	Ⓨ Ⓝ	Ⓨ Ⓝ
Places axillary pad approximately 1 to 1.5 inches below axilla	Ⓨ Ⓝ	Ⓨ Ⓝ	Ⓨ Ⓝ
Places elbow in approximately 30 degrees flexion	Ⓨ Ⓝ	Ⓨ Ⓝ	Ⓨ Ⓝ
Tester instructs athlete in walking with ambulatory device	**Test 1**	**Test 2**	**Test 3**
Weight evenly distributed on crutches	Ⓨ Ⓝ	Ⓨ Ⓝ	Ⓨ Ⓝ
Athlete places one crutch tip forward	Ⓨ Ⓝ	Ⓨ Ⓝ	Ⓨ Ⓝ
Athlete steps forward with opposite foot	Ⓨ Ⓝ	Ⓨ Ⓝ	Ⓨ Ⓝ
Athlete places other crutch tip forward	Ⓨ Ⓝ	Ⓨ Ⓝ	Ⓨ Ⓝ
Athlete steps forward with other foot	Ⓨ Ⓝ	Ⓨ Ⓝ	Ⓨ Ⓝ

The psychomotor skill was performed completely and in the appropriate order   **0 1 2 3 4 5**

The tester had control of the subject and the situation (showed confidence)   **0 1 2 3 4 5**

Method of performing the skill allowed the tester the ability to determine:
severity, proper progression, and the *fit* in the overall picture (Oral)   **0 1 2 3 4 5**

In order for a grade of *minimum standard* to be given, the total must be ≥11   **TOTAL = _____**

```
 1    2    3    4    5    6    7    8    9   10   11   12   13   14   15
 |____|____|____|____|____|____|____|____|____|____|____|____|____|____|
```

Not Acceptable   **Meets**   **Exceeds**
                                        Minimum Standards   **Minimum Standards**

TEST ENVIRONMENTS	**SKILL TEST INFORMATION**	
L: Laboratory/Classroom Testing	**Positive Finding:**	N/A
C: Clinical/Field Testing	**Involved Structure:**	N/A
P: Practicum Testing	**Special Considerations:**	N/A
A: Assessment/Mock Exam Testing	**Reference(s):**	Houglum; Prentice (2003)
S: Self-Reporting	**Supplies Needed:**	Crutches of various sizes

AMBULATION ASSISTS/MISCELLANEOUS
(AA-Test 6)

Peer Review_____   Peer Review _____

Skill Acquisition: _____   Practice Opportunities: _____

This task allows you the opportunity to demonstrate the **use of a sling psychrometer to measure heat and humidity.** *You have 2 minutes to complete this task.*

Tester places measuring device in appropriate position	Test 1	Test 2	Test 3
Moistens web bulb	Ⓨ Ⓝ	Ⓨ Ⓝ	Ⓨ Ⓝ
Slides instrument into measuring position	Ⓨ Ⓝ	Ⓨ Ⓝ	Ⓨ Ⓝ
Tester follows correct procedures for using measuring device	**Test 1**	**Test 2**	**Test 3**
Stands in the center of the practice area, out of shade	Ⓨ Ⓝ	Ⓨ Ⓝ	Ⓨ Ⓝ
Twirls sling psychrometer for about 2 minutes	Ⓨ Ⓝ	Ⓨ Ⓝ	Ⓨ Ⓝ
Slides instrument into in proper position to read	Ⓨ Ⓝ	Ⓨ Ⓝ	Ⓨ Ⓝ
Tester uses measurement according to accepted guidelines	**Test 1**	**Test 2**	**Test 3**
Records measurements correctly	Ⓨ Ⓝ	Ⓨ Ⓝ	Ⓨ Ⓝ

The psychomotor skill was performed completely and in the appropriate order   **0 1 2 3 4 5**

The tester had control of the subject and the situation (showed confidence)   **0 1 2 3 4 5**

Method of performing the skill allowed the tester the ability to determine:
severity, proper progression, and the *fit* in the overall picture (Oral)   **0 1 2 3 4 5**

In order for a grade of *minimum standard* to be given, the total must be ≥11   **TOTAL = _____**

```
  1    2    3    4    5    6    7    8    9   10   11   12   13   14   15
  |    |    |    |    |    |    |    |    |    |    |    |    |    |    |
```
Not Acceptable   **Meets**   **Exceeds**
                                          Minimum Standards   **Minimum Standards**

TEST ENVIRONMENTS

L: Laboratory/Classroom Testing
C: Clinical/Field Testing
P: Practicum Testing
A: Assessment/Mock Exam Testing
S: Self-Reporting

SKILL TEST INFORMATION

Positive Finding: Temperature/humidity
Involved Structure: N/A
Special Considerations: N/A
Reference(s): Manufacturer's recommendations
Supplies Needed: Sling psychrometer, water source, pencil/paper

AMBULATION ASSISTS/MISCELLANEOUS
(AA-Test 7)

Peer Review_____   Peer Review _____

Skill Acquisition: _____   Practice Opportunities: _____

This problem allows you the opportunity to demonstrate the proper technique for **using a bag-valve mask (BVM) to ventilate a nonbreathing spectator.** *This person is not suspected of having a spinal injury. You have 2 minutes to complete this task.*

Tester places patient in appropriate position	Test 1	Test 2	Test 3
Supine (flat surface)	Ⓨ Ⓝ	Ⓨ Ⓝ	Ⓨ Ⓝ
Tester performs test according to accepted guidelines	**Test 1**	**Test 2**	**Test 3**
Tester positioned at the patient's head (kneeling)	Ⓨ Ⓝ	Ⓨ Ⓝ	Ⓨ Ⓝ
Checks for breathing by listening over nose and mouth	Ⓨ Ⓝ	Ⓨ Ⓝ	Ⓨ Ⓝ
Once lack of breathing has been established: Opens patient's airway (Head-Tilt, Chin-Lift Maneuver)	Ⓨ Ⓝ	Ⓨ Ⓝ	Ⓨ Ⓝ
Selects appropriately sized mask	Ⓨ Ⓝ	Ⓨ Ⓝ	Ⓨ Ⓝ
Places BVM on the patient's face (bridge of the nose to mouth/upper chin)	Ⓨ Ⓝ	Ⓨ Ⓝ	Ⓨ Ⓝ
One hand supports the mask to the face and jaw	Ⓨ Ⓝ	Ⓨ Ⓝ	Ⓨ Ⓝ
Other hand squeezes the bag once every 5 seconds	Ⓨ Ⓝ	Ⓨ Ⓝ	Ⓨ Ⓝ

The psychomotor skill was performed completely and in the appropriate order   0 1 2 3 4 5

The tester had control of the subject and the situation (showed confidence)   0 1 2 3 4 5

Method of performing the skill allowed the tester the ability to determine:
severity, proper progression, and the *fit* in the overall picture (Oral)   0 1 2 3 4 5

In order for a grade of *minimum standard* to be given, the total must be ≥11   TOTAL = _____

```
1    2    3    4    5    6    7    8    9    10   11   12   13   14   15
|    |    |    |    |    |    |    |    |    |    |    |    |    |    |
```

Not Acceptable   **Meets**   **Exceeds**
                                      Minimum Standards   **Minimum Standards**

TEST ENVIRONMENTS

L: Laboratory/Classroom Testing
C: Clinical/Field Testing
P: Practicum Testing
A: Assessment/Mock Exam Testing
S: Self-Reporting

SKILL TEST INFORMATION

Purpose:	Provide ventilation
Involved Structure:	Airway
Special Considerations:	May be used to assist ventilation; may be used to administer oxygen; best used with two persons
Reference(s):	Limmer et al
Supplies Needed:	Bag-valve mask

Chapter 4

LIGAMENTOUS STRESS TESTS

LIGAMENTOUS STRESS TESTS
(LST-U-Test 1)

Peer Review_____   Peer Review _____

Skill Acquisition: _____   Practice Opportunities: _____

Please demonstrate how you would perform the orthopedic test known as the **Acromioclavicular Joint Distraction Test** *for the shoulder. You have 2 minutes to complete this task.*

Tester places athlete and limb in appropriate position	Test 1	Test 2	Test 3
Seated or standing	Ⓨ Ⓝ	Ⓨ Ⓝ	Ⓨ Ⓝ
Arm relaxed at side, elbow at 90 degrees flexion	Ⓨ Ⓝ	Ⓨ Ⓝ	Ⓨ Ⓝ
Tester placed in proper position	**Test 1**	**Test 2**	**Test 3**
Stands on involved side	Ⓨ Ⓝ	Ⓨ Ⓝ	Ⓨ Ⓝ
Holds subject's arm just above elbow	Ⓨ Ⓝ	Ⓨ Ⓝ	Ⓨ Ⓝ
Places other hand over involved AC joint	Ⓨ Ⓝ	Ⓨ Ⓝ	Ⓨ Ⓝ
Tester performs test according to accepted guidelines	**Test 1**	**Test 2**	**Test 3**
Applies gentle downward pressure on the arm	Ⓨ Ⓝ	Ⓨ Ⓝ	Ⓨ Ⓝ
Maintains relaxation of the limb	Ⓨ Ⓝ	Ⓨ Ⓝ	Ⓨ Ⓝ
Performs assessment bilaterally	Ⓨ Ⓝ	Ⓨ Ⓝ	Ⓨ Ⓝ

The psychomotor skill was performed completely and in the appropriate order   0 1 2 3 4 5

The tester had control of the subject and the situation (showed confidence)   0 1 2 3 4 5

Method of performing the skill allowed the tester the ability to determine:
severity, proper progression, and the *fit* in the overall picture (Oral)   0 1 2 3 4 5

In order for a grade of *minimum standard* to be given, the total must be ≥11   **TOTAL = _____**

```
 1    2    3    4    5    6    7    8    9    10   11   12   13   14   15
 |    |    |    |    |    |    |    |    |    |    |    |    |    |    |
```
Not Acceptable   **Meets**   **Exceeds**
                                        Minimum Standards   **Minimum Standards**

TEST ENVIRONMENTS
L: Laboratory/Classroom Testing
C: Clinical/Field Testing
P: Practicum Testing
A: Assessment/Mock Exam Testing
S: Self-Reporting

SKILL TEST INFORMATION

Positive Finding: Pain; step deformity/movement of the AC joint

Involved Structure: AC joint; AC/coracoclavicular ligaments (sprain)

Special Considerations: N/A

Reference(s): Konin et al (2002); Starkey et al (2002)

Supplies Needed: N/A

LIGAMENTOUS STRESS TESTS
(LST-U-Test 2)

Peer Review_____   Peer Review _____

Skill Acquisition: _____.   Practice Opportunities: _____

Please demonstrate how you would perform the orthopedic test known as the **Acromioclavicular Shear Test (AC Joint Compression Test)** *for the shoulder. You have 2 minutes to complete this task.*

Tester places athlete and limb in appropriate position	Test 1	Test 2	Test 3
Seated or standing	Ⓨ Ⓝ	Ⓨ Ⓝ	Ⓨ Ⓝ
Arm relaxed at side (hanging naturally to the side)	Ⓨ Ⓝ	Ⓨ Ⓝ	Ⓨ Ⓝ
Tester placed in proper position	**Test 1**	**Test 2**	**Test 3**
Stands on involved side	Ⓨ Ⓝ	Ⓨ Ⓝ	Ⓨ Ⓝ
Places one hand on the subject's clavicle	Ⓨ Ⓝ	Ⓨ Ⓝ	Ⓨ Ⓝ
Places other hand on the spine of the scapula	Ⓨ Ⓝ	Ⓨ Ⓝ	Ⓨ Ⓝ
Tester performs test according to accepted guidelines	**Test 1**	**Test 2**	**Test 3**
Gently squeezes the hands together (cupping motion)	Ⓨ Ⓝ	Ⓨ Ⓝ	Ⓨ Ⓝ
Maintains relaxation of the limb	Ⓨ Ⓝ	Ⓨ Ⓝ	Ⓨ Ⓝ
Performs assessment bilaterally	Ⓨ Ⓝ	Ⓨ Ⓝ	Ⓨ Ⓝ

The psychomotor skill was performed completely and in the appropriate order   **0 1 2 3 4 5**

The tester had control of the subject and the situation (showed confidence)   **0 1 2 3 4 5**

Method of performing the skill allowed the tester the ability to determine:
severity, proper progression, and the *fit* in the overall picture (Oral)   **0 1 2 3 4 5**

In order for a grade of *minimum standard* to be given, the total must be ≥11   **TOTAL = _____**

```
  1    2    3    4    5    6    7    8    9   10   11   12   13   14   15
  |    |    |    |    |    |    |    |    |    |    |    |    |    |    |
```

Not Acceptable   **Meets**   **Exceeds**
                                          Minimum Standards   **Minimum Standards**

TEST ENVIRONMENTS

L: Laboratory/Classroom Testing
C: Clinical/Field Testing
P: Practicum Testing
A: Assessment/Mock Exam Testing
S: Self-Reporting

SKILL TEST INFORMATION

Positive Finding: Pain; movement of the clavicle
Involved Structure: AC joint; AC/coracoclavicular ligaments (sprain)
Special Considerations: Do not perform if obvious AC joint deformity
Reference(s): Konin et al (2002); Magee; Starkey et al (2002)
Supplies Needed: N/A

LIGAMENTOUS STRESS TESTS
(LST-U-Test 3)

Peer Review_____   Peer Review _____

Skill Acquisition: _____   Practice Opportunities: _____

*Please demonstrate how you would perform the orthopedic test known as the **Anterior Drawer Test for the Shoulder** to help rule out joint laxity. You have 2 minutes to complete this task.*

Tester places athlete and limb in appropriate position	Test 1	Test 2	Test 3
Supine	Ⓨ Ⓝ	Ⓨ Ⓝ	Ⓨ Ⓝ
Places arm in:			
Abduction	Ⓨ Ⓝ	Ⓨ Ⓝ	Ⓨ Ⓝ
Forward flexion (horizontal flexion); around 10 degrees	Ⓨ Ⓝ	Ⓨ Ⓝ	Ⓨ Ⓝ
Lateral rotation	Ⓨ Ⓝ	Ⓨ Ⓝ	Ⓨ Ⓝ
Tester placed in proper position	**Test 1**	**Test 2**	**Test 3**
Places on hand in the axilla area (holding athlete's arm)	Ⓨ Ⓝ	Ⓨ Ⓝ	Ⓨ Ⓝ
Stabilizes the athlete's scapula with the opposite hand	Ⓨ Ⓝ	Ⓨ Ⓝ	Ⓨ Ⓝ
Applies counterpressure to the athlete's coracoid process with thumb	Ⓨ Ⓝ	Ⓨ Ⓝ	Ⓨ Ⓝ
Tester performs test according to accepted guidelines	**Test 1**	**Test 2**	**Test 3**
Instructs the athlete to relax	Ⓨ Ⓝ	Ⓨ Ⓝ	Ⓨ Ⓝ
Appropriate pressure administered (direction and intensity, forward displacement of the humerus)	Ⓨ Ⓝ	Ⓨ Ⓝ	Ⓨ Ⓝ
Maintains relaxation of the limb	Ⓨ Ⓝ	Ⓨ Ⓝ	Ⓨ Ⓝ
Performs assessment bilaterally	Ⓨ Ⓝ	Ⓨ Ⓝ	Ⓨ Ⓝ

The psychomotor skill was performed completely and in the appropriate order   0 1 2 3 4 5

The tester had control of the subject and the situation (showed confidence)   0 1 2 3 4 5

Method of performing the skill allowed the tester the ability to determine:
severity, proper progression, and the *fit* in the overall picture (Oral)   0 1 2 3 4 5

In order for a grade of *minimum standard* to be given, the total must be ≥11   **TOTAL = _____**

```
1    2    3    4    5    6    7    8    9    10   11   12   13   14   15
|____|____|____|____|____|____|____|____|____|____|____|____|____|____|
```

Not Acceptable   **Meets**   **Exceeds**
                                    Minimum Standards   **Minimum Standards**

TEST ENVIRONMENTS

L: Laboratory/Classroom Testing
C: Clinical/Field Testing
P: Practicum Testing
A: Assessment/Mock Exam Testing
S: Self-Reporting

SKILL TEST INFORMATION

Positive Finding: Anterior displacement; clicking/apprehension
Involved Structure: Anterior instability of the shoulder
Special Considerations: N/A
Reference(s): Konin et al (2002); Magee
Supplies Needed: N/A

LIGAMENTOUS STRESS TESTS
(LST-U-Test 4)

Peer Review_____   Peer Review _____

Skill Acquisition: _____   Practice Opportunities: _____

Please demonstrate how you would perform the orthopedic test known as the **Clunk Test for the Shoulder.** *You have 2 minutes to complete this task.*

Tester places athlete and limb in appropriate position	Test 1	Test 2	Test 3
Supine	Y N	Y N	Y N
Arm in full abduction/external rotation (passive)	Y N	Y N	Y N
Tester placed in proper position	**Test 1**	**Test 2**	**Test 3**
Standing behind athlete's head	Y N	Y N	Y N
Supports posterior humeral head with one hand	Y N	Y N	Y N
Grips posterior humerus just proximal to elbow with other hand	Y N	Y N	Y N
Tester performs test according to accepted guidelines	**Test 1**	**Test 2**	**Test 3**
Pushes anteriorly on humeral head	Y N	Y N	Y N
Rotates humerus in a lateral rotation with other hand (may continue by internally rotating and circumducting the humeral head)	Y N	Y N	Y N
Maintains relaxation of the limb	Y N	Y N	Y N
Performs assessment bilaterally	Y N	Y N	Y N

The psychomotor skill was performed completely and in the appropriate order   **0 1 2 3 4 5**

The tester had control of the subject and the situation (showed confidence)   **0 1 2 3 4 5**

Method of performing the skill allowed the tester the ability to determine:
severity, proper progression, and the *fit* in the overall picture (Oral)   **0 1 2 3 4 5**

In order for a grade of *minimum standard* to be given, the total must be ≥11   **TOTAL = _____**

```
 1    2    3    4    5    6    7    8    9   10   11   12   13   14   15
 |    |    |    |    |    |    |    |    |    |    |    |    |    |    |
```
Not Acceptable   **Meets**   **Exceeds**
                              Minimum Standards   **Minimum Standards**

TEST ENVIRONMENTS	**SKILL TEST INFORMATION**	
L: Laboratory/Classroom Testing	**Positive Finding:**	Grinding, clunking
C: Clinical/Field Testing	**Involved Structure:**	Glenoid labrum tear
P: Practicum Testing	**Special Considerations:**	N/A
A: Assessment/Mock Exam Testing	**Reference(s):**	Konin et al (2002); Magee
S: Self-Reporting	**Supplies Needed:**	Table

LIGAMENTOUS STRESS TESTS
(LST-U-Test 5)

Peer Review_____   Peer Review _____

Skill Acquisition: _____   Practice Opportunities: _____

Please demonstrate how you would perform the orthopedic test known as the **Feagin Test for the Shoulder.** *You have 2 minutes to complete this task.*

Tester places athlete and limb in appropriate position	Test 1	Test 2	Test 3
Standing	Ⓨ Ⓝ	Ⓨ Ⓝ	Ⓨ Ⓝ
Shoulder abducted to 90 degrees, with elbow fully extended	Ⓨ Ⓝ	Ⓨ Ⓝ	Ⓨ Ⓝ
Forearm resting on examiner's shoulder	Ⓨ Ⓝ	Ⓨ Ⓝ	Ⓨ Ⓝ
Tester placed in proper position	**Test 1**	**Test 2**	**Test 3**
Stands to the side of athlete, faces the athlete	Ⓨ Ⓝ	Ⓨ Ⓝ	Ⓨ Ⓝ
Hands clasped together around upper and middle third of humerus	Ⓨ Ⓝ	Ⓨ Ⓝ	Ⓨ Ⓝ
Tester performs test according to accepted guidelines	**Test 1**	**Test 2**	**Test 3**
Pushes humerus down and forward	Ⓨ Ⓝ	Ⓨ Ⓝ	Ⓨ Ⓝ
Maintains relaxation of the limb	Ⓨ Ⓝ	Ⓨ Ⓝ	Ⓨ Ⓝ
Performs assessment bilaterally	Ⓨ Ⓝ	Ⓨ Ⓝ	Ⓨ Ⓝ

The psychomotor skill was performed completely and in the appropriate order   **0 1 2 3 4 5**

The tester had control of the subject and the situation (showed confidence)   **0 1 2 3 4 5**

Method of performing the skill allowed the tester the ability to determine: severity, proper progression, and the *fit* in the overall picture (Oral)   **0 1 2 3 4 5**

In order for a grade of *minimum standard* to be given, the total must be ≥11   **TOTAL = _____**

```
   1    2    3    4    5    6    7    8    9    10   11   12   13   14   15
   |    |    |    |    |    |    |    |    |    |    |    |    |    |    |
```

Not Acceptable   **Meets**   **Exceeds**
                                   Minimum Standards   **Minimum Standards**

TEST ENVIRONMENTS

L: Laboratory/Classroom Testing
C: Clinical/Field Testing
P: Practicum Testing
A: Assessment/Mock Exam Testing
S: Self-Reporting

SKILL TEST INFORMATION

Positive Finding:	Apprehension
Involved Structure:	Anteroinferior instability
Special Considerations:	Modification of the sulcus sign test
Reference(s):	Magee
Supplies Needed:	N/A

LIGAMENTOUS STRESS TESTS
(LST-U-Test 6)

Peer Review_____   Peer Review _____

Skill Acquisition: _____   Practice Opportunities: _____

*Please demonstrate how you would perform the orthopedic test known as the **Sternoclavicular Joint Stress Test** in order to rule out ligamentous damage. You have 2 minutes to complete this task.*

Tester places athlete and limb in appropriate position	Test 1	Test 2	Test 3
Seated or standing	Ⓨ Ⓝ	Ⓨ Ⓝ	Ⓨ Ⓝ
Arm relaxed at side	Ⓨ Ⓝ	Ⓨ Ⓝ	Ⓨ Ⓝ
Tester placed in proper position	**Test 1**	**Test 2**	**Test 3**
Stands in front of the athlete	Ⓨ Ⓝ	Ⓨ Ⓝ	Ⓨ Ⓝ
Places one hand on the proximal end of the athlete's clavicle	Ⓨ Ⓝ	Ⓨ Ⓝ	Ⓨ Ⓝ
Places the other hand on the spine of the scapula	Ⓨ Ⓝ	Ⓨ Ⓝ	Ⓨ Ⓝ
Tester performs test according to accepted guidelines	**Test 1**	**Test 2**	**Test 3**
Applies gentle downward and inward pressure on the clavicle	Ⓨ Ⓝ	Ⓨ Ⓝ	Ⓨ Ⓝ
Notes any movement at the sternoclavicular joint	Ⓨ Ⓝ	Ⓨ Ⓝ	Ⓨ Ⓝ
Maintains relaxation of the involved limb	Ⓨ Ⓝ	Ⓨ Ⓝ	Ⓨ Ⓝ
Performs assessment bilaterally	Ⓨ Ⓝ	Ⓨ Ⓝ	Ⓨ Ⓝ

The psychomotor skill was performed completely and in the appropriate order   **0 1 2 3 4 5**

The tester had control of the subject and the situation (showed confidence)   **0 1 2 3 4 5**

Method of performing the skill allowed the tester the ability to determine:
severity, proper progression, and the *fit* in the overall picture (Oral)   **0 1 2 3 4 5**

In order for a grade of *minimum standard* to be given, the total must be ≥11   **TOTAL = _____**

```
 1    2    3    4    5    6    7    8    9   10   11   12   13   14   15
 |    |    |    |    |    |    |    |    |    |    |    |    |    |    |
```
Not Acceptable   **Meets**   **Exceeds**
                                            Minimum Standards   **Minimum Standards**

TEST ENVIRONMENTS

L: Laboratory/Classroom Testing
C: Clinical/Field Testing
P: Practicum Testing
A: Assessment/Mock Exam Testing
S: Self-Reporting

SKILL TEST INFORMATION

Positive Finding: Pain and/or movement
Involved Structure: Clavicle; SC ligament sprain, possibly involving the costo-clavicular ligament
Special Considerations: N/A
Reference(s): Konin et al (2002)
Supplies Needed: N/A

LIGAMENTOUS STRESS TESTS
(LST-U-Test 7)

Peer Review_____   Peer Review _____

Skill Acquisition: _____   Practice Opportunities: _____

Please demonstrate how you would perform the orthopedic test known as the **Posterior Drawer Test for the Shoulder**. *You have 2 minutes to complete this task.*

Tester places athlete and limb in appropriate position	Test 1	Test 2	Test 3
Supine	Ⓨ Ⓝ	Ⓨ Ⓝ	Ⓨ Ⓝ
Arm passively placed in the 90-90 position	Ⓨ Ⓝ	Ⓨ Ⓝ	Ⓨ Ⓝ
Tester placed in proper position	**Test 1**	**Test 2**	**Test 3**
Stands next to the involved shoulder	Ⓨ Ⓝ	Ⓨ Ⓝ	Ⓨ Ⓝ
Places one hand on the athlete's distal humerus	Ⓨ Ⓝ	Ⓨ Ⓝ	Ⓨ Ⓝ
Places the other hand posterior to shoulder capsule to stabilize the scapula (thumb on the coracoid process)	Ⓨ Ⓝ	Ⓨ Ⓝ	Ⓨ Ⓝ
Tester performs test according to accepted guidelines	Ⓨ Ⓝ	Ⓨ Ⓝ	Ⓨ Ⓝ
Moves the shoulder to about 30 degrees of horizontal flexion	**Test 1**	**Test 2**	**Test 3**
Applies passive internal rotation to the shoulder	Ⓨ Ⓝ	Ⓨ Ⓝ	Ⓨ Ⓝ
Applies downward pressure (forcing the head of humerus posteriorly)	Ⓨ Ⓝ	Ⓨ Ⓝ	Ⓨ Ⓝ
Maintains relaxation of the limb	Ⓨ Ⓝ	Ⓨ Ⓝ	Ⓨ Ⓝ
Performs assessment bilaterally	Ⓨ Ⓝ	Ⓨ Ⓝ	Ⓨ Ⓝ

The psychomotor skill was performed completely and in the appropriate order   **0 1 2 3 4 5**

The tester had control of the subject and the situation (showed confidence)   **0 1 2 3 4 5**

Method of performing the skill allowed the tester the ability to determine:
severity, proper progression, and the *fit* in the overall picture (Oral)   **0 1 2 3 4 5**

In order for a grade of *minimum standard* to be given, the total must be ≥11   **TOTAL = _____**

| 1 | 2 | 3 | 4 | 5 | 6 | 7 | 8 | 9 | 10 | 11 | 12 | 13 | 14 | 15 |

Not Acceptable   **Meets**   **Exceeds**
                          Minimum Standards   **Minimum Standards**

TEST ENVIRONMENTS
L: Laboratory/Classroom Testing
C: Clinical/Field Testing
P: Practicum Testing
A: Assessment/Mock Exam Testing
S: Self-Reporting

SKILL TEST INFORMATION
Positive Finding: Posterior instability of the humeral head; apprehension
Involved Structure: Posterior structures
Special Considerations: N/A
Reference(s): Konin et al (2002); Magee
Supplies Needed: Table

LIGAMENTOUS STRESS TESTS
(LST-U-Test 8)

Peer Review_____   Peer Review _____

Skill Acquisition: _____   Practice Opportunities: _____

Please demonstrate how you would perform the orthopedic test known as the **Jobe Relocation Test (Fowler Sign/Fowler Test/Relocation Test)** *for the shoulder. You have 2 minutes to complete this task.*

Tester places athlete and limb in appropriate position	Test 1	Test 2	Test 3
Supine	Y N	Y N	Y N
Shoulder in 90 degrees abduction	Y N	Y N	Y N
Shoulder in full external rotation	Y N	Y N	Y N
Tester placed in proper position	**Test 1**	**Test 2**	**Test 3**
Stands next the involved shoulder	Y N	Y N	Y N
Places distal hand on the subject's wrist	Y N	Y N	Y N
Places the other hand over subject's humeral head (anterior)	Y N	Y N	Y N
Tester performs test according to accepted guidelines	**Test 1**	**Test 2**	**Test 3**
Applies posterior force to the humeral head	Y N	Y N	Y N
Applies passive external rotation to the shoulder	Y N	Y N	Y N
Maintains relaxation of the limb	Y N	Y N	Y N
Performs assessment bilaterally	Y N	Y N	Y N

The psychomotor skill was performed completely and in the appropriate order   **0 1 2 3 4 5**

The tester had control of the subject and the situation (showed confidence)   **0 1 2 3 4 5**

Method of performing the skill allowed the tester the ability to determine:
severity, proper progression, and the *fit* in the overall picture (Oral)   **0 1 2 3 4 5**

In order for a grade of *minimum standard* to be given, the total must be ≥11   **TOTAL = _____**

```
   1    2    3    4    5    6    7    8    9   10   11   12   13   14   15
   |----|----|----|----|----|----|----|----|----|----|----|----|----|----|
```

Not Acceptable   **Meets**   **Exceeds**
                                   Minimum Standards   **Minimum Standards**

TEST ENVIRONMENTS

L: Laboratory/Classroom Testing
C: Clinical/Field Testing
P: Practicum Testing
A: Assessment/Mock Exam Testing
S: Self-Reporting

SKILL TEST INFORMATION

Positive Finding: Reduction of pain; apprehension
Involved Structure: Anterior structures of the shoulder
Special Considerations: Should be performed immediately following the apprehension test (anterior)
Reference(s): Konin et al (2002); Magee
Supplies Needed: Table

LIGAMENTOUS STRESS TESTS
(LST-U-Test 9)

Peer Review_____   Peer Review _____

Skill Acquisition: _____   Practice Opportunities: _____

Please demonstrate how you would perform the orthopedic test known as the **Apprehension Test (Crank Test)** *for an anterior shoulder dislocation. You have 2 minutes to complete this task.*

Tester places athlete and limb in appropriate position	Test 1	Test 2	Test 3
Supine	Ⓨ Ⓝ	Ⓨ Ⓝ	Ⓨ Ⓝ
Shoulder placed in 90 degrees abduction	Ⓨ Ⓝ	Ⓨ Ⓝ	Ⓨ Ⓝ
Elbow placed in 90 degrees of flexion	Ⓨ Ⓝ	Ⓨ Ⓝ	Ⓨ Ⓝ
Tester placed in proper position	**Test 1**	**Test 2**	**Test 3**
Stands next to the involved shoulder	Ⓨ Ⓝ	Ⓨ Ⓝ	Ⓨ Ⓝ
Places one hand on the subject's wrist	Ⓨ Ⓝ	Ⓨ Ⓝ	Ⓨ Ⓝ
Post the other hand under the distal humerus	Ⓨ Ⓝ	Ⓨ Ⓝ	Ⓨ Ⓝ
Tester performs test according to accepted guidelines	**Test 1**	**Test 2**	**Test 3**
Moves the limb slowly into external rotation	Ⓨ Ⓝ	Ⓨ Ⓝ	Ⓨ Ⓝ
Maintains relaxation of the limb	Ⓨ Ⓝ	Ⓨ Ⓝ	Ⓨ Ⓝ
Performs assessment bilaterally	Ⓨ Ⓝ	Ⓨ Ⓝ	Ⓨ Ⓝ

The psychomotor skill was performed completely and in the appropriate order   0 1 2 3 4 5

The tester had control of the subject and the situation (showed confidence)   0 1 2 3 4 5

Method of performing the skill allowed the tester the ability to determine:
severity, proper progression, and the *fit* in the overall picture (Oral)   0 1 2 3 4 5

In order for a grade of *minimum standard* to be given, the total must be ≥11   **TOTAL = _____**

```
   1    2    3    4    5    6    7    8    9   10   11   12   13   14   15
   |    |    |    |    |    |    |    |    |    |    |    |    |    |    |
```
Not Acceptable   **Meets**   **Exceeds**
                                         Minimum Standards   **Minimum Standards**

TEST ENVIRONMENTS

L: Laboratory/Classroom Testing
C: Clinical/Field Testing
P: Practicum Testing
A: Assessment/Mock Exam Testing
S: Self-Reporting

SKILL TEST INFORMATION

Positive Finding: Apprehension, pain
Involved Structure: Anterior structures
Special Considerations: Do not perform when there is obvious deformity
Reference(s): Konin et al (2002); Magee; Starkey et al (2002)
Supplies Needed: Table

LIGAMENTOUS STRESS TESTS
(LST-U-Test 10)

Peer Review_____   Peer Review _____

Skill Acquisition: _____   Practice Opportunities: _____

This problem allows you the opportunity to demonstrate the **Test for Inferior Shoulder Instability (Sulcus Sign/ Sulcus Test).** *You have 2 minutes to complete this task.*

Tester places athlete and limb in appropriate position	Test 1	Test 2	Test 3
Seated or standing	Ⓨ Ⓝ	Ⓨ Ⓝ	Ⓨ Ⓝ
Arms relaxed by side; elbow flexed to 90 degrees (resting in lap)	Ⓨ Ⓝ	Ⓨ Ⓝ	Ⓨ Ⓝ
Tester placed in proper position	**Test 1**	**Test 2**	**Test 3**
Sits perpendicular to the athlete	Ⓨ Ⓝ	Ⓨ Ⓝ	Ⓨ Ⓝ
Places one hand on the scapula	Ⓨ Ⓝ	Ⓨ Ⓝ	Ⓨ Ⓝ
Places the other hand on the elbow or forearm	Ⓨ Ⓝ	Ⓨ Ⓝ	Ⓨ Ⓝ
Tester performs test according to accepted guidelines	**Test 1**	**Test 2**	**Test 3**
Inferiorly distracts the humerus (pulls distally)	Ⓨ Ⓝ	Ⓨ Ⓝ	Ⓨ Ⓝ
Maintains relaxation of the limb	Ⓨ Ⓝ	Ⓨ Ⓝ	Ⓨ Ⓝ
Performs assessment bilaterally	Ⓨ Ⓝ	Ⓨ Ⓝ	Ⓨ Ⓝ

The psychomotor skill was performed completely and in the appropriate order   **0 1 2 3 4 5**

The tester had control of the subject and the situation (showed confidence)   **0 1 2 3 4 5**

Method of performing the skill allowed the tester the ability to determine: severity, proper progression, and the *fit* in the overall picture (Oral)   **0 1 2 3 4 5**

In order for a grade of *minimum standard* to be given, the total must be ≥11   **TOTAL = _____**

```
  1     2     3     4     5     6     7     8     9     10     11     12     13     14     15
  |__|__|__|__|__|__|__|__|__|__|__|__|__|__|__|__|__|__|__|__|__|__|__|__|__|__|__|__|__|
```

Not Acceptable   **Meets**   **Exceeds**
                                          Minimum Standards   **Minimum Standards**

TEST ENVIRONMENTS

L: Laboratory/Classroom Testing
C: Clinical/Field Testing
P: Practicum Testing
A: Assessment/Mock Exam Testing
S: Self-Reporting

SKILL TEST INFORMATION

Positive Finding:	Step-off deformity; sunken area
Involved Structure:	Superior glenohumeral ligament
Special Considerations:	N/A
Reference(s):	Konin et al (2002); Magee; Starkey et al (2002)
Supplies Needed:	N/A

LIGAMENTOUS STRESS TESTS
(LST-U-Test 11)

Peer Review_____   Peer Review _____

Skill Acquisition: _____   Practice Opportunities: _____

This problem allows you the opportunity to demonstrate the **Posterior Apprehension Test (Posterior Stress Test) for the Shoulder**. *You have 2 minutes to complete this task.*

Tester places athlete and limb in appropriate position	Test 1	Test 2	Test 3
Supine	Ⓨ Ⓝ	Ⓨ Ⓝ	Ⓨ Ⓝ
Shoulder positioned in 90 degrees of flexion	Ⓨ Ⓝ	Ⓨ Ⓝ	Ⓨ Ⓝ
Elbow positioned in 90 degrees of flexion	Ⓨ Ⓝ	Ⓨ Ⓝ	Ⓨ Ⓝ
Tester placed in proper position	**Test 1**	**Test 2**	**Test 3**
Stands beside the athlete	Ⓨ Ⓝ	Ⓨ Ⓝ	Ⓨ Ⓝ
Stabilizes the shoulder with one hand	Ⓨ Ⓝ	Ⓨ Ⓝ	Ⓨ Ⓝ
Places the other hand on the elbow or forearm	Ⓨ Ⓝ	Ⓨ Ⓝ	Ⓨ Ⓝ
Tester performs test according to accepted guidelines	Ⓨ Ⓝ	Ⓨ Ⓝ	Ⓨ Ⓝ
Positions the shoulder in internal rotation	Ⓨ Ⓝ	Ⓨ Ⓝ	Ⓨ Ⓝ
Applies a posterior force through the long axis (push down toward the floor)	Ⓨ Ⓝ	Ⓨ Ⓝ	Ⓨ Ⓝ
Maintains relaxation of the limb	Ⓨ Ⓝ	Ⓨ Ⓝ	Ⓨ Ⓝ
Performs assessment bilaterally	Ⓨ Ⓝ	Ⓨ Ⓝ	Ⓨ Ⓝ

The psychomotor skill was performed completely and in the appropriate order   **0 1 2 3 4 5**

The tester had control of the subject and the situation (showed confidence)   **0 1 2 3 4 5**

Method of performing the skill allowed the tester the ability to determine:
severity, proper progression, and the *fit* in the overall picture (Oral)   **0 1 2 3 4 5**

In order for a grade of *minimum standard* to be given, the total must be ≥11   **TOTAL = _____**

```
  1    2    3    4    5    6    7    8    9   10   11   12   13   14   15
  |    |    |    |    |    |    |    |    |    |    |    |    |    |    |
```
Not Acceptable   **Meets**   **Exceeds**
                                            Minimum Standards   **Minimum Standards**

TEST ENVIRONMENTS
L: Laboratory/Classroom Testing
C: Clinical/Field Testing
P: Practicum Testing
A: Assessment/Mock Exam Testing
S: Self-Reporting

SKILL TEST INFORMATION
Positive Finding: Apprehension, guarding
Involved Structure: Posterior capsule, posterior structures
Special Considerations: N/A
Reference(s): Konin et al (2002); Magee; Starkey et al (2002)
Supplies Needed: Table

LIGAMENTOUS STRESS TESTS
(LST-U-Test 12)

Peer Review_____   Peer Review _____

Skill Acquisition: _____   Practice Opportunities: _____

This problem allows you the opportunity to demonstrate the orthopedic test known as the **Valgus Stress Test for the Elbow**. *You have 2 minutes to complete this task.*

Tester places athlete and limb in appropriate position	Test 1	Test 2	Test 3
Stands or sits facing the examiner	Ⓨ Ⓝ	Ⓨ Ⓝ	Ⓨ Ⓝ
Arms relaxed, elbow flexed to 20 to 30 degrees flexion	Ⓨ Ⓝ	Ⓨ Ⓝ	Ⓨ Ⓝ
Tester placed in proper position	**Test 1**	**Test 2**	**Test 3**
Grasps distal forearm with one hand	Ⓨ Ⓝ	Ⓨ Ⓝ	Ⓨ Ⓝ
Places other hand over the lateral epicondyle of the elbow	Ⓨ Ⓝ	Ⓨ Ⓝ	Ⓨ Ⓝ
Tester performs test according to accepted guidelines	**Test 1**	**Test 2**	**Test 3**
Applies a valgus stress to the lateral epicondyle of the elbow	Ⓨ Ⓝ	Ⓨ Ⓝ	Ⓨ Ⓝ
Maintains relaxation of the limb	Ⓨ Ⓝ	Ⓨ Ⓝ	Ⓨ Ⓝ
Performs assessment bilaterally	Ⓨ Ⓝ	Ⓨ Ⓝ	Ⓨ Ⓝ

The psychomotor skill was performed completely and in the appropriate order   **0 1 2 3 4 5**

The tester had control of the subject and the situation (showed confidence)   **0 1 2 3 4 5**

Method of performing the skill allowed the tester the ability to determine:
severity, proper progression, and the *fit* in the overall picture (Oral)   **0 1 2 3 4 5**

In order for a grade of *minimum standard* to be given, the total must be ≥11   **TOTAL = _____**

```
  1     2     3     4     5     6     7     8     9    10    11    12    13    14    15
  |_____|_____|_____|_____|_____|_____|_____|_____|_____|_____|_____|_____|_____|_____|
```
Not Acceptable   **Meets**   **Exceeds**
                                    Minimum Standards   **Minimum Standards**

TEST ENVIRONMENTS

L: Laboratory/Classroom Testing
C: Clinical/Field Testing
P: Practicum Testing
A: Assessment/Mock Exam Testing
S: Self-Reporting

SKILL TEST INFORMATION

Positive Finding: Pain and laxity
Involved Structure: Ulnar collateral ligament
Special Considerations: N/A
Reference(s): Konin et al (2002); Starkey et al (2002)
Supplies Needed: N/A

LIGAMENTOUS STRESS TESTS
(LST-U-Test 13)

Peer Review_____   Peer Review _____

Skill Acquisition: _____   Practice Opportunities: _____

This problem allows you the opportunity to demonstrate the orthopedic test known as the **Varus Stress Test for the Elbow**. *You have 2 minutes to complete this task.*

Tester places athlete and limb in appropriate position	Test 1	Test 2	Test 3
Stands or sits facing the examiner	Ⓨ Ⓝ	Ⓨ Ⓝ	Ⓨ Ⓝ
Arms relaxed, elbow flexed to 20 to 30 degrees flexion	Ⓨ Ⓝ	Ⓨ Ⓝ	Ⓨ Ⓝ
Tester placed in proper position	**Test 1**	**Test 2**	**Test 3**
Grasps distal forearm with one hand	Ⓨ Ⓝ	Ⓨ Ⓝ	Ⓨ Ⓝ
Places other hand over the medial epicondyle of the elbow	Ⓨ Ⓝ	Ⓨ Ⓝ	Ⓨ Ⓝ
Tester performs test according to accepted guidelines	**Test 1**	**Test 2**	**Test 3**
Applies a varus stress to the medial epicondyle of the elbow	Ⓨ Ⓝ	Ⓨ Ⓝ	Ⓨ Ⓝ
Maintains relaxation of the limb	Ⓨ Ⓝ	Ⓨ Ⓝ	Ⓨ Ⓝ
Performs assessment bilaterally	Ⓨ Ⓝ	Ⓨ Ⓝ	Ⓨ Ⓝ

The psychomotor skill was performed completely and in the appropriate order   **0 1 2 3 4 5**

The tester had control of the subject and the situation (showed confidence)   **0 1 2 3 4 5**

Method of performing the skill allowed the tester the ability to determine:
severity, proper progression, and the *fit* in the overall picture (Oral)   **0 1 2 3 4 5**

In order for a grade of *minimum standard* to be given, the total must be ≥11   **TOTAL = _____**

```
 1    2    3    4    5    6    7    8    9    10   11   12   13   14   15
 |____|____|____|____|____|____|____|____|____|____|____|____|____|____|
```

Not Acceptable   **Meets**   **Exceeds**
                               Minimum Standards   **Minimum Standards**

TEST ENVIRONMENTS

L: Laboratory/Classroom Testing
C: Clinical/Field Testing
P: Practicum Testing
A: Assessment/Mock Exam Testing
S: Self-Reporting

SKILL TEST INFORMATION

Positive Finding: Pain and laxity
Involved Structure: Radial collateral ligament
Special Considerations: N/A
Reference(s): Konin et al (2002); Starkey et al (2002)
Supplies Needed: N/A

LIGAMENTOUS STRESS TESTS
(LST-U-Test 14)

Peer Review_____   Peer Review _____

Skill Acquisition: _____   Practice Opportunities: _____

This problem allows you the opportunity to demonstrate the orthopedic test known as the **Valgus Stress Test for the Second Proximal Interphalangeal (PIP) Joint**. *You have 2 minutes to complete this task.*

Tester places athlete and limb in appropriate position	Test 1	Test 2	Test 3
Stands or sits facing the examiner	Ⓨ Ⓝ	Ⓨ Ⓝ	Ⓨ Ⓝ
Second PIP is flexed (15 to 30 degrees)	Ⓨ Ⓝ	Ⓨ Ⓝ	Ⓨ Ⓝ
Tester placed in proper position	**Test 1**	**Test 2**	**Test 3**
Grasps the distal end of the proximal phalanx with one hand (thumb and index finger	Ⓨ Ⓝ	Ⓨ Ⓝ	Ⓨ Ⓝ
Places other hand over the middle phalanx (thumb and index finger)	Ⓨ Ⓝ	Ⓨ Ⓝ	Ⓨ Ⓝ
Tester performs test according to accepted guidelines	**Test 1**	**Test 2**	**Test 3**
Applies a valgus stress to the joint (second proximal interphalangeal joint)	Ⓨ Ⓝ	Ⓨ Ⓝ	Ⓨ Ⓝ
Maintains relaxation of the limb	Ⓨ Ⓝ	Ⓨ Ⓝ	Ⓨ Ⓝ
Performs assessment bilaterally	Ⓨ Ⓝ	Ⓨ Ⓝ	Ⓨ Ⓝ

The psychomotor skill was performed completely and in the appropriate order   **0 1 2 3 4 5**

The tester had control of the subject and the situation (showed confidence)   **0 1 2 3 4 5**

Method of performing the skill allowed the tester the ability to determine:
severity, proper progression, and the *fit* in the overall picture (Oral)   **0 1 2 3 4 5**

In order for a grade of *minimum standard* to be given, the total must be ≥11   **TOTAL = _____**

```
1     2     3     4     5     6     7     8     9     10    11    12    13    14    15
|_____|_____|_____|_____|_____|_____|_____|_____|_____|_____|_____|_____|_____|_____|
```

Not Acceptable   **Meets**   **Exceeds**
                               Minimum Standards   **Minimum Standards**

TEST ENVIRONMENTS

L: Laboratory/Classroom Testing
C: Clinical/Field Testing
P: Practicum Testing
A: Assessment/Mock Exam Testing
S: Self-Reporting

SKILL TEST INFORMATION

Positive Finding: Pain and laxity
Involved Structure: Medial collateral ligament (finger)
Special Considerations: N/A
Reference(s): Magee; Starkey et al (2002)
Supplies Needed: N/A

LIGAMENTOUS STRESS TESTS
(LST-U-Test 15)

Peer Review_____   Peer Review _____

Skill Acquisition: _____   Practice Opportunities: _____

This problem allows you the opportunity to demonstrate the orthopedic test known as the **Varus Stress Test for the Third Distal Interphalangeal (DIP) Joint**. *You have 2 minutes to complete this task.*

Tester places athlete and limb in appropriate position	Test 1	Test 2	Test 3
Stands or sits facing the examiner	Ⓨ Ⓝ	Ⓨ Ⓝ	Ⓨ Ⓝ
Third DIP is flexed (15 to 30 degrees)	Ⓨ Ⓝ	Ⓨ Ⓝ	Ⓨ Ⓝ
Tester placed in proper position	**Test 1**	**Test 2**	**Test 3**
Grasps the distal end of the middle phalanx with one hand (thumb & index finger)	Ⓨ Ⓝ	Ⓨ Ⓝ	Ⓨ Ⓝ
Places other hand over the distal phalanx (thumb & index finger)	Ⓨ Ⓝ	Ⓨ Ⓝ	Ⓨ Ⓝ
Tester performs test according to accepted guidelines	**Test 1**	**Test 2**	**Test 3**
Applies a varus stress to the joint (third PIP joint)	Ⓨ Ⓝ	Ⓨ Ⓝ	Ⓨ Ⓝ
Maintains relaxation of the limb	Ⓨ Ⓝ	Ⓨ Ⓝ	Ⓨ Ⓝ
Performs assessment bilaterally	Ⓨ Ⓝ	Ⓨ Ⓝ	Ⓨ Ⓝ

The psychomotor skill was performed completely and in the appropriate order   **0 1 2 3 4 5**

The tester had control of the subject and the situation (showed confidence)   **0 1 2 3 4 5**

Method of performing the skill allowed the tester the ability to determine:
severity, proper progression, and the *fit* in the overall picture (Oral)   **0 1 2 3 4 5**

In order for a grade of *minimum standard* to be given, the total must be ≥11   **TOTAL = _____**

```
  1    2    3    4    5    6    7    8    9    10   11   12   13   14   15
  |----|----|----|----|----|----|----|----|----|----|----|----|----|----|
```

Not Acceptable   **Meets**   **Exceeds**
                                   Minimum Standards   **Minimum Standards**

TEST ENVIRONMENTS

L: Laboratory/Classroom Testing
C: Clinical/Field Testing
P: Practicum Testing
A: Assessment/Mock Exam Testing
S: Self-Reporting

SKILL TEST INFORMATION

Positive Finding: Pain and laxity
Involved Structure: Lateral collateral ligament (finger)
Special Considerations: N/A
Reference(s): Magee; Starkey et al (2002)
Supplies Needed: N/A

LIGAMENTOUS STRESS TESTS
(LST-L-Test 1)

Peer Review_____   Peer Review _____

Skill Acquisition: _____   Practice Opportunities: _____

Please demonstrate how you would perform the ligamentous stress test for the ankle known as the **Anterior Drawer Test for the Ankle**. *You have 2 minutes to complete this task.*

Tester places athlete and limb in appropriate position	Test 1	Test 2	Test 3
Supine or sitting with feet relaxed over edge of table	Ⓨ Ⓝ	Ⓨ Ⓝ	Ⓨ Ⓝ
Knee flexed to 90 degrees	Ⓨ Ⓝ	Ⓨ Ⓝ	Ⓨ Ⓝ
Tester placed in proper position	**Test 1**	**Test 2**	**Test 3**
Stabilizes tibia and fibula with one hand	Ⓨ Ⓝ	Ⓨ Ⓝ	Ⓨ Ⓝ
Holds foot in 20 degrees of plantar flexion	Ⓨ Ⓝ	Ⓨ Ⓝ	Ⓨ Ⓝ
Tester performs test according to accepted guidelines	**Test 1**	**Test 2**	**Test 3**
Maintains relaxation of the limb	Ⓨ Ⓝ	Ⓨ Ⓝ	Ⓨ Ⓝ
Draws talus forward (anterior displacement) on lower leg	Ⓨ Ⓝ	Ⓨ Ⓝ	Ⓨ Ⓝ
Performs assessment bilaterally	Ⓨ Ⓝ	Ⓨ Ⓝ	Ⓨ Ⓝ

The psychomotor skill was performed completely and in the appropriate order   **0 1 2 3 4 5**

The tester had control of the subject and the situation (showed confidence)   **0 1 2 3 4 5**

Method of performing the skill allowed the tester the ability to determine:
severity, proper progression, and the *fit* in the overall picture (Oral)   **0 1 2 3 4 5**

In order for a grade of *minimum standard* to be given, the total must be ≥11   **TOTAL = _____**

```
 1     2     3     4     5     6     7     8     9    10    11    12    13    14    15
 |     |     |     |     |     |     |     |     |     |     |     |     |     |     |
```

Not Acceptable   **Meets**   **Exceeds**
                                              Minimum Standards   **Minimum Standards**

TEST ENVIRONMENTS

L: Laboratory/Classroom Testing
C: Clinical/Field Testing
P: Practicum Testing
A: Assessment/Mock Exam Testing
S: Self-Reporting

SKILL TEST INFORMATION

Positive Finding:	Anterior translation; clunk
Involved Structure:	Anterior talofibular ligament
Special Considerations:	N/A
Reference(s):	Konin et al (2002); Magee; Starkey et al (2002)
Supplies Needed:	Table or chair

LIGAMENTOUS STRESS TESTS
(LST-L-Test 2)

Peer Review_____   Peer Review _____

Skill Acquisition: _____   Practice Opportunities: _____

This problem allows you the opportunity to demonstrate a ligamentous stress test known as the **Talar Tilt Test (Inversion Stress Test)**. *You have 2 minutes to complete this task.*

Tester places athlete and limb in appropriate position	Test 1	Test 2	Test 3
Seated/supine (may be done side lying on the uninvolved side)	Ⓨ Ⓝ	Ⓨ Ⓝ	Ⓨ Ⓝ
Foot over the edge of the table	Ⓨ Ⓝ	Ⓨ Ⓝ	Ⓨ Ⓝ
Knee flexed to 90 degrees	Ⓨ Ⓝ	Ⓨ Ⓝ	Ⓨ Ⓝ
Tester placed in proper position	**Test 1**	**Test 2**	**Test 3**
Stabilizes tibia and fibula with one hand	Ⓨ Ⓝ	Ⓨ Ⓝ	Ⓨ Ⓝ
Holds foot in neutral position with other hand	Ⓨ Ⓝ	Ⓨ Ⓝ	Ⓨ Ⓝ
Tester performs test according to accepted guidelines	**Test 1**	**Test 2**	**Test 3**
Maintains relaxation of the limb	Ⓨ Ⓝ	Ⓨ Ⓝ	Ⓨ Ⓝ
Passively inverts the calcaneus	Ⓨ Ⓝ	Ⓨ Ⓝ	Ⓨ Ⓝ
Performs assessment bilaterally	Ⓨ Ⓝ	Ⓨ Ⓝ	Ⓨ Ⓝ

The psychomotor skill was performed completely and in the appropriate order   0 1 2 3 4 5

The tester had control of the subject and the situation (showed confidence)   0 1 2 3 4 5

Method of performing the skill allowed the tester the ability to determine:
severity, proper progression, and the *fit* in the overall picture (Oral)   0 1 2 3 4 5

In order for a grade of *minimum standard* to be given, the total must be ≥11   TOTAL = _____

```
 1    2    3    4    5    6    7    8    9   10   11   12   13   14   15
 |____|____|____|____|____|____|____|____|____|____|____|____|____|____|
Not Acceptable                          Meets                  Exceeds
                                  Minimum Standards      Minimum Standards
```

TEST ENVIRONMENTS

L: Laboratory/Classroom Testing
C: Clinical/Field Testing
P: Practicum Testing
A: Assessment/Mock Exam Testing
S: Self-Reporting

SKILL TEST INFORMATION

Positive Finding: Inversion greater than the uninvolved limb; pain, laxity

Involved Structure: Calcaneofibular ligament

Special Considerations: N/A

Reference(s): Konin et al (2002); Magee; Starkey et al (2002)

Supplies Needed: Table or chair

LIGAMENTOUS STRESS TESTS
(LST-L-Test 3)

Peer Review_____   Peer Review _____

Skill Acquisition: _____   Practice Opportunities: _____

Please demonstrate how you would do the ligamentous stress test known as the **Kleiger Test (External Rotation Test)***. You have 2 minutes to complete this task.*

Tester places athlete and limb in appropriate position	Test 1	Test 2	Test 3
Seated	Ⓨ Ⓝ	Ⓨ Ⓝ	Ⓨ Ⓝ
Knee flexed to 90 degrees (legs over the edge of the table)	Ⓨ Ⓝ	Ⓨ Ⓝ	Ⓨ Ⓝ
Foot placed in a neutral position (0 degrees dorsiflexion)	Ⓨ Ⓝ	Ⓨ Ⓝ	Ⓨ Ⓝ
Tester placed in proper position	**Test 1**	**Test 2**	**Test 3**
Stabilizes tibia (do not compress the fibula) with one hand	Ⓨ Ⓝ	Ⓨ Ⓝ	Ⓨ Ⓝ
Grasps the foot (medial aspect) with the other hand	Ⓨ Ⓝ	Ⓨ Ⓝ	Ⓨ Ⓝ
Tester performs test according to accepted guidelines	**Test 1**	**Test 2**	**Test 3**
Maintains relaxation of the limb	Ⓨ Ⓝ	Ⓨ Ⓝ	Ⓨ Ⓝ
Rotates the foot laterally (calcaneus and talus)	Ⓨ Ⓝ	Ⓨ Ⓝ	Ⓨ Ⓝ
Performs assessment bilaterally	Ⓨ Ⓝ	Ⓨ Ⓝ	Ⓨ Ⓝ

The psychomotor skill was performed completely and in the appropriate order   **0 1 2 3 4 5**

The tester had control of the subject and the situation (showed confidence)   **0 1 2 3 4 5**

Method of performing the skill allowed the tester the ability to determine:
severity, proper progression, and the *fit* in the overall picture (Oral)   **0 1 2 3 4 5**

In order for a grade of *minimum standard* to be given, the total must be ≥11   **TOTAL = _____**

```
   1    2    3    4    5    6    7    8    9   10   11   12   13   14   15
   |    |    |    |    |    |    |    |    |    |    |    |    |    |    |
```
Not Acceptable   **Meets**   **Exceeds**
                                       Minimum Standards   **Minimum Standards**

TEST ENVIRONMENTS

L: Laboratory/Classroom Testing
C: Clinical/Field Testing
P: Practicum Testing
A: Assessment/Mock Exam Testing
S: Self-Reporting

SKILL TEST INFORMATION

Positive Finding: Pain
Involved Structure: Deltoid ligament; syndesmosis
Special Considerations: Pay close attention to the location of the pain
Reference(s): Magee; Starkey et al (2002)
Supplies Needed: Table or chair

LIGAMENTOUS STRESS TESTS
(LST-L-Test 4)

Peer Review_____   Peer Review _____

Skill Acquisition: _____   Practice Opportunities: _____

*This problem allows you the opportunity to demonstrate a ligamentous stress test known as the **Eversion Stress Test (Eversion Talar Tilt Test)**. You have 2 minutes to complete this task.*

Tester places athlete and limb in appropriate position	Test 1	Test 2	Test 3
Seated/supine	Y N	Y N	Y N
Foot over the edge of the table	Y N	Y N	Y N
Knee flexed to 90 degrees	Y N	Y N	Y N
Tester placed in proper position	**Test 1**	**Test 2**	**Test 3**
Stabilizes tibia and fibula with one hand	Y N	Y N	Y N
Holds foot in neutral position with other hand	Y N	Y N	Y N
Tester performs test according to accepted guidelines	**Test 1**	**Test 2**	**Test 3**
Maintains relaxation of the limb	Y N	Y N	Y N
Passively everts the calcaneus	Y N	Y N	Y N
Performs assessment bilaterally	Y N	Y N	Y N

The psychomotor skill was performed completely and in the appropriate order   0 1 2 3 4 5

The tester had control of the subject and the situation (showed confidence)   0 1 2 3 4 5

Method of performing the skill allowed the tester the ability to determine: severity, proper progression, and the *fit* in the overall picture (Oral)   0 1 2 3 4 5

In order for a grade of *minimum standard* to be given, the total must be ≥11   TOTAL = _____

```
 1    2    3    4    5    6    7    8    9    10   11   12   13   14   15
 |----|----|----|----|----|----|----|----|----|----|----|----|----|----|
```
Not Acceptable   **Meets**   **Exceeds**
                                    Minimum Standards   **Minimum Standards**

TEST ENVIRONMENTS
L: Laboratory/Classroom Testing
C: Clinical/Field Testing
P: Practicum Testing
A: Assessment/Mock Exam Testing
S: Self-Reporting

SKILL TEST INFORMATION
Positive Finding: Eversion greater than the uninvolved limb
Involved Structure: Deltoid ligament
Special Considerations: N/A
Reference(s): Starkey et al (2002)
Supplies Needed: Table

LIGAMENTOUS STRESS TESTS
(LST-L-Test 5)

Peer Review_____   Peer Review _____

Skill Acquisition: _____   Practice Opportunities: _____

This problem allows you the opportunity to demonstrate an orthopedic test known as the **Valgus Stress Test for the Knee**. *You have 2 minutes to complete this task.*

Tester places athlete and limb in appropriate position	Test 1	Test 2	Test 3
Supine	Y N	Y N	Y N
Knee in 20 to 30 degrees of flexion (superficial MCL)	Y N	Y N	Y N
Knee in 0 degrees of extension (deep MCL)	Y N	Y N	Y N
Tester placed in proper position	**Test 1**	**Test 2**	**Test 3**
Places one hand on distal, medial tibia	Y N	Y N	Y N
Places the other hand on distal, lateral femur	Y N	Y N	Y N
Tester performs test according to accepted guidelines	**Test 1**	**Test 2**	**Test 3**
Maintains relaxation of the limb	Y N	Y N	Y N
Applies valgus stress to the knee joint	Y N	Y N	Y N
Prevents the tibia and femur from rotating during the test	Y N	Y N	Y N
Performs assessment bilaterally	Y N	Y N	Y N

The psychomotor skill was performed completely and in the appropriate order   **0 1 2 3 4 5**

The tester had control of the subject and the situation (showed confidence)   **0 1 2 3 4 5**

Method of performing the skill allowed the tester the ability to determine:
severity, proper progression, and the *fit* in the overall picture (Oral)   **0 1 2 3 4 5**

In order for a grade of *minimum standard* to be given, the total must be ≥11   **TOTAL = _____**

```
  1     2     3     4     5     6     7     8     9    10    11    12    13    14    15
  |     |     |     |     |     |     |     |     |     |     |     |     |     |     |
```
Not Acceptable   **Meets**   **Exceeds**
                                          Minimum Standards   **Minimum Standards**

TEST ENVIRONMENTS

L: Laboratory/Classroom Testing
C: Clinical/Field Testing
P: Practicum Testing
A: Assessment/Mock Exam Testing
S: Self-Reporting

SKILL TEST INFORMATION

Positive Finding: Laxity; pain
Involved Structure: Medial collateral ligament
Special Considerations: 0 degrees extension = deep MCL;
20 to 30 degrees extension =
superficial portion of the MCL
Reference(s): Konin et al (2002); Starkey et al (2002)
Supplies Needed: Table

LIGAMENTOUS STRESS TESTS
(LST-L-Test 6)

Peer Review _____   Peer Review _____

Skill Acquisition: _____   Practice Opportunities: _____

This problem allows you the opportunity to demonstrate an orthopedic test known as the **Varus Stress Test for the Knee**. *You have 2 minutes to complete this task.*

Tester places athlete and limb in appropriate position	Test 1	Test 2	Test 3
Supine	Ⓨ Ⓝ	Ⓨ Ⓝ	Ⓨ Ⓝ
Knee in 20 to 30 degrees of flexion	Ⓨ Ⓝ	Ⓨ Ⓝ	Ⓨ Ⓝ
Tester placed in proper position	**Test 1**	**Test 2**	**Test 3**
Places one hand on distal, lateral tibia	Ⓨ Ⓝ	Ⓨ Ⓝ	Ⓨ Ⓝ
Places the other hand on distal, medial femur	Ⓨ Ⓝ	Ⓨ Ⓝ	Ⓨ Ⓝ
Tester performs test according to accepted guidelines	**Test 1**	**Test 2**	**Test 3**
Maintains relaxation of the limb	Ⓨ Ⓝ	Ⓨ Ⓝ	Ⓨ Ⓝ
Applies varus stress to the knee joint	Ⓨ Ⓝ	Ⓨ Ⓝ	Ⓨ Ⓝ
Prevents the tibia and femur from rotating during the test	Ⓨ Ⓝ	Ⓨ Ⓝ	Ⓨ Ⓝ
Performs assessment bilaterally	Ⓨ Ⓝ	Ⓨ Ⓝ	Ⓨ Ⓝ

The psychomotor skill was performed completely and in the appropriate order   **0 1 2 3 4 5**

The tester had control of the subject and the situation (showed confidence)   **0 1 2 3 4 5**

Method of performing the skill allowed the tester the ability to determine:
severity, proper progression, and the *fit* in the overall picture (Oral)   **0 1 2 3 4 5**

In order for a grade of *minimum standard* to be given, the total must be ≥11   **TOTAL = _____**

```
  1    2    3    4    5    6    7    8    9   10   11   12   13   14   15
  |____|____|____|____|____|____|____|____|____|____|____|____|____|____|
```

Not Acceptable	Meets Minimum Standards	Exceeds Minimum Standards

TEST ENVIRONMENTS

L: Laboratory/Classroom Testing
C: Clinical/Field Testing
P: Practicum Testing
A: Assessment/Mock Exam Testing
S: Self-Reporting

SKILL TEST INFORMATION

Positive Finding: Laxity, pain
Involved Structure: Lateral collateral ligament
Special Considerations: N/A
Reference(s): Konin et al (2002); Starkey et al (2002)
Supplies Needed: Table

LIGAMENTOUS STRESS TESTS
(LST-L-Test 7)

Peer Review_____   Peer Review _____

Skill Acquisition: _____   Practice Opportunities: _____

This problem allows you the opportunity to demonstrate the **Lachman Test (Anterior Lachman/Ritchie/Trillat/ Lachman-Trillat Test)**. *You have 2 minutes to complete this task.*

Tester places athlete and limb in appropriate position	Test 1	Test 2	Test 3
Supine	Ⓨ Ⓝ	Ⓨ Ⓝ	Ⓨ Ⓝ
Knee in 10 to 25 degrees of flex on	Ⓨ Ⓝ	Ⓨ Ⓝ	Ⓨ Ⓝ
Tester placed in proper position	**Test 1**	**Test 2**	**Test 3**
Stabilizes posteriorly on calf with one hand	Ⓨ Ⓝ	Ⓨ Ⓝ	Ⓨ Ⓝ
Stabilizes anteriorly on distal femur with other hand (just proximal to the patella)	Ⓨ Ⓝ	Ⓨ Ⓝ	Ⓨ Ⓝ
Tester performs test according to accepted guidelines	**Test 1**	**Test 2**	**Test 3**
Maintains relaxation of the limb	Ⓨ Ⓝ	Ⓨ Ⓝ	Ⓨ Ⓝ
Attempts to anteriorly displace tibia on femur (draws anteriorly)	Ⓨ Ⓝ	Ⓨ Ⓝ	Ⓨ Ⓝ
Performs assessment bilaterally	Ⓨ Ⓝ	Ⓨ Ⓝ	Ⓨ Ⓝ

The psychomotor skill was performed completely and in the appropriate order   **0 1 2 3 4 5**

The tester had control of the subject and the situation (showed confidence)   **0 1 2 3 4 5**

Method of performing the skill allowed the tester the ability to determine:
severity, proper progression, and the *fit* in the overall picture (Oral)   **0 1 2 3 4 5**

In order for a grade of *minimum standard* to be given, the total must be ≥11   **TOTAL = _____**

```
  1    2    3    4    5    6    7    8    9   10   11   12   13   14   15
  |    |    |    |    |    |    |    |    |    |    |    |    |    |    |
```
Not Acceptable   **Meets**   **Exceeds**
                                    Minimum Standards   **Minimum Standards**

TEST ENVIRONMENTS

L: Laboratory/Classroom Testing
C: Clinical/Field Testing
P: Practicum Testing
A: Assessment/Mock Exam Testing
S: Self-Reporting

SKILL TEST INFORMATION

Positive Finding: Excessive anterior translation
Involved Structure: ACL
Special Considerations: Many variations to this test
Reference(s): Konin et al (2002); Magee; Starkey et al (2002)
Supplies Needed: Table

LIGAMENTOUS STRESS TESTS
(LST-L-Test 8)

Peer Review_____   Peer Review _____

Skill Acquisition: _____   Practice Opportunities: _____

This problem allows you the opportunity to demonstrate the **Anterior Drawer Test (Drawer Sign) for the Knee**. *You have 2 minutes to complete this task.*

Tester places athlete and limb in appropriate position	Test 1	Test 2	Test 3
Supine	Ⓨ Ⓝ	Ⓨ Ⓝ	Ⓨ Ⓝ
Hip is flexed to 45 degrees	Ⓨ Ⓝ	Ⓨ Ⓝ	Ⓨ Ⓝ
Knee is flexed to 90 degrees (foot in neutral)	Ⓨ Ⓝ	Ⓨ Ⓝ	Ⓨ Ⓝ
Tester placed in proper position	**Test 1**	**Test 2**	**Test 3**
Sits on athlete's involved foot	Ⓨ Ⓝ	Ⓨ Ⓝ	Ⓨ Ⓝ
Cups the hands around the proximal (posterior) aspect of the lower leg, thumbs on the tibial plateau	Ⓨ Ⓝ	Ⓨ Ⓝ	Ⓨ Ⓝ
Tester performs test according to accepted guidelines	**Test 1**	**Test 2**	**Test 3**
Applies an anterior force to the proximal aspect of the lower leg	Ⓨ Ⓝ	Ⓨ Ⓝ	Ⓨ Ⓝ
Maintains relaxation of the limb	Ⓨ Ⓝ	Ⓨ Ⓝ	Ⓨ Ⓝ
Performs assessment bilaterally	Ⓨ Ⓝ	Ⓨ Ⓝ	Ⓨ Ⓝ

The psychomotor skill was performed completely and in the appropriate order   0 1 2 3 4 5

The tester had control of the subject and the situation (showed confidence)   0 1 2 3 4 5

Method of performing the skill allowed the tester the ability to determine:
severity, proper progression, and the *fit* in the overall picture (Oral)   0 1 2 3 4 5

In order for a grade of *minimum standard* to be given, the total must be ≥11   **TOTAL = _____**

```
 1    2    3    4    5    6    7    8    9    10   11   12   13   14   15
 |    |    |    |    |    |    |    |    |    |    |    |    |    |    |
```
Not Acceptable   **Meets**   **Exceeds**
                                          Minimum Standards   **Minimum Standards**

SKILL TEST INFORMATION

TEST ENVIRONMENTS

L: Laboratory/Classroom Testing
C: Clinical/Field Testing
P: Practicum Testing
A: Assessment/Mock Exam Testing
S: Self-Reporting

Positive Finding: Anterior displacement
Involved Structure: ACL
Special Considerations: Check posterior cruciate ligament first; relax hamstrings
Reference(s): Konin et al (2002); Magee; Starkey et al (2002)
Supplies Needed: Table

LIGAMENTOUS STRESS TESTS
(LST-L-Test 9)

Peer Review_____   Peer Review _____

Skill Acquisition: _____   Practice Opportunities: _____

This problem allows you the opportunity to demonstrate the **Posterior Drawer Test for the Knee**. *You have 2 minutes to complete this task.*

Tester places athlete and limb in appropriate position	Test 1	Test 2	Test 3
Supine	Ⓨ Ⓝ	Ⓨ Ⓝ	Ⓨ Ⓝ
Hip is flexed to 45 degrees	Ⓨ Ⓝ	Ⓨ Ⓝ	Ⓨ Ⓝ
Knee is flexed to 90 degrees (foot in neutral)	Ⓨ Ⓝ	Ⓨ Ⓝ	Ⓨ Ⓝ
Tester placed in proper position	**Test 1**	**Test 2**	**Test 3**
Sits on athlete's involved foot	Ⓨ Ⓝ	Ⓨ Ⓝ	Ⓨ Ⓝ
Cups the hands around the proximal (posterior) aspect of the lower leg, thumbs on the tibial plateau	Ⓨ Ⓝ	Ⓨ Ⓝ	Ⓨ Ⓝ
Tester performs test according to accepted guidelines	**Test 1**	**Test 2**	**Test 3**
Applies a posterior force to the proximal aspect of the lower leg	Ⓨ Ⓝ	Ⓨ Ⓝ	Ⓨ Ⓝ
Maintains relaxation of the limb	Ⓨ Ⓝ	Ⓨ Ⓝ	Ⓨ Ⓝ
Performs assessment bilaterally	Ⓨ Ⓝ	Ⓨ Ⓝ	Ⓨ Ⓝ

The psychomotor skill was performed completely and in the appropriate order   0 1 2 3 4 5

The tester had control of the subject and the situation (showed confidence)   0 1 2 3 4 5

Method of performing the skill allowed the tester the ability to determine: severity, proper progression, and the *fit* in the overall picture (Oral)   0 1 2 3 4 5

In order for a grade of *minimum standard* to be given, the total must be ≥11   TOTAL = _____

```
  1    2    3    4    5    6    7    8    9   10   11   12   13   14   15
```
Not Acceptable   **Meets**   **Exceeds**
                                        Minimum Standards   **Minimum Standards**

TEST ENVIRONMENTS
L: Laboratory/Classroom Testing
C: Clinical/Field Testing
P: Practicum Testing
A: Assessment/Mock Exam Testing
S: Self-Reporting

SKILL TEST INFORMATION
Positive Finding: Posterior displacement
Involved Structure: PCL
Special Considerations: N/A
Reference(s): Konin et al (2002); Starkey et al (2002)
Supplies Needed: Table

LIGAMENTOUS STRESS TESTS
(LST-L-Test 10)

Peer Review_____   Peer Review _____

Skill Acquisition: _____   Practice Opportunities: _____

This problem allows you the opportunity to demonstrate the **Slocum Test (Internal Tibial Rotation) for the Knee.** *You have 2 minutes to complete this task.*

Tester places athlete and limb in appropriate position	Test 1	Test 2	Test 3
Supine	Ⓨ Ⓝ	Ⓨ Ⓝ	Ⓨ Ⓝ
Hip is flexed to 45 degrees	Ⓨ Ⓝ	Ⓨ Ⓝ	Ⓨ Ⓝ
Knee is flexed to 90 degrees (foot in neutral)	Ⓨ Ⓝ	Ⓨ Ⓝ	Ⓨ Ⓝ
Tibia internally rotated 15 to 30 degrees	Ⓨ Ⓝ	Ⓨ Ⓝ	Ⓨ Ⓝ

Tester placed in proper position	Test 1	Test 2	Test 3
Sits on athlete's involved foot	Ⓨ Ⓝ	Ⓨ Ⓝ	Ⓨ Ⓝ
Cups the hands around the proximal (posterior) aspect of the lower leg, thumbs on the tibial plateau	Ⓨ Ⓝ	Ⓨ Ⓝ	Ⓨ Ⓝ

Tester performs test according to accepted guidelines	Test 1	Test 2	Test 3
Applies an anterior force to the proximal aspect of the lower leg	Ⓨ Ⓝ	Ⓨ Ⓝ	Ⓨ Ⓝ
Maintains relaxation of the limb	Ⓨ Ⓝ	Ⓨ Ⓝ	Ⓨ Ⓝ
Performs assessment bilaterally	Ⓨ Ⓝ	Ⓨ Ⓝ	Ⓨ Ⓝ

The psychomotor skill was performed completely and in the appropriate order   **0 1 2 3 4 5**

The tester had control of the subject and the situation (showed confidence)   **0 1 2 3 4 5**

Method of performing the skill allowed the tester the ability to determine:
severity, proper progression, and the *fit* in the overall picture (Oral)   **0 1 2 3 4 5**

In order for a grade of *minimum standard* to be given, the total must be ≥11   **TOTAL = _____**

```
 1    2    3    4    5    6    7    8    9    10   11   12   13   14   15
 |    |    |    |    |    |    |    |    |    |    |    |    |    |    |
```

Not Acceptable   **Meets**   **Exceeds**
                                    Minimum Standards   **Minimum Standards**

TEST ENVIRONMENTS

L: Laboratory/Classroom Testing
C: Clinical/Field Testing
P: Practicum Testing
A: Assessment/Mock Exam Testing
S: Self-Reporting

SKILL TEST INFORMATION

Positive Finding: Anterior displacement
Involved Structure: ACL; posterolateral capsule
Special Considerations: Hamstring guarding
Reference(s): Konin et al (2002); Magee
Supplies Needed: Table

LIGAMENTOUS STRESS TESTS
(LST-L-Test 11)

Peer Review_____   Peer Review _____

Skill Acquisition: _____   Practice Opportunities: _____

This problem allows you the opportunity to demonstrate the **Slocum Test (External Tibial Rotation) for the Knee.** *You have 2 minutes to complete this task.*

Tester places athlete and limb in appropriate position	Test 1	Test 2	Test 3
Supine	Ⓨ Ⓝ	Ⓨ Ⓝ	Ⓨ Ⓝ
Hip is flexed to 45 degrees	Ⓨ Ⓝ	Ⓨ Ⓝ	Ⓨ Ⓝ
Knee is flexed to 90 degrees (foot in neutral)	Ⓨ Ⓝ	Ⓨ Ⓝ	Ⓨ Ⓝ
Tibia externally rotated 15 to 20 degrees	Ⓨ Ⓝ	Ⓨ Ⓝ	Ⓨ Ⓝ
Tester placed in proper position	**Test 1**	**Test 2**	**Test 3**
Sits on athlete's involved foot	Ⓨ Ⓝ	Ⓨ Ⓝ	Ⓨ Ⓝ
Cups the hands around the proximal (posterior) aspect of the lower leg, thumbs on the tibial plateau	Ⓨ Ⓝ	Ⓨ Ⓝ	Ⓨ Ⓝ
Tester performs test according to accepted guidelines	**Test 1**	**Test 2**	**Test 3**
Applies an anterior force to the proximal aspect of the lower leg	Ⓨ Ⓝ	Ⓨ Ⓝ	Ⓨ Ⓝ
Maintains relaxation of the limb	Ⓨ Ⓝ	Ⓨ Ⓝ	Ⓨ Ⓝ
Performs assessment bilaterally	Ⓨ Ⓝ	Ⓨ Ⓝ	Ⓨ Ⓝ

The psychomotor skill was performed completely and in the appropriate order   **0 1 2 3 4 5**

The tester had control of the subject and the situation (showed confidence)   **0 1 2 3 4 5**

Method of performing the skill allowed the tester the ability to determine:
severity, proper progression, and the *fit* in the overall picture (Oral)   **0 1 2 3 4 5**

In order for a grade of *minimum standard* to be given, the total must be ≥11   **TOTAL = _____**

```
 1    2    3    4    5    6    7    8    9    10   11   12   13   14   15
 |    |    |    |    |    |    |    |    |    |    |    |    |    |    |
```
Not Acceptable   **Meets**   **Exceeds**
                                     Minimum Standards   **Minimum Standards**

TEST ENVIRONMENTS
L: Laboratory/Classroom Testing
C: Clinical/Field Testing
P: Practicum Testing
A: Assessment/Mock Exam Testing
S: Self-Reporting

SKILL TEST INFORMATION
Positive Finding: Anterior displacement
Involved Structure: ACL; posteromedial capsule
Special Considerations: Hamstring guarding
Reference(s): Konin et al (2002); Magee
Supplies Needed: Table

LIGAMENTOUS STRESS TESTS
(LST-L-Test 12)

Peer Review_____   Peer Review _____

Skill Acquisition: _____   Practice Opportunities: _____

This problem allows you the opportunity to demonstrate the **Hughston Posteromedial Drawer Test for the Knee.** *You have 2 minutes to complete this task.*

Tester places athlete and limb in appropriate position	Test 1	Test 2	Test 3
Supine	Ⓨ Ⓝ	Ⓨ Ⓝ	Ⓨ Ⓝ
Hip is flexed to 45 degrees	Ⓨ Ⓝ	Ⓨ Ⓝ	Ⓨ Ⓝ
Knee is flexed to 90 degrees (foot in neutral)	Ⓨ Ⓝ	Ⓨ Ⓝ	Ⓨ Ⓝ
Tibia internally rotated 15 to 30 degrees	Ⓨ Ⓝ	Ⓨ Ⓝ	Ⓨ Ⓝ
Tester placed in proper position	**Test 1**	**Test 2**	**Test 3**
Sits on athlete's involved foot	Ⓨ Ⓝ	Ⓨ Ⓝ	Ⓨ Ⓝ
Cups the hands around the proximal (posterior) aspect of the lower leg, thumbs on the tibial plateau	Ⓨ Ⓝ	Ⓨ Ⓝ	Ⓨ Ⓝ
Tester performs test according to accepted guidelines	**Test 1**	**Test 2**	**Test 3**
Applies a posterior force to the proximal aspect of the lower leg	Ⓨ Ⓝ	Ⓨ Ⓝ	Ⓨ Ⓝ
Maintains relaxation of the limb	Ⓨ Ⓝ	Ⓨ Ⓝ	Ⓨ Ⓝ
Performs assessment bilaterally	Ⓨ Ⓝ	Ⓨ Ⓝ	Ⓨ Ⓝ

The psychomotor skill was performed completely and in the appropriate order   **0 1 2 3 4 5**

The tester had control of the subject and the situation (showed confidence)   **0 1 2 3 4 5**

Method of performing the skill allowed the tester the ability to determine:
severity, proper progression, and the *fit* in the overall picture (Oral)   **0 1 2 3 4 5**

In order for a grade of *minimum standard* to be given, the total must be ≥11   **TOTAL = _____**

```
  1     2     3     4     5     6     7     8     9    10    11    12    13    14    15
  |     |     |     |     |     |     |     |     |     |     |     |     |     |     |
```
Not Acceptable   **Meets**   **Exceeds**
                                               Minimum Standards   **Minimum Standards**

TEST ENVIRONMENTS
L: Laboratory/Classroom Testing
C: Clinical/Field Testing
P: Practicum Testing
A: Assessment/Mock Exam Testing
S: Self-Reporting

SKILL TEST INFORMATION
Positive Finding: Posterior displacement
Involved Structure: PCL; posteromedial capsule
Special Considerations: N/A
Reference(s): Konin et al (2002); Magee
Supplies Needed: Table

LIGAMENTOUS STRESS TESTS
(LST-L-Test 13)

Peer Review_____   Peer Review _____

Skill Acquisition: _____   Practice Opportunities: _____

This problem allows you the opportunity to demonstrate the **Hughston Posterolateral Drawer Test for the Knee.**
You have 2 minutes to complete this task.

Tester places athlete and limb in appropriate position	Test 1	Test 2	Test 3
Supine	Ⓨ Ⓝ	Ⓨ Ⓝ	Ⓨ Ⓝ
Hip is flexed to 45 degrees	Ⓨ Ⓝ	Ⓨ Ⓝ	Ⓨ Ⓝ
Knee is flexed to 90 degrees (foot in neutral)	Ⓨ Ⓝ	Ⓨ Ⓝ	Ⓨ Ⓝ
Tibia externally rotated 15 to 20 degrees	Ⓨ Ⓝ	Ⓨ Ⓝ	Ⓨ Ⓝ
Tester placed in proper position	**Test 1**	**Test 2**	**Test 3**
Sits on athlete's involved foot	Ⓨ Ⓝ	Ⓨ Ⓝ	Ⓨ Ⓝ
Cups the hands around the proximal (anterior) aspect of the lower leg, thumbs on the tibial plateau	Ⓨ Ⓝ	Ⓨ Ⓝ	Ⓨ Ⓝ
Tester performs test according to accepted guidelines	**Test 1**	**Test 2**	**Test 3**
Applies an posterior force to the proximal aspect of the lower leg	Ⓨ Ⓝ	Ⓨ Ⓝ	Ⓨ Ⓝ
Maintains relaxation of the limb	Ⓨ Ⓝ	Ⓨ Ⓝ	Ⓨ Ⓝ
Performs assessment bilaterally	Ⓨ Ⓝ	Ⓨ Ⓝ	Ⓨ Ⓝ

The psychomotor skill was performed completely and in the appropriate order   **0 1 2 3 4 5**

The tester had control of the subject and the situation (showed confidence)   **0 1 2 3 4 5**

Method of performing the skill allowed the tester the ability to determine:
severity, proper progression, and the *fit* in the overall picture (Oral)   **0 1 2 3 4 5**

In order for a grade of *minimum standard* to be given, the total must be ≥11   **TOTAL = _____**

```
  1    2    3    4    5    6    7    8    9   10   11   12   13   14   15
  |    |    |    |    |    |    |    |    |    |    |    |    |    |    |
```
Not Acceptable   **Meets**   **Exceeds**
                                            Minimum Standards   **Minimum Standards**

TEST ENVIRONMENTS
L: Laboratory/Classroom Testing
C: Clinical/Field Testing
P: Practicum Testing
A: Assessment/Mock Exam Testing
S: Self-Reporting

SKILL TEST INFORMATION
Positive Finding: Posterior displacement
Involved Structure: PCL; posterolateral capsule
Special Considerations: N/A
Reference(s):   Konin et al (2002); Magee
Supplies Needed: Table

LIGAMENTOUS STRESS TESTS
(LST-L-Test 14)

Peer Review_____   Peer Review _____

Skill Acquisition: _____   Practice Opportunities: _____

This problem allows you the opportunity to demonstrate the **Posterior Sag Test (Gravity Drawer Test) for the Knee**. *You have 2 minutes to complete this task.*

Tester places athlete and limb in appropriate position	Test 1	Test 2	Test 3
Supine	Ⓨ Ⓝ	Ⓨ Ⓝ	Ⓨ Ⓝ
Hips flexed to 45 degrees	Ⓨ Ⓝ	Ⓨ Ⓝ	Ⓨ Ⓝ
Knee is flexed to 90 degrees (foot in neutral)	Ⓨ Ⓝ	Ⓨ Ⓝ	Ⓨ Ⓝ
Tester placed in proper position	**Test 1**	**Test 2**	**Test 3**
Stands to the side of the athlete	Ⓨ Ⓝ	Ⓨ Ⓝ	Ⓨ Ⓝ
Tester performs test according to accepted guidelines	**Test 1**	**Test 2**	**Test 3**
Observes tibial tubercles for posterior displacement of the tibia on the femur	Ⓨ Ⓝ	Ⓨ Ⓝ	Ⓨ Ⓝ
Maintains relaxation of the limb	Ⓨ Ⓝ	Ⓨ Ⓝ	Ⓨ Ⓝ
Observes bilaterally	Ⓨ Ⓝ	Ⓨ Ⓝ	Ⓨ Ⓝ

The psychomotor skill was performed completely and in the appropriate order   0 1 2 3 4 5

The tester had control of the subject and the situation (showed confidence)   0 1 2 3 4 5

Method of performing the skill allowed the tester the ability to determine:
severity, proper progression, and the *fit* in the overall picture (Oral)   0 1 2 3 4 5

In order for a grade of *minimum standard* to be given, the total must be ≥11   TOTAL = _____

```
 1    2    3    4    5    6    7    8    9   10   11   12   13   14   15
 |    |    |    |    |    |    |    |    |    |    |    |    |    |    |
```

Not Acceptable   **Meets**   **Exceeds**
                              Minimum Standards   **Minimum Standards**

TEST ENVIRONMENTS

L: Laboratory/Classroom Testing
C: Clinical/Field Testing
P: Practicum Testing
A: Assessment/Mock Exam Testing
S: Self-Reporting

SKILL TEST INFORMATION

Positive Finding: Posterior displacement (looking for a "sag")

Involved Structure: PCL

Special Considerations: Adding active contraction of the quad is the voluntary anterior draw sign

Reference(s): Konin et al (2002); Magee

Supplies Needed: Table

LIGAMENTOUS STRESS TESTS
(LST-L-Test 15)

Peer Review_____   Peer Review _____

Skill Acquisition: _____   Practice Opportunities: _____

This problem allows you the opportunity to demonstrate the **Godfrey Test (Godfrey 90/90/Godfrey Gravity Test) for the Knee.** *You have 2 minutes to complete this task.*

Tester places athlete and limb in appropriate position	Test 1	Test 2	Test 3
Supine	Ⓨ Ⓝ	Ⓨ Ⓝ	Ⓨ Ⓝ
Passively flexes the athlete's hips and knee to 90 degrees (90/90 position)	Ⓨ Ⓝ	Ⓨ Ⓝ	Ⓨ Ⓝ
Tester placed in proper position	**Test 1**	**Test 2**	**Test 3**
Stands to the side of the athlete	Ⓨ Ⓝ	Ⓨ Ⓝ	Ⓨ Ⓝ
Places both hands under the distal aspect of both lower legs (stabilizes the femur)	Ⓨ Ⓝ	Ⓨ Ⓝ	Ⓨ Ⓝ
Tester performs test according to accepted guidelines	**Test 1**	**Test 2**	**Test 3**
Observes tibial tubercles for posterior displacement of the tibia on the femur	Ⓨ Ⓝ	Ⓨ Ⓝ	Ⓨ Ⓝ
Maintains relaxation of the limb	Ⓨ Ⓝ	Ⓨ Ⓝ	Ⓨ Ⓝ
Observes bilaterally	Ⓨ Ⓝ	Ⓨ Ⓝ	Ⓨ Ⓝ

The psychomotor skill was performed completely and in the appropriate order   0 1 2 3 4 5

The tester had control of the subject and the situation (showed confidence)   0 1 2 3 4 5

Method of performing the skill allowed the tester the ability to determine:
severity, proper progression, and the *fit* in the overall picture (Oral)   0 1 2 3 4 5

In order for a grade of *minimum standard* to be given, the total must be ≥11   TOTAL = _____

```
 1     2     3     4     5     6     7     8     9    10    11    12    13    14    15
 |     |     |     |     |     |     |     |     |     |     |     |     |     |     |
```

Not Acceptable   **Meets**   **Exceeds**
                                    Minimum Standards   **Minimum Standards**

TEST ENVIRONMENTS

L: Laboratory/Classroom Testing
C: Clinical/Field Testing
P: Practicum Testing
A: Assessment/Mock Exam Testing
S: Self-Reporting

SKILL TEST INFORMATION

Positive Finding:	Downward displacement of the involved tibia
Involved Structure:	PCL
Special Considerations:	N/A
Reference(s):	Konin et al (2002); Magee; Starkey et al (2002)
Supplies Needed:	Table

LIGAMENTOUS STRESS TESTS
(LST-L-Test 16)

Peer Review_____   Peer Review _____

Skill Acquisition: _____   Practice Opportunities: _____

This problem allows you the opportunity to demonstrate the **Lateral Pivot-Shift (MacIntosh Test/Lamaire Test) for the Knee**. *You have 2 minutes to complete this task.*

Tester places athlete and limb in appropriate position	Test 1	Test 2	Test 3
Supine	Ⓨ Ⓝ	Ⓨ Ⓝ	Ⓨ Ⓝ
Hips flexed to 20 to 40 degrees	Ⓨ Ⓝ	Ⓨ Ⓝ	Ⓨ Ⓝ
Knee in full extension (bounce home reinforces full extension)	Ⓨ Ⓝ	Ⓨ Ⓝ	Ⓨ Ⓝ
Tester placed in proper position	**Test 1**	**Test 2**	**Test 3**
Stands to the side of the athlete	Ⓨ Ⓝ	Ⓨ Ⓝ	Ⓨ Ⓝ
Grasps the distal aspect of the lower leg with one hand	Ⓨ Ⓝ	Ⓨ Ⓝ	Ⓨ Ⓝ
Places the other hand laterally over the fibular head	Ⓨ Ⓝ	Ⓨ Ⓝ	Ⓨ Ⓝ
Tester performs test according to accepted guidelines	**Test 1**	**Test 2**	**Test 3**
Applies a valgus stress over the knee	Ⓨ Ⓝ	Ⓨ Ⓝ	Ⓨ Ⓝ
Maintains internal rotation of the tibia	Ⓨ Ⓝ	Ⓨ Ⓝ	Ⓨ Ⓝ
Passively flexes the athlete's knee through 90 degrees, slowly	Ⓨ Ⓝ	Ⓨ Ⓝ	Ⓨ Ⓝ
Palpates for a backward shift of the tibia	Ⓨ Ⓝ	Ⓨ Ⓝ	Ⓨ Ⓝ
Maintains relaxation of the limb	Ⓨ Ⓝ	Ⓨ Ⓝ	Ⓨ Ⓝ
Performs assessment bilaterally	Ⓨ Ⓝ	Ⓨ Ⓝ	Ⓨ Ⓝ

The psychomotor skill was performed completely and in the appropriate order   0 1 2 3 4 5

The tester had control of the subject and the situation (showed confidence)   0 1 2 3 4 5

Method of performing the skill allowed the tester the ability to determine:
severity, proper progression, and the *fit* in the overall picture (Oral)   0 1 2 3 4 5

In order for a grade of *minimum standard* to be given, the total must be ≥11   TOTAL = _____

```
  1     2     3     4     5     6     7     8     9    10    11    12    13    14    15
  |     |     |     |     |     |     |     |     |     |     |     |     |     |     |
```

Not Acceptable   **Meets**   **Exceeds**
                                          Minimum Standards   **Minimum Standards**

SKILL TEST INFORMATION

Positive Finding: "Clunk"; posterior displacement of the tibia; slight external rotation of the tibia

TEST ENVIRONMENTS

L: Laboratory/Classroom Testing
C: Clinical/Field Testing
P: Practicum Testing
A: Assessment/Mock Exam Testing
S: Self-Reporting

Involved Structure: ACL; posterolateral capsule
Special Considerations: Positive sign occurs around 25 degrees
Reference(s): Magee; Starkey et al (2002)
Supplies Needed: Table

LIGAMENTOUS STRESS TESTS
(LST-L-Test 17)

Peer Review_____   Peer Review _____

Skill Acquisition: _____   Practice Opportunities: _____

This problem allows you the opportunity to demonstrate the **Jerk Test (Jerk Test of Hughston) for the Knee**. *You have 2 minutes to complete this task.*

Tester places athlete and limb in appropriate position	Test 1	Test 2	Test 3
Supine	Y N	Y N	Y N
Hip flexed to 45 degrees	Y N	Y N	Y N
Knee in full flexion	Y N	Y N	Y N
Tester placed in proper position	**Test 1**	**Test 2**	**Test 3**
Stands to the side of the athlete	Y N	Y N	Y N
Grasps the distal aspect of the lower leg with one hand	Y N	Y N	Y N
Places the other hand laterally over the fibular head	Y N	Y N	Y N
Tester performs test according to accepted guidelines	**Test 1**	**Test 2**	**Test 3**
Applies a valgus stress over the knee	Y N	Y N	Y N
Maintains internal rotation of the tibia	Y N	Y N	Y N
Passively extends the athlete's knee from 90 degrees to full extension, slowly	Y N	Y N	Y N
Maintains relaxation of the limb	Y N	Y N	Y N
Performs assessment bilaterally	Y N	Y N	Y N

The psychomotor skill was performed completely and in the appropriate order   **0 1 2 3 4 5**

The tester had control of the subject and the situation (showed confidence)   **0 1 2 3 4 5**

Method of performing the skill allowed the tester the ability to determine:
severity, proper progression, and the *fit* in the overall picture (Oral)   **0 1 2 3 4 5**

In order for a grade of *minimum standard* to be given, the total must be ≥11   **TOTAL = _____**

```
 1    2    3    4    5    6    7    8    9   10   11   12   13   14   15
 |    |    |    |    |    |    |    |    |    |    |    |    |    |    |
```

Not Acceptable   **Meets**   **Exceeds**
                                              Minimum Standards   **Minimum Standards**

TEST ENVIRONMENTS

L: Laboratory/Classroom Testing
C: Clinical/Field Testing
P: Practicum Testing
A: Assessment/Mock Exam Testing
S: Self-Reporting

SKILL TEST INFORMATION

Positive Finding:	"Clunk/jerk"; anterior subluxation or displacement of the tibia; slight internal rotation of the tibia
Involved Structure:	ACL; posterolateral capsule
Special Considerations:	Positive sign occurs around 25 degrees
Reference(s):	Konin et al (2002); Magee
Supplies Needed:	Table

Chapter 5

MANUAL MUSCLE TESTING

Manual Muscle Testing
(MMT-U-Test 1)

Peer Review_____   Peer Review _____

Skill Acquisition: _____   Practice Opportunities: _____

*This problem allows you the opportunity to demonstrate a manual muscle test for the **latissimus dorsi** muscle. You have 2 minutes to complete this task.*

Tester places athlete and limb in appropriate position	Test 1	Test 2	Test 3
Prone	Ⓨ Ⓝ	Ⓨ Ⓝ	Ⓨ Ⓝ
Shoulder placed in slight extension and adduction (palm facing body)	Ⓨ Ⓝ	Ⓨ Ⓝ	Ⓨ Ⓝ
Tester placed in proper position	**Test 1**	**Test 2**	**Test 3**
Stands to the side of the athlete	Ⓨ Ⓝ	Ⓨ Ⓝ	Ⓨ Ⓝ
Places one hand on the medial forearm	Ⓨ Ⓝ	Ⓨ Ⓝ	Ⓨ Ⓝ
Tester performs test according to accepted guidelines	**Test 1**	**Test 2**	**Test 3**
Instructs the athlete to hold this position	Ⓨ Ⓝ	Ⓨ Ⓝ	Ⓨ Ⓝ
Applies resistance in the direction of extension and adduction	Ⓨ Ⓝ	Ⓨ Ⓝ	Ⓨ Ⓝ
Holds resistance for 5 seconds	Ⓨ Ⓝ	Ⓨ Ⓝ	Ⓨ Ⓝ
Performs assessment bilaterally	Ⓨ Ⓝ	Ⓨ Ⓝ	Ⓨ Ⓝ

The psychomotor skill was performed completely and in the appropriate order   0 1 2 3 4 5

The tester had control of the subject and the situation (showed confidence)   0 1 2 3 4 5

Method of performing the skill allowed the tester the ability to determine:
severity, proper progression, and the *fit* in the overall picture (Oral)   0 1 2 3 4 5

In order for a grade of *minimum standard* to be given, the total must be ≥11   TOTAL = _____

```
  1    2    3    4    5    6    7    8    9   10   11   12   13   14   15
  |    |    |    |    |    |    |    |    |    |    |    |    |    |    |
```

Not Acceptable   **Meets**   **Exceeds**
                                    Minimum Standards   **Minimum Standards**

TEST ENVIRONMENTS	**SKILL TEST INFORMATION**

TEST ENVIRONMENTS

L: Laboratory/Classroom Testing
C: Clinical/Field Testing
P: Practicum Testing
A: Assessment/Mock Exam Testing
S: Self-Reporting

SKILL TEST INFORMATION

Positive Finding: Decreased ability to hold contraction
Involved Structure: Latissimus dorsi
Special Considerations: N/A
Reference(s): Kendall et al
Supplies Needed: Table

Manual Muscle Testing
(MMT-U-Test 2)

Peer Review_____   Peer Review _____

Skill Acquisition: _____   Practice Opportunities: _____

This problem allows you the opportunity to demonstrate a manual muscle test for the **pectoralis major (upper portion)** *muscle. You have 2 minutes to complete this task.*

Tester places athlete and limb in appropriate position	Test 1	Test 2	Test 3
Supine	Ⓨ Ⓝ	Ⓨ Ⓝ	Ⓨ Ⓝ
Shoulder placed in 90 degrees of flexion with slight medial rotation	Ⓨ Ⓝ	Ⓨ Ⓝ	Ⓨ Ⓝ
Elbow placed in full extension	Ⓨ Ⓝ	Ⓨ Ⓝ	Ⓨ Ⓝ
Tester placed in proper position	**Test 1**	**Test 2**	**Test 3**
Stands at the end of table, above the athlete's head	Ⓨ Ⓝ	Ⓨ Ⓝ	Ⓨ Ⓝ
Places one hand on the medial forearm	Ⓨ Ⓝ	Ⓨ Ⓝ	Ⓨ Ⓝ
Places other hand on the athlete's opposite shoulder (stabilizes body)	Ⓨ Ⓝ	Ⓨ Ⓝ	Ⓨ Ⓝ
Tester performs test according to accepted guidelines	**Test 1**	**Test 2**	**Test 3**
Instructs the athlete to hold this position	Ⓨ Ⓝ	Ⓨ Ⓝ	Ⓨ Ⓝ
Applies resistance in the direction of horizontal abduction (horizontal extension)	Ⓨ Ⓝ	Ⓨ Ⓝ	Ⓨ Ⓝ
Holds resistance for 5 seconds	Ⓨ Ⓝ	Ⓨ Ⓝ	Ⓨ Ⓝ
Performs assessment bilaterally	Ⓨ Ⓝ	Ⓨ Ⓝ	Ⓨ Ⓝ

The psychomotor skill was performed completely and in the appropriate order   **0 1 2 3 4 5**

The tester had control of the subject and the situation (showed confidence)   **0 1 2 3 4 5**

Method of performing the skill allowed the tester the ability to determine:
severity, proper progression, and the *fit* in the overall picture (Oral)   **0 1 2 3 4 5**

In order for a grade of *minimum standard* to be given, the total must be ≥11   **TOTAL = _____**

```
  1    2    3    4    5    6    7    8    9    10   11   12   13   14   15
  |____|____|____|____|____|____|____|____|____|____|____|____|____|____|
```

Not Acceptable   **Meets**   **Exceeds**
                                 Minimum Standards   **Minimum Standards**

TEST ENVIRONMENTS

L: Laboratory/Classroom Testing
C: Clinical/Field Testing
P: Practicum Testing
A: Assessment/Mock Exam Testing
S: Self-Reporting

SKILL TEST INFORMATION

Positive Finding: Decreased ability to hold contraction
Involved Structure: Pectoralis major (upper portion)
Special Considerations: N/A
Reference(s): Kendall et al
Supplies Needed: Table

MANUAL MUSCLE TESTING
(MMT-U-Test 3)

Peer Review_____   Peer Review _____

Skill Acquisition: _____   Practice Opportunities: _____

This problem allows you the opportunity to demonstrate a manual muscle test for the **pectoralis major (lower portion)** *muscle. You have 2 minutes to complete this task.*

Tester places athlete and limb in appropriate position	Test 1	Test 2	Test 3
Supine	Ⓨ Ⓝ	Ⓨ Ⓝ	Ⓨ Ⓝ
Shoulder placed in 90 degrees of flexion, slight medial rotation (moves the shoulder obliquely toward the opposite iliac crest)	Ⓨ Ⓝ	Ⓨ Ⓝ	Ⓨ Ⓝ
Elbow placed in full extension	Ⓨ Ⓝ	Ⓨ Ⓝ	Ⓨ Ⓝ
Tester placed in proper position	**Test 1**	**Test 2**	**Test 3**
Stands at the end of table, above the athlete's head	Ⓨ Ⓝ	Ⓨ Ⓝ	Ⓨ Ⓝ
Places one hand on the medial forearm	Ⓨ Ⓝ	Ⓨ Ⓝ	Ⓨ Ⓝ
Places other hand on the athlete's opposite iliac crest (stabilizes body)	Ⓨ Ⓝ	Ⓨ Ⓝ	Ⓨ Ⓝ
Tester performs test according to accepted guidelines	**Test 1**	**Test 2**	**Test 3**
Instructs the athlete to hold this position	Ⓨ Ⓝ	Ⓨ Ⓝ	Ⓨ Ⓝ
Applies resistance obliquely in the direction of horizontal abduction (horizontal extension)	Ⓨ Ⓝ	Ⓨ Ⓝ	Ⓨ Ⓝ
Holds resistance for 5 seconds	Ⓨ Ⓝ	Ⓨ Ⓝ	Ⓨ Ⓝ
Performs assessment bilaterally	Ⓨ Ⓝ	Ⓨ Ⓝ	Ⓨ Ⓝ

The psychomotor skill was performed completely and in the appropriate order   **0 1 2 3 4 5**

The tester had control of the subject and the situation (showed confidence)   **0 1 2 3 4 5**

Method of performing the skill allowed the tester the ability to determine:
severity, proper progression, and the *fit* in the overall picture (Oral)   **0 1 2 3 4 5**

In order for a grade of *minimum standard* to be given, the total must be ≥11   **TOTAL = _____**

```
 1     2     3     4     5     6     7     8     9    10    11    12    13    14    15
 |     |     |     |     |     |     |     |     |     |     |     |     |     |     |
```

Not Acceptable   **Meets**   **Exceeds**
                                    Minimum Standards   **Minimum Standards**

TEST ENVIRONMENTS

L: Laboratory/Classroom Testing
C: Clinical/Field Testing
P: Practicum Testing
A: Assessment/Mock Exam Testing
S: Self-Reporting

SKILL TEST INFORMATION

Positive Finding: Decreased ability to hold contraction
Involved Structure: Pectoralis major (lower portion)
Special Considerations: N/A
Reference(s): Kendall et al
Supplies Needed: Table

MANUAL MUSCLE TESTING
(MMT-U-Test 4)

Peer Review _____   Peer Review _____

Skill Acquisition: _____   Practice Opportunities: _____

This problem allows you the opportunity to demonstrate a manual muscle test for the **pectoralis minor** *muscle. You have 2 minutes to complete this task.*

Tester places athlete and limb in appropriate position	Test 1	Test 2	Test 3
Supine (head at the end of the table)	Y N	Y N	Y N
Arm at the side	Y N	Y N	Y N
Tester placed in proper position	**Test 1**	**Test 2**	**Test 3**
Stands to the side, facing the athlete	Y N	Y N	Y N
Places one hand on the anterior aspect of the shoulder	Y N	Y N	Y N
Tester performs test according to accepted guidelines	**Test 1**	**Test 2**	**Test 3**
Has the athlete actively thrust the shoulder forward (lift off the table)	Y N	Y N	Y N
Applies downward resistance against anterior shoulder (toward the table)	Y N	Y N	Y N
Holds resistance for 5 seconds	Y N	Y N	Y N
Performs assessment bilaterally	Y N	Y N	Y N

The psychomotor skill was performed completely and in the appropriate order   0 1 2 3 4 5

The tester had control of the subject and the situation (showed confidence)   0 1 2 3 4 5

Method of performing the skill allowed the tester the ability to determine: severity, proper progression, and the *fit* in the overall picture (Oral)   0 1 2 3 4 5

In order for a grade of *minimum standard* to be given, the total must be ≥11   **TOTAL = _____**

1	2	3	4	5	6	7	8	9	10	11	12	13	14	15

Not Acceptable   **Meets Minimum Standards**   **Exceeds Minimum Standards**

TEST ENVIRONMENTS

L: Laboratory/Classroom Testing
C: Clinical/Field Testing
P: Practicum Testing
A: Assessment/Mock Exam Testing
S: Self-Reporting

SKILL TEST INFORMATION

Positive Finding:	Decreased ability to hold contraction
Involved Structure:	Pectoralis minor
Special Considerations:	N/A
Reference(s):	Kendall et al
Supplies Needed:	Table

MANUAL MUSCLE TESTING
(MMT-U-Test 5)

Peer Review_____   Peer Review _____

Skill Acquisition: _____   Practice Opportunities: _____

This problem allows you the opportunity to demonstrate a manual muscle test for the **middle deltoid** *muscle. You have 2 minutes to complete this task.*

Tester places athlete and limb in appropriate position	Test 1	Test 2	Test 3
Seated	Ⓨ Ⓝ	Ⓨ Ⓝ	Ⓨ Ⓝ
Shoulder abducted to 90 degrees	Ⓨ Ⓝ	Ⓨ Ⓝ	Ⓨ Ⓝ
Elbow flexed to 90 degrees (palm facing downward)	Ⓨ Ⓝ	Ⓨ Ⓝ	Ⓨ Ⓝ
Tester placed in proper position	**Test 1**	**Test 2**	**Test 3**
Stands behind or to the side of the athlete	Ⓨ Ⓝ	Ⓨ Ⓝ	Ⓨ Ⓝ
Places one hand around the distal humerus	Ⓨ Ⓝ	Ⓨ Ⓝ	Ⓨ Ⓝ
Tester performs test according to accepted guidelines	**Test 1**	**Test 2**	**Test 3**
Instructs the athlete to hold this position	Ⓨ Ⓝ	Ⓨ Ⓝ	Ⓨ Ⓝ
Applies resistance downward in the direction of adduction	Ⓨ Ⓝ	Ⓨ Ⓝ	Ⓨ Ⓝ
Holds resistance for 5 seconds	Ⓨ Ⓝ	Ⓨ Ⓝ	Ⓨ Ⓝ
Performs assessment bilaterally	Ⓨ Ⓝ	Ⓨ Ⓝ	Ⓨ Ⓝ

The psychomotor skill was performed completely and in the appropriate order   0 1 2 3 4 5

The tester had control of the subject and the situation (showed confidence)   0 1 2 3 4 5

Method of performing the skill allowed the tester the ability to determine:
severity, proper progression, and the *fit* in the overall picture (Oral)   0 1 2 3 4 5

In order for a grade of *minimum standard* to be given, the total must be ≥11   TOTAL = _____

```
 1    2    3    4    5    6    7    8    9    10   11   12   13   14   15
 |    |    |    |    |    |    |    |    |    |    |    |    |    |    |
```
Not Acceptable   **Meets**   **Exceeds**
                                                    Minimum Standards   **Minimum Standards**

TEST ENVIRONMENTS

L: Laboratory/Classroom Testing
C: Clinical/Field Testing
P: Practicum Testing
A: Assessment/Mock Exam Testing
S: Self-Reporting

SKILL TEST INFORMATION

Positive Finding: Decreased ability to hold contraction
Involved Structure: Middle deltoid
Special Considerations: Elbow may be placed into an extended position for greater leverage
Reference(s): Kendall et al
Supplies Needed: Chair

MANUAL MUSCLE TESTING
(MMT-U-Test 6)

Peer Review_____   Peer Review _____

Skill Acquisition: _____   Practice Opportunities: _____

This problem allows you the opportunity to demonstrate a manual muscle test in a seated position for the **anterior deltoid** *muscle. You have 2 minutes to complete this task.*

Tester places athlete and limb in appropriate position	Test 1	Test 2	Test 3
Seated	Y N	Y N	Y N
Shoulder abducted to 90 degrees (slight flexion)	Y N	Y N	Y N
Shoulder placed in slight external rotation	Y N	Y N	Y N
Elbow flexed to 90 degrees (palm facing downward)	Y N	Y N	Y N
Tester placed in proper position	**Test 1**	**Test 2**	**Test 3**
Stands facing the athlete	Y N	Y N	Y N
Places one hand around the distal humerus	Y N	Y N	Y N
Applies counterpressure posteriorly to the shoulder girdle with the other hand	Y N	Y N	Y N
Tester performs test according to accepted guidelines	**Test 1**	**Test 2**	**Test 3**
Instructs the athlete to hold this position	Y N	Y N	Y N
Applies resistance downward in the direction of adduction and slight extension	Y N	Y N	Y N
Holds resistance for 5 seconds	Y N	Y N	Y N
Performs assessment bilaterally	Y N	Y N	Y N

The psychomotor skill was performed completely and in the appropriate order   **0 1 2 3 4 5**

The tester had control of the subject and the situation (showed confidence)   **0 1 2 3 4 5**

Method of performing the skill allowed the tester the ability to determine:
severity, proper progression, and the *fit* in the overall picture (Oral)   **0 1 2 3 4 5**

In order for a grade of *minimum standard* to be given, the total must be ≥11   **TOTAL = _____**

1	2	3	4	5	6	7	8	9	10	11	12	13	14	15

Not Acceptable   **Meets**   **Exceeds**
                          Minimum Standards   **Minimum Standards**

TEST ENVIRONMENTS

L: Laboratory/Classroom Testing
C: Clinical/Field Testing
P: Practicum Testing
A: Assessment/Mock Exam Testing
S: Self-Reporting

SKILL TEST INFORMATION

Positive Finding: Decreased ability to hold contraction
Involved Structure: Anterior deltoid
Special Considerations: Elbow may be placed into an extended position for greater leverage
Reference(s): Kendall et al
Supplies Needed: Chair

MANUAL MUSCLE TESTING
(MMT-U-Test 7)

Peer Review_____   Peer Review _____

Skill Acquisition: _____   Practice Opportunities: _____

This problem allows you the opportunity to demonstrate a manual muscle test in a seated position for the **posterior deltoid** *muscle. You have 2 minutes to complete this task.*

Tester places athlete and limb in appropriate position	Test 1	Test 2	Test 3
Seated	Ⓨ Ⓝ	Ⓨ Ⓝ	Ⓨ Ⓝ
Shoulder abducted to 90 degrees (slight extension)	Ⓨ Ⓝ	Ⓨ Ⓝ	Ⓨ Ⓝ
Shoulder placed in slight medial rotation	Ⓨ Ⓝ	Ⓨ Ⓝ	Ⓨ Ⓝ
Elbow flexed to 90 degrees (palm facing downward)	Ⓨ Ⓝ	Ⓨ Ⓝ	Ⓨ Ⓝ
Tester placed in proper position	**Test 1**	**Test 2**	**Test 3**
Stands behind the athlete	Ⓨ Ⓝ	Ⓨ Ⓝ	Ⓨ Ⓝ
Places one hand on the posterolateral surface of the distal humerus	Ⓨ Ⓝ	Ⓨ Ⓝ	Ⓨ Ⓝ
Applies counter pressure anteriorly to the shoulder girdle with the other hand	Ⓨ Ⓝ	Ⓨ Ⓝ	Ⓨ Ⓝ
Tester performs test according to accepted guidelines	**Test 1**	**Test 2**	**Test 3**
Instructs the athlete to hold his position	Ⓨ Ⓝ	Ⓨ Ⓝ	Ⓨ Ⓝ
Applies resistance downward in the direction of adduction and slight flexion	Ⓨ Ⓝ	Ⓨ Ⓝ	Ⓨ Ⓝ
Holds resistance for 5 seconds	Ⓨ Ⓝ	Ⓨ Ⓝ	Ⓨ Ⓝ
Performs assessment bilaterally	Ⓨ Ⓝ	Ⓨ Ⓝ	Ⓨ Ⓝ

The psychomotor skill was performed completely and in the appropriate order   0 1 2 3 4 5

The tester had control of the subject and the situation (showed confidence)   0 1 2 3 4 5

Method of performing the skill allowed the tester the ability to determine:
severity, proper progression, and the *fit* in the overall picture (Oral)   0 1 2 3 4 5

In order for a grade of *minimum standard* to be given, the total must be ≥11   TOTAL = _____

```
 1     2     3     4     5     6     7     8     9    10    11    12    13    14    15
 |──┴──|──┴──|──┴──|──┴──|──┴──|──┴──|──┴──|──┴──|──┴──|──┴──|──┴──|──┴──|──┴──|──┴──|
```

Not Acceptable   **Meets**   **Exceeds**
                                     Minimum Standards   **Minimum Standards**

TEST ENVIRONMENTS

L: Laboratory/Classroom Testing
C: Clinical/Field Testing
P: Practicum Testing
A: Assessment/Mock Exam Testing
S: Self-Reporting

SKILL TEST INFORMATION

Positive Finding:	Decreased ability to hold contraction
Involved Structure:	Posterior deltoid
Special Considerations:	Elbow may be placed into an extended position for greater leverage
Reference(s):	Kendall et al
Supplies Needed:	Chair

MANUAL MUSCLE TESTING
(MMT-U-Test 8)

Peer Review_____   Peer Review _____

Skill Acquisition: _____   Practice Opportunities: _____

This problem allows you the opportunity to demonstrate a manual muscle test for the **teres major** *muscle. You have 2 minutes to complete this task.*

Tester places athlete and limb in appropriate position	Test 1	Test 2	Test 3
Prone (head facing the test arm)	Ⓨ Ⓝ	Ⓨ Ⓝ	Ⓨ Ⓝ
Shoulder extended, adducted, and medially rotated (hand on the posterior iliac crest)	Ⓨ Ⓝ	Ⓨ Ⓝ	Ⓨ Ⓝ
Tester placed in proper position	**Test 1**	**Test 2**	**Test 3**
Stands on the side of the test arm	Ⓨ Ⓝ	Ⓨ Ⓝ	Ⓨ Ⓝ
Places hand on the distal humerus just above the elbow	Ⓨ Ⓝ	Ⓨ Ⓝ	Ⓨ Ⓝ
Tester performs test according to accepted guidelines	**Test 1**	**Test 2**	**Test 3**
Instructs the athlete to hold this position	Ⓨ Ⓝ	Ⓨ Ⓝ	Ⓨ Ⓝ
Applies resistance downward in the direction of abduction and flexion	Ⓨ Ⓝ	Ⓨ Ⓝ	Ⓨ Ⓝ
Holds resistance for 5 seconds	Ⓨ Ⓝ	Ⓨ Ⓝ	Ⓨ Ⓝ
Performs assessment bilaterally	Ⓨ Ⓝ	Ⓨ Ⓝ	Ⓨ Ⓝ

The psychomotor skill was performed completely and in the appropriate order   0 1 2 3 4 5

The tester had control of the subject and the situation (showed confidence)   0 1 2 3 4 5

Method of performing the skill allowed the tester the ability to determine:
severity, proper progression, and the *fit* in the overall picture (Oral)   0 1 2 3 4 5

In order for a grade of *minimum standard* to be given, the total must be ≥11   **TOTAL =** _____

```
  1     2     3     4     5     6     7     8     9    10    11    12    13    14    15
  |     |     |     |     |     |     |     |     |     |     |     |     |     |     |
```

Not Acceptable   **Meets**   **Exceeds**
                              Minimum Standards   **Minimum Standards**

TEST ENVIRONMENTS

L: Laboratory/Classroom Testing
C: Clinical/Field Testing
P: Practicum Testing
A: Assessment/Mock Exam Testing
S: Self-Reporting

SKILL TEST INFORMATION

Positive Finding:	Decreased ability to hold contraction
Involved Structure:	Teres major
Special Considerations:	N/A
Reference(s):	Kendall et al
Supplies Needed:	Table

MANUAL MUSCLE TESTING
(MMT-U-Test 9)

Peer Review_____   Peer Review _____

Skill Acquisition: _____   Practice Opportunities: _____

This problem allows you the opportunity to demonstrate a manual muscle test for the **coracobrachialis** *muscle. You have 2 minutes to complete this task.*

Tester places athlete and limb in appropriate position	Test 1	Test 2	Test 3
Seated or supine	Ⓨ Ⓝ	Ⓨ Ⓝ	Ⓨ Ⓝ
Shoulder flexed to approximately 75 degrees	Ⓨ Ⓝ	Ⓨ Ⓝ	Ⓨ Ⓝ
Shoulder placed in lateral rotation	Ⓨ Ⓝ	Ⓨ Ⓝ	Ⓨ Ⓝ
Elbow flexed to 90 degrees and supinated	Ⓨ Ⓝ	Ⓨ Ⓝ	Ⓨ Ⓝ
Tester placed in proper position	**Test 1**	**Test 2**	**Test 3**
Stands to the side of the athlete	Ⓨ Ⓝ	Ⓨ Ⓝ	Ⓨ Ⓝ
Places one hand on the anteromedial surface of the distal humerus	Ⓨ Ⓝ	Ⓨ Ⓝ	Ⓨ Ⓝ
Tester performs test according to accepted guidelines	**Test 1**	**Test 2**	**Test 3**
Instructs the athlete to hold this position	Ⓨ Ⓝ	Ⓨ Ⓝ	Ⓨ Ⓝ
Applies resistance downward in the direction of extension	Ⓨ Ⓝ	Ⓨ Ⓝ	Ⓨ Ⓝ
Holds resistance for 5 seconds	Ⓨ Ⓝ	Ⓨ Ⓝ	Ⓨ Ⓝ
Performs assessment bilaterally	Ⓨ Ⓝ	Ⓨ Ⓝ	Ⓨ Ⓝ

The psychomotor skill was performed completely and in the appropriate order   0 1 2 3 4 5

The tester had control of the subject and the situation (showed confidence)   0 1 2 3 4 5

Method of performing the skill allowed the tester the ability to determine:
severity, proper progression, and the *fit* in the overall picture (Oral)   0 1 2 3 4 5

In order for a grade of *minimum standard* to be given, the total must be ≥11   TOTAL = _____

| 1 | 2 | 3 | 4 | 5 | 6 | 7 | 8 | 9 | 10 | 11 | 12 | 13 | 14 | 15 |

Not Acceptable   **Meets**   **Exceeds**
                                      Minimum Standards   **Minimum Standards**

TEST ENVIRONMENTS

L: Laboratory/Classroom Testing
C: Clinical/Field Testing
P: Practicum Testing
A: Assessment/Mock Exam Testing
S: Self-Reporting

SKILL TEST INFORMATION

Positive Finding: Decreased ability to hold contraction
Involved Structure: Coracobrachialis
Special Considerations: N/A
Reference(s): Kendall et al
Supplies Needed: Chair

MANUAL MUSCLE TESTING
(MMT-U-Test 10)

Peer Review_____   Peer Review _____

Skill Acquisition: _____   Practice Opportunities: _____

This problem allows you the opportunity to demonstrate a manual muscle test for the **rhomboid/levator** *muscle. You have 2 minutes to complete this task.*

Tester places athlete and limb in appropriate position	Test 1	Test 2	Test 3
Prone (shoulder at the edge of the table)	Ⓨ Ⓝ	Ⓨ Ⓝ	Ⓨ Ⓝ
Shoulder extended (hyperextended)/slight lateral rotation/full adduction	Ⓨ Ⓝ	Ⓨ Ⓝ	Ⓨ Ⓝ
Elbow flexed to 90 degrees	Ⓨ Ⓝ	Ⓨ Ⓝ	Ⓨ Ⓝ
Tester placed in proper position	**Test 1**	**Test 2**	**Test 3**
Stands to the side, facing the athlete	Ⓨ Ⓝ	Ⓨ Ⓝ	Ⓨ Ⓝ
Places one hand on the shoulder/scapula	Ⓨ Ⓝ	Ⓨ Ⓝ	Ⓨ Ⓝ
Places the other hand against the medial aspect of the elbow	Ⓨ Ⓝ	Ⓨ Ⓝ	Ⓨ Ⓝ
Tester performs test according to accepted guidelines	**Test 1**	**Test 2**	**Test 3**
Has the athlete actively attain the position	Ⓨ Ⓝ	Ⓨ Ⓝ	Ⓨ Ⓝ
Applies resistance against the arm in the direction of abduction/lateral rotation of the inferior angle of the scapula	Ⓨ Ⓝ	Ⓨ Ⓝ	Ⓨ Ⓝ
Applies a depressive force to the shoulder with the other hand	Ⓨ Ⓝ	Ⓨ Ⓝ	Ⓨ Ⓝ
Holds resistance for 5 seconds	Ⓨ Ⓝ	Ⓨ Ⓝ	Ⓨ Ⓝ
Performs assessment bilaterally	Ⓨ Ⓝ	Ⓨ Ⓝ	Ⓨ Ⓝ

The psychomotor skill was performed completely and in the appropriate order   **0 1 2 3 4 5**

The tester had control of the subject and the situation (showed confidence)   **0 1 2 3 4 5**

Method of performing the skill allowed the tester the ability to determine: severity, proper progression, and the *fit* in the overall picture (Oral)   **0 1 2 3 4 5**

In order for a grade of *minimum standard* to be given, the total must be ≥11   **TOTAL = _____**

| 1 | 2 | 3 | 4 | 5 | 6 | 7 | 8 | 9 | 10 | 11 | 12 | 13 | 14 | 15 |

Not Acceptable   **Meets**   **Exceeds**
                                       Minimum Standards   **Minimum Standards**

TEST ENVIRONMENTS

L: Laboratory/Classroom Testing
C: Clinical/Field Testing
P: Practicum Testing
A: Assessment/Mock Exam Testing
S: Self-Reporting

SKILL TEST INFORMATION

Positive Finding: Decreased ability to hold contraction
Involved Structure: Rhomboid/levator
Special Considerations: N/A
Reference(s): Kendall et al
Supplies Needed: Table

MANUAL MUSCLE TESTING
(MMT-U-Test 11)

Peer Review_____   Peer Review _____

Skill Acquisition: _____   Practice Opportunities: _____

This problem allows you the opportunity to demonstrate a manual muscle test for the **rhomboid (Alternate Test)** *muscle. You have 2 minutes to complete this task.*

Tester places athlete and limb in appropriate position	Test 1	Test 2	Test 3
Prone	Ⓨ Ⓝ	Ⓨ Ⓝ	Ⓨ Ⓝ
Shoulder abducted to 90 degrees	Ⓨ Ⓝ	Ⓨ Ⓝ	Ⓨ Ⓝ
Shoulder medially rotated with thumb pointing downward	Ⓨ Ⓝ	Ⓨ Ⓝ	Ⓨ Ⓝ
Tester placed in proper position	**Test 1**	**Test 2**	**Test 3**
Stands to the side, facing the athlete	Ⓨ Ⓝ	Ⓨ Ⓝ	Ⓨ Ⓝ
Places one hand on the opposite scapula	Ⓨ Ⓝ	Ⓨ Ⓝ	Ⓨ Ⓝ
Places the other hand against the distal forearm (radius/ulna)	Ⓨ Ⓝ	Ⓨ Ⓝ	Ⓨ Ⓝ
Tester performs test according to accepted guidelines	**Test 1**	**Test 2**	**Test 3**
Has the athlete actively horizontally extend the shoulder	Ⓨ Ⓝ	Ⓨ Ⓝ	Ⓨ Ⓝ
Applies resistance against the arm in the direction of horizontal flexion (downward direction toward the table)	Ⓨ Ⓝ	Ⓨ Ⓝ	Ⓨ Ⓝ
Holds resistance for 5 seconds	Ⓨ Ⓝ	Ⓨ Ⓝ	Ⓨ Ⓝ
Performs assessment bilaterally	Ⓨ Ⓝ	Ⓨ Ⓝ	Ⓨ Ⓝ

The psychomotor skill was performed completely and in the appropriate order   **0 1 2 3 4 5**

The tester had control of the subject and the situation (showed confidence)   **0 1 2 3 4 5**

Method of performing the skill allowed the tester the ability to determine:
severity, proper progression, and the *fit* in the overall picture (Oral)   **0 1 2 3 4 5**

In order for a grade of *minimum standard* to be given, the total must be ≥11   **TOTAL = _____**

1	2	3	4	5	6	7	8	9	10	11	12	13	14	15

Not Acceptable   **Meets**   **Exceeds**
                          Minimum Standards   **Minimum Standards**

TEST ENVIRONMENTS

L: Laboratory/Classroom Testing
C: Clinical/Field Testing
P: Practicum Testing
A: Assessment/Mock Exam Testing
S: Self-Reporting

SKILL TEST INFORMATION

Positive Finding: Decreased ability to hold contraction
Involved Structure: Rhomboid (alternate)
Special Considerations: N/A
Reference(s): Kendall et al
Supplies Needed: Table

MANUAL MUSCLE TESTING
(MMT-U-Test 12)

Peer Review_____   Peer Review _____

Skill Acquisition: _____   Practice Opportunities: _____

*This problem allows you the opportunity to demonstrate a manual muscle test for the **serratus anterior** muscle. You have 2 minutes to complete this task.*

Tester places athlete and limb in appropriate position	Test 1	Test 2	Test 3
Supine	Ⓨ Ⓝ	Ⓨ Ⓝ	Ⓨ Ⓝ
Shoulder flexed to 90 degrees	Ⓨ Ⓝ	Ⓨ Ⓝ	Ⓨ Ⓝ
Shoulder elevated off the table (abduction of the scapula/as if punching)	Ⓨ Ⓝ	Ⓨ Ⓝ	Ⓨ Ⓝ
Fingers clenched in a fist	Ⓨ Ⓝ	Ⓨ Ⓝ	Ⓨ Ⓝ
Tester placed in proper position	**Test 1**	**Test 2**	**Test 3**
Stands to the side, facing the athlete (may need a stool to stand on)	Ⓨ Ⓝ	Ⓨ Ⓝ	Ⓨ Ⓝ
Clasps one or both hands over the elevated fist	Ⓨ Ⓝ	Ⓨ Ⓝ	Ⓨ Ⓝ
Tester performs test according to accepted guidelines	**Test 1**	**Test 2**	**Test 3**
Instructs the athlete to maintain the elevated position	Ⓨ Ⓝ	Ⓨ Ⓝ	Ⓨ Ⓝ
Applies a downward resistance against the clenched fist (axial pressure pushing shoulder back down to the table)	Ⓨ Ⓝ	Ⓨ Ⓝ	Ⓨ Ⓝ
Holds resistance for 5 seconds	Ⓨ Ⓝ	Ⓨ Ⓝ	Ⓨ Ⓝ
Performs assessment bilaterally	Ⓨ Ⓝ	Ⓨ Ⓝ	Ⓨ Ⓝ

The psychomotor skill was performed completely and in the appropriate order   0 1 2 3 4 5

The tester had control of the subject and the situation (showed confidence)   0 1 2 3 4 5

Method of performing the skill allowed the tester the ability to determine:
severity, proper progression, and the *fit* in the overall picture (Oral)   0 1 2 3 4 5

In order for a grade of *minimum standard* to be given, the total must be ≥11   TOTAL = _____

```
 1    2    3    4    5    6    7    8    9   10   11   12   13   14   15
 |    |    |    |    |    |    |    |    |    |    |    |    |    |    |
```

Not Acceptable   **Meets**   **Exceeds**
                          Minimum Standards   **Minimum Standards**

TEST ENVIRONMENTS

L: Laboratory/Classroom Testing
C: Clinical/Field Testing
P: Practicum Testing
A: Assessment/Mock Exam Testing
S: Self-Reporting

SKILL TEST INFORMATION

Positive Finding: Decreased ability to hold contraction
Involved Structure: Serratus anterior
Special Considerations: N/A
Reference(s): Kendall et al
Supplies Needed: Table

MANUAL MUSCLE TESTING
(MMT-U-Test 13)

Peer Review_____   Peer Review _____

Skill Acquisition: _____   Practice Opportunities: _____

*This problem allows you the opportunity to demonstrate a manual muscle test for the **middle trapezius** muscle. You have 2 minutes to complete this task.*

Tester places athlete and limb in appropriate position	Test 1	Test 2	Test 3
Prone	Ⓨ Ⓝ	Ⓨ Ⓝ	Ⓨ Ⓝ
Shoulder abducted to 90 degrees	Ⓨ Ⓝ	Ⓨ Ⓝ	Ⓨ Ⓝ
Shoulder laterally rotated with thumb pointing upward	Ⓨ Ⓝ	Ⓨ Ⓝ	Ⓨ Ⓝ
Tester placed in proper position	**Test 1**	**Test 2**	**Test 3**
Stands to the side, facing the athlete	Ⓨ Ⓝ	Ⓨ Ⓝ	Ⓨ Ⓝ
Places one hand on the opposite scapula	Ⓨ Ⓝ	Ⓨ Ⓝ	Ⓨ Ⓝ
Places the other hand against the distal forearm (radius/ulna)	Ⓨ Ⓝ	Ⓨ Ⓝ	Ⓨ Ⓝ
Tester performs test according to accepted guidelines	**Test 1**	**Test 2**	**Test 3**
Has the athlete actively horizontally extend the shoulder	Ⓨ Ⓝ	Ⓨ Ⓝ	Ⓨ Ⓝ
Applies resistance against the arm in the direction of horizontal flexion (downward direction toward the table)	Ⓨ Ⓝ	Ⓨ Ⓝ	Ⓨ Ⓝ
Holds resistance for 5 seconds	Ⓨ Ⓝ	Ⓨ Ⓝ	Ⓨ Ⓝ
Performs assessment bilaterally	Ⓨ Ⓝ	Ⓨ Ⓝ	Ⓨ Ⓝ

The psychomotor skill was performed completely and in the appropriate order   0 1 2 3 4 5

The tester had control of the subject and the situation (showed confidence)   0 1 2 3 4 5

Method of performing the skill allowed the tester the ability to determine:
severity, proper progression, and the *fit* in the overall picture (Oral)   0 1 2 3 4 5

In order for a grade of *minimum standard* to be given, the total must be ≥11   TOTAL = _____

```
 1    2    3    4    5    6    7    8    9   10   11   12   13   14   15
 |    |    |    |    |    |    |    |    |    |    |    |    |    |    |
```

Not Acceptable   **Meets**   **Exceeds**
                              Minimum Standards   **Minimum Standards**

TEST ENVIRONMENT

L: Laboratory/Classroom Testing
C: Clinical/Field Testing
P: Practicum Testing
A: Assessment/Mock Exam Testing
S: Self-Reporting

SKILL TEST INFORMATION

Positive Finding:	Decreased ability to hold contraction
Involved Structure:	Middle trapezius
Special Considerations:	N/A
Reference(s):	Kendall et al
Supplies Needed:	Table

MANUAL MUSCLE TESTING
(MMT-U-Test 14)

Peer Review_____   Peer Review _____

Skill Acquisition: _____   Practice Opportunities: _____

This problem allows you the opportunity to demonstrate a manual muscle test for the **lower trapezius** *muscle. You have 2 minutes to complete this task.*

Tester places athlete and limb in appropriate position	Test 1	Test 2	Test 3
Prone (shoulder at the edge of the table)	Ⓨ Ⓝ	Ⓨ Ⓝ	Ⓨ Ⓝ
Shoulder abducted to 130 degrees	Ⓨ Ⓝ	Ⓨ Ⓝ	Ⓨ Ⓝ
Shoulder laterally rotated with thumb pointing upward	Ⓨ Ⓝ	Ⓨ Ⓝ	Ⓨ Ⓝ

Tester placed in proper position	Test 1	Test 2	Test 3
Stands to the side, facing the athlete	Ⓨ Ⓝ	Ⓨ Ⓝ	Ⓨ Ⓝ
Places one hand on the opposite scapula	Ⓨ Ⓝ	Ⓨ Ⓝ	Ⓨ Ⓝ
Places the other hand against the distal forearm (radius/ulna)	Ⓨ Ⓝ	Ⓨ Ⓝ	Ⓨ Ⓝ

Tester performs test according to accepted guidelines	Test 1	Test 2	Test 3
Has the athlete actively horizontally extend the shoulder	Ⓨ Ⓝ	Ⓨ Ⓝ	Ⓨ Ⓝ
Applies resistance against the arm in the direction of horizontal flexion (downward direction toward the table)	Ⓨ Ⓝ	Ⓨ Ⓝ	Ⓨ Ⓝ
Holds resistance for 5 seconds	Ⓨ Ⓝ	Ⓨ Ⓝ	Ⓨ Ⓝ
Performs assessment bilaterally	Ⓨ Ⓝ	Ⓨ Ⓝ	Ⓨ Ⓝ

The psychomotor skill was performed completely and in the appropriate order   **0 1 2 3 4 5**

The tester had control of the subject and the situation (showed confidence)   **0 1 2 3 4 5**

Method of performing the skill allowed the tester the ability to determine: severity, proper progression, and the *fit* in the overall picture (Oral)   **0 1 2 3 4 5**

In order for a grade of *minimum standard* to be given, the total must be ≥11   **TOTAL = _____**

1	2	3	4	5	6	7	8	9	10	11	12	13	14	15

Not Acceptable   **Meets Minimum Standards**   **Exceeds Minimum Standards**

TEST ENVIRONMENTS

L: Laboratory/Classroom Testing
C: Clinical/Field Testing
P: Practicum Testing
A: Assessment/Mock Exam Testing
S: Self-Reporting

SKILL TEST INFORMATION

Positive Finding: Decreased ability to hold contraction
Involved Structure: Lower trapezius
Special Considerations: N/A
Reference(s): Kendall et al
Supplies Needed: Table

MANUAL MUSCLE TESTING
(MMT-U-Test 15)

Peer Review_____   Peer Review _____

Skill Acquisition: _____   Practice Opportunities: _____

This problem allows you the opportunity to demonstrate a manual muscle test for the **upper trapezius** *muscle. You have 2 minutes to complete this task.*

Tester places athlete and limb in appropriate position	Test 1	Test 2	Test 3
Seated	Ⓨ Ⓝ	Ⓨ Ⓝ	Ⓨ Ⓝ
Elevates acrominal end of clavicle toward the head	Ⓨ Ⓝ	Ⓨ Ⓝ	Ⓨ Ⓝ
Brings the head toward the elevated clavicle (lateral flexion)	Ⓨ Ⓝ	Ⓨ Ⓝ	Ⓨ Ⓝ
Laterally rotates the head toward the opposite side	Ⓨ Ⓝ	Ⓨ Ⓝ	Ⓨ Ⓝ
Tester placed in proper position	**Test 1**	**Test 2**	**Test 3**
Stands facing the back of the athlete	Ⓨ Ⓝ	Ⓨ Ⓝ	Ⓨ Ⓝ
Places one hand on the side of the head	Ⓨ Ⓝ	Ⓨ Ⓝ	Ⓨ Ⓝ
Places the other hand against the shoulder	Ⓨ Ⓝ	Ⓨ Ⓝ	Ⓨ Ⓝ
Tester performs test according to accepted guidelines	**Test 1**	**Test 2**	**Test 3**
Instructs the athlete to hold the position	Ⓨ Ⓝ	Ⓨ Ⓝ	Ⓨ Ⓝ
Applies resistance against the head in the direction of lateral flexion to the opposite side	Ⓨ Ⓝ	Ⓨ Ⓝ	Ⓨ Ⓝ
Applies resistance against the shoulder in the direction of depression (downward pressure)	Ⓨ Ⓝ	Ⓨ Ⓝ	Ⓨ Ⓝ
Holds resistance for 5 seconds	Ⓨ Ⓝ	Ⓨ Ⓝ	Ⓨ Ⓝ
Performs assessment bilaterally	Ⓨ Ⓝ	Ⓨ Ⓝ	Ⓨ Ⓝ

The psychomotor skill was performed completely and in the appropriate order   0 1 2 3 4 5

The tester had control of the subject and the situation (showed confidence)   0 1 2 3 4 5

Method of performing the skill allowed the tester the ability to determine:
severity, proper progression, and the *fit* in the overall picture (Oral)   0 1 2 3 4 5

In order for a grade of *minimum standard* to be given, the total must be ≥11   TOTAL = _____

```
   1     2     3     4     5     6     7     8     9    10    11    12    13    14    15
   |     |     |     |     |     |     |     |     |     |     |     |     |     |     |
```
   Not Acceptable   **Meets**   **Exceeds**
                                                   Minimum Standards   **Minimum Standards**

TEST ENVIRONMENTS
L: Laboratory/Classroom Testing
C: Clinical/Field Testing
P: Practicum Testing
A: Assessment/Mock Exam Testing
S: Self-Reporting

SKILL TEST INFORMATION
Positive Finding: Decreased ability to hold contraction
Involved Structure: Upper trapezius
Special Considerations: N/A
Reference(s): Kendall et al
Supplies Needed: Stool/chair

MANUAL MUSCLE TESTING
(MMT-U-Test 16)

Peer Review_____   Peer Review _____

Skill Acquisition: _____   Practice Opportunities: _____

This problem allows you the opportunity to demonstrate a manual muscle test for the **supraspinatus** *muscle. You have 2 minutes to complete this task.*

Tester places athlete and limb in appropriate position	Test 1	Test 2	Test 3
Seated or standing	Ⓨ Ⓝ	Ⓨ Ⓝ	Ⓨ Ⓝ
Arm placed at the side (palm flat against the side)	Ⓨ Ⓝ	Ⓨ Ⓝ	Ⓨ Ⓝ
Head and neck extended and laterally flexed	Ⓨ Ⓝ	Ⓨ Ⓝ	Ⓨ Ⓝ
Neck/face laterally rotated to the opposite side	Ⓨ Ⓝ	Ⓨ Ⓝ	Ⓨ Ⓝ

Tester placed in proper position	Test 1	Test 2	Test 3
Stands facing the athlete	Ⓨ Ⓝ	Ⓨ Ⓝ	Ⓨ Ⓝ
Stabilizes the opposite shoulder with one hand	Ⓨ Ⓝ	Ⓨ Ⓝ	Ⓨ Ⓝ
Places the other hand against the distal forearm	Ⓨ Ⓝ	Ⓨ Ⓝ	Ⓨ Ⓝ

Tester performs test according to accepted guidelines	Test 1	Test 2	Test 3
Instructs the athlete to initiate abduction of the shoulder	Ⓨ Ⓝ	Ⓨ Ⓝ	Ⓨ Ⓝ
Applies resistance in the direction of adduction	Ⓨ Ⓝ	Ⓨ Ⓝ	Ⓨ Ⓝ
Holds resistance for 5 seconds	Ⓨ Ⓝ	Ⓨ Ⓝ	Ⓨ Ⓝ
Performs assessment bilaterally	Ⓨ Ⓝ	Ⓨ Ⓝ	Ⓨ Ⓝ

The psychomotor skill was performed completely and in the appropriate order   **0 1 2 3 4 5**

The tester had control of the subject and the situation (showed confidence)   **0 1 2 3 4 5**

Method of performing the skill allowed the tester the ability to determine:
severity, proper progression, and the *fit* in the overall picture (Oral)   **0 1 2 3 4 5**

In order for a grade of *minimum standard* to be given, the total must be ≥11   **TOTAL = _____**

```
 1    2    3    4    5    6    7    8    9   10   11   12   13   14   15
 |____|____|____|____|____|____|____|____|____|____|____|____|____|____|
```

Not Acceptable   **Meets**   **Exceeds**
                                    Minimum Standards   **Minimum Standards**

TEST ENVIRONMENTS
L: Laboratory/Classroom Testing
C: Clinical/Field Testing
P: Practicum Testing
A: Assessment/Mock Exam Testing
S: Self-Reporting

SKILL TEST INFORMATION
Positive Finding: Decreased ability to hold contraction
Involved Structure: N/A
Special Considerations: Supraspinatus
Reference(s): Kendall et al
Supplies Needed: N/A

MANUAL MUSCLE TESTING
(MMT-U-Test 17)

Peer Review_____   Peer Review _____

Skill Acquisition: _____   Practice Opportunities: _____

This problem allows you the opportunity to demonstrate a manual muscle test in a prone position for the **infraspinatus** *muscle. You have 2 minutes to complete this task.*

Tester places athlete and limb in appropriate position	Test 1	Test 2	Test 3
Prone (head facing away from the test arm)	Y N	Y N	Y N
Shoulder flexed to 90 degrees and externally rotated to approximately 90 degrees	Y N	Y N	Y N
Elbow flexed to 90 degrees (elbow off the edge of table)	Y N	Y N	Y N
Tester placed in proper position	**Test 1**	**Test 2**	**Test 3**
Stands on the side of the test arm	Y N	Y N	Y N
Places one hand under the arm near the elbow to stabilize the humerus	Y N	Y N	Y N
Places the other hand on the distal forearm	Y N	Y N	Y N
Tester performs test according to accepted guidelines	**Test 1**	**Test 2**	**Test 3**
Instructs the athlete to hold this position	Y N	Y N	Y N
Applies resistance downward in the direction of medial rotation	Y N	Y N	Y N
Holds resistance for 5 seconds	Y N	Y N	Y N
Performs assessment bilaterally	Y N	Y N	Y N

The psychomotor skill was performed completely and in the appropriate order   **0 1 2 3 4 5**

The tester had control of the subject and the situation (showed confidence)   **0 1 2 3 4 5**

Method of performing the skill allowed the tester the ability to determine:
severity, proper progression, and the *fit* in the overall picture (Oral)   **0 1 2 3 4 5**

In order for a grade of *minimum standard* to be given, the total must be ≥11   **TOTAL = _____**

1	2	3	4	5	6	7	8	9	10	11	12	13	14	15

Not Acceptable   **Meets**   **Exceeds**
                                  Minimum Standards   **Minimum Standards**

TEST ENVIRONMENTS

L: Laboratory/Classroom Testing
C: Clinical/Field Testing
P: Practicum Testing
A: Assessment/Mock Exam Testing
S: Self-Reporting

SKILL TEST INFORMATION

Positive Finding:	Decreased ability to hold contraction
Involved Structure:	Infraspinatus
Special Considerations:	Same as for teres minor
Reference(s):	Kendall et al
Supplies Needed:	Table

MANUAL MUSCLE TESTING
(MMT-U-Test 18)

Peer Review_____   Peer Review _____

Skill Acquisition: _____   Practice Opportunities: _____

This problem allows you the opportunity to demonstrate a manual muscle test in a prone position for the **teres minor** *muscle. You have 2 minutes to complete this task.*

Tester places athlete and limb in appropriate position	Test 1	Test 2	Test 3
Prone (head facing away from the test arm)	Y N	Y N	Y N
Shoulder flexed to 90 degrees and externally rotated to approximately 90 degrees	Y N	Y N	Y N
Elbow flexed to 90 degrees (elbow off the edge of the table)	Y N	Y N	Y N
Tester placed in proper position	**Test 1**	**Test 2**	**Test 3**
Stands on the side of the test arm	Y N	Y N	Y N
Places one hand under the arm near the elbow to stabilize the humerus	Y N	Y N	Y N
Places the other hand on the distal forearm	Y N	Y N	Y N
Tester performs test according to accepted guidelines	**Test 1**	**Test 2**	**Test 3**
Instructs the athlete to hold this position	Y N	Y N	Y N
Applies resistance downward in the direction of medial rotation	Y N	Y N	Y N
Holds resistance for 5 seconds	Y N	Y N	Y N
Performs assessment bilaterally	Y N	Y N	Y N

The psychomotor skill was performed completely and in the appropriate order   0 1 2 3 4 5

The tester had control of the subject and the situation (showed confidence)   0 1 2 3 4 5

Method of performing the skill allowed the tester the ability to determine:
severity, proper progression, and the *fit* in the overall picture (Oral)   0 1 2 3 4 5

In order for a grade of *minimum standard* to be given, the total must be ≥11   TOTAL = _____

```
  1    2    3    4    5    6    7    8    9    10   11   12   13   14   15
  |____|____|____|____|____|____|____|____|____|____|____|____|____|____|
```

Not Acceptable   **Meets**   **Exceeds**
                                    Minimum Standards   **Minimum Standards**

TEST ENVIRONMENTS

L: Laboratory/Classroom Testing
C: Clinical/Field Testing
P: Practicum Testing
A: Assessment/Mock Exam Testing
S: Self-Reporting

SKILL TEST INFORMATION

Positive Finding: Decreased ability to hold contraction
Involved Structure: Teres minor
Special Considerations: Same as for Infraspinatus
Reference(s): Kendall et al
Supplies Needed: Table

MANUAL MUSCLE TESTING
(MMT-U-Test 19)

Skill Acquisition: _____   Practice Opportunities: _____

This problem allows you the opportunity to demonstrate a manual muscle test in a prone position for the **subscapularis** *muscle. You have 2 minutes to complete this task.*

Tester places athlete and limb in appropriate position	Test 1	Test 2	Test 3
Prone (head facing away from the test arm)	Ⓨ Ⓝ	Ⓨ Ⓝ	Ⓨ Ⓝ
Shoulder abducted to 90 degrees and internally rotated to approximately 45 degrees	Ⓨ Ⓝ	Ⓨ Ⓝ	Ⓨ Ⓝ
Elbow flexed to 90 degrees (elbow off the edge of the table)	Ⓨ Ⓝ	Ⓨ Ⓝ	Ⓨ Ⓝ
Tester placed in proper position	**Test 1**	**Test 2**	**Test 3**
Stands on the side of the test arm	Ⓨ Ⓝ	Ⓨ Ⓝ	Ⓨ Ⓝ
Places one hand under the arm near the elbow to stabilize the humerus	Ⓨ Ⓝ	Ⓨ Ⓝ	Ⓨ Ⓝ
Places other hand at the distal forearm	Ⓨ Ⓝ	Ⓨ Ⓝ	Ⓨ Ⓝ
Tester performs test according to accepted guidelines	**Test 1**	**Test 2**	**Test 3**
Instructs the athlete to hold this position	Ⓨ Ⓝ	Ⓨ Ⓝ	Ⓨ Ⓝ
Applies resistance downward in the direction of lateral rotation	Ⓨ Ⓝ	Ⓨ Ⓝ	Ⓨ Ⓝ
Holds resistance for 5 seconds	Ⓨ Ⓝ	Ⓨ Ⓝ	Ⓨ Ⓝ
Performs assessment bilaterally	Ⓨ Ⓝ	Ⓨ Ⓝ	Ⓨ Ⓝ

The psychomotor skill was performed completely and in the appropriate order   **0 1 2 3 4 5**

The tester had control of the subject and the situation (showed confidence)   **0 1 2 3 4 5**

Method of performing the skill allowed the tester the ability to determine:
severity, proper progression, and the *fit* in the overall picture (Oral)   **0 1 2 3 4 5**

In order for a grade of *minimum standard* to be given, the total must be ≥11   **TOTAL = _____**

1	2	3	4	5	6	7	8	9	10	11	12	13	14	15

Not Acceptable   **Meets**   **Exceeds**
                              Minimum Standards   **Minimum Standards**

TEST ENVIRONMENTS

L: Laboratory/Classroom Testing
C: Clinical/Field Testing
P: Practicum Testing
A: Assessment/Mock Exam Testing
S: Self-Reporting

SKILL TEST INFORMATION

Positive Finding: Decreased ability to hold contraction
Involved Structure: Subscapularis
Special Considerations: N/A
Reference(s): Kendall et al
Supplies Needed: Table

MANUAL MUSCLE TESTING
(MMT-U-Test 20)

Peer Review_____   Peer Review _____

Skill Acquisition: _____   Practice Opportunities: _____

This problem allows you the opportunity to demonstrate a manual muscle test for the **triceps brachii (supine)** *muscle. You have 2 minutes to complete this task.*

Tester places athlete and limb in appropriate position	Test 1	Test 2	Test 3
Supine	Ⓨ Ⓝ	Ⓨ Ⓝ	Ⓨ Ⓝ
Shoulder flexed to 90 degrees (arm perpendicular to the table)	Ⓨ Ⓝ	Ⓨ Ⓝ	Ⓨ Ⓝ
Elbow extended to about 10 degrees (slightly less than full extension)	Ⓨ Ⓝ	Ⓨ Ⓝ	Ⓨ Ⓝ
Tester placed in proper position	**Test 1**	**Test 2**	**Test 3**
Stands to the side, facing the athlete	Ⓨ Ⓝ	Ⓨ Ⓝ	Ⓨ Ⓝ
Places one hand on the biceps to stabilize the humerus	Ⓨ Ⓝ	Ⓨ Ⓝ	Ⓨ Ⓝ
Places the other hand around the distal forearm	Ⓨ Ⓝ	Ⓨ Ⓝ	Ⓨ Ⓝ
Tester performs test according to accepted guidelines	**Test 1**	**Test 2**	**Test 3**
Instructs the athlete to hold this position	Ⓨ Ⓝ	Ⓨ Ⓝ	Ⓨ Ⓝ
Applies resistance in the direction of flexion	Ⓨ Ⓝ	Ⓨ Ⓝ	Ⓨ Ⓝ
Holds resistance for 5 seconds	Ⓨ Ⓝ	Ⓨ Ⓝ	Ⓨ Ⓝ
Performs assessment bilaterally	Ⓨ Ⓝ	Ⓨ Ⓝ	Ⓨ Ⓝ

The psychomotor skill was performed completely and in the appropriate order   **0 1 2 3 4 5**

The tester had control of the subject and the situation (showed confidence)   **0 1 2 3 4 5**

Method of performing the skill allowed the tester the ability to determine:
severity, proper progression, and the *fit* in the overall picture (Oral)   **0 1 2 3 4 5**

In order for a grade of *minimum standard* to be given, the total must be ≥11   **TOTAL = _____**

| 1 | 2 | 3 | 4 | 5 | 6 | 7 | 8 | 9 | 10 | 11 | 12 | 13 | 14 | 15 |

Not Acceptable   **Meets**   **Exceeds**
                      Minimum Standards   **Minimum Standards**

TEST ENVIRONMENTS

L: Laboratory/Classroom Testing
C: Clinical/Field Testing
P: Practicum Testing
A: Assessment/Mock Exam Testing
S: Self-Reporting

SKILL TEST INFORMATION

Positive Finding:	Decreased ability to hold contraction
Involved Structure:	Triceps brachii
Special Considerations:	N/A
Reference(s):	Kendall et al
Supplies Needed:	Table

MANUAL MUSCLE TESTING
(MMT-U-Test 21)

Peer Review_____   Peer Review _____

Skill Acquisition: _____   Practice Opportunities: _____

This problem allows you the opportunity to demonstrate a manual muscle test for the **triceps brachii (prone)** *muscle. You have 2 minutes to complete this task.*

Tester places athlete and limb in appropriate position	Test 1	Test 2	Test 3
Prone	Ⓨ Ⓝ	Ⓨ Ⓝ	Ⓨ Ⓝ
Shoulder abducted to 90 degrees (arm supported by the table)	Ⓨ Ⓝ	Ⓨ Ⓝ	Ⓨ Ⓝ
Elbow placed in a slightly flexed position	Ⓨ Ⓝ	Ⓨ Ⓝ	Ⓨ Ⓝ
Tester placed in proper position	**Test 1**	**Test 2**	**Test 3**
Stands to the side, facing the athlete	Ⓨ Ⓝ	Ⓨ Ⓝ	Ⓨ Ⓝ
Places one hand under the arm near the elbow	Ⓨ Ⓝ	Ⓨ Ⓝ	Ⓨ Ⓝ
Places the other hand around the distal forearm	Ⓨ Ⓝ	Ⓨ Ⓝ	Ⓨ Ⓝ
Tester performs test according to accepted guidelines	**Test 1**	**Test 2**	**Test 3**
Instructs the athlete to hold this position	Ⓨ Ⓝ	Ⓨ Ⓝ	Ⓨ Ⓝ
Applies resistance in the direction of flexion	Ⓨ Ⓝ	Ⓨ Ⓝ	Ⓨ Ⓝ
Holds resistance for 5 seconds	Ⓨ Ⓝ	Ⓨ Ⓝ	Ⓨ Ⓝ
Performs assessment bilaterally	Ⓨ Ⓝ	Ⓨ Ⓝ	Ⓨ Ⓝ

The psychomotor skill was performed completely and in the appropriate order   **0 1 2 3 4 5**

The tester had control of the subject and the situation (showed confidence)   **0 1 2 3 4 5**

Method of performing the skill allowed the tester the ability to determine:
severity, proper progression, and the *fit* in the overall picture (Oral)   **0 1 2 3 4 5**

In order for a grade of *minimum standard* to be given, the total must be ≥11   **TOTAL = _____**

```
  1    2    3    4    5    6    7    8    9    10   11   12   13   14   15
  |    |    |    |    |    |    |    |    |    |    |    |    |    |    |
```
   Not Acceptable   **Meets**   **Exceeds**
                                        Minimum Standards   **Minimum Standards**

TEST ENVIRONMENTS

L: Laboratory/Classroom Testing
C: Clinical/Field Testing
P: Practicum Testing
A: Assessment/Mock Exam Testing
S: Self-Reporting

SKILL TEST INFORMATION

Positive Finding:	Decreased ability to hold contraction
Involved Structure:	Triceps brachii/anconeus
Special Considerations:	N/A
Reference(s):	Kendall et al
Supplies Needed:	Table

MANUAL MUSCLE TESTING
(MMT-U-Test 22)

Peer Review_____   Peer Review _____

Skill Acquisition: _____   Practice Opportunities: _____

This problem allows you the opportunity to demonstrate a manual muscle test for the **biceps brachii** *muscle. You have 2 minutes to complete this task.*

Tester places athlete and limb in appropriate position	Test 1	Test 2	Test 3
Supine or seated	Ⓨ Ⓝ	Ⓨ Ⓝ	Ⓨ Ⓝ
Places the elbow in 30 to 45 degrees flexion	Ⓨ Ⓝ	Ⓨ Ⓝ	Ⓨ Ⓝ
Places forearm in a supinated position	Ⓨ Ⓝ	Ⓨ Ⓝ	Ⓨ Ⓝ
Tester placed in proper position	**Test 1**	**Test 2**	**Test 3**
Stands to the side, facing the athlete	Ⓨ Ⓝ	Ⓨ Ⓝ	Ⓨ Ⓝ
Places one hand under the elbow	Ⓨ Ⓝ	Ⓨ Ⓝ	Ⓨ Ⓝ
Places the other hand against the distal forearm (radius/ulna)	Ⓨ Ⓝ	Ⓨ Ⓝ	Ⓨ Ⓝ
Tester performs test according to accepted guidelines	**Test 1**	**Test 2**	**Test 3**
Instructs the athlete to maintain the flexed position	Ⓨ Ⓝ	Ⓨ Ⓝ	Ⓨ Ⓝ
Applies resistance against the arm in the direction of extension	Ⓨ Ⓝ	Ⓨ Ⓝ	Ⓨ Ⓝ
Holds resistance for 5 seconds	Ⓨ Ⓝ	Ⓨ Ⓝ	Ⓨ Ⓝ
Performs assessment bilaterally	Ⓨ Ⓝ	Ⓨ Ⓝ	Ⓨ Ⓝ

The psychomotor skill was performed completely and in the appropriate order   0 1 2 3 4 5

The tester had control of the subject and the situation (showed confidence)   0 1 2 3 4 5

Method of performing the skill allowed the tester the ability to determine:
severity, proper progression, and the *fit* in the overall picture (Oral)   0 1 2 3 4 5

In order for a grade of *minimum standard* to be given, the total must be ≥11   TOTAL = _____

```
  1    2    3    4    5    6    7    8    9   10   11   12   13   14   15
  |    |    |    |    |    |    |    |    |    |    |    |    |    |    |
```
Not Acceptable   **Meets**   **Exceeds**
                                        Minimum Standards   **Minimum Standards**

TEST ENVIRONMENTS
L: Laboratory/Classroom Testing
C: Clinical/Field Testing
P: Practicum Testing
A: Assessment/Mock Exam Testing
S: Self-Reporting

SKILL TEST INFORMATION
Positive Finding: Decreased ability to hold contraction
Involved Structure: Biceps brachii
Special Considerations: N/A
Reference(s): Kendall et al
Supplies Needed: N/A

MANUAL MUSCLE TESTING
(MMT-U-Test 23)

Peer Review_____   Peer Review _____

Skill Acquisition: _____   Practice Opportunities: _____

*Please demonstrate a manual muscle test for the **brachialis** muscle. You have 2 minutes to complete this task.*

Tester places athlete and limb in appropriate position	Test 1	Test 2	Test 3
Supine or seated	Ⓨ Ⓝ	Ⓨ Ⓝ	Ⓨ Ⓝ
Tester placed in proper position	**Test 1**	**Test 2**	**Test 3**
Supports the elbow with one hand applied under the olecranon process	Ⓨ Ⓝ	Ⓨ Ⓝ	Ⓨ Ⓝ
Tester performs test according to accepted guidelines	**Test 1**	**Test 2**	**Test 3**
Has athlete actively flex the elbow slightly less than 90 degrees (with forearm in supination)	Ⓨ Ⓝ	Ⓨ Ⓝ	Ⓨ Ⓝ
Applies resistance against the lower forearm (in the direction of extension of the elbow)	Ⓨ Ⓝ	Ⓨ Ⓝ	Ⓨ Ⓝ
Holds resistance for 5 seconds	Ⓨ Ⓝ	Ⓨ Ⓝ	Ⓨ Ⓝ
Performs assessment bilaterally	Ⓨ Ⓝ	Ⓨ Ⓝ	Ⓨ Ⓝ

The psychomotor skill was performed completely and in the appropriate order   **0 1 2 3 4 5**

The tester had control of the subject and the situation (showed confidence)   **0 1 2 3 4 5**

Method of performing the skill allowed the tester the ability to determine:
severity, proper progression, and the *fit* in the overall picture (Oral)   **0 1 2 3 4 5**

In order for a grade of *minimum standard* to be given, the total must be ≥11   **TOTAL = _____**

1	2	3	4	5	6	7	8	9	10	11	12	13	14	15

Not Acceptable   **Meets**   **Exceeds**
                              Minimum Standards   **Minimum Standards**

TEST ENVIRONMENTS

L: Laboratory/Classroom Testing
C: Clinical/Field Testing
P: Practicum Testing
A: Assessment/Mock Exam Testing
S: Self-Reporting

SKILL TEST INFORMATION

Positive Finding: Decreased ability to hold contraction
Involved Structure: Brachialis
Special Considerations: N/A
Reference(s): Kendall et al
Supplies Needed: Table

MANUAL MUSCLE TESTING
(MMT-U-Test 24)

Peer Review_____   Peer Review _____

Skill Acquisition: _____   Practice Opportunities: _____

This problem allows you the opportunity to demonstrate a manual muscle test for the **brachioradialis** *muscle. You have 2 minutes to complete this task.*

Tester places athlete and limb in appropriate position	Test 1	Test 2	Test 3
Supine or seated	Ⓨ Ⓝ	Ⓨ Ⓝ	Ⓨ Ⓝ
Elbow placed in slight flexion (resting on the table)	Ⓨ Ⓝ	Ⓨ Ⓝ	Ⓨ Ⓝ
Forearm placed in a neutral position (between supination and pronation)	Ⓨ Ⓝ	Ⓨ Ⓝ	Ⓨ Ⓝ
Tester placed in proper position	**Test 1**	**Test 2**	**Test 3**
Places one hand under the elbow (to cushion from table pressure)	Ⓨ Ⓝ	Ⓨ Ⓝ	Ⓨ Ⓝ
Places other hand around the distal forearm	Ⓨ Ⓝ	Ⓨ Ⓝ	Ⓨ Ⓝ
Tester performs test according to accepted guidelines	**Test 1**	**Test 2**	**Test 3**
Instructs the athlete to hold this position	Ⓨ Ⓝ	Ⓨ Ⓝ	Ⓨ Ⓝ
Applies resistance in the direction of extension	Ⓨ Ⓝ	Ⓨ Ⓝ	Ⓨ Ⓝ
Holds resistance for 5 seconds	Ⓨ Ⓝ	Ⓨ Ⓝ	Ⓨ Ⓝ
Performs assessment bilaterally	Ⓨ Ⓝ	Ⓨ Ⓝ	Ⓨ Ⓝ

The psychomotor skill was performed completely and in the appropriate order   0 1 2 3 4 5

The tester had control of the subject and the situation (showed confidence)   0 1 2 3 4 5

Method of performing the skill allowed the tester the ability to determine:
severity, proper progression, and the *fit* in the overall picture (Oral)   0 1 2 3 4 5

In order for a grade of *minimum standard* to be given, the total must be ≥11   TOTAL = _____

```
  1    2    3    4    5    6    7    8    9    10   11   12   13   14   15
  |____|____|____|____|____|____|____|____|____|____|____|____|____|____|
```

Not Acceptable   **Meets**   **Exceeds**
                              Minimum Standards   **Minimum Standards**

TEST ENVIRONMENTS

L: Laboratory/Classroom Testing
C: Clinical/Field Testing
P: Practicum Testing
A: Assessment/Mock Exam Testing
S: Self-Reporting

SKILL TEST INFORMATION

Positive Finding: Decreased ability to hold contraction
Involved Structure: Brachioradialis
Special Considerations: N/A
Reference(s): Kendall et al
Supplies Needed: Chair, table

MANUAL MUSCLE TESTING
(MMT-U-Test 25)

Peer Review_____   Peer Review _____

Skill Acquisition: _____   Practice Opportunities: _____

This problem allows you the opportunity to demonstrate a manual muscle test for the **pronator quadratus** *muscle. You have 2 minutes to complete this task.*

Tester places athlete and limb in appropriate position	Test 1	Test 2	Test 3
Seated or supine	Ⓨ Ⓝ	Ⓨ Ⓝ	Ⓨ Ⓝ
Elbow placed in full flexion	Ⓨ Ⓝ	Ⓨ Ⓝ	Ⓨ Ⓝ
Elbow/forearm placed in full pronation	Ⓨ Ⓝ	Ⓨ Ⓝ	Ⓨ Ⓝ
Elbow placed against athlete's side (avoid shoulder abduction)	Ⓨ Ⓝ	Ⓨ Ⓝ	Ⓨ Ⓝ
Tester placed in proper position	**Test 1**	**Test 2**	**Test 3**
Stands to the side, facing the athlete	Ⓨ Ⓝ	Ⓨ Ⓝ	Ⓨ Ⓝ
Stabilizes the elbow against the side with one hand	Ⓨ Ⓝ	Ⓨ Ⓝ	Ⓨ Ⓝ
Places the other hand around the distal forearm	Ⓨ Ⓝ	Ⓨ Ⓝ	Ⓨ Ⓝ
Tester performs test according to accepted guidelines	**Test 1**	**Test 2**	**Test 3**
Instructs the athlete to hold the position	Ⓨ Ⓝ	Ⓨ Ⓝ	Ⓨ Ⓝ
Applies resistance in a rotating motion against the distal forearm in the direction of supination	Ⓨ Ⓝ	Ⓨ Ⓝ	Ⓨ Ⓝ
Holds resistance for 5 seconds	Ⓨ Ⓝ	Ⓨ Ⓝ	Ⓨ Ⓝ
Performs assessment bilaterally	Ⓨ Ⓝ	Ⓨ Ⓝ	Ⓨ Ⓝ

The psychomotor skill was performed completely and in the appropriate order   0 1 2 3 4 5

The tester had control of the subject and the situation (showed confidence)   0 1 2 3 4 5

Method of performing the skill allowed the tester the ability to determine:
severity, proper progression, and the *fit* in the overall picture (Oral)   0 1 2 3 4 5

In order for a grade of *minimum standard* to be given, the total must be ≥11   TOTAL = _____

```
  1     2     3     4     5     6     7     8     9    10    11    12    13    14    15
  |_____|_____|_____|_____|_____|_____|_____|_____|_____|_____|_____|_____|_____|_____|
```

Not Acceptable   **Meets**   **Exceeds**
                              Minimum Standards   **Minimum Standards**

TEST ENVIRONMENTS

L: Laboratory/Classroom Testing
C: Clinical/Field Testing
P: Practicum Testing
A: Assessment/Mock Exam Testing
S: Self-Reporting

SKILL TEST INFORMATION

Positive Finding:	Decreased ability to hold contraction
Involved Structure:	Pronator quadratus
Special Considerations:	N/A
Reference(s):	Kendall et al
Supplies Needed:	Table

Manual Muscle Testing
(MMT-U-Test 26)

Peer Review_____   Peer Review _____

Skill Acquisition: _____   Practice Opportunities: _____

This problem allows you the opportunity to demonstrate a manual muscle test for the **supinator (biceps elongated)** *muscle. You have 2 minutes to complete this task.*

Tester places athlete and limb in appropriate position	Test 1	Test 2	Test 3
Seated or standing	Ⓨ Ⓝ	Ⓨ Ⓝ	Ⓨ Ⓝ
Shoulder placed in extension	Ⓨ Ⓝ	Ⓨ Ⓝ	Ⓨ Ⓝ
Elbow placed in full extension	Ⓨ Ⓝ	Ⓨ Ⓝ	Ⓨ Ⓝ
Tester placed in proper position	**Test 1**	**Test 2**	**Test 3**
Stands behind the athlete	Ⓨ Ⓝ	Ⓨ Ⓝ	Ⓨ Ⓝ
Stabilizes the elbow with one hand	Ⓨ Ⓝ	Ⓨ Ⓝ	Ⓨ Ⓝ
Places the other hand around the distal forearm	Ⓨ Ⓝ	Ⓨ Ⓝ	Ⓨ Ⓝ
Tester performs test according to accepted guidelines	**Test 1**	**Test 2**	**Test 3**
Instructs the athlete to hold the position	Ⓨ Ⓝ	Ⓨ Ⓝ	Ⓨ Ⓝ
Applies resistance in a rotating motion against the distal forearm in the direction of pronation	Ⓨ Ⓝ	Ⓨ Ⓝ	Ⓨ Ⓝ
Holds resistance for 5 seconds	Ⓨ Ⓝ	Ⓨ Ⓝ	Ⓨ Ⓝ
Performs assessment bilaterally	Ⓨ Ⓝ	Ⓨ Ⓝ	Ⓨ Ⓝ

The psychomotor skill was performed completely and in the appropriate order   0 1 2 3 4 5

The tester had control of the subject and the situation (showed confidence)   0 1 2 3 4 5

Method of performing the skill allowed the tester the ability to determine:
severity, proper progression, and the *fit* in the overall picture (Oral)   0 1 2 3 4 5

In order for a grade of *minimum standard* to be given, the total must be ≥11   TOTAL = _____

```
  1     2     3     4     5     6     7     8     9    10    11    12    13    14    15
  |     |     |     |     |     |     |     |     |     |     |     |     |     |     |
```
Not Acceptable   **Meets**   **Exceeds**
                                              Minimum Standards   **Minimum Standards**

TEST ENVIRONMENTS

L: Laboratory/Classroom Testing
C: Clinical/Field Testing
P: Practicum Testing
A: Assessment/Mock Exam Testing
S: Self-Reporting

SKILL TEST INFORMATION

Positive Finding: Decreased ability to hold contraction
Involved Structure: Supinator (biceps elongated)
Special Considerations: N/A
Reference(s): Kendall et al
Supplies Needed: Stool/chair

MANUAL MUSCLE TESTING
(MMT-U-Test 27)

Peer Review_____   Peer Review _____

Skill Acquisition: _____   Practice Opportunities: _____

This problem allows you the opportunity to demonstrate a manual muscle test for the **flexor carpi radialis** *muscle. You have 2 minutes to complete this task.*

Tester places athlete and limb in appropriate position	Test 1	Test 2	Test 3
Seated or supine	Ⓨ Ⓝ	Ⓨ Ⓝ	Ⓨ Ⓝ
Forearm placed in slightly less than full supination	Ⓨ Ⓝ	Ⓨ Ⓝ	Ⓨ Ⓝ
Tester placed in proper position	**Test 1**	**Test 2**	**Test 3**
Stands in front, facing the athlete	Ⓨ Ⓝ	Ⓨ Ⓝ	Ⓨ Ⓝ
Places one hand on the underside of the wrist	Ⓨ Ⓝ	Ⓨ Ⓝ	Ⓨ Ⓝ
Places the other hand on the thenar eminence	Ⓨ Ⓝ	Ⓨ Ⓝ	Ⓨ Ⓝ
Tester performs test according to accepted guidelines	**Test 1**	**Test 2**	**Test 3**
Has the athlete actively flex the wrist	Ⓨ Ⓝ	Ⓨ Ⓝ	Ⓨ Ⓝ
Applies resistance against the thenar eminence in the direction of extension (toward the ulnar side)	Ⓨ Ⓝ	Ⓨ Ⓝ	Ⓨ Ⓝ
Holds resistance for 5 seconds	Ⓨ Ⓝ	Ⓨ Ⓝ	Ⓨ Ⓝ
Performs assessment bilaterally	Ⓨ Ⓝ	Ⓨ Ⓝ	Ⓨ Ⓝ

The psychomotor skill was performed completely and in the appropriate order   **0 1 2 3 4 5**

The tester had control of the subject and the situation (showed confidence)   **0 1 2 3 4 5**

Method of performing the skill allowed the tester the ability to determine:
severity, proper progression, and the *fit* in the overall picture (Oral)   **0 1 2 3 4 5**

In order for a grade of *minimum standard* to be given, the total must be ≥11   **TOTAL = _____**

```
  1    2    3    4    5    6    7    8    9    10   11   12   13   14   15
  |    |    |    |    |    |    |    |    |    |    |    |    |    |    |
```

Not Acceptable   **Meets**   **Exceeds**
                                     Minimum Standards   **Minimum Standards**

TEST ENVIRONMENTS

L: Laboratory/Classroom Testing
C: Clinical/Field Testing
P: Practicum Testing
A: Assessment/Mock Exam Testing
S: Self-Reporting

SKILL TEST INFORMATION

Positive Finding: Decreased ability to hold contraction
Involved Structure: Flexor carpi radialis
Special Considerations: N/A
Reference(s): Kendall et al
Supplies Needed: N/A

MANUAL MUSCLE TESTING
(MMT-U-Test 28)

Peer Review_____   Peer Review _____

Skill Acquisition: _____   Practice Opportunities: _____

This problem allows you the opportunity to demonstrate a manual muscle test for the **flexor carpi ulnaris** *muscle. You have 2 minutes to complete this task.*

Tester places athlete and limb in appropriate position	Test 1	Test 2	Test 3
Seated or supine	Ⓨ Ⓝ	Ⓨ Ⓝ	Ⓨ Ⓝ
Forearm placed in full supination	Ⓨ Ⓝ	Ⓨ Ⓝ	Ⓨ Ⓝ
Tester placed in proper position	**Test 1**	**Test 2**	**Test 3**
Stands in front, facing the athlete	Ⓨ Ⓝ	Ⓨ Ⓝ	Ⓨ Ⓝ
Places one hand on the underside of the wrist	Ⓨ Ⓝ	Ⓨ Ⓝ	Ⓨ Ⓝ
Places the other hand on the hypothenar eminence	Ⓨ Ⓝ	Ⓨ Ⓝ	Ⓨ Ⓝ
Tester performs test according to accepted guidelines	**Test 1**	**Test 2**	**Test 3**
Has the athlete actively flex the wrist	Ⓨ Ⓝ	Ⓨ Ⓝ	Ⓨ Ⓝ
Applies resistance against the hypothenar eminence in the direction of extension (toward the radial side)	Ⓨ Ⓝ	Ⓨ Ⓝ	Ⓨ Ⓝ
Holds resistance for 5 seconds	Ⓨ Ⓝ	Ⓨ Ⓝ	Ⓨ Ⓝ
Performs assessment bilaterally	Ⓨ Ⓝ	Ⓨ Ⓝ	Ⓨ Ⓝ

The psychomotor skill was performed completely and in the appropriate order   **0 1 2 3 4 5**

The tester had control of the subject and the situation (showed confidence)   **0 1 2 3 4 5**

Method of performing the skill allowed the tester the ability to determine:
severity, proper progression, and the *fit* in the overall picture (Oral)   **0 1 2 3 4 5**

In order for a grade of *minimum standard* to be given, the total must be ≥11   **TOTAL = _____**

| 1 | 2 | 3 | 4 | 5 | 6 | 7 | 8 | 9 | 10 | 11 | 12 | 13 | 14 | 15 |

Not Acceptable   **Meets**   **Exceeds**
                                Minimum Standards   **Minimum Standards**

TEST ENVIRONMENTS

L: Laboratory/Classroom Testing
C: Clinical/Field Testing
P: Practicum Testing
A: Assessment/Mock Exam Testing
S: Self-Reporting

SKILL TEST INFORMATION

Positive Finding: Decreased ability to hold contraction
Involved Structure: Flexor carpi ulnaris
Special Considerations: N/A
Reference(s):   Kendall et al
Supplies Needed: N/A

MANUAL MUSCLE TESTING
(MMT-U-Test 29)

Peer Review _____ Peer Review _____

Skill Acquisition: _____   Practice Opportunities: _____

This problem allows you the opportunity to demonstrate a manual muscle test for the **extensor carpi ulnaris** *muscle. You have 2 minutes to complete this task.*

Tester places athlete and limb in appropriate position	Test 1	Test 2	Test 3
Seated or supine	Y N	Y N	Y N
Forearm placed in full pronation	Y N	Y N	Y N
Tester placed in proper position	**Test 1**	**Test 2**	**Test 3**
Stands in front, facing the athlete	Y N	Y N	Y N
Places one hand on the underside of the forearm/wrist	Y N	Y N	Y N
Places the other hand against the dorsum of the fifth metacarpal	Y N	Y N	Y N
Tester performs test according to accepted guidelines	**Test 1**	**Test 2**	**Test 3**
Has the athlete actively extend the wrist	Y N	Y N	Y N
Applies resistance against the dorsum of the fifth metacarpal in the direction of flexion (toward the radial side)	Y N	Y N	Y N
Holds resistance for 5 seconds	Y N	Y N	Y N
Performs assessment bilaterally	Y N	Y N	Y N

The psychomotor skill was performed completely and in the appropriate order   **0 1 2 3 4 5**

The tester had control of the subject and the situation (showed confidence)   **0 1 2 3 4 5**

Method of performing the skill allowed the tester the ability to determine:
severity, proper progression, and the *fit* in the overall picture (Oral)   **0 1 2 3 4 5**

In order for a grade of *minimum standard* to be given, the total must be ≥11   **TOTAL = _____**

```
    1    2    3    4    5    6    7    8    9   10   11   12   13   14   15
    |____|____|____|____|____|____|____|____|____|____|____|____|____|____|
  Not Acceptable                        Meets                   Exceeds
                                   Minimum Standards        Minimum Standards
```

TEST ENVIRONMENTS

L: Laboratory/Classroom Testing
C: Clinical/Field Testing
P: Practicum Testing
A: Assessment/Mock Exam Testing
S: Self-Reporting

SKILL TEST INFORMATION

Positive Finding: Decreased ability to hold contraction
Involved Structure: Extensor carpi ulnaris
Special Considerations: N/A
Reference(s): Kendall et al
Supplies Needed: N/A

MANUAL MUSCLE TESTING
(MMT-U-Test 30)

Peer Review _____ Peer Review _____

Skill Acquisition: _____   Practice Opportunities: _____

Please demonstrate a manual muscle test for the **extensor carpi radialis longus** *muscle. You have 2 minutes to complete this task.*

Tester places athlete and limb in appropriate position	Test 1	Test 2	Test 3
Seated with elbow flexed to 30 degrees	Ⓨ Ⓝ	Ⓨ Ⓝ	Ⓨ Ⓝ
Tester placed in proper position	**Test 1**	**Test 2**	**Test 3**
Forearm resting on the table at almost full pronation	Ⓨ Ⓝ	Ⓨ Ⓝ	Ⓨ Ⓝ
Tester performs test according to accepted guidelines	**Test 1**	**Test 2**	**Test 3**
Has athlete actively extend the wrist toward the radial side (allowing the fingers to flex)	Ⓨ Ⓝ	Ⓨ Ⓝ	Ⓨ Ⓝ
Applies resistance against the dorsal surface of the hand along the second and third metacarpals (in the direction of flexion of the wrist toward the ulnar side)	Ⓨ Ⓝ	Ⓨ Ⓝ	Ⓨ Ⓝ
Holds resistance for 5 seconds	Ⓨ Ⓝ	Ⓨ Ⓝ	Ⓨ Ⓝ
Performs assessment bilaterally	Ⓨ Ⓝ	Ⓨ Ⓝ	Ⓨ Ⓝ

The psychomotor skill was performed completely and in the appropriate order   0 1 2 3 4 5

The tester had control of the subject and the situation (showed confidence)   0 1 2 3 4 5

Method of performing the skill allowed the tester the ability to determine: severity, proper progression, and the *fit* in the overall picture (Oral)   0 1 2 3 4 5

In order for a grade of *minimum standard* to be given, the total must be ≥11   TOTAL = _____

```
 1    2    3    4    5    6    7    8    9   10   11   12   13   14   15
 |    |    |    |    |    |    |    |    |    |    |    |    |    |    |
```

Not Acceptable   **Meets**   **Exceeds**
                                     Minimum Standards   **Minimum Standards**

TEST ENVIRONMENTS
L: Laboratory/Classroom Testing
C: Clinical/Field Testing
P: Practicum Testing
A: Assessment/Mock Exam Testing
S: Self-Reporting

SKILL TEST INFORMATION
Positive Finding: Decreased ability to hold contraction
Involved Structure: Extensor carpi radialis longus
Special Considerations: N/A
Reference(s): Kendall et al
Supplies Needed: Table

MANUAL MUSCLE TESTING
(MMT-U-Test 31)

Peer Review _____ Peer Review _____

Skill Acquisition: _____   Practice Opportunities: _____

Please demonstrate a manual muscle test for the **palmaris longus** *muscle. You have 2 minutes to complete this task.*

Tester places athlete and limb in appropriate position	Test 1	Test 2	Test 3
Supine or seated	Ⓨ Ⓝ	Ⓨ Ⓝ	Ⓨ Ⓝ
Tester placed in proper position	Ⓨ Ⓝ	Ⓨ Ⓝ	Ⓨ Ⓝ
Directs athlete to rest forearm on the table in supinated position	Ⓨ Ⓝ	Ⓨ Ⓝ	Ⓨ Ⓝ
Tester performs test according to accepted guidelines	**Test 1**	**Test 2**	**Test 3**
Has athlete actively "cup" the hand and flex the wrist	Ⓨ Ⓝ	Ⓨ Ⓝ	Ⓨ Ⓝ
Applies resistance against the thenar and the hypothenar eminences (in the direction of flattening the palm)	Ⓨ Ⓝ	Ⓨ Ⓝ	Ⓨ Ⓝ
Applies resistance against the hand (direction of extending the wrist)	Ⓨ Ⓝ	Ⓨ Ⓝ	Ⓨ Ⓝ
Holds resistance for 5 seconds	Ⓨ Ⓝ	Ⓨ Ⓝ	Ⓨ Ⓝ
Performs assessment bilaterally	Ⓨ Ⓝ	Ⓨ Ⓝ	Ⓨ Ⓝ

The psychomotor skill was performed completely and in the appropriate order   0 1 2 3 4 5

The tester had control of the subject and the situation (showed confidence)   0 1 2 3 4 5

Method of performing the skill allowed the tester the ability to determine:
severity, proper progression, and the *fit* in the overall picture (Oral)   0 1 2 3 4 5

In order for a grade of *minimum standard* to be given, the total must be ≥11   TOTAL = _____

```
  1    2    3    4    5    6    7    8    9   10   11   12   13   14   15
  |    |    |    |    |    |    |    |    |    |    |    |    |    |    |
```

Not Acceptable   **Meets**   **Exceeds**
                                              Minimum Standards   **Minimum Standards**

TEST ENVIRONMENTS

L: Laboratory/Classroom Testing
C: Clinical/Field Testing
P: Practicum Testing
A: Assessment/Mock Exam Testing
S: Self-Reporting

SKILL TEST INFORMATION

Positive Finding: Decreased ability to hold contraction
Involved Structure: Palmaris longus
Special Considerations: N/A
Reference(s): Kendall et al
Supplies Needed: Table

MANUAL MUSCLE TESTING
(MMT-U-Test 32)

Peer Review _____ Peer Review _____

Skill Acquisition: _____   Practice Opportunities: _____

This problem allows you the opportunity to demonstrate a manual muscle test for the **extensor pollicis longus** *muscle. You have 2 minutes to complete this task.*

Tester places athlete and limb in appropriate position	Test 1	Test 2	Test 3
Seated or standing	Ⓨ Ⓝ	Ⓨ Ⓝ	Ⓨ Ⓝ

Tester placed in proper position	Test 1	Test 2	Test 3
Stands to the side, facing the athlete	Ⓨ Ⓝ	Ⓨ Ⓝ	Ⓨ Ⓝ
Places one hand on the under side of the hand and wrist	Ⓨ Ⓝ	Ⓨ Ⓝ	Ⓨ Ⓝ
Places the other hand against the dorsal surface of the distal phalanx of the thumb	Ⓨ Ⓝ	Ⓨ Ⓝ	Ⓨ Ⓝ

Tester performs test according to accepted guidelines	Test 1	Test 2	Test 3
Has the athlete actively extend the thumb	Ⓨ Ⓝ	Ⓨ Ⓝ	Ⓨ Ⓝ
Applies resistance against the thumb (distal phalanx) in the direction of flexion	Ⓨ Ⓝ	Ⓨ Ⓝ	Ⓨ Ⓝ
Holds resistance for 5 seconds	Ⓨ Ⓝ	Ⓨ Ⓝ	Ⓨ Ⓝ
Performs assessment bilaterally	Ⓨ Ⓝ	Ⓨ Ⓝ	Ⓨ Ⓝ

The psychomotor skill was performed completely and in the appropriate order   0 1 2 3 4 5

The tester had control of the subject and the situation (showed confidence)   0 1 2 3 4 5

Method of performing the skill allowed the tester the ability to determine:
severity, proper progression, and the *fit* in the overall picture (Oral)   0 1 2 3 4 5

In order for a grade of *minimum standard* to be given, the total must be ≥11   **TOTAL** = _____

```
  1   2   3   4   5   6   7   8   9   10   11   12   13   14   15
  |   |   |   |   |   |   |   |   |   |    |    |    |    |    |
```

Not Acceptable   **Meets**   **Exceeds**
                              Minimum Standards   **Minimum Standards**

TEST ENVIRONMENTS

L: Laboratory/Classroom Testing
C: Clinical/Field Testing
P: Practicum Testing
A: Assessment/Mock Exam Testing
S: Self-Reporting

SKILL TEST INFORMATION

Positive Finding: Decreased ability to hold contraction
Involved Structure: Extensor pollicis longus
Special Considerations: N/A
Reference(s): Kendall et al
Supplies Needed: N/A

Manual Muscle Testing
(MMT-U-Test 33)

Skill Acquisition: _____   Practice Opportunities: _____

This problem allows you the opportunity to demonstrate a manual muscle test for the **extensor pollicis brevis** *muscle. You have 2 minutes to complete this task.*

Tester places athlete and limb in appropriate position	Test 1	Test 2	Test 3
Seated or standing	Ⓨ Ⓝ	Ⓨ Ⓝ	Ⓨ Ⓝ
Tester placed in proper position	**Test 1**	**Test 2**	**Test 3**
Stands to the side, facing the athlete	Ⓨ Ⓝ	Ⓨ Ⓝ	Ⓨ Ⓝ
Places one hand on the underside of the hand and wrist	Ⓨ Ⓝ	Ⓨ Ⓝ	Ⓨ Ⓝ
Places the other hand against the dorsal surface of the proximal phalanx of the thumb	Ⓨ Ⓝ	Ⓨ Ⓝ	Ⓨ Ⓝ
Tester performs test according to accepted guidelines	**Test 1**	**Test 2**	**Test 3**
Has the athlete actively extend the thumb	Ⓨ Ⓝ	Ⓨ Ⓝ	Ⓨ Ⓝ
Applies resistance against the thumb (proximal phalanx) in the direction of flexion	Ⓨ Ⓝ	Ⓨ Ⓝ	Ⓨ Ⓝ
Holds resistance for 5 seconds	Ⓨ Ⓝ	Ⓨ Ⓝ	Ⓨ Ⓝ
Performs assessment bilaterally	Ⓨ Ⓝ	Ⓨ Ⓝ	Ⓨ Ⓝ

The psychomotor skill was performed completely and in the appropriate order   **0 1 2 3 4 5**

The tester had control of the subject and the situation (showed confidence)   **0 1 2 3 4 5**

Method of performing the skill allowed the tester the ability to determine:
severity, proper progression, and the *fit* in the overall picture (Oral)   **0 1 2 3 4 5**

In order for a grade of *minimum standard* to be given, the total must be ≥11   **TOTAL = _____**

```
 1    2    3    4    5    6    7    8    9    10   11   12   13   14   15
 |    |    |    |    |    |    |    |    |    |    |    |    |    |    |
```
Not Acceptable   **Meets**   **Exceeds**
                                    Minimum Standards   **Minimum Standards**

TEST ENVIRONMENTS

L: Laboratory/Classroom Testing
C: Clinical/Field Testing
P: Practicum Testing
A: Assessment/Mock Exam Testing
S: Self-Reporting

SKILL TEST INFORMATION

Positive Finding: Decreased ability to hold contraction
Involved Structure: Extensor pollicis brevis
Special Considerations: N/A
Reference(s): Kendall et al
Supplies Needed: N/A

MANUAL MUSCLE TESTING
(MMT-U-Test 34)

Peer Review _____ Peer Review _____

Skill Acquisition: _____   Practice Opportunities: _____

Please demonstrate how you would perform the ligamentous stress test for the ankle known as the **abductor pollicis brevis** *muscle. You have 2 minutes to complete this task.*

Tester places athlete and limb in appropriate position	Test 1	Test 2	Test 3
Seated or standing	Ⓨ Ⓝ	Ⓨ Ⓝ	Ⓨ Ⓝ
Tester placed in proper position	**Test 1**	**Test 2**	**Test 3**
Stands to the side, facing the athlete	Ⓨ Ⓝ	Ⓨ Ⓝ	Ⓨ Ⓝ
Places one hand on the underside of the hand and wrist	Ⓨ Ⓝ	Ⓨ Ⓝ	Ⓨ Ⓝ
Places the other hand against the dorsal surface of the proximal phalanx of the thumb	Ⓨ Ⓝ	Ⓨ Ⓝ	Ⓨ Ⓝ
Tester performs test according to accepted guidelines	**Test 1**	**Test 2**	**Test 3**
Has the athlete actively abduct the thumb	Ⓨ Ⓝ	Ⓨ Ⓝ	Ⓨ Ⓝ
Applies resistance against thumb (proximal phalanx) in the direction of adduction (toward the palm)	Ⓨ Ⓝ	Ⓨ Ⓝ	Ⓨ Ⓝ
Holds resistance for 5 seconds	Ⓨ Ⓝ	Ⓨ Ⓝ	Ⓨ Ⓝ
Performs assessment bilaterally	Ⓨ Ⓝ	Ⓨ Ⓝ	Ⓨ Ⓝ

The psychomotor skill was performed completely and in the appropriate order   **0 1 2 3 4 5**

The tester had control of the subject and the situation (showed confidence)   **0 1 2 3 4 5**

Method of performing the skill allowed the tester the ability to determine:
severity, proper progression, and the *fit* in the overall picture (Oral)   **0 1 2 3 4 5**

In order for a grade of *minimum standard* to be given, the total must be ≥11   **TOTAL = _____**

```
  1    2    3    4    5    6    7    8    9   10   11   12   13   14   15
  |----|----|----|----|----|----|----|----|----|----|----|----|----|----|
```
Not Acceptable   **Meets**   **Exceeds**
                                    Minimum Standards   **Minimum Standards**

TEST ENVIRONMENTS
L: Laboratory/Classroom Testing
C: Clinical/Field Testing
P: Practicum Testing
A: Assessment/Mock Exam Testing
S: Self-Reporting

SKILL TEST INFORMATION
Positive Finding: Decreased ability to hold contraction
Involved Structure: Abductor pollicis brevis
Special Considerations: N/A
Reference(s): Kendall et al
Supplies Needed: N/A

MANUAL MUSCLE TESTING
(MMT-U-Test 35)

Peer Review _____ Peer Review _____

Skill Acquisition: _____   Practice Opportunities: _____

This problem allows you the opportunity to demonstrate a manual muscle test for the **flexor pollicis longus** **muscle.** *You have 2 minutes to complete this task.*

Tester places athlete and limb in appropriate position	Test 1	Test 2	Test 3
Seated or supine	Ⓨ Ⓝ	Ⓨ Ⓝ	Ⓨ Ⓝ
Tester placed in proper position	**Test 1**	**Test 2**	**Test 3**
Stands to the side, facing the athlete	Ⓨ Ⓝ	Ⓨ Ⓝ	Ⓨ Ⓝ
Places one hand on the underside of the hand and wrist (stabilizing the metacarpal and proximal phalanx)	Ⓨ Ⓝ	Ⓨ Ⓝ	Ⓨ Ⓝ
Places the other hand against the palmar surface of the distal phalanx of the thumb	Ⓨ Ⓝ	Ⓨ Ⓝ	Ⓨ Ⓝ
Tester performs test according to accepted guidelines	**Test 1**	**Test 2**	**Test 3**
Has the athlete actively flex the thumb	Ⓨ Ⓝ	Ⓨ Ⓝ	Ⓨ Ⓝ
Applies resistance against the thumb (distal phalanx) in the direction of flexion	Ⓨ Ⓝ	Ⓨ Ⓝ	Ⓨ Ⓝ
Holds resistance for 5 seconds	Ⓨ Ⓝ	Ⓨ Ⓝ	Ⓨ Ⓝ
Performs assessment bilaterally	Ⓨ Ⓝ	Ⓨ Ⓝ	Ⓨ Ⓝ

The psychomotor skill was performed completely and in the appropriate order   **0 1 2 3 4 5**

The tester had control of the subject and the situation (showed confidence)   **0 1 2 3 4 5**

Method of performing the skill allowed the tester the ability to determine:
severity, proper progression, and the *fit* in the overall picture (Oral)   **0 1 2 3 4 5**

In order for a grade of *minimum standard* to be given, the total must be ≥11   **TOTAL = _____**

```
  1    2    3    4    5    6    7    8    9   10   11   12   13   14   15
  |    |    |    |    |    |    |    |    |    |    |    |    |    |    |
```

Not Acceptable   **Meets**   **Exceeds**
                                     Minimum Standards   **Minimum Standards**

TEST ENVIRONMENTS	**SKILL TEST INFORMATION**

TEST ENVIRONMENTS

L: Laboratory/Classroom Testing
C: Clinical/Field Testing
P: Practicum Testing
A: Assessment/Mock Exam Testing
S: Self-Reporting

SKILL TEST INFORMATION

Positive Finding:	Decreased ability to hold contraction
Involved Structure:	Flexor pollicis longus and brevis
Special Considerations:	N/A
Reference(s):	Kendall et al
Supplies Needed:	N/A

MANUAL MUSCLE TESTING
(MMT-U-Test 36)

Skill Acquisition: _____   Practice Opportunities: _____

Please demonstrate a manual muscle test for the **flexor pollicus brevis** *muscle. You have 2 minutes to complete this task.*

Tester places athlete and limb in appropriate position	Test 1	Test 2	Test 3
Supine or seated	Ⓨ Ⓝ	Ⓨ Ⓝ	Ⓨ Ⓝ
Tester placed in proper position	Ⓨ Ⓝ	Ⓨ Ⓝ	Ⓨ Ⓝ
Stabilizes the hand	Ⓨ Ⓝ	Ⓨ Ⓝ	Ⓨ Ⓝ

Tester performs test according to accepted guidelines	Test 1	Test 2	Test 3
Has athlete actively flex the metacarpophalangeal joint (without flexion of interphalangeal joint)	Ⓨ Ⓝ	Ⓨ Ⓝ	Ⓨ Ⓝ
Applies resistance against the palmar surface of the proximal phalanx (in the direction of extension of the thumb)	Ⓨ Ⓝ	Ⓨ Ⓝ	Ⓨ Ⓝ
Holds resistance for 5 seconds	Ⓨ Ⓝ	Ⓨ Ⓝ	Ⓨ Ⓝ
Performs assessment bilaterally	Ⓨ Ⓝ	Ⓨ Ⓝ	Ⓨ Ⓝ

The psychomotor skill was performed completely and in the appropriate order   0 1 2 3 4 5

The tester had control of the subject and the situation (showed confidence)   0 1 2 3 4 5

Method of performing the skill allowed the tester the ability to determine: severity, proper progression, and the *fit* in the overall picture (Oral)   0 1 2 3 4 5

In order for a grade of *minimum standard* to be given, the total must be ≥11   **TOTAL = _____**

```
  1    2    3    4    5    6    7    8    9   10   11   12   13   14   15
  |    |    |    |    |    |    |    |    |    |    |    |    |    |    |
```
Not Acceptable   **Meets**   **Exceeds**
                                      Minimum Standards   **Minimum Standards**

TEST ENVIRONMENTS

L: Laboratory/Classroom Testing
C: Clinical/Field Testing
P: Practicum Testing
A: Assessment/Mock Exam Testing
S: Self-Reporting

SKILL TEST INFORMATION

Positive Finding:	Decreased ability to hold contraction
Involved Structure:	Flexor pollicus brevis
Special Considerations:	N/A
Reference(s):	Kendall et al
Supplies Needed:	Table

MANUAL MUSCLE TESTING
(MMT-U-Test 37)

Peer Review _____ Peer Review _____

Skill Acquisition: _____   Practice Opportunities: _____

Please demonstrate a manual muscle test for the **opponens pollicus** *muscle. You have 2 minutes to complete this task.*

Tester places athlete and limb in appropriate position	Test 1	Test 2	Test 3
Supine or seated	Ⓨ Ⓝ	Ⓨ Ⓝ	Ⓨ Ⓝ
Tester placed in proper position	Ⓨ Ⓝ	Ⓨ Ⓝ	Ⓨ Ⓝ
Stabilizes the hand	Ⓨ Ⓝ	Ⓨ Ⓝ	Ⓨ Ⓝ
Tester performs test according to accepted guidelines	**Test 1**	**Test 2**	**Test 3**
Has athlete actively flex, abduct, and medially rotate the metacarpal bone (so that the thumbnail shows in the palmar view)	Ⓨ Ⓝ	Ⓨ Ⓝ	Ⓨ Ⓝ
Applies resistance against the metacarpal bone (in the direction of extension, adduction and lateral rotation of the thumb)	Ⓨ Ⓝ	Ⓨ Ⓝ	Ⓨ Ⓝ
Holds resistance for 5 seconds	Ⓨ Ⓝ	Ⓨ Ⓝ	Ⓨ Ⓝ
Performs assessment bilaterally	Ⓨ Ⓝ	Ⓨ Ⓝ	Ⓨ Ⓝ

The psychomotor skill was performed completely and in the appropriate order   **0 1 2 3 4 5**

The tester had control of the subject and the situation (showed confidence)   **0 1 2 3 4 5**

Method of performing the skill allowed the tester the ability to determine: severity, proper progression, and the *fit* in the overall picture (Oral)   **0 1 2 3 4 5**

In order for a grade of *minimum standard* to be given, the total must be ≥11   **TOTAL = _____**

```
    1    2    3    4    5    6    7    8    9    10    11    12    13    14    15
    |____|____|____|____|____|____|____|____|____|____|____|____|____|____|
```

Not Acceptable   **Meets**   **Exceeds**
                                          Minimum Standards   **Minimum Standards**

TEST ENVIRONMENTS

L: Laboratory/Classroom Testing
C: Clinical/Field Testing
P: Practicum Testing
A: Assessment/Mock Exam Testing
S: Self-Reporting

SKILL TEST INFORMATION

Positive Finding: Decreased ability to hold contraction
Involved Structure: Opponens pollicus
Special Considerations: N/A
Reference(s): Kendall et al
Supplies Needed: Table

MANUAL MUSCLE TESTING
(MMT-U-Test 38)

Peer Review _____ Peer Review _____

Skill Acquisition: _____   Practice Opportunities: _____

Please demonstrate a manual muscle test for the **adductor pollicus** *muscle. You have 2 minutes to complete this task.*

Tester places athlete and limb in appropriate position	Test 1	Test 2	Test 3
Supine or seated	Ⓨ Ⓝ	Ⓨ Ⓝ	Ⓨ Ⓝ
Tester placed in proper position	**Test 1**	**Test 2**	**Test 3**
Stabilizes hand or directs the athlete to rest hand on table	Ⓨ Ⓝ	Ⓨ Ⓝ	Ⓨ Ⓝ
Tester performs test according to accepted guidelines	**Test 1**	**Test 2**	**Test 3**
Has athlete actively adduct the thumb toward the palm	Ⓨ Ⓝ	Ⓨ Ⓝ	Ⓨ Ⓝ
Applies resistance against the medial surface of the thumb (in the direction of abduction of the thumb)	Ⓨ Ⓝ	Ⓨ Ⓝ	Ⓨ Ⓝ
Holds resistance for 5 seconds	Ⓨ Ⓝ	Ⓨ Ⓝ	Ⓨ Ⓝ
Performs assessment bilaterally	Ⓨ Ⓝ	Ⓨ Ⓝ	Ⓨ Ⓝ

The psychomotor skill was performed completely and in the appropriate order   **0 1 2 3 4 5**

The tester had control of the subject and the situation (showed confidence)   **0 1 2 3 4 5**

Method of performing the skill allowed the tester the ability to determine: severity, proper progression, and the *fit* in the overall picture (Oral)   **0 1 2 3 4 5**

In order for a grade of *minimum standard* to be given, the total must be ≥11   **TOTAL = _____**

1	2	3	4	5	6	7	8	9	10	11	12	13	14	15

Not Acceptable   **Meets**   **Exceeds**
                         Minimum Standards   **Minimum Standards**

TEST ENVIRONMENTS

L: Laboratory/Classroom Testing
C: Clinical/Field Testing
P: Practicum Testing
A: Assessment/Mock Exam Testing
S: Self-Reporting

SKILL TEST INFORMATION

Positive Finding: Decreased ability to hold contraction
Involved Structure: Adductor pollicus
Special Considerations: N/A
Reference(s): Kendall et al
Supplies Needed Table

MANUAL MUSCLE TESTING
(MMT-U-Test 39)

Peer Review _____ Peer Review _____

Skill Acquisition: _____   Practice Opportunities: _____

*Please demonstrate a manual muscle test for the **abductor pollicus longus** muscle. You have 2 minutes to complete this task.*

Tester places athlete and limb in appropriate position	Test 1	Test 2	Test 3
Supine or seated	Ⓨ Ⓝ	Ⓨ Ⓝ	Ⓨ Ⓝ
Tester placed in proper position	**Test 1**	**Test 2**	**Test 3**
Stabilizes wrist-forearm with lateral side up	Ⓨ Ⓝ	Ⓨ Ⓝ	Ⓨ Ⓝ
Tester performs test according to accepted guidelines	**Test 1**	**Test 2**	**Test 3**
Has athlete actively abduct and slightly extend the first metacarpal bone	Ⓨ Ⓝ	Ⓨ Ⓝ	Ⓨ Ⓝ
Applies resistance against the lateral aspect of the thumb (in the direction of adduction and flexion of the thumb)	Ⓨ Ⓝ	Ⓨ Ⓝ	Ⓨ Ⓝ
Holds resistance for 5 seconds	Ⓨ Ⓝ	Ⓨ Ⓝ	Ⓨ Ⓝ
Performs assessment bilaterally	Ⓨ Ⓝ	Ⓨ Ⓝ	Ⓨ Ⓝ

The psychomotor skill was performed completely and in the appropriate order   0 1 2 3 4 5

The tester had control of the subject and the situation (showed confidence)   0 1 2 3 4 5

Method of performing the skill allowed the tester the ability to determine:
severity, proper progression, and the *fit* in the overall picture (Oral)   0 1 2 3 4 5

In order for a grade of *minimum standard* to be given, the total must be ≥11   TOTAL = _____

```
   1    2    3    4    5    6    7    8    9   10   11   12   13   14   15
   |    |    |    |    |    |    |    |    |    |    |    |    |    |    |
```

Not Acceptable   Meets   Exceeds
                                  Minimum Standards   Minimum Standards

TEST ENVIRONMENTS

L: Laboratory/Classroom Testing
C: Clinical/Field Testing
P: Practicum Testing
A: Assessment/Mock Exam Testing
S: Self-Reporting

SKILL TEST INFORMATION

Positive Finding: Decreased ability to hold contraction
Involved Structure: Abductor pollicus longus
Special Considerations: N/A
Reference(s) Kendall et al
Supplies Needed: Table

MANUAL MUSCLE TESTING
(MMT-U-Test 40)

Peer Review _____ Peer Review _____

Skill Acquisition: _____   Practice Opportunities: _____

*This problem allows you the opportunity to demonstrate a manual muscle test for the **opponens digiti minimi** muscle. You have 2 minutes to complete this task.*

Tester places athlete and limb in appropriate position	Test 1	Test 2	Test 3
Seated or supine	Ⓨ Ⓝ	Ⓨ Ⓝ	Ⓨ Ⓝ
Wrist placed in full supination	Ⓨ Ⓝ	Ⓨ Ⓝ	Ⓨ Ⓝ
Tester placed in proper position	**Test 1**	**Test 2**	**Test 3**
Stands in front, facing the athlete	Ⓨ Ⓝ	Ⓨ Ⓝ	Ⓨ Ⓝ
Places one hand on the underside of the hand (first metacarpal is gripped firmly)	Ⓨ Ⓝ	Ⓨ Ⓝ	Ⓨ Ⓝ
Places the other hand against the palmar surface of the fifth metacarpal	Ⓨ Ⓝ	Ⓨ Ⓝ	Ⓨ Ⓝ
Tester performs test according to accepted guidelines	**Test 1**	**Test 2**	**Test 3**
Has the athlete actively oppose the fifth metacarpal/finger (moves toward the thumb)	Ⓨ Ⓝ	Ⓨ Ⓝ	Ⓨ Ⓝ
Applies resistance against palmar surface of the fifth metacarpal (attempting to flatten the hand)	Ⓨ Ⓝ	Ⓨ Ⓝ	Ⓨ Ⓝ
Holds resistance for 5 seconds	Ⓨ Ⓝ	Ⓨ Ⓝ	Ⓨ Ⓝ
Performs assessment bilaterally	Ⓨ Ⓝ	Ⓨ Ⓝ	Ⓨ Ⓝ

The psychomotor skill was performed completely and in the appropriate order   0 1 2 3 4 5

The tester had control of the subject and the situation (showed confidence)   0 1 2 3 4 5

Method of performing the skill allowed the tester the ability to determine:
severity, proper progression, and the *fit* in the overall picture (Oral)   0 1 2 3 4 5

In order for a grade of *minimum standard* to be given, the total must be ≥11   **TOTAL = _____**

```
   1    2    3    4    5    6    7    8    9   10   11   12   13   14   15
   |    |    |    |    |    |    |    |    |    |    |    |    |    |    |
```

Not Acceptable   **Meets**   **Exceeds**
                                      Minimum Standards   **Minimum Standards**

TEST ENVIRONMENTS

L: Laboratory/Classroom Testing
C: Clinical/Field Testing
P: Practicum Testing
A: Assessment/Mock Exam Testing
S: Self-Reporting

SKILL TEST INFORMATION

Positive Finding:	Decreased ability to hold contraction
Involved Structure:	Opponens digiti minimi
Special Considerations:	N/A
Reference(s):	Kendall et al
Supplies Needed:	N/A

Manual Muscle Testing
(MMT-U-Test 41)

Peer Review _____ Peer Review _____

Skill Acquisition: _____   Practice Opportunities: _____

This problem allows you the opportunity to demonstrate a manual muscle test for the **flexor digitorum profundus** *muscle. You have 2 minutes to complete this task.*

Tester places athlete and limb in appropriate position	Test 1	Test 2	Test 3
Seated or supine	Ⓨ Ⓝ	Ⓨ Ⓝ	Ⓨ Ⓝ
Wrist placed in full supination (slight extension)	Ⓨ Ⓝ	Ⓨ Ⓝ	Ⓨ Ⓝ
Tester placed in proper position	**Test 1**	**Test 2**	**Test 3**
Stands in front, facing the athlete	Ⓨ Ⓝ	Ⓨ Ⓝ	Ⓨ Ⓝ
Stabilizes the proximal and middle phalanges with one hand	Ⓨ Ⓝ	Ⓨ Ⓝ	Ⓨ Ⓝ
Places the other hand against the palmar surface of the distal phalanx (2, 3, 4, 5)	Ⓨ Ⓝ	Ⓨ Ⓝ	Ⓨ Ⓝ
Tester performs test according to accepted guidelines	**Test 1**	**Test 2**	**Test 3**
Has the athlete actively flex the DIP joints of the second to fifth phalanges	Ⓨ Ⓝ	Ⓨ Ⓝ	Ⓨ Ⓝ
Applies resistance against the palmar surface of each phalange in the direction of extension	Ⓨ Ⓝ	Ⓨ Ⓝ	Ⓨ Ⓝ
Isolates each phalange separately (2, 3, 4, 5)	Ⓨ Ⓝ	Ⓨ Ⓝ	Ⓨ Ⓝ
Holds resistance for 5 seconds	Ⓨ Ⓝ	Ⓨ Ⓝ	Ⓨ Ⓝ
Performs assessment bilaterally	Ⓨ Ⓝ	Ⓨ Ⓝ	Ⓨ Ⓝ

The psychomotor skill was performed completely and in the appropriate order   0 1 2 3 4 5

The tester had control of the subject and the situation (showed confidence)   0 1 2 3 4 5

Method of performing the skill allowed the tester the ability to determine:
severity, proper progression, and the *fit* in the overall picture (Oral)   0 1 2 3 4 5

In order for a grade of *minimum standard* to be given, the total must be ≥11   TOTAL = _____

```
   1    2    3    4    5    6    7    8    9   10   11   12   13   14   15
   |    |    |    |    |    |    |    |    |    |    |    |    |    |    |
```

Not Acceptable   **Meets**   **Exceeds**
                                  Minimum Standards   **Minimum Standards**

TEST ENVIRONMENTS

L: Laboratory/Classroom Testing
C: Clinical/Field Testing
P: Practicum Testing
A: Assessment/Mock Exam Testing
S: Self-Reporting

SKILL TEST INFORMATION

Positive Finding: Decreased ability to hold contraction
Involved Structure: Flexor digitorum profundus
Special Considerations: N/A
Reference(s): Kendall et al
Supplies Needed: N/A

MANUAL MUSCLE TESTING
(MMT-U-Test 42)

Peer Review _____ Peer Review _____

Skill Acquisition: _____   Practice Opportunities: _____

Please demonstrate a manual muscle test for the **flexor digiti minimi** *muscle. You have 2 minutes to complete this task.*

Tester places athlete and limb in appropriate position	Test 1	Test 2	Test 3
Supine or seated	Ⓨ Ⓝ	Ⓨ Ⓝ	Ⓨ Ⓝ
Tester placed in proper position	**Test 1**	**Test 2**	**Test 3**
Stabilizes the hand or directs the athlete to rest hand on the table	Ⓨ Ⓝ	Ⓨ Ⓝ	Ⓨ Ⓝ
Tester performs test according to accepted guidelines	**Test 1**	**Test 2**	**Test 3**
Has athlete actively flex the metacarpophalangeal joint (maintaining extension of the interphalangeal joint)	Ⓨ Ⓝ	Ⓨ Ⓝ	Ⓨ Ⓝ
Applies resistance against the palmer surface of the proximal phalanx (in the direction of extension of the metacarpophalangeal joint)	Ⓨ Ⓝ	Ⓨ Ⓝ	Ⓨ Ⓝ
Holds resistance for 5 seconds	Ⓨ Ⓝ	Ⓨ Ⓝ	Ⓨ Ⓝ
Performs assessment bilaterally	Ⓨ Ⓝ	Ⓨ Ⓝ	Ⓨ Ⓝ

The psychomotor skill was performed completely and in the appropriate order   **0 1 2 3 4 5**

The tester had control of the subject and the situation (showed confidence)   **0 1 2 3 4 5**

Method of performing the skill allowed the tester the ability to determine:
severity, proper progression, and the *fit* in the overall picture (Oral)   **0 1 2 3 4 5**

In order for a grade of *minimum standard* to be given, the total must be ≥11   **TOTAL = _____**

```
  1    2    3    4    5    6    7    8    9   10   11   12   13   14   15
  |____|____|____|____|____|____|____|____|____|____|____|____|____|____|
```

Not Acceptable   **Meets**   **Exceeds**
                                      Minimum Standards   **Minimum Standards**

TEST ENVIRONMENTS

L: Laboratory/Classroom Testing
C: Clinical/Field Testing
P: Practicum Testing
A: Assessment/Mock Exam Testing
S: Self-Reporting

SKILL TEST INFORMATION

Positive Finding: Decreased ability to hold contraction
Involved Structure: Flexor digiti minimi
Special Considerations: N/A
Reference(s): Kendall et al
Supplies Needed: Table

MANUAL MUSCLE TESTING
(MMT-U-Test 43)

Peer Review _____ Peer Review _____

Skill Acquisition: _____   Practice Opportunities: _____

*Please demonstrate a manual muscle test for the **abductor digiti minimi** muscle. You have 2 minutes to complete this task.*

Tester places athlete and limb in appropriate position	Test 1	Test 2	Test 3
Supine or seated	Ⓨ Ⓝ	Ⓨ Ⓝ	Ⓨ Ⓝ
Tester placed in proper position	**Test 1**	**Test 2**	**Test 3**
Stabilizes the hand or directs the athlete to rest hand on the table	Ⓨ Ⓝ	Ⓨ Ⓝ	Ⓨ Ⓝ
Tester performs test according to accepted guidelines	**Test 1**	**Test 2**	**Test 3**
Has athlete actively abduct the fifth digit	Ⓨ Ⓝ	Ⓨ Ⓝ	Ⓨ Ⓝ
Applies resistance against the ulnar side of the fifth digit (in the direction of adduction toward the midline of the hand)	Ⓨ Ⓝ	Ⓨ Ⓝ	Ⓨ Ⓝ
Holds resistance for 5 seconds	Ⓨ Ⓝ	Ⓨ Ⓝ	Ⓨ Ⓝ
Performs assessment bilaterally	Ⓨ Ⓝ	Ⓨ Ⓝ	Ⓨ Ⓝ

The psychomotor skill was performed completely and in the appropriate order   **0 1 2 3 4 5**

The tester had control of the subject and the situation (showed confidence)   **0 1 2 3 4 5**

Method of performing the skill allowed the tester the ability to determine:
severity, proper progression, and the *fit* in the overall picture (Oral)   **0 1 2 3 4 5**

In order for a grade of *minimum standard* to be given, the total must be ≥11   **TOTAL = _____**

```
 1    2    3    4    5    6    7    8    9    10   11   12   13   14   15
 |----|----|----|----|----|----|----|----|----|----|----|----|----|----|
```
Not Acceptable   Meets   Exceeds
                                          Minimum Standards   Minimum Standards

TEST ENVIRONMENTS

L: Laboratory/Classroom Testing
C: Clinical/Field Testing
P: Practicum Testing
A: Assessment/Mock Exam Testing
S: Self-Reporting

SKILL TEST INFORMATION

Positive Finding: Decreased ability to hold contraction
Involved Structure: Abductor digiti minimi
Special Considerations: N/A
Reference(s): Kendall et al
Supplies Needed: Table

Manual Muscle Testing
(MMT-U-Test 44)

Peer Review _____ Peer Review _____

Skill Acquisition: _____ Practice Opportunities: _____

Please demonstrate a manual muscle test for the **extensor digitorum** *muscle. You have 2 minutes to complete this task.*

Tester places athlete and limb in appropriate position	Test 1	Test 2	Test 3
Supine or seated	Ⓨ Ⓝ	Ⓨ Ⓝ	Ⓨ Ⓝ
Tester placed in proper position	**Test 1**	**Test 2**	**Test 3**
Stabilizes the wrist avoiding full extension	Ⓨ Ⓝ	Ⓨ Ⓝ	Ⓨ Ⓝ
Tester performs test according to accepted guidelines	**Test 1**	**Test 2**	**Test 3**
Has athlete actively extend the metacarpophalangeal joints of digits 2 to 5 (with interphalangeal joints relaxed)	Ⓨ Ⓝ	Ⓨ Ⓝ	Ⓨ Ⓝ
Applies resistance against the dorsal surface or proximal phalanges (in the direction of flexion of the metacarpophalangeal joints)	Ⓨ Ⓝ	Ⓨ Ⓝ	Ⓨ Ⓝ
Holds resistance for 5 seconds	Ⓨ Ⓝ	Ⓨ Ⓝ	Ⓨ Ⓝ
Performs assessment bilaterally	Ⓨ Ⓝ	Ⓨ Ⓝ	Ⓨ Ⓝ

The psychomotor skill was performed completely and in the appropriate order   **0 1 2 3 4 5**

The tester had control of the subject and the situation (showed confidence)   **0 1 2 3 4 5**

Method of performing the skill allowed the tester the ability to determine:
severity, proper progression, and the *fit* in the overall picture (Oral)   **0 1 2 3 4 5**

In order for a grade of *minimum standard* to be given, the total must be ≥11   **TOTAL = _____**

```
  1     2     3     4     5     6     7     8     9    10    11    12    13    14    15
  |     |     |     |     |     |     |     |     |     |     |     |     |     |     |
```

Not Acceptable   **Meets**   **Exceeds**
                                          Minimum Standards   **Minimum Standards**

TEST ENVIRONMENTS

L: Laboratory/Classroom Testing
C: Clinical/Field Testing
P: Practicum Testing
A: Assessment/Mock Exam Testing
S: Self-Reporting

SKILL TEST INFORMATION

Positive Finding: Decreased ability to hold contraction
Involved Structure: Extensor digitorum
Special Considerations: N/A
Reference(s): Kendall et al
Supplies Needed: Table

MANUAL MUSCLE TESTING
(MMT-U-Test 45)

Peer Review _____ Peer Review _____

Skill Acquisition: _____   Practice Opportunities: _____

This problem allows you the opportunity to demonstrate a **Myotome Assessment** *in order to rule out damage to nerve root* **C5**. *You have 2 minutes to complete this task.*

Tester places athlete and limb in appropriate position	Test 1	Test 2	Test 3
Seated or standing	Ⓨ Ⓝ	Ⓨ Ⓝ	Ⓨ Ⓝ
Tester performs test according to accepted guidelines	**Test 1**	**Test 2**	**Test 3**
Instructs the athlete to abduct the shoulder against resistance (deltoid) and/or	Ⓨ Ⓝ	Ⓨ Ⓝ	Ⓨ Ⓝ
Instructs the athlete to flex the elbow against resistance (biceps)	Ⓨ Ⓝ	Ⓨ Ⓝ	Ⓨ Ⓝ
Performs a break test at some point in the range of motion	Ⓨ Ⓝ	Ⓨ Ⓝ	Ⓨ Ⓝ
Holds resistance for 5 seconds	Ⓨ Ⓝ	Ⓨ Ⓝ	Ⓨ Ⓝ
Performs assessment bilaterally	Ⓨ Ⓝ	Ⓨ Ⓝ	Ⓨ Ⓝ

The psychomotor skill was performed completely and in the appropriate order   0 1 2 3 4 5

The tester had control of the subject and the situation (showed confidence)   0 1 2 3 4 5

Method of performing the skill allowed the tester the ability to determine:
severity, proper progression, and the *fit* in the overall picture (Oral)   0 1 2 3 4 5

In order for a grade of *minimum standard* to be given, the total must be ≥11   TOTAL = _____

```
  1    2    3    4    5    6    7    8    9    10   11   12   13   14   15
  |    |    |    |    |    |    |    |    |    |    |    |    |    |    |
```

Not Acceptable   **Meets**   **Exceeds**
                                   Minimum Standards   **Minimum Standards**

TEST ENVIRONMENTS

L: Laboratory/Classroom Testing
C: Clinical/Field Testing
P: Practicum Testing
A: Assessment/Mock Exam Testing
S: Self-Reporting

SKILL TEST INFORMATION

Positive Finding: Unable to maintain position against resistance
Involved Structure: Nerve root C5
Special Considerations: Rule out nerve root damage
Reference(s): Hoppenfeld
Supplies Needed: N/A

MANUAL MUSCLE TESTING
(MMT-U-Test 46)

Peer Review _____ Peer Review _____

Skill Acquisition: _____   Practice Opportunities: _____

This problem allows you the opportunity to demonstrate a **Myotome Assessment** *in order to rule out damage to nerve root* **C6**. *You have 2 minutes to complete this task.*

Tester places athlete and limb in appropriate position	Test 1	Test 2	Test 3
Seated or standing	Ⓨ Ⓝ	Ⓨ Ⓝ	Ⓨ Ⓝ

Tester performs test according to accepted guidelines	Test 1	Test 2	Test 3
Instructs the athlete to extend the wrist against resistance (exterior carpi radialis longus and brevis) and/or	Ⓨ Ⓝ	Ⓨ Ⓝ	Ⓨ Ⓝ
Instructs the athlete to flex the elbow against resistance (biceps)	Ⓨ Ⓝ	Ⓨ Ⓝ	Ⓨ Ⓝ
Performs a break test at some point in the range of motion	Ⓨ Ⓝ	Ⓨ Ⓝ	Ⓨ Ⓝ
Holds resistance for 5 seconds	Ⓨ Ⓝ	Ⓨ Ⓝ	Ⓨ Ⓝ
Performs assessment bilaterally	Ⓨ Ⓝ	Ⓨ Ⓝ	Ⓨ Ⓝ

The psychomotor skill was performed completely and in the appropriate order   **0 1 2 3 4 5**

The tester had control of the subject and the situation (showed confidence)   **0 1 2 3 4 5**

Method of performing the skill allowed the tester the ability to determine: severity, proper progression, and the *fit* in the overall picture (Oral)   **0 1 2 3 4 5**

In order for a grade of *minimum standard* to be given, the total must be ≥11   **TOTAL = _____**

| 1 | 2 | 3 | 4 | 5 | 6 | 7 | 8 | 9 | 10 | 11 | 12 | 13 | 14 | 15 |

Not Acceptable   **Meets**   **Exceeds**
                                       Minimum Standards   **Minimum Standards**

TEST ENVIRONMENTS
L: Laboratory/Classroom Testing
C: Clinical/Field Testing
P: Practicum Testing
A: Assessment/Mock Exam Testing
S: Self-Reporting

SKILL TEST INFORMATION
Positive Finding: Unable to maintain position against resistance
Involved Structure: Nerve root C6
Special Considerations: Rule out nerve root damage
Reference(s): Hoppenfeld
Supplies Needed: N/A

Manual Muscle Testing
(MMT-U-Test 47)

Peer Review _____ Peer Review _____

Skill Acquisition: _____   Practice Opportunities: _____

This problem allows you the opportunity to demonstrate a **Myotome Assessment** *in order to rule out damage to nerve root* **C7**. *You have 2 minutes to complete this task.*

Tester places athlete and limb in appropriate position	Test 1	Test 2	Test 3
Seated or standing	Ⓨ Ⓝ	Ⓨ Ⓝ	Ⓨ Ⓝ
Tester performs test according to accepted guidelines	**Test 1**	**Test 2**	**Test 3**
Instructs the athlete to flex the wrist against resistance and/or	Ⓨ Ⓝ	Ⓨ Ⓝ	Ⓨ Ⓝ
Instructs the athlete to extend the elbow against resistance	Ⓨ Ⓝ	Ⓨ Ⓝ	Ⓨ Ⓝ
Performs a break test at some point in the range of motion	Ⓨ Ⓝ	Ⓨ Ⓝ	Ⓨ Ⓝ
Holds resistance for 5 seconds	Ⓨ Ⓝ	Ⓨ Ⓝ	Ⓨ Ⓝ
Performs assessment bilaterally	Ⓨ Ⓝ	Ⓨ Ⓝ	Ⓨ Ⓝ

The psychomotor skill was performed completely and in the appropriate order   0 1 2 3 4 5

The tester had control of the subject and the situation (showed confidence)   0 1 2 3 4 5

Method of performing the skill allowed the tester the ability to determine:
severity, proper progression, and the *fit* in the overall picture (Oral)   0 1 2 3 4 5

In order for a grade of *minimum standard* to be given, the total must be ≥11   TOTAL = _____

```
  1    2    3    4    5    6    7    8    9   10   11   12   13   14   15
  |    |    |    |    |    |    |    |    |    |    |    |    |    |    |
```

Not Acceptable   **Meets**   **Exceeds**
                               Minimum Standards   **Minimum Standards**

TEST ENVIRONMENTS

L: Laboratory/Classroom Testing
C: Clinical/Field Testing
P: Practicum Testing
A: Assessment/Mock Exam Testing
S: Self-Reporting

SKILL TEST INFORMATION

Positive Finding:	Unable to maintain position against resistance
Involved Structure:	Nerve root C7
Special Considerations:	Rule out nerve root damage
Reference(s):	Hoppenfeld
Supplies Needed:	N/A

MANUAL MUSCLE TESTING
(MMT-U-Test 48)

Peer Review _____ Peer Review _____

Skill Acquisition: _____   Practice Opportunities: _____

This problem allows you the opportunity to demonstrate a **Myotome Assessment** *in order to rule out damage to nerve root* **C8**. *You have 2 minutes to complete this task.*

Tester places athlete and limb in appropriate position	Test 1	Test 2	Test 3
Seated or standing	Y N	Y N	Y N
Tester performs test according to accepted guidelines	**Test 1**	**Test 2**	**Test 3**
Instructs the athlete to flex the fingers against resistance and/or	Y N	Y N	Y N
Instructs the athlete to abduct the fingers against resistance	Y N	Y N	Y N
Performs a break test at some point in the range of motion	Y N	Y N	Y N
Holds resistance for 5 seconds	Y N	Y N	Y N
Performs assessment bilaterally	Y N	Y N	Y N

The psychomotor skill was performed completely and in the appropriate order   0 1 2 3 4 5

The tester had control of the subject and the situation (showed confidence)   0 1 2 3 4 5

Method of performing the skill allowed the tester the ability to determine:
severity, proper progression, and the *fit* in the overall picture (Oral)   0 1 2 3 4 5

In order for a grade of *minimum standard* to be given, the total must be ≥11   TOTAL = _____

```
   1    2    3    4    5    6    7    8    9    10   11   12   13   14   15
   |----|----|----|----|----|----|----|----|----|----|----|----|----|----|
 Not Acceptable                            Meets                 Exceeds
                                     Minimum Standards      Minimum Standards
```

TEST ENVIRONMENTS
L: Laboratory/Classroom Testing
C: Clinical/Field Testing
P: Practicum Testing
A: Assessment/Mock Exam Testing
S: Self-Reporting

SKILL TEST INFORMATION
Positive Finding: Unable to maintain position against resistance
Involved Structure: Nerve root C8
Special Considerations: Rule out nerve root damage
Reference(s): Hoppenfeld; Magee
Supplies Needed: N/A

MANUAL MUSCLE TESTING
(MMT-U-Test 49)

Peer Review _____ Peer Review _____

Skill Acquisition: _____   Practice Opportunities: _____

This problem allows you the opportunity to demonstrate a **Myotome Assessment** *in order to rule out damage to nerve root* **T1**. *You have 2 minutes to complete this task.*

Tester places athlete and limb in appropriate position	Test 1	Test 2	Test 3
Seated or standing	Ⓨ Ⓝ	Ⓨ Ⓝ	Ⓨ Ⓝ
Tester performs test according to accepted guidelines	**Test 1**	**Test 2**	**Test 3**
Instructs the athlete to abduct the fingers against resistance (interossei muscles)	Ⓨ Ⓝ	Ⓨ Ⓝ	Ⓨ Ⓝ
Performs a break test at some point in the range of motion	Ⓨ Ⓝ	Ⓨ Ⓝ	Ⓨ Ⓝ
Holds resistance for 5 seconds	Ⓨ Ⓝ	Ⓨ Ⓝ	Ⓨ Ⓝ
Performs assessment bilaterally	Ⓨ Ⓝ	Ⓨ Ⓝ	Ⓨ Ⓝ

The psychomotor skill was performed completely and in the appropriate order   0 1 2 3 4 5

The tester had control of the subject and the situation (showed confidence)   0 1 2 3 4 5

Method of performing the skill allowed the tester the ability to determine:
severity, proper progression, and the *fit* in the overall picture (Oral)   0 1 2 3 4 5

In order for a grade of *minimum standard* to be given, the total must be ≥11   TOTAL = _____

```
  1    2    3    4    5    6    7    8    9   10   11   12   13   14   15
  |    |    |    |    |    |    |    |    |    |    |    |    |    |    |
```

Not Acceptable   **Meets**   **Exceeds**
                              Minimum Standards   **Minimum Standards**

TEST ENVIRONMENTS

L: Laboratory/Classroom Testing
C: Clinical/Field Testing
P: Practicum Testing
A: Assessment/Mock Exam Testing
S: Self-Reporting

SKILL TEST INFORMATION

Positive Finding: Unable to maintain position against resistance
Involved Structure: Nerve root T1
Special Considerations: Rule out nerve root damage
Reference(s): Hoppenfeld
Supplies Needed: N/A

MANUAL MUSCLE TESTING
(MMT-L-Test 1)

Peer Review _____ Peer Review _____

Skill Acquisition: _____   Practice Opportunities: _____

Please demonstrate a manual muscle test for the **gluteus medius** *muscle. You have 2 minutes to complete this task.*

Tester places athlete and limb in appropriate position	Test 1	Test 2	Test 3
Side lying (bottom leg flexed at the hip and knee)	Ⓨ Ⓝ	Ⓨ Ⓝ	Ⓨ Ⓝ
Pelvis slightly rotated forward	Ⓨ Ⓝ	Ⓨ Ⓝ	Ⓨ Ⓝ
Tester placed in proper position	**Test 1**	**Test 2**	**Test 3**
Stands behind the athlete halfway between the hips and knees	Ⓨ Ⓝ	Ⓨ Ⓝ	Ⓨ Ⓝ
Stabilizes the pelvis (iliac crest) with one hand	Ⓨ Ⓝ	Ⓨ Ⓝ	Ⓨ Ⓝ
Places other hand on the distal tibia/fibula	Ⓨ Ⓝ	Ⓨ Ⓝ	Ⓨ Ⓝ
Tester performs test according to accepted guidelines	**Test 1**	**Test 2**	**Test 3**
Has athlete actively abduct the hip (slight extension and external rotation)	Ⓨ Ⓝ	Ⓨ Ⓝ	Ⓨ Ⓝ
Applies resistance against the lower leg in the direction of adduction and flexion	Ⓨ Ⓝ	Ⓨ Ⓝ	Ⓨ Ⓝ
Holds resistance for 5 seconds	Ⓨ Ⓝ	Ⓨ Ⓝ	Ⓨ Ⓝ
Performs assessment bilaterally	Ⓨ Ⓝ	Ⓨ Ⓝ	Ⓨ Ⓝ

The psychomotor skill was performed completely and in the appropriate order   0 1 2 3 4 5

The tester had control of the subject and the situation (showed confidence)   0 1 2 3 4 5

Method of performing the skill allowed the tester the ability to determine:
severity, proper progression, and the *fit* in the overall picture (Oral)   0 1 2 3 4 5

In order for a grade of *minimum standard* to be given, the total must be ≥11   **TOTAL =** _____

```
 1    2    3    4    5    6    7    8    9   10   11   12   13   14   15
 |    |    |    |    |    |    |    |    |    |    |    |    |    |    |
```

Not Acceptable   **Meets**   **Exceeds**
                                     Minimum Standards   **Minimum Standards**

TEST ENVIRONMENTS

L: Laboratory/Classroom Testing
C: Clinical/Field Testing
P: Practicum Testing
A: Assessment/Mock Exam Testing
S: Self-Reporting

SKILL TEST INFORMATION

Positive Finding:	Decreased ability to hold contraction
Involved Structure:	Gluteus medius
Special Considerations:	N/A
Reference(s):	Kendall et al
Supplies Needed:	Table

MANUAL MUSCLE TESTING
(MMT-L-Test 2)

Peer Review _____ Peer Review _____

Skill Acquisition: _____   Practice Opportunities: _____

*Please demonstrate a manual muscle test for the **gluteus minimus** muscle. You have 2 minutes to complete this task.*

Tester places athlete and limb in appropriate position	Test 1	Test 2	Test 3
Side lying (bottom leg flexed at the hip and knee)	Ⓨ Ⓝ	Ⓨ Ⓝ	Ⓨ Ⓝ
Tester placed in proper position	Test 1	Test 2	Test 3
Stands behind the athlete halfway between the hips and knees	Ⓨ Ⓝ	Ⓨ Ⓝ	Ⓨ Ⓝ
Stabilizes the pelvis (iliac crest) with one hand	Ⓨ Ⓝ	Ⓨ Ⓝ	Ⓨ Ⓝ
Places the other hand on the distal tibia/fibula	Ⓨ Ⓝ	Ⓨ Ⓝ	Ⓨ Ⓝ
Tester performs test according to accepted guidelines	Test 1	Test 2	Test 3
Has athlete actively abduct hip (neutral, no external rotation)	Ⓨ Ⓝ	Ⓨ Ⓝ	Ⓨ Ⓝ
Applies resistance to the lower leg in the direction of adduction and extension	Ⓨ Ⓝ	Ⓨ Ⓝ	Ⓨ Ⓝ
Holds resistance for 5 seconds	Ⓨ Ⓝ	Ⓨ Ⓝ	Ⓨ Ⓝ
Performs assessment bilaterally	Ⓨ Ⓝ	Ⓨ Ⓝ	Ⓨ Ⓝ

The psychomotor skill was performed completely and in the appropriate order   0 1 2 3 4 5

The tester had control of the subject and the situation (showed confidence)   0 1 2 3 4 5

Method of performing the skill allowed the tester the ability to determine:
severity, proper progression, and the *fit* in the overall picture (Oral)   0 1 2 3 4 5

In order for a grade of *minimum standard* to be given, the total must be ≥11   TOTAL = _____

```
1   2   3   4   5   6   7   8   9   10   11   12   13   14   15
|   |   |   |   |   |   |   |   |   |    |    |    |    |    |
```
Not Acceptable   **Meets**   **Exceeds**
                                    Minimum Standards   **Minimum Standards**

TEST ENVIRONMENTS
L: Laboratory/Classroom Testing
C: Clinical/Field Testing
P: Practicum Testing
A: Assessment/Mock Exam Testing
S: Self-Reporting

SKILL TEST INFORMATION
Positive Finding: Decreased ability to hold contraction
Involved Structure: Gluteus minimus
Special Considerations: N/A
Reference(s): Kendall et al
Supplies Needed: Table

MANUAL MUSCLE TESTING
(MMT-L-Test 3)

Peer Review _____ Peer Review _____

Skill Acquisition: _____   Practice Opportunities: _____

*Please demonstrate a manual muscle test for the **gluteus maximus** muscle. You have 2 minutes to complete this task.*

Tester places athlete and limb in appropriate position	Test 1	Test 2	Test 3
Prone	Y N	Y N	Y N
Knee flexed at or greater than 90 degrees	Y N	Y N	Y N
Tester placed in proper position	**Test 1**	**Test 2**	**Test 3**
Stands near the affected side	Y N	Y N	Y N
Stabilizes the pelvis with one hand	Y N	Y N	Y N
Places the other hand on the posterior aspect of the thigh (distal hamstrings)	Y N	Y N	Y N
Tester performs test according to accepted guidelines	**Test 1**	**Test 2**	**Test 3**
Has athlete actively extend the hip	Y N	Y N	Y N
Applies resistance to the leg in the direction of flexion	Y N	Y N	Y N
Holds resistance for 5 seconds	Y N	Y N	Y N
Performs assessment bilaterally	Y N	Y N	Y N

The psychomotor skill was performed completely and in the appropriate order   **0 1 2 3 4 5**

The tester had control of the subject and the situation (showed confidence)   **0 1 2 3 4 5**

Method of performing the skill allowed the tester the ability to determine:
severity, proper progression, and the *fit* in the overall picture (Oral)   **0 1 2 3 4 5**

In order for a grade of *minimum standard* to be given, the total must be ≥11   **TOTAL = _____**

1	2	3	4	5	6	7	8	9	10	11	12	13	14	15

Not Acceptable   **Meets**   **Exceeds**
Minimum Standards   **Minimum Standards**

TEST ENVIRONMENTS

L: Laboratory/Classroom Testing
C: Clinical/Field Testing
P: Practicum Testing
A: Assessment/Mock Exam Testing
S: Self-Reporting

SKILL TEST INFORMATION

Positive Finding: Decreased ability to hold contraction
Involved Structure: Gluteus maximus
Special Considerations: N/A
Reference(s): Kendall et al
Supplies Needed: Table

MANUAL MUSCLE TESTING
(MMT-L-Test 4)

Peer Review _____ Peer Review _____

Skill Acquisition: _____   Practice Opportunities: _____

Please demonstrate a manual muscle test for the **medial rotators of the hip** *muscles. You have 2 minutes to complete this task.*

Tester places athlete and limb in appropriate position	Test 1	Test 2	Test 3
Seated	Ⓨ Ⓝ	Ⓨ Ⓝ	Ⓨ Ⓝ
Knees hanging over the edge of the table	Ⓨ Ⓝ	Ⓨ Ⓝ	Ⓨ Ⓝ
Tester placed in proper position	**Test 1**	**Test 2**	**Test 3**
Stabilized trunk	Ⓨ Ⓝ	Ⓨ Ⓝ	Ⓨ Ⓝ
Tester performs test according to accepted guidelines	**Test 1**	**Test 2**	**Test 3**
Athlete actively medially rotate the hip	Ⓨ Ⓝ	Ⓨ Ⓝ	Ⓨ Ⓝ
Applies counterpressure against the medial side of the lower thigh with one hand and pressure to the lateral side of the leg above the ankle, pushing the leg inward to laterally rotate the thigh	Ⓨ Ⓝ	Ⓨ Ⓝ	Ⓨ Ⓝ
Holds resistance for 5 seconds	Ⓨ Ⓝ	Ⓨ Ⓝ	Ⓨ Ⓝ
Performs assessment bilaterally	Ⓨ Ⓝ	Ⓨ Ⓝ	Ⓨ Ⓝ

The psychomotor skill was performed completely and in the appropriate order   **0 1 2 3 4 5**

The tester had control of the subject and the situation (showed confidence)   **0 1 2 3 4 5**

Method of performing the skill allowed the tester the ability to determine:
severity, proper progression, and the *fit* in the overall picture (Oral)   **0 1 2 3 4 5**

In order for a grade of *minimum standard* to be given, the total must be ≥11   **TOTAL = _____**

1	2	3	4	5	6	7	8	9	10	11	12	13	14	15

Not Acceptable   **Meets**   **Exceeds**
                          Minimum Standards   **Minimum Standards**

TEST ENVIRONMENTS

L: Laboratory/Classroom Testing
C: Clinical/Field Testing
P: Practicum Testing
A: Assessment/Mock Exam Testing
S: Self-Reporting

SKILL TEST INFORMATION

Positive Finding: Decreased ability to hold contraction
Involved Structure: Medial rotators of the hip
Special Considerations: N/A
Reference(s): Kendall et al
Supplies Needed: Table

MANUAL MUSCLE TESTING
(MMT-L-Test 5)

Peer Review _____ Peer Review _____

Skill Acquisition: _____   Practice Opportunities: _____

Please demonstrate a manual muscle test for the **lateral rotators of the hip** *muscles. You have 2 minutes to complete this task.*

Tester places athlete and limb in appropriate position	Test 1	Test 2	Test 3
Seated	Ⓨ Ⓝ	Ⓨ Ⓝ	Ⓨ Ⓝ
Knees hanging over the edge of the table	Ⓨ Ⓝ	Ⓨ Ⓝ	Ⓨ Ⓝ
Tester placed in proper position	**Test 1**	**Test 2**	**Test 3**
Stabilized trunk	Ⓨ Ⓝ	Ⓨ Ⓝ	Ⓨ Ⓝ
Tester performs test according to accepted guidelines	**Test 1**	**Test 2**	**Test 3**
Has athlete actively laterally rotate the thigh	Ⓨ Ⓝ	Ⓨ Ⓝ	Ⓨ Ⓝ
Applies counterpressure against the lateral side of the lower thigh with one hand and pressure to the medial side of the leg above the ankle, pushing the leg inward to medially rotate the thigh	Ⓨ Ⓝ	Ⓨ Ⓝ	Ⓨ Ⓝ
Holds resistance for 5 seconds	Ⓨ Ⓝ	Ⓨ Ⓝ	Ⓨ Ⓝ
Performs assessment bilaterally	Ⓨ Ⓝ	Ⓨ Ⓝ	Ⓨ Ⓝ

The psychomotor skill was performed completely and in the appropriate order   **0 1 2 3 4 5**

The tester had control of the subject and the situation (showed confidence)   **0 1 2 3 4 5**

Method of performing the skill allowed the tester the ability to determine: severity, proper progression, and the *fit* in the overall picture (Oral)   **0 1 2 3 4 5**

In order for a grade of *minimum standard* to be given, the total must be ≥11   **TOTAL = _____**

```
 1    2    3    4    5    6    7    8    9   10   11   12   13   14   15
 |____|____|____|____|____|____|____|____|____|____|____|____|____|____|
```

Not Acceptable   **Meets**   **Exceeds**
                            Minimum Standards   **Minimum Standards**

TEST ENVIRONMENTS

L: Laboratory/Classroom Testing
C: Clinical/Field Testing
P: Practicum Testing
A: Assessment/Mock Exam Testing
S: Self-Reporting

SKILL TEST INFORMATION

Positive Finding: Decreased ability to hold contraction
Involved Structure: Lateral rotators of the hip
Special Considerations: N/A
Reference(s): Kendall et al
Supplies Needed Table

MANUAL MUSCLE TESTING
(MMT-L-Test 6)

Peer Review _____ Peer Review _____

Skill Acquisition: _____   Practice Opportunities: _____

Please demonstrate a manual muscle test for the **hip adductors** *muscles. You have 2 minutes to complete this task.*

Tester places athlete and limb in appropriate position	Test 1	Test 2	Test 3
Lying on the side of the involved limb	Ⓨ Ⓝ	Ⓨ Ⓝ	Ⓨ Ⓝ
Legs and lumbar spine in a straight line	Ⓨ Ⓝ	Ⓨ Ⓝ	Ⓨ Ⓝ
Tester placed in proper position	**Test 1**	**Test 2**	**Test 3**
Holds the upper leg in abduction	Ⓨ Ⓝ	Ⓨ Ⓝ	Ⓨ Ⓝ
Tester performs test according to accepted guidelines	**Test 1**	**Test 2**	**Test 3**
Athlete actively abducts the leg nearest the table straight up (prevents extension, rotation, or flexion of the hip)	Ⓨ Ⓝ	Ⓨ Ⓝ	Ⓨ Ⓝ
Applies resistance against the medial aspect of the distal end of the thigh (direction of abduction)	Ⓨ Ⓝ	Ⓨ Ⓝ	Ⓨ Ⓝ
Holds resistance for 5 seconds	Ⓨ Ⓝ	Ⓨ Ⓝ	Ⓨ Ⓝ
Performs assessment bilaterally	Ⓨ Ⓝ	Ⓨ Ⓝ	Ⓨ Ⓝ

The psychomotor skill was performed completely and in the appropriate order   **0 1 2 3 4 5**

The tester had control of the subject and the situation (showed confidence)   **0 1 2 3 4 5**

Method of performing the skill allowed the tester the ability to determine:
severity, proper progression, and the *fit* in the overall picture (Oral)   **0 1 2 3 4 5**

In order for a grade of *minimum standard* to be given, the total must be ≥11   **TOTAL = _____**

1	2	3	4	5	6	7	8	9	10	11	12	13	14	15

Not Acceptable   **Meets**   **Exceeds**
                                   Minimum Standards   **Minimum Standards**

TEST ENVIRONMENTS

L: Laboratory/Classroom Testing
C: Clinical/Field Testing
P: Practicum Testing
A: Assessment/Mock Exam Testing
S: Self-Reporting

SKILL TEST INFORMATION

Positive Finding: Decreased ability to hold contraction
Involved Structure: Hip adductors
Special Considerations: N/A
Reference(s): Kendall et al
Supplies Needed: Table

MANUAL MUSCLE TESTING
(MMT-L-Test 7)

Peer Review _____ Peer Review _____

Skill Acquisition: _____   Practice Opportunities: _____

Please demonstrate a manual muscle test for the **quadratus lumborum** *muscle. You have 2 minutes to complete this task.*

Tester places athlete and limb in appropriate position	Test 1	Test 2	Test 3
Prone	Ⓨ Ⓝ	Ⓨ Ⓝ	Ⓨ Ⓝ
Leg abducted to approximately 30 degrees	Ⓨ Ⓝ	Ⓨ Ⓝ	Ⓨ Ⓝ
Tester placed in proper position	**Test 1**	**Test 2**	**Test 3**
Standing at the end of the table, holding the affected leg at the ankle	Ⓨ Ⓝ	Ⓨ Ⓝ	Ⓨ Ⓝ
Tester performs test according to accepted guidelines	**Test 1**	**Test 2**	**Test 3**
Athlete actively laterally elevate the pelvis	Ⓨ Ⓝ	Ⓨ Ⓝ	Ⓨ Ⓝ
Applies resistance as traction on the extremity (directly opposing the line of pull of the muscle)	Ⓨ Ⓝ	Ⓨ Ⓝ	Ⓨ Ⓝ
Holds resistance for 5 seconds	Ⓨ Ⓝ	Ⓨ Ⓝ	Ⓨ Ⓝ
Performs assessment bilaterally	Ⓨ Ⓝ	Ⓨ Ⓝ	Ⓨ Ⓝ

The psychomotor skill was performed completely and in the appropriate order   0 1 2 3 4 5

The tester had control of the subject and the situation (showed confidence)   0 1 2 3 4 5

Method of performing the skill allowed the tester the ability to determine:
severity, proper progression, and the *fit* in the overall picture (Oral)   0 1 2 3 4 5

In order for a grade of *minimum standard* to be given, the total must be ≥ 11 TOTAL = _____

```
 1    2    3    4    5    6    7    8    9   10   11   12   13   14   15
 |    |    |    |    |    |    |    |    |    |    |    |    |    |    |
```
Not Acceptable   **Meets**   **Exceeds**
                              Minimum Standards   **Minimum Standards**

TEST ENVIRONMENTS
L: Laboratory/Classroom Testing
C: Clinical/Field Testing
P: Practicum Testing
A: Assessment/Mock Exam Testing
S: Self-Reporting

SKILL TEST INFORMATION
Positive Finding: Decreased ability to hold contraction
Involved Structure: Quadratus lumborum
Special Considerations: N/A
Reference(s): Kendall et al
Supplies Needed: Table

MANUAL MUSCLE TESTING
(MMT-L-Test 8)

Peer Review _____ Peer Review _____

Skill Acquisition: _____   Practice Opportunities: _____

Please demonstrate a manual muscle test for the **iliopsoas (with emphasis on the psoas minor)** *muscle. You have 2 minutes to complete this task.*

Tester places athlete and limb in appropriate position	Test 1	Test 2	Test 3
Supine	Ⓨ Ⓝ	Ⓨ Ⓝ	Ⓨ Ⓝ
Tester placed in proper position	**Test 1**	**Test 2**	**Test 3**
Stabilizes the opposite iliac crest	Ⓨ Ⓝ	Ⓨ Ⓝ	Ⓨ Ⓝ
Places the other hand on the distal tibia/fibula	Ⓨ Ⓝ	Ⓨ Ⓝ	Ⓨ Ⓝ
Tester performs test according to accepted guidelines	**Test 1**	**Test 2**	**Test 3**
Has the athlete actively flex the hip (slight abduction and lateral rotation)	Ⓨ Ⓝ	Ⓨ Ⓝ	Ⓨ Ⓝ
Applies resistance to the anteromedial aspect of the leg (direction of extension and slight abduction)	Ⓨ Ⓝ	Ⓨ Ⓝ	Ⓨ Ⓝ
Holds resistance for 5 seconds	Ⓨ Ⓝ	Ⓨ Ⓝ	Ⓨ Ⓝ
Performs assessment bilaterally	Ⓨ Ⓝ	Ⓨ Ⓝ	Ⓨ Ⓝ

The psychomotor skill was performed completely and in the appropriate order   **0 1 2 3 4 5**

The tester had control of the subject and the situation (showed confidence)   **0 1 2 3 4 5**

Method of performing the skill allowed the tester the ability to determine: severity, proper progression, and the *fit* in the overall picture (Oral)   **0 1 2 3 4 5**

In order for a grade of *minimum standard* to be given, the total must be ≥11   **TOTAL = _____**

```
  1    2    3    4    5    6    7    8    9   10   11   12   13   14   15
  |    |    |    |    |    |    |    |    |    |    |    |    |    |    |
```
Not Acceptable   Meets   Exceeds
                                        Minimum Standards   Minimum Standards

TEST ENVIRONMENTS

L: Laboratory/Classroom Testing
C: Clinical/Field Testing
P: Practicum Testing
A: Assessment/Mock Exam Testing
S: Self-Reporting

SKILL TEST INFORMATION

Positive Finding:	Decreased ability to hold contraction
Involved Structure:	Iliopsoas, psoas minor
Special Considerations:	Seated hip flexion (knee flexed) isolates the iliopsoas
Reference(s):	Kendall et al
Supplies Needed:	Table

MANUAL MUSCLE TESTING
(MMT-L-Test 9)

Peer Review _____ Peer Review _____

Skill Acquisition: _____   Practice Opportunities: _____

Please demonstrate a manual muscle test for the **tensor fasciae latae** *muscle. You have 2 minutes to complete this task.*

Tester places athlete and limb in appropriate position	Test 1	Test 2	Test 3
Supine	Ⓨ Ⓝ	Ⓨ Ⓝ	Ⓨ Ⓝ
Tester placed in proper position	**Test 1**	**Test 2**	**Test 3**
Stabilizes the opposite iliac crest (if needed)	Ⓨ Ⓝ	Ⓨ Ⓝ	Ⓨ Ⓝ
Places the other hand on the distal tibia/fibula	Ⓨ Ⓝ	Ⓨ Ⓝ	Ⓨ Ⓝ
Tester performs test according to accepted guidelines	**Test 1**	**Test 2**	**Test 3**
Has athlete actively abduct/flex hip (medially rotate the hip with the knee extended)	Ⓨ Ⓝ	Ⓨ Ⓝ	Ⓨ Ⓝ
Applies resistance to the leg in the direction of extension and adduction	Ⓨ Ⓝ	Ⓨ Ⓝ	Ⓨ Ⓝ
Holds resistance for 5 seconds	Ⓨ Ⓝ	Ⓨ Ⓝ	Ⓨ Ⓝ
Performs assessment bilaterally	Ⓨ Ⓝ	Ⓨ Ⓝ	Ⓨ Ⓝ

The psychomotor skill was performed completely and in the appropriate order   **0 1 2 3 4 5**

The tester had control of the subject and the situation (showed confidence)   **0 1 2 3 4 5**

Method of performing the skill allowed the tester the ability to determine:
severity, proper progression, and the *fit* in the overall picture (Oral)   **0 1 2 3 4 5**

In order for a grade of *minimum standard* to be given, the total must be ≥11   **TOTAL = _____**

```
   1    2    3    4    5    6    7    8    9   10   11   12   13   14   15
   |    |    |    |    |    |    |    |    |    |    |    |    |    |    |
```

Not Acceptable   **Meets**   **Exceeds**
                               Minimum Standards   **Minimum Standards**

TEST ENVIRONMENTS

L: Laboratory/Classroom Testing
C: Clinical/Field Testing
P: Practicum Testing
A: Assessment/Mock Exam Testing
S: Self-Reporting

SKILL TEST INFORMATION

Positive Finding:	Decreased ability to hold contraction
Involved Structure:	Tensor fasciae latae
Special Considerations:	N/A
Reference(s):	Kendall et al
Supplies Needed:	Table

Manual Muscle Testing
(MMT-L-Test 10)

Peer Review _____ Peer Review _____

Skill Acquisition: _____   Practice Opportunities: _____

Please demonstrate a manual muscle test for the **sartorius** *muscle. You have 2 minutes to complete this task.*

Tester places athlete and limb in appropriate position	Test 1	Test 2	Test 3
Supine	Y N	Y N	Y N
Places thigh in lateral rotation, abduction, and flexion	Y N	Y N	Y N
Places knee in a flexed position	Y N	Y N	Y N
Tester placed in proper position	**Test 1**	**Test 2**	**Test 3**
Stands in front and to the side of the athlete	Y N	Y N	Y N
Places hand on the anterolateral surface of the lower thigh	Y N	Y N	Y N
Places other hand at the distal end of the tibia/fibula	Y N	Y N	Y N
Tester performs test according to accepted guidelines	**Test 1**	**Test 2**	**Test 3**
Applies resistance to hip flexion/abduction and lateral rotation	Y N	Y N	Y N
Applies resistance to knee flexion	Y N	Y N	Y N
Holds resistance for 5 seconds	Y N	Y N	Y N
Performs assessment bilaterally	Y N	Y N	Y N

The psychomotor skill was performed completely and in the appropriate order   0 1 2 3 4 5

The tester had control of the subject and the situation (showed confidence)   0 1 2 3 4 5

Method of performing the skill allowed the tester the ability to determine:
severity, proper progression, and the *fit* in the overall picture (Oral)   0 1 2 3 4 5

In order for a grade of *minimum standard* to be given, the total must be ≥11   TOTAL = _____

1   2   3   4   5   6   7   8   9   10   11   12   13   14   15

Not Acceptable   **Meets**   **Exceeds**
                                    Minimum Standards   **Minimum Standards**

TEST ENVIRONMENTS

L: Laboratory/Classroom Testing
C: Clinical/Field Testing
P: Practicum Testing
A: Assessment/Mock Exam Testing
S: Self-Reporting

SKILL TEST INFORMATION

Positive Finding:	Decreased ability to hold contraction
Involved Structure:	Sartorius
Special Considerations:	Must resist multiple actions
Reference(s):	Kendall et al
Supplies Needed:	Table

MANUAL MUSCLE TESTING
(MMT-L-Test 11)

Peer Review _____ Peer Review _____

Skill Acquisition: _____   Practice Opportunities: _____

Please demonstrate a manual muscle test for the **semitendinosus/semimembranosus** *muscle. You have 2 minutes to complete this task.*

Tester places athlete and limb in appropriate position	Test 1	Test 2	Test 3
Prone	Y N	Y N	Y N
Tester placed in proper position	**Test 1**	**Test 2**	**Test 3**
Holds the thigh firmly against the table	Y N	Y N	Y N
Places the other hand against the distal tibia/fibula (posterior aspect)	Y N	Y N	Y N
Tester performs test according to accepted guidelines	**Test 1**	**Test 2**	**Test 3**
Has athlete actively flex the knee between 50 and 70 degrees	Y N	Y N	Y N
Thigh and leg placed in medial rotation	Y N	Y N	Y N
Applies resistance to the leg proximal to the ankle, in the direction of knee extension	Y N	Y N	Y N
Holds resistance for 5 seconds	Y N	Y N	Y N
Performs assessment bilaterally	Y N	Y N	Y N

The psychomotor skill was performed completely and in the appropriate order   0 1 2 3 4 5

The tester had control of the subject and the situation (showed confidence)   0 1 2 3 4 5

Method of performing the skill allowed the tester the ability to determine: severity, proper progression, and the *fit* in the overall picture (Oral)   0 1 2 3 4 5

In order for a grade of *minimum standard* to be given, the total must be ≥11   TOTAL = _____

1 2 3 4 5 6 7 8 9 10 11 12 13 14 15

Not Acceptable   **Meets Minimum Standards**   **Exceeds Minimum Standards**

TEST ENVIRONMENTS

L: Laboratory/Classroom Testing
C: Clinical/Field Testing
P: Practicum Testing
A: Assessment/Mock Exam Testing
S: Self-Reporting

SKILL TEST INFORMATION

Positive Finding: Decreased ability to hold contraction
Involved Structure: Semitendinosus, semimembranosus
Special Considerations: N/A
Reference(s): Kendall et al
Supplies Needed: Table

MANUAL MUSCLE TESTING
(MMT-L-Test 12)

Peer Review _____ Peer Review _____

Skill Acquisition: _____   Practice Opportunities: _____

Please demonstrate a manual muscle test for the **biceps femoris** *muscle. You have 2 minutes to complete this task.*

Tester places athlete and limb in appropriate position	Test 1	Test 2	Test 3
Prone	Ⓨ Ⓝ	Ⓨ Ⓝ	Ⓨ Ⓝ
Tester placed in proper position	**Test 1**	**Test 2**	**Test 3**
Holds the thigh firmly against the table	Ⓨ Ⓝ	Ⓨ Ⓝ	Ⓨ Ⓝ
Places the other hand against the distal tibia/fibula (posterior aspect)	Ⓨ Ⓝ	Ⓨ Ⓝ	Ⓨ Ⓝ
Tester performs test according to accepted guidelines	**Test 1**	**Test 2**	**Test 3**
Has athlete actively flex the knee between 50 and 70 degrees	Ⓨ Ⓝ	Ⓨ Ⓝ	Ⓨ Ⓝ
Thigh and leg are placed in lateral rotation	Ⓨ Ⓝ	Ⓨ Ⓝ	Ⓨ Ⓝ
Applies resistance to] the leg proximal to the ankle, in the direction of knee extension	Ⓨ Ⓝ	Ⓨ Ⓝ	Ⓨ Ⓝ
Holds resistance for 5 seconds	Ⓨ Ⓝ	Ⓨ Ⓝ	Ⓨ Ⓝ
Performs assessment bilaterally	Ⓨ Ⓝ	Ⓨ Ⓝ	Ⓨ Ⓝ

The psychomotor skill was performed completely and in the appropriate order   0 1 2 3 4 5

The tester had control of the subject and the situation (showed confidence)   0 1 2 3 4 5

Method of performing the skill allowed the tester the ability to determine:
severity, proper progression, and the *fit* in the overall picture (Oral)   0 1 2 3 4 5

In order for a grade of *minimum standard* to be given, the total must be ≥11   TOTAL = _____

```
 1    2    3    4    5    6    7    8    9   10   11   12   13   14   15
 |    |    |    |    |    |    |    |    |    |    |    |    |    |    |
```

Not Acceptable   **Meets**   **Exceeds**
                              Minimum Standards   **Minimum Standards**

TEST ENVIRONMENTS

L: Laboratory/Classroom Testing
C: Clinical/Field Testing
P: Practicum Testing
A: Assessment/Mock Exam Testing
S: Self-Reporting

SKILL TEST INFORMATION

Positive Finding:	Decreased ability to hold contraction
Involved Structure:	Biceps femoris
Special Considerations:	N/A
Reference(s):	Kendall et al
Supplies Needed:	Table

MANUAL MUSCLE TESTING
(MMT-L-Test 13)

Peer Review _____ Peer Review _____

Skill Acquisition: _____   Practice Opportunities: _____

Please demonstrate a manual muscle test for the **quadriceps femoris** *muscle. You have 2 minutes to complete this task.*

Tester places athlete and limb in appropriate position	Test 1	Test 2	Test 3
Seated	Ⓨ Ⓝ	Ⓨ Ⓝ	Ⓨ Ⓝ
Knees over the side of the table (holding onto the table)	Ⓨ Ⓝ	Ⓨ Ⓝ	Ⓨ Ⓝ
Tester placed in proper position	**Test 1**	**Test 2**	**Test 3**
Holds the thigh firmly down on the table	Ⓨ Ⓝ	Ⓨ Ⓝ	Ⓨ Ⓝ
Places the other hand against the distal tibia/fibula (anterior aspect)	Ⓨ Ⓝ	Ⓨ Ⓝ	Ⓨ Ⓝ
Tester performs test according to accepted guidelines	**Test 1**	**Test 2**	**Test 3**
Has the athlete actively extend the knee joint (without rotation of the thigh)	Ⓨ Ⓝ	Ⓨ Ⓝ	Ⓨ Ⓝ
Applies resistance to the leg above the ankle, in the direction of flexion	Ⓨ Ⓝ	Ⓨ Ⓝ	Ⓨ Ⓝ
Holds resistance for 5 seconds	Ⓨ Ⓝ	Ⓨ Ⓝ	Ⓨ Ⓝ
Performs assessment bilaterally	Ⓨ Ⓝ	Ⓨ Ⓝ	Ⓨ Ⓝ

The psychomotor skill was performed completely and in the appropriate order   **0 1 2 3 4 5**

The tester had control of the subject and the situation (showed confidence)   **0 1 2 3 4 5**

Method of performing the skill allowed the tester the ability to determine:
severity, proper progression, and the *fit* in the overall picture (Oral)   **0 1 2 3 4 5**

In order for a grade of *minimum standard* to be given, the total must be ≥11   **TOTAL = _____**

```
1    2    3    4    5    6    7    8    9    10    11    12    13    14    15
|    |    |    |    |    |    |    |    |    |     |     |     |     |     |
```

Not Acceptable   **Meets**   **Exceeds**
                                   Minimum Standards   **Minimum Standards**

TEST ENVIRONMENTS
L: Laboratory/Classroom Testing
C: Clinical/Field Testing
P: Practicum Testing
A: Assessment/Mock Exam Testing
S: Self-Reporting

SKILL TEST INFORMATION

Positive Finding: Decreased ability to hold contraction
Involved Structure: Rectus femoris, vastus lateralis, vastus intermedius, vastus medialis
Special Considerations: N/A
Reference(s): Kendall et al
Supplies Needed: Table

MANUAL MUSCLE TESTING
(MMT-L-Test 14)

Peer Review _____ Peer Review _____

Skill Acquisition: _____   Practice Opportunities: _____

Please demonstrate a manual muscle test for the **tibialis anterior** *muscle. You have 2 minutes to complete this task*

Tester places athlete and limb in appropriate position	Test 1	Test 2	Test 3
Supine or seated	(Y) (N)	(Y) (N)	(Y) (N)
Tester placed in proper position	**Test 1**	**Test 2**	**Test 3**
Supports the leg just above the ankle joint (stabilizes)	(Y) (N)	(Y) (N)	(Y) (N)
Tester performs test according to accepted guidelines	**Test 1**	**Test 2**	**Test 3**
Has athlete actively dorsiflex the ankle joint and invert the foot (without extension of the great toe)	(Y) (N)	(Y) (N)	(Y) (N)
Applies resistance to the medial side, dorsal surface of the foot (direction of plantar flexion of the ankle joint and eversion of the foot)	(Y) (N)	(Y) (N)	(Y) (N)
Holds resistance for 5 seconds	(Y) (N)	(Y) (N)	(Y) (N)
Performs assessment bilaterally	(Y) (N)	(Y) (N)	(Y) (N)

The psychomotor skill was performed completely and in the appropriate order   0 1 2 3 4 5

The tester had control of the subject and the situation (showed confidence)   0 1 2 3 4 5

Method of performing the skill allowed the tester the ability to determine:
severity, proper progression, and the *fit* in the overall picture (Oral)   0 1 2 3 4 5

In order for a grade of *minimum standard* to be given, the total must be ≥11   **TOTAL = _____**

```
 1    2    3    4    5    6    7    8    9   10   11   12   13   14   15
 |    |    |    |    |    |    |    |    |    |    |    |    |    |    |
```
Not Acceptable   **Meets**   **Exceeds**
                                            Minimum Standards   **Minimum Standards**

TEST ENVIRONMENTS

L: Laboratory/Classroom Testing
C: Clinical/Field Testing
P: Practicum Testing
A: Assessment/Mock Exam Testing
S: Self-Reporting

SKILL TEST INFORMATION

Positive Finding:	Decreased ability to hold contraction; may be seen as a partial "drop foot"
Involved Structure:	Tibialis anterior
Special Considerations:	N/A
Reference(s):	Kendall et al
Supplies Needed:	Table

MANUAL MUSCLE TESTING
(MMT-L-Test 15)

Peer Review _____ Peer Review _____

Skill Acquisition: _____   Practice Opportunities: _____

*Please demonstrate a manual muscle test for the **tibialis posterior** muscle. You have 2 minutes to complete this task.*

Tester places athlete and limb in appropriate position	Test 1	Test 2	Test 3
Supine with involved extremity in lateral rotation	Ⓨ Ⓝ	Ⓨ Ⓝ	Ⓨ Ⓝ
Tester placed in proper position	**Test 1**	**Test 2**	**Test 3**
Supports the leg just above the ankle joint	Ⓨ Ⓝ	Ⓨ Ⓝ	Ⓨ Ⓝ
Tester performs test according to accepted guidelines	**Test 1**	**Test 2**	**Test 3**
Athlete actively invert the foot and plantar flex the ankle	Ⓨ Ⓝ	Ⓨ Ⓝ	Ⓨ Ⓝ
Applies resistance against the medial side and plantar surface of the foot (direction of dorsiflexion of the ankle joint & eversion of the foot)	Ⓨ Ⓝ	Ⓨ Ⓝ	Ⓨ Ⓝ
Holds resistance for 5 seconds	Ⓨ Ⓝ	Ⓨ Ⓝ	Ⓨ Ⓝ
Performs assessment bilaterally	Ⓨ Ⓝ	Ⓨ Ⓝ	Ⓨ Ⓝ

The psychomotor skill was performed completely and in the appropriate order   **0 1 2 3 4 5**

The tester had control of the subject and the situation (showed confidence)   **0 1 2 3 4 5**

Method of performing the skill allowed the tester the ability to determine: severity, proper progression, and the *fit* in the overall picture (Oral)   **0 1 2 3 4 5**

In order for a grade of *minimum standard* to be given, the total must be ≥11   **TOTAL = _____**

```
  1   2   3   4   5   6   7   8   9   10   11   12   13   14   15
  |   |   |   |   |   |   |   |   |   |    |    |    |    |    |
```

Not Acceptable   **Meets**   **Exceeds**
                                   Minimum Standards   **Minimum Standards**

TEST ENVIRONMENTS

L: Laboratory/Classroom Testing
C: Clinical/Field Testing
P: Practicum Testing
A: Assessment/Mock Exam Testing
S: Self-Reporting

SKILL TEST INFORMATION

Positive Finding: Decreased ability to hold contraction
Involved Structure: Tibialis posterior
Special Considerations: N/A
Reference(s): Kendall et al
Supplies Needed: Table

MANUAL MUSCLE TESTING
(MMT-L-Test 16)

Peer Review _____ Peer Review _____

Skill Acquisition: _____   Practice Opportunities: _____

Please demonstrate a manual muscle test for the **soleus** *muscle. You have 2 minutes to complete this task.*

Tester places athlete and limb in appropriate position	Test 1	Test 2	Test 3
Prone	Y N	Y N	Y N
Knee flexed to 90 degrees	Y N	Y N	Y N
Tester placed in proper position	**Test 1**	**Test 2**	**Test 3**
Supports the leg proximal to the ankle	Y N	Y N	Y N
Places the other hand on the calcaneus	Y N	Y N	Y N
Tester performs test according to accepted guidelines	**Test 1**	**Test 2**	**Test 3**
Has the athlete actively plantar flex the ankle joint (without inversion and/or eversion)	Y N	Y N	Y N
Applies resistance to the calcaneus, pulling the heel in the direction of dorsiflexion	Y N	Y N	Y N
Holds resistance for 5 seconds	Y N	Y N	Y N
Performs assessment bilaterally	Y N	Y N	Y N

The psychomotor skill was performed completely and in the appropriate order   0 1 2 3 4 5

The tester had control of the subject and the situation (showed confidence)   0 1 2 3 4 5

Method of performing the skill allowed the tester the ability to determine:
severity, proper progression, and the *fit* in the overall picture (Oral)   0 1 2 3 4 5

In order for a grade of *minimum standard* to be given, the total must be ≥11   TOTAL = _____

1 2 3 4 5 6 7 8 9 10 11 12 13 14 15

Not Acceptable   **Meets Minimum Standards**   **Exceeds Minimum Standards**

TEST ENVIRONMENTS

L: Laboratory/Classroom Testing
C: Clinical/Field Testing
P: Practicum Testing
A: Assessment/Mock Exam Testing
S: Self-Reporting

SKILL TEST INFORMATION

Positive Finding: Inability to point the toes
Involved Structure: Soleus
Special Considerations: N/A
Reference(s): Kendall et al
Supplies Needed: Table

MANUAL MUSCLE TESTING
(MMT-L-Test 17)

Peer Review _____ Peer Review _____

Skill Acquisition: _____   Practice Opportunities: _____

Please demonstrate a manual muscle test for the **gastrocnemius** *muscle. You have 2 minutes to complete this task.*

Tester places athlete and limb in appropriate position	Test 1	Test 2	Test 3
Prone	Ⓨ Ⓝ	Ⓨ Ⓝ	Ⓨ Ⓝ
Knee extended with foot over the edge of the table	Ⓨ Ⓝ	Ⓨ Ⓝ	Ⓨ Ⓝ
Tester placed in proper position	**Test 1**	**Test 2**	**Test 3**
No fixation/stabilization needed	Ⓨ Ⓝ	Ⓨ Ⓝ	Ⓨ Ⓝ
Places one hand on the calcaneus (heel)	Ⓨ Ⓝ	Ⓨ Ⓝ	Ⓨ Ⓝ
Places other hand on the plantar surface of the forefoot	Ⓨ Ⓝ	Ⓨ Ⓝ	Ⓨ Ⓝ
Tester performs test according to accepted guidelines	**Test 1**	**Test 2**	**Test 3**
Had athlete actively plantar flex the foot	Ⓨ Ⓝ	Ⓨ Ⓝ	Ⓨ Ⓝ
Applies resistance to the forefoot and calcaneus	Ⓨ Ⓝ	Ⓨ Ⓝ	Ⓨ Ⓝ
Holds resistance for 5 seconds	Ⓨ Ⓝ	Ⓨ Ⓝ	Ⓨ Ⓝ
Performs assessment bilaterally	Ⓨ Ⓝ	Ⓨ Ⓝ	Ⓨ Ⓝ

The psychomotor skill was performed completely and in the appropriate order   **0 1 2 3 4 5**

The tester had control of the subject and the situation (showed confidence)   **0 1 2 3 4 5**

Method of performing the skill allowed the tester the ability to determine:
severity, proper progression, and the *fit* in the overall picture (Oral)   **0 1 2 3 4 5**

In order for a grade of *minimum standard* to be given, the total must be ≥11   **TOTAL = _____**

1	2	3	4	5	6	7	8	9	10	11	12	13	14	15

Not Acceptable   **Meets**   **Exceeds**
                          Minimum Standards   **Minimum Standards**

TEST ENVIRONMENTS

L: Laboratory/Classroom Testing
C: Clinical/Field Testing
P: Practicum Testing
A: Assessment/Mock Exam Testing
S: Self-Reporting

SKILL TEST INFORMATION

Positive Finding: Decreased ability to hold contraction
Involved Structure: Gastrocnemius, plantaris
Special Considerations: May be done standing on one leg (rise on toes, heel off the ground)
Reference(s): Kendall et al
Supplies Needed: Table

Manual Muscle Testing
(MMT-L-Test 18)

Peer Review _____ Peer Review _____

Skill Acquisition: _____   Practice Opportunities: _____

Please demonstrate a manual muscle test for the **peroneus longus** *muscle. You have 2 minutes to complete this task.*

Tester places athlete and limb in appropriate position	Test 1	Test 2	Test 3
Supine (lower leg internally rotated) or side lying	Ⓨ Ⓝ	Ⓨ Ⓝ	Ⓨ Ⓝ
Places foot in inverted position	Ⓨ Ⓝ	Ⓨ Ⓝ	Ⓨ Ⓝ
Tester placed in proper position	**Test 1**	**Test 2**	**Test 3**
Stands at the end of the table facing the athlete	Ⓨ Ⓝ	Ⓨ Ⓝ	Ⓨ Ⓝ
Stabilizes the lower leg with one hand	Ⓨ Ⓝ	Ⓨ Ⓝ	Ⓨ Ⓝ
Places the other hand on the lateral aspect of the metatarsals	Ⓨ Ⓝ	Ⓨ Ⓝ	Ⓨ Ⓝ
Tester performs test according to accepted guidelines	**Test 1**	**Test 2**	**Test 3**
Has athlete actively evert the foot	Ⓨ Ⓝ	Ⓨ Ⓝ	Ⓨ Ⓝ
Applies resistance to the foot in the direction of inversion and dorsiflexion	Ⓨ Ⓝ	Ⓨ Ⓝ	Ⓨ Ⓝ
Holds resistance for 5 seconds	Ⓨ Ⓝ	Ⓨ Ⓝ	Ⓨ Ⓝ
Performs assessment bilaterally	Ⓨ Ⓝ	Ⓨ Ⓝ	Ⓨ Ⓝ

The psychomotor skill was performed completely and in the appropriate order   **0 1 2 3 4 5**

The tester had control of the subject and the situation (showed confidence)   **0 1 2 3 4 5**

Method of performing the skill allowed the tester the ability to determine:
severity, proper progression, and the *fit* in the overall picture (Oral)   **0 1 2 3 4 5**

In order for a grade of *minimum standard* to be given, the total must be ≥11   **TOTAL = _____**

```
  1    2    3    4    5    6    7    8    9   10   11   12   13   14   15
  |____|____|____|____|____|____|____|____|____|____|____|____|____|____|
```

Not Acceptable   **Meets**   **Exceeds**
                                          Minimum Standards   **Minimum Standards**

TEST ENVIRONMENTS

L: Laboratory/Classroom Testing
C: Clinical/Field Testing
P: Practicum Testing
A: Assessment/Mock Exam Testing
S: Self-Reporting

SKILL TEST INFORMATION

Positive Finding:	Decreased ability to hold contraction
Involved Structure:	Peroneus longus, peroneus brevis
Special Considerations:	Assists in plantar flexion
Reference(s):	Kendall et al
Supplies Needed:	Table

MANUAL MUSCLE TESTING
(MMT-L-Test 19)

Peer Review _____ Peer Review _____

Skill Acquisition: _____   Practice Opportunities: _____

Please demonstrate a manual muscle test for the **peroneus tertius** *muscle. You have 2 minutes to complete this task.*

Tester places athlete and limb in appropriate position	Test 1	Test 2	Test 3
Supine or seated	Ⓨ Ⓝ	Ⓨ Ⓝ	Ⓨ Ⓝ
Tester placed in proper position	**Test 1**	**Test 2**	**Test 3**
Supports the leg just above the ankle joint	Ⓨ Ⓝ	Ⓨ Ⓝ	Ⓨ Ⓝ
Tester performs test according to accepted guidelines	**Test 1**	**Test 2**	**Test 3**
Instructs the athlete to actively dorsiflex the ankle joint, with eversion of the foot	Ⓨ Ⓝ	Ⓨ Ⓝ	Ⓨ Ⓝ
Applies resistance against the lateral side, dorsal surface of the foot (direction of plantar flexion of the ankle joint & inversion of the foot)	Ⓨ Ⓝ	Ⓨ Ⓝ	Ⓨ Ⓝ
Holds resistance for 5 seconds	Ⓨ Ⓝ	Ⓨ Ⓝ	Ⓨ Ⓝ
Performs assessment bilaterally	Ⓨ Ⓝ	Ⓨ Ⓝ	Ⓨ Ⓝ

The psychomotor skill was performed completely and in the appropriate order   **0 1 2 3 4 5**

The tester had control of the subject and the situation (showed confidence)   **0 1 2 3 4 5**

Method of performing the skill allowed the tester the ability to determine:
severity, proper progression, and the *fit* in the overall picture (Oral)   **0 1 2 3 4 5**

In order for a grade of *minimum standard* to be given, the total must be ≥11   **TOTAL = _____**

```
 1     2     3     4     5     6     7     8     9    10    11    12    13    14    15
 |     |     |     |     |     |     |     |     |     |     |     |     |     |     |
```

Not Acceptable   **Meets**   **Exceeds**
                                    Minimum Standards   **Minimum Standards**

TEST ENVIRONMENTS

L: Laboratory/Classroom Testing
C: Clinical/Field Testing
P: Practicum Testing
A: Assessment/Mock Exam Testing
S: Self-Reporting

SKILL TEST INFORMATION

Positive Finding: Decreased ability to hold contraction
Involved Structure: Peroneus tertius
Special Considerations: N/A
Reference(s): Kendall et al
Supplies Needed: Table

Manual Muscle Testing
(MMT-L-Test 20)

Please demonstrate a manual muscle test for the **flexor hallucis longus** *muscle. You have 2 minutes to complete this task.*

Tester places athlete and limb in appropriate position	Test 1	Test 2	Test 3
Supine or seated	Ⓨ Ⓝ	Ⓨ Ⓝ	Ⓨ Ⓝ
Tester placed in proper position	**Test 1**	**Test 2**	**Test 3**
Stabilizes the metatarsophalangeal joint in neutral position (0 degrees)	Ⓨ Ⓝ	Ⓨ Ⓝ	Ⓨ Ⓝ
Maintains the ankle joint approximately midway between dorsal and plantar flexion (25 degrees)	Ⓨ Ⓝ	Ⓨ Ⓝ	Ⓨ Ⓝ
Tester performs test according to accepted guidelines	**Test 1**	**Test 2**	**Test 3**
Has athlete actively flex the interphalangeal joint of the great toe	Ⓨ Ⓝ	Ⓨ Ⓝ	Ⓨ Ⓝ
Applies resistance to the plantar surface of the distal phalanx in the direction of extension	Ⓨ Ⓝ	Ⓨ Ⓝ	Ⓨ Ⓝ
Holds resistance for 5 seconds	Ⓨ Ⓝ	Ⓨ Ⓝ	Ⓨ Ⓝ
Performs assessment bilaterally	Ⓨ Ⓝ	Ⓨ Ⓝ	Ⓨ Ⓝ

The psychomotor skill was performed completely and in the appropriate order   0 1 2 3 4 5

The tester had control of the subject and the situation (showed confidence)   0 1 2 3 4 5

Method of performing the skill allowed the tester the ability to determine:
severity, proper progression, and the *fit* in the overall picture (Oral)   0 1 2 3 4 5

In order for a grade of *minimum standard* to be given, the total must be ≥11   TOTAL = _____

```
  1    2    3    4    5    6    7    8    9   10   11   12   13   14   15
  |    |    |    |    |    |    |    |    |    |    |    |    |    |    |
```
Not Acceptable   **Meets**   **Exceeds**
                                    Minimum Standards   **Minimum Standards**

TEST ENVIRONMENTS

L: Laboratory/Classroom Testing
C: Clinical/Field Testing
P: Practicum Testing
A: Assessment/Mock Exam Testing
S: Self-Reporting

SKILL TEST INFORMATION

Positive Finding: Decreased ability to hold contraction
Involved Structure: Flexor hallucis longus
Special Considerations: N/A
Reference(s): Kendall et al
Supplies Needed: Table

MANUAL MUSCLE TESTING
(MMT-L-Test 21)

Peer Review _____ Peer Review _____

Skill Acquisition: _____   Practice Opportunities: _____

Please demonstrate a manual muscle test for the **flexor hallicus brevis** *muscle. You have 2 minutes to complete this task.*

Tester places athlete and limb in appropriate position	Test 1	Test 2	Test 3
Supine or seated	Ⓨ Ⓝ	Ⓨ Ⓝ	Ⓨ Ⓝ
Tester placed in proper position	Ⓨ Ⓝ	Ⓨ Ⓝ	Ⓨ Ⓝ
Stabilizes the foot proximal to the metatarsophalangeal joint, maintaining neutral	Ⓨ Ⓝ	Ⓨ Ⓝ	Ⓨ Ⓝ
Tester performs test according to accepted guidelines	**Test 1**	**Test 2**	**Test 3**
Instruct the athlete actively to flex the metatarsophalangeal joint of the great toe (without extension of the great toe)	Ⓨ Ⓝ	Ⓨ Ⓝ	Ⓨ Ⓝ
Applies resistance against the plantar surface of the proximal phalanx (direction of great toe extension)	Ⓨ Ⓝ	Ⓨ Ⓝ	Ⓨ Ⓝ
Holds resistance for 5 seconds	Ⓨ Ⓝ	Ⓨ Ⓝ	Ⓨ Ⓝ
Performs assessment bilaterally	Ⓨ Ⓝ	Ⓨ Ⓝ	Ⓨ Ⓝ

The psychomotor skill was performed completely and in the appropriate order   0 1 2 3 4 5

The tester had control of the subject and the situation (showed confidence)   0 1 2 3 4 5

Method of performing the skill allowed the tester the ability to determine:
severity, proper progression, and the *fit* in the overall picture (Oral)   0 1 2 3 4 5

In order for a grade of *minimum standard* to be given, the total must be ≥11   TOTAL = _____

```
 1    2    3    4    5    6    7    8    9    10   11   12   13   14   15
 |    |    |    |    |    |    |    |    |    |    |    |    |    |    |
```
Not Acceptable   **Meets**   **Exceeds**
                                          Minimum Standards   **Minimum Standards**

TEST ENVIRONMENTS

L: Laboratory/Classroom Testing
C: Clinical/Field Testing
P: Practicum Testing
A: Assessment/Mock Exam Testing
S: Self-Reporting

SKILL TEST INFORMATION

Positive Finding:	Decreased ability to hold contraction
Involved Structure:	Flexor hallicus brevis
Special Considerations:	N/A
Reference(s):	Kendall et al
Supplies Needed:	Table

MANUAL MUSCLE TESTING
(MMT-L-Test 22)

Peer Review _____ Peer Review _____

Skill Acquisition: _____   Practice Opportunities: _____

Please demonstrate a manual muscle test for the **adductor hallucis** *muscle. You have 2 minutes to complete this task.*

Tester places athlete and limb in appropriate position	Test 1	Test 2	Test 3
Supine or seated	Ⓨ Ⓝ	Ⓨ Ⓝ	Ⓨ Ⓝ
Tester placed in proper position	**Test 1**	**Test 2**	**Test 3**
Supports the leg by gripping the heel firmly	Ⓨ Ⓝ	Ⓨ Ⓝ	Ⓨ Ⓝ
Tester performs test according to accepted guidelines	**Test 1**	**Test 2**	**Test 3**
Athlete actively abduct the great toe	Ⓨ Ⓝ	Ⓨ Ⓝ	Ⓨ Ⓝ
Applies resistance against the medial side of the first metatarsal and proximal phalanx	Ⓨ Ⓝ	Ⓨ Ⓝ	Ⓨ Ⓝ
Holds resistance for 5 seconds	Ⓨ Ⓝ	Ⓨ Ⓝ	Ⓨ Ⓝ
Performs assessment bilaterally	Ⓨ Ⓝ	Ⓨ Ⓝ	Ⓨ Ⓝ

The psychomotor skill was performed completely and in the appropriate order   0 1 2 3 4 5

The tester had control of the subject and the situation (showed confidence)   0 1 2 3 4 5

Method of performing the skill allowed the tester the ability to determine: severity, proper progression, and the *fit* in the overall picture (Oral)   0 1 2 3 4 5

In order for a grade of *minimum standard* to be given, the total must be ≥11   TOTAL = _____

```
  1    2    3    4    5    6    7    8    9   10   11   12   13   14   15
  |    |    |    |    |    |    |    |    |    |    |    |    |    |    |
```
Not Acceptable   **Meets**   **Exceeds**
                                               Minimum Standards   **Minimum Standards**

TEST ENVIRONMENTS

L: Laboratory/Classroom Testing
C: Clinical/Field Testing
P: Practicum Testing
A: Assessment/Mock Exam Testing
S: Self-Reporting

SKILL TEST INFORMATION

Positive Finding: Decreased ability to hold contraction
Involved Structure: Adductor hallucis
Special Considerations: N/A
Reference(s): Kendall et al
Supplies Needed: Table

MANUAL MUSCLE TESTING
(MMT-L-Test 23)

Peer Review _____ Peer Review _____

Skill Acquisition: _____ Practice Opportunities: _____

Please demonstrate a manual muscle test for the **extensor hallucis longus** *muscle. You have 2 minutes to complete this task.*

Tester places athlete and limb in appropriate position	Test 1	Test 2	Test 3
Supine or seated	Ⓨ Ⓝ	Ⓨ Ⓝ	Ⓨ Ⓝ
Tester placed in proper position	**Test 1**	**Test 2**	**Test 3**
Stabilize the foot in slight plantar flexion	Ⓨ Ⓝ	Ⓨ Ⓝ	Ⓨ Ⓝ
Tester performs test according to accepted guidelines	**Test 1**	**Test 2**	**Test 3**
Instructs the athlete to actively extend the metatarsophalangeal and interphalangeal joints of the great toe	Ⓨ Ⓝ	Ⓨ Ⓝ	Ⓨ Ⓝ
Applies resistance against the dorsal surface of the distal and proximal phalanges of the great toe (in the direction of the flexion of the great toe)	Ⓨ Ⓝ	Ⓨ Ⓝ	Ⓨ Ⓝ
Holds resistance for 5 seconds	Ⓨ Ⓝ	Ⓨ Ⓝ	Ⓨ Ⓝ
Performs assessment bilaterally	Ⓨ Ⓝ	Ⓨ Ⓝ	Ⓨ Ⓝ

The psychomotor skill was performed completely and in the appropriate order   **0 1 2 3 4 5**

The tester had control of the subject and the situation (showed confidence)   **0 1 2 3 4 5**

Method of performing the skill allowed the tester the ability to determine:
severity, proper progression, and the *fit* in the overall picture (Oral)   **0 1 2 3 4 5**

In order for a grade of *minimum standard* to be given, the total must be ≥11   **TOTAL = _____**

```
  1     2     3     4     5     6     7     8     9    10    11    12    13    14    15
  |_____|_____|_____|_____|_____|_____|_____|_____|_____|_____|_____|_____|_____|_____|
```

Not Acceptable   **Meets**   **Exceeds**
                                      Minimum Standards   **Minimum Standards**

TEST ENVIRONMENTS

L: Laboratory/Classroom Testing
C: Clinical/Field Testing
P: Practicum Testing
A: Assessment/Mock Exam Testing
S: Self-Reporting

SKILL TEST INFORMATION

Positive Finding: Decreased ability to hold contraction
Involved Structure: Extensor hallucis longus
Special Considerations: N/A
Reference(s): Kendall et al
Supplies Needed: Table

MANUAL MUSCLE TESTING
(MMT-L-Test 24)

Peer Review _____ Peer Review _____

Skill Acquisition: _____   Practice Opportunities: _____

Please demonstrate a manual muscle test for the **extensor digitorum longus/brevis** *muscle. You have 2 minutes to complete this task.*

	Test 1	Test 2	Test 3
Tester places athlete and limb in appropriate position	Test 1	Test 2	Test 3
Supine or seated	Ⓨ Ⓝ	Ⓨ Ⓝ	Ⓨ Ⓝ
Tester placed in proper position	Test 1	Test 2	Test 3
Stabilizes the foot in slight plantar flexion	Ⓨ Ⓝ	Ⓨ Ⓝ	Ⓨ Ⓝ
Tester performs test according to accepted guidelines	Test 1	Test 2	Test 3
Instructs the athlete to actively dorsiflex the ankle, with eversion of the foot	Ⓨ Ⓝ	Ⓨ Ⓝ	Ⓨ Ⓝ
Applies resistance against the lateral side, dorsal surface of the foot (in the direction of plantar flexion of the ankle joint & inversion of the foot)	Ⓨ Ⓝ	Ⓨ Ⓝ	Ⓨ Ⓝ
Holds resistance for 5 seconds	Ⓨ Ⓝ	Ⓨ Ⓝ	Ⓨ Ⓝ
Performs assessment bilaterally	Ⓨ Ⓝ	Ⓨ Ⓝ	Ⓨ Ⓝ

The psychomotor skill was performed completely and in the appropriate order   0 1 2 3 4 5

The tester had control of the subject and the situation (showed confidence)   0 1 2 3 4 5

Method of performing the skill allowed the tester the ability to determine:
severity, proper progression, and the *fit* in the overall picture (Oral)   0 1 2 3 4 5

In order for a grade of *minimum standard* to be given, the total must be ≥11   TOTAL = _____

```
  1    2    3    4    5    6    7    8    9   10   11   12   13   14   15
  |    |    |    |    |    |    |    |    |    |    |    |    |    |    |
```

Not Acceptable   **Meets**   **Exceeds**
                              Minimum Standards   **Minimum Standards**

TEST ENVIRONMENTS

L: Laboratory/Classroom Testing
C: Clinical/Field Testing
P: Practicum Testing
A: Assessment/Mock Exam Testing
S: Self-Reporting

SKILL TEST INFORMATION

Positive Finding:	Decreased ability to hold contraction
Involved Structure:	Extensor digitorum longus/brevis
Special Considerations:	N/A
Reference(s):	Kendall et al
Supplies Needed:	Table

MANUAL MUSCLE TESTING
(MMT-L-Test 25)

Peer Review _____ Peer Review _____

Skill Acquisition: _____   Practice Opportunities: _____

Please demonstrate a manual muscle test for the **flexor digitorum longus** *muscle. You have 2 minutes to complete this task.*

Tester places athlete and limb in appropriate position	Test 1	Test 2	Test 3
Supine or seated	Ⓨ Ⓝ	Ⓨ Ⓝ	Ⓨ Ⓝ
Knee flexed to permit neutral position of the foot	Ⓨ Ⓝ	Ⓨ Ⓝ	Ⓨ Ⓝ
Tester placed in proper position	**Test 1**	**Test 2**	**Test 3**
Stabilizes the metatarsals	Ⓨ Ⓝ	Ⓨ Ⓝ	Ⓨ Ⓝ
Maintains neutral position of the foot and ankle	Ⓨ Ⓝ	Ⓨ Ⓝ	Ⓨ Ⓝ
Tester performs test according to accepted guidelines	**Test 1**	**Test 2**	**Test 3**
Athlete actively flex the distal interphalangeal joints of the second to fifth digits	Ⓨ Ⓝ	Ⓨ Ⓝ	Ⓨ Ⓝ
Applies resistance against the plantar surface of the distal phalanges of the four toes (direction of extension of the digits)	Ⓨ Ⓝ	Ⓨ Ⓝ	Ⓨ Ⓝ
Holds resistance for 5 seconds	Ⓨ Ⓝ	Ⓨ Ⓝ	Ⓨ Ⓝ
Performs assessment bilaterally	Ⓨ Ⓝ	Ⓨ Ⓝ	Ⓨ Ⓝ

The psychomotor skill was performed completely and in the appropriate order   **0 1 2 3 4 5**

The tester had control of the subject and the situation (showed confidence)   **0 1 2 3 4 5**

Method of performing the skill allowed the tester the ability to determine:
severity, proper progression, and the *fit* in the overall picture (Oral)   **0 1 2 3 4 5**

In order for a grade of *minimum standard* to be given, the total must be ≥11   **TOTAL = _____**

```
 1    2    3    4    5    6    7    8    9    10   11   12   13   14   15
 |    |    |    |    |    |    |    |    |    |    |    |    |    |    |
```

Not Acceptable   **Meets**   **Exceeds**
                              Minimum Standards   **Minimum Standards**

TEST ENVIRONMENTS

L: Laboratory/Classroom Testing
C: Clinical/Field Testing
P: Practicum Testing
A: Assessment/Mock Exam Testing
S: Self-Reporting

SKILL TEST INFORMATION

Positive Finding: Decreased ability to hold contraction
Involved Structure: Flexor digitorum longus
Special Considerations: N/A
Reference(s): Kendall et al
Supplies Needed: Table

Manual Muscle Testing
(MMT-L-Test 26)

Peer Review _____ Peer Review _____

Skill Acquisition: _____   Practice Opportunities: _____

Please demonstrate a manual muscle test for the **flexor digitorum brevis** *muscle. You have 2 minutes to complete this task.*

Tester places athlete and limb in appropriate position	Test 1	Test 2	Test 3
Supine or seated	Ⓨ Ⓝ	Ⓨ Ⓝ	Ⓨ Ⓝ
Tester placed in proper position	**Test 1**	**Test 2**	**Test 3**
Stabilizes the proximal phalanges and maintains a neutral position of foot and ankle	Ⓨ Ⓝ	Ⓨ Ⓝ	Ⓨ Ⓝ
Tester performs test according to accepted guidelines	**Test 1**	**Test 2**	**Test 3**
Athlete actively flex the proximal interphalangeal joints of the second to fifth digits	Ⓨ Ⓝ	Ⓨ Ⓝ	Ⓨ Ⓝ
Applies resistance against the plantar surface of the middle phalanx of the four toes (direction of extension)	Ⓨ Ⓝ	Ⓨ Ⓝ	Ⓨ Ⓝ
Holds resistance for 5 seconds	Ⓨ Ⓝ	Ⓨ Ⓝ	Ⓨ Ⓝ
Performs assessment bilaterally	Ⓨ Ⓝ	Ⓨ Ⓝ	Ⓨ Ⓝ

The psychomotor skill was performed completely and in the appropriate order   0 1 2 3 4 5

The tester had control of the subject and the situation (showed confidence)   0 1 2 3 4 5

Method of performing the skill allowed the tester the ability to determine:
severity, proper progression, and the *fit* in the overall picture (Oral)   0 1 2 3 4 5

In order for a grade of *minimum standard* to be given, the total must be ≥11   TOTAL = _____

```
  1    2    3    4    5    6    7    8    9   10   11   12   13   14   15
  |    |    |    |    |    |    |    |    |    |    |    |    |    |    |
```
Not Acceptable   **Meets**   **Exceeds**
                                           Minimum Standards   **Minimum Standards**

TEST ENVIRONMENTS

L: Laboratory/Classroom Testing
C: Clinical/Field Testing
P: Practicum Testing
A: Assessment/Mock Exam Testing
S: Self-Reporting

SKILL TEST INFORMATION

Positive Finding:	Decreased ability to hold contraction
Involved Structure:	Flexor digitorum brevis
Special Considerations:	N/A
Reference(s):	Kendall et al
Supplies Needed:	Table

MANUAL MUSCLE TESTING
(MMT-L-Test 27)

Peer Review _____ Peer Review _____

Skill Acquisition: _____   Practice Opportunities: _____

This problem allows you the opportunity to demonstrate a **Myotome Assessment** *in order to rule out damage to nerve root* **L3**. *You have 2 minutes to complete this task.*

Tester places athlete and limb in appropriate position	Test 1	Test 2	Test 3
Seated	Ⓨ Ⓝ	Ⓨ Ⓝ	Ⓨ Ⓝ
Tester performs test according to accepted guidelines	**Test 1**	**Test 2**	**Test 3**
Instructs the athlete to flex the hip against resistance (iliopsoas)	Ⓨ Ⓝ	Ⓨ Ⓝ	Ⓨ Ⓝ
Performs a break test at some point in the range of motion	Ⓨ Ⓝ	Ⓨ Ⓝ	Ⓨ Ⓝ
Holds resistance for 5 seconds	Ⓨ Ⓝ	Ⓨ Ⓝ	Ⓨ Ⓝ
Performs assessment bilaterally	Ⓨ Ⓝ	Ⓨ Ⓝ	Ⓨ Ⓝ

The psychomotor skill was performed completely and in the appropriate order   0 1 2 3 4 5

The tester had control of the subject and the situation (showed confidence)   0 1 2 3 4 5

Method of performing the skill allowed the tester the ability to determine:
severity, proper progression, and the *fit* in the overall picture (Oral)   0 1 2 3 4 5

In order for a grade of *minimum standard* to be given, the total must be ≥11   TOTAL = _____

```
  1    2    3    4    5    6    7    8    9   10   11   12   13   14   15
  |    |    |    |    |    |    |    |    |    |    |    |    |    |    |
```

Not Acceptable   **Meets**   **Exceeds**
                                    Minimum Standards   **Minimum Standards**

TEST ENVIRONMENTS

L: Laboratory/Classroom Testing
C: Clinical/Field Testing
P: Practicum Testing
A: Assessment/Mock Exam Testing
S: Self-Reporting

SKILL TEST INFORMATION

Positive Finding: Unable to maintain proper position against resistance
Involved Structure: Nerve root L3
Special Considerations: Rule out nerve root damage
Reference(s): Magee
Supplies Needed: N/A

Manual Muscle Testing
(MMT-L-Test 28)

Peer Review _____ Peer Review _____

Skill Acquisition: _____   Practice Opportunities: _____

This problem allows you the opportunity to demonstrate a **Myotome Assessment** *in order to rule out damage to nerve root* **L4**. *You have 2 minutes to complete this task.*

Tester places athlete and limb in appropriate position	Test 1	Test 2	Test 3
Seated or standing	Ⓨ Ⓝ	Ⓨ Ⓝ	Ⓨ Ⓝ
Tester performs test according to accepted guidelines	**Test 1**	**Test 2**	**Test 3**
Instructs the athlete to invert the ankle against resistance (tibialis anterior)	Ⓨ Ⓝ	Ⓨ Ⓝ	Ⓨ Ⓝ
Performs a break test at some point in the range of motion	Ⓨ Ⓝ	Ⓨ Ⓝ	Ⓨ Ⓝ
Holds resistance for 5 seconds	Ⓨ Ⓝ	Ⓨ Ⓝ	Ⓨ Ⓝ
Performs assessment bilaterally	Ⓨ Ⓝ	Ⓨ Ⓝ	Ⓨ Ⓝ

The psychomotor skill was performed completely and in the appropriate order   0 1 2 3 4 5

The tester had control of the subject and the situation (showed confidence)   0 1 2 3 4 5

Method of performing the skill allowed the tester the ability to determine:
severity, proper progression, and the *fit* in the overall picture (Oral)   0 1 2 3 4 5

In order for a grade of *minimum standard* to be given, the total must be ≥11   TOTAL = _____

```
  1    2    3    4    5    6    7    8    9   10   11   12   13   14   15
  |    |    |    |    |    |    |    |    |    |    |    |    |    |    |
```

Not Acceptable   **Meets**   **Exceeds**
                                    Minimum Standards   **Minimum Standards**

TEST ENVIRONMENTS

L: Laboratory/Classroom Testing
C: Clinical/Field Testing
P: Practicum Testing
A: Assessment/Mock Exam Testing
S: Self-Reporting

SKILL TEST INFORMATION

Positive Finding:	Unable to maintain proper position against resistance
Involved Structure:	Nerve root L4
Special Considerations:	Rule out nerve root damage
Reference(s):	Hoppenfeld
Supplies Needed:	N/A

MANUAL MUSCLE TESTING
(MMT-L-Test 29)

Peer Review _____ Peer Review _____

Skill Acquisition: _____   Practice Opportunities: _____

*This problem allows you the opportunity to demonstrate a **Myotome Assessment** in order to rule out damage to nerve root **L5**. You have 2 minutes to complete this task.*

Tester places athlete and limb in appropriate position	Test 1	Test 2	Test 3
Seated or standing	Ⓨ Ⓝ	Ⓨ Ⓝ	Ⓨ Ⓝ

Tester performs test according to accepted guidelines	Test 1	Test 2	Test 3
Instructs the athlete to extend the great toe against resistance (interossei muscles)	Ⓨ Ⓝ	Ⓨ Ⓝ	Ⓨ Ⓝ
Performs a break test at some point in the range of motion	Ⓨ Ⓝ	Ⓨ Ⓝ	Ⓨ Ⓝ
Holds resistance for 5 seconds	Ⓨ Ⓝ	Ⓨ Ⓝ	Ⓨ Ⓝ
Performs assessment bilaterally	Ⓨ Ⓝ	Ⓨ Ⓝ	Ⓨ Ⓝ

The psychomotor skill was performed completely and in the appropriate order   **0 1 2 3 4 5**

The tester had control of the subject and the situation (showed confidence)   **0 1 2 3 4 5**

Method of performing the skill allowed the tester the ability to determine:
severity, proper progression, and the *fit* in the overall picture (Oral)   **0 1 2 3 4 5**

In order for a grade of *minimum standard* to be given, the total must be ≥11   **TOTAL = _____**

```
  1    2    3    4    5    6    7    8    9   10   11   12   13   14   15
  |    |    |    |    |    |    |    |    |    |    |    |    |    |    |
```

Not Acceptable   **Meets**   **Exceeds**
                                        Minimum Standards   **Minimum Standards**

TEST ENVIRONMENTS

L: Laboratory/Classroom Testing
C: Clinical/Field Testing
P: Practicum Testing
A: Assessment/Mock Exam Testing
S: Self-Reporting

SKILL TEST INFORMATION

Positive Finding: Unable to maintain proper position against resistance
Involved Structure: Nerve root L5
Special Considerations: Rule out nerve root damage
Reference(s): Hoppenfeld
Supplies Needed: N/A

MANUAL MUSCLE TESTING
(MMT-L-Test 30)

Peer Review _____ Peer Review _____

Skill Acquisition: _____   Practice Opportunities: _____

This problem allows you the opportunity to demonstrate a **Myotome Assessment** *in order to rule out damage to nerve root* **S1**. *You have 2 minutes to complete this task.*

Tester places athlete and limb in appropriate position	Test 1	Test 2	Test 3
Seated	Ⓨ Ⓝ	Ⓨ Ⓝ	Ⓨ Ⓝ
Tester performs test according to accepted guidelines	**Test 1**	**Test 2**	**Test 3**
Instructs the athlete to evert the ankle against resistance (peroneus longus and brevis)	Ⓨ Ⓝ	Ⓨ Ⓝ	Ⓨ Ⓝ
Performs a break test at some point in the range of motion	Ⓨ Ⓝ	Ⓨ Ⓝ	Ⓨ Ⓝ
Holds resistance for 5 seconds	Ⓨ Ⓝ	Ⓨ Ⓝ	Ⓨ Ⓝ
Performs assessment bilaterally	Ⓨ Ⓝ	Ⓨ Ⓝ	Ⓨ Ⓝ

The psychomotor skill was performed completely and in the appropriate order   0 1 2 3 4 5

The tester had control of the subject and the situation (showed confidence)   0 1 2 3 4 5

Method of performing the skill allowed the tester the ability to determine:
severity, proper progression, and the *fit* in the overall picture (Oral)   0 1 2 3 4 5

In order for a grade of *minimum standard* to be given, the total must be ≥11   TOTAL = _____

| 1 | 2 | 3 | 4 | 5 | 6 | 7 | 8 | 9 | 10 | 11 | 12 | 13 | 14 | 15 |

Not Acceptable   **Meets**   **Exceeds**
                            Minimum Standards   **Minimum Standards**

TEST ENVIRONMENTS

L: Laboratory/Classroom Testing
C: Clinical/Field Testing
P: Practicum Testing
A: Assessment/Mock Exam Testing
S: Self-Reporting

SKILL TEST INFORMATION

Positive Finding: Unable to maintain proper position against resistance
Involved Structure: Nerve root S1
Special Considerations: Rule out nerve root damage
Reference(s): Hoppenfeld
Supplies Needed: N/A

MANUAL MUSCLE TESTING
(MMT-L-Test 31)

Peer Review _____ Peer Review _____

Skill Acquisition: _____   Practice Opportunities: _____

This problem allows you the opportunity to demonstrate a **Myotome Assessment** *in order to rule out damage to nerve root* **S2**. *You have 2 minutes to complete this task.*

Tester places athlete and limb in appropriate position	Test 1	Test 2	Test 3
Seated	Ⓨ Ⓝ	Ⓨ Ⓝ	Ⓨ Ⓝ
Tester performs test according to accepted guidelines	**Test 1**	**Test 2**	**Test 3**
Instructs the athlete to flex the knee against resistance (hamstring)	Ⓨ Ⓝ	Ⓨ Ⓝ	Ⓨ Ⓝ
Performs a break test at some point in the range of motion	Ⓨ Ⓝ	Ⓨ Ⓝ	Ⓨ Ⓝ
Holds resistance for 5 seconds	Ⓨ Ⓝ	Ⓨ Ⓝ	Ⓨ Ⓝ
Performs assessment bilaterally	Ⓨ Ⓝ	Ⓨ Ⓝ	Ⓨ Ⓝ

The psychomotor skill was performed completely and in the appropriate order   **0 1 2 3 4 5**

The tester had control of the subject and the situation (showed confidence)   **0 1 2 3 4 5**

Method of performing the skill allowed the tester the ability to determine:
severity, proper progression, and the *fit* in the overall picture (Oral)   **0 1 2 3 4 5**

In order for a grade of *minimum standard* to be given, the total must be ≥11   **TOTAL = _____**

```
  1     2     3     4     5     6     7     8     9    10    11    12    13    14    15
  |     |     |     |     |     |     |     |     |     |     |     |     |     |     |
```

Not Acceptable   **Meets**   **Exceeds**
                                    Minimum Standards   **Minimum Standards**

TEST ENVIRONMENTS

L: Laboratory/Classroom Testing
C: Clinical/Field Testing
P: Practicum Testing
A: Assessment/Mock Exam Testing
S: Self-Reporting

SKILL TEST INFORMATION

Positive Finding:	Unable to maintain proper position against resistance
Involved Structure:	Nerve root S2
Special Considerations:	Rule out nerve root damage
Reference(s):	Magee
Supplies Needed:	N/A

Chapter 6

REFLEX TESTING

REFLEX TESTING
(RT-U-Test 1)

Peer Review _____ Peer Review _____

Skill Acquisition: _____   Practice Opportunities: _____

Please demonstrate how you would perform a test to check the **C5 reflex (biceps)**. *You have 2 minutes to complete this task.*

Tester places athlete and limb in appropriate position	Test 1	Test 2	Test 3
Seated or standing	Ⓨ Ⓝ	Ⓨ Ⓝ	Ⓨ Ⓝ
Places the athlete's arm over the tester's opposite arm (support under the medial elbow)	Ⓨ Ⓝ	Ⓨ Ⓝ	Ⓨ Ⓝ
Elbow resting at approximately a 90 degree angle	Ⓨ Ⓝ	Ⓨ Ⓝ	Ⓨ Ⓝ
Tester performs test according to accepted guidelines	**Test 1**	**Test 2**	**Test 3**
Places thumb over the biceps tendon (in the cubital fossa)	Ⓨ Ⓝ	Ⓨ Ⓝ	Ⓨ Ⓝ
Maintains relaxation of the limb	Ⓨ Ⓝ	Ⓨ Ⓝ	Ⓨ Ⓝ
Strikes the thumbnail over the biceps tendon	Ⓨ Ⓝ	Ⓨ Ⓝ	Ⓨ Ⓝ
Uses the pointed end of the neurological hammer	Ⓨ Ⓝ	Ⓨ Ⓝ	Ⓨ Ⓝ
Elicits reflex	Ⓨ Ⓝ	Ⓨ Ⓝ	Ⓨ Ⓝ
Performs assessment bilaterally	Ⓨ Ⓝ	Ⓨ Ⓝ	Ⓨ Ⓝ

The psychomotor skill was performed completely and in the appropriate order   **0 1 2 3 4 5**

The tester had control of the subject and the situation (showed confidence)   **0 1 2 3 4 5**

Method of performing the skill allowed the tester the ability to determine:
severity, proper progression, and the *fit* in the overall picture (Oral)   **0 1 2 3 4 5**

In order for a grade of *minimum standard* to be given, the total must be ≥11   **TOTAL = _____**

```
 1    2    3    4    5    6    7    8    9   10   11   12   13   14   15
 |____|____|____|____|____|____|____|____|____|____|____|____|____|____|
```

Not Acceptable   **Meets**   **Exceeds**
                                    Minimum Standards   **Minimum Standards**

TEST ENVIRONMENTS

L: Laboratory/Classroom Testing
C: Clinical/Field Testing
P: Practicum Testing
A: Assessment/Mock Exam Testing
S: Self-Reporting

SKILL TEST INFORMATION

Positive Finding: No reflex or abnormal movement (hyper/hypo)
Involved Structure: Nerve root coming off C5
Special Considerations: C6 may be involved
Reference(s): Hoppenfeld
Supplies Needed: Table/chair, reflex hammer

Reflex Testing
(RT-U-Test 2)

Skill Acquisition: _____   Practice Opportunities: _____

Please demonstrate how you would perform a test to check the **C6 reflex (brachioradialis)**. *You have 2 minutes to complete this task*

Tester places athlete and limb in appropriate position	Test 1	Test 2	Test 3
Seated	Y N	Y N	Y N
Places the athlete's arm over the tester's opposite arm (support under the medial elbow)	Y N	Y N	Y N
Elbow resting at approximately 90 degree angle	Y N	Y N	Y N
Tester performs test according to accepted guidelines	**Test 1**	**Test 2**	**Test 3**
Maintains relaxation of the limb	Y N	Y N	Y N
Strikes the brachioradialis tendon at the distal end of the radius	Y N	Y N	Y N
Uses the flat end of the neurological hammer	Y N	Y N	Y N
Elicits reflex	Y N	Y N	Y N
Performs assessment bilaterally	Y N	Y N	Y N

The psychomotor skill was performed completely and in the appropriate order   **0 1 2 3 4 5**

The tester had control of the subject and the situation (showed confidence)   **0 1 2 3 4 5**

Method of performing the skill allowed the tester the ability to determine: severity, proper progression, and the fit in the overall picture (Oral)   **0 1 2 3 4 5**

In order for a grade of minimum standard to be given, the total must be >11   **TOTAL = _____**

```
  1    2    3    4    5    6    7    8    9   10   11   12   13   14   15
  |    |    |    |    |    |    |    |    |    |    |    |    |    |    |
```

Not Acceptable   **Meets**   **Exceeds**
                                    Minimum Standards   **Minimum Standards**

TEST ENVIRONMENTS

L: Laboratory/Classroom Testing
C: Clinical/Field Testing
P: Practicum Testing
A: Assessment/Mock Exam Testing
S: Self-Reporting

SKILL TEST INFORMATION

Positive Finding:	No reflex or abnormal movement (hyper/hypo)
Involved Structure:	Nerve root coming off C6
Special Considerations:	C5 may be involved
Reference(s):	Hoppenfeld
Supplies Needed:	Table/chair, reflex hammer

REFLEX TESTING
(RT-U-Test 3)

Peer Review _____ Peer Review _____

Skill Acquisition: _____   Practice Opportunities: _____

Please demonstrate how you would perform a test to check the **C7 reflex (triceps)**. *You have 2 minutes to complete this task.*

Tester places athlete and limb in appropriate position	Test 1	Test 2	Test 3
Seated	Y N	Y N	Y N
Places the athlete's arm over the tester's opposite arm (support under the medial elbow)	Y N	Y N	Y N
Elbow resting at approximately 90 degree angle	Y N	Y N	Y N
Tester performs test according to accepted guidelines	**Test 1**	**Test 2**	**Test 3**
Maintains relaxation of the limb	Y N	Y N	Y N
Strikes the triceps tendon where it crosses the olecranon fossa	Y N	Y N	Y N
Uses the pointed end of the neurological hammer	Y N	Y N	Y N
Elicits reflex	Y N	Y N	Y N
Performs assessment bilaterally	Y N	Y N	Y N

The psychomotor skill was performed completely and in the appropriate order   **0 1 2 3 4 5**

The tester had control of the subject and the situation (showed confidence)   **0 1 2 3 4 5**

Method of performing the skill allowed the tester the ability to determine:
severity, proper progression, and the *fit* in the overall picture (Oral)   **0 1 2 3 4 5**

In order for a grade of *minimum standard* to be given, the total must be ≥11   **TOTAL = _____**

```
  1    2    3    4    5    6    7    8    9   10   11   12   13   14   15
  |    |    |    |    |    |    |    |    |    |    |    |    |    |    |
```

Not Acceptable   **Meets**   **Exceeds**
                                      Minimum Standards   **Minimum Standards**

TEST ENVIRONMENTS

L: Laboratory/Classroom Testing
C: Clinical/Field Testing
P: Practicum Testing
A: Assessment/Mock Exam Testing
S: Self-Reporting

SKILL TEST INFORMATION

Positive Finding: No reflex or abnormal movement (hyper/hypo)
Involved Structure: Nerve root coming off C7
Special Considerations: C8 may be involved
Reference(s): Hoppenfeld
Supplies Needed: Table/chair, reflex hammer

REFLEX TESTING
(RT-L-Test 1)

Peer Review _____ Peer Review _____

Skill Acquisition: _____ Practice Opportunities: _____

Please demonstrate how you would perform a test to check the **S1 reflex (Achilles' tendon)**. *You have 2 minutes to complete this task.*

Tester places athlete and limb in appropriate position	Test 1	Test 2	Test 3
Prone or seated	Ⓨ Ⓝ	Ⓨ Ⓝ	Ⓨ Ⓝ
Foot hanging over the edge of the table (prone) or	Ⓨ Ⓝ	Ⓨ Ⓝ	Ⓨ Ⓝ
Foot dangling off the edge of the table (seated)	Ⓨ Ⓝ	Ⓨ Ⓝ	Ⓨ Ⓝ
Tester performs test according to accepted guidelines	**Test 1**	**Test 2**	**Test 3**
Applies slight stretch (gently dorsiflex the foot)	Ⓨ Ⓝ	Ⓨ Ⓝ	Ⓨ Ⓝ
Maintains relaxation of the limb	Ⓨ Ⓝ	Ⓨ Ⓝ	Ⓨ Ⓝ
Strikes the Achilles' tendon	Ⓨ Ⓝ	Ⓨ Ⓝ	Ⓨ Ⓝ
Uses the flat end of the neurological hammer (some texts use pointed end)	Ⓨ Ⓝ	Ⓨ Ⓝ	Ⓨ Ⓝ
Elicits reflex	Ⓨ Ⓝ	Ⓨ Ⓝ	Ⓨ Ⓝ
Performs assessment bilaterally	Ⓨ Ⓝ	Ⓨ Ⓝ	Ⓨ Ⓝ

The psychomotor skill was performed completely and in the appropriate order   **0 1 2 3 4 5**

The tester had control of the subject and the situation (showed confidence)   **0 1 2 3 4 5**

Method of performing the skill allowed the tester the ability to determine:
severity, proper progression, and the *fit* in the overall picture (Oral)   **0 1 2 3 4 5**

In order for a grade of *minimum standard* to be given, the total must be ≥11   **TOTAL = _____**

```
 1    2    3    4    5    6    7    8    9    10   11   12   13   14   15
 |    |    |    |    |    |    |    |    |    |    |    |    |    |    |
```
Not Acceptable   **Meets**   **Exceeds**
                                    Minimum Standards   **Minimum Standards**

TEST ENVIRONMENTS

L: Laboratory/Classroom Testing
C: Clinical/Field Testing
P: Practicum Testing
A: Assessment/Mock Exam Testing
S: Self-Reporting

SKILL TEST INFORMATION

Positive Finding:	No reflex or abnormal movement (hyper/hypo)
Involved Structure:	Nerve root coming off S1
Special Considerations:	S2 may be involved
Reference(s):	Hoppenfeld
Supplies Needed:	Table/chair, reflex hammer

REFLEX TESTING
(RT-L-Test 2)

Peer Review _____   Peer Review _____

Skill Acquisition: _____   Practice Opportunities: _____

Please demonstrate how you would perform a test to check the **L4 reflex (patellar)**. *You have 2 minutes to complete this task.*

Tester places athlete and limb in appropriate position	Test 1	Test 2	Test 3
Seated	Ⓨ Ⓝ	Ⓨ Ⓝ	Ⓨ Ⓝ
Legs hanging over the edge of the table (knees at 90 degrees)	Ⓨ Ⓝ	Ⓨ Ⓝ	Ⓨ Ⓝ
Tester performs test according to accepted guidelines	**Test 1**	**Test 2**	**Test 3**
Maintains relaxation of the limb	Ⓨ Ⓝ	Ⓨ Ⓝ	Ⓨ Ⓝ
Strikes the patella tendon	Ⓨ Ⓝ	Ⓨ Ⓝ	Ⓨ Ⓝ
Uses the pointed end of the neurological hammer (some texts use flat end)	Ⓨ Ⓝ	Ⓨ Ⓝ	Ⓨ Ⓝ
Elicits reflex	Ⓨ Ⓝ	Ⓨ Ⓝ	Ⓨ Ⓝ
Performs assessment bilaterally	Ⓨ Ⓝ	Ⓨ Ⓝ	Ⓨ Ⓝ

The psychomotor skill was performed completely and in the appropriate order   0 1 2 3 4 5

The tester had control of the subject and the situation (showed confidence)   0 1 2 3 4 5

Method of performing the skill allowed the tester the ability to determine:
severity, proper progression, and the *fit* in the overall picture (Oral)   0 1 2 3 4 5

In order for a grade of *minimum standard* to be given, the total must be ≥11   TOTAL = _____

```
 1     2     3     4     5     6     7     8     9    10    11    12    13    14    15
 |_____|_____|_____|_____|_____|_____|_____|_____|_____|_____|_____|_____|_____|_____|
```

Not Acceptable   **Meets**   **Exceeds**
                                    Minimum Standards   **Minimum Standards**

TEST ENVIRONMENTS

L: Laboratory/Classroom Testing
C: Clinical/Field Testing
P: Practicum Testing
A: Assessment/Mock Exam Testing
S: Self-Reporting

SKILL TEST INFORMATION

Positive Finding:	No reflex or abnormal movement (hyper/hypo)
Involved Structure:	Nerve root coming off L4
Special Considerations:	L2/L3 may be involved
Reference(s):	Hoppenfeld
Supplies Needed:	Table/chair, reflex hammer

REFLEX TESTING
(RT-L-Test 3)

Peer Review _____ Peer Review _____

Skill Acquisition: _____   Practice Opportunities: _____

Please demonstrate how you would perform a test for the pathological reflex known as **Babinski's Reflex** *to rule out an upper motor neuron lesion. You have 2 minutes to complete this task.*

Tester places athlete and limb in appropriate position	Test 1	Test 2	Test 3
Supine	Ⓨ Ⓝ	Ⓨ Ⓝ	Ⓨ Ⓝ
Tester performs test according to accepted guidelines	**Test 1**	**Test 2**	**Test 3**
Maintains relaxation of the limb	Ⓨ Ⓝ	Ⓨ Ⓝ	Ⓨ Ⓝ
Uses a pointed object to stroke the plantar surface of the foot:			
Lateral border	Ⓨ Ⓝ	Ⓨ Ⓝ	Ⓨ Ⓝ
Proximal to distal	Ⓨ Ⓝ	Ⓨ Ⓝ	Ⓨ Ⓝ
Even/appropriate pressure	Ⓨ Ⓝ	Ⓨ Ⓝ	Ⓨ Ⓝ
Performs assessment bilaterally	Ⓨ Ⓝ	Ⓨ Ⓝ	Ⓨ Ⓝ

The psychomotor skill was performed completely and in the appropriate order   **0 1 2 3 4 5**

The tester had control of the subject and the situation (showed confidence)   **0 1 2 3 4 5**

Method of performing the skill allowed the tester the ability to determine:
severity, proper progression, and the *fit* in the overall picture (Oral)   **0 1 2 3 4 5**

In order for a grade of *minimum standard* to be given, the total must be ≥11   **TOTAL = _____**

| 1 | 2 | 3 | 4 | 5 | 6 | 7 | 8 | 9 | 10 | 11 | 12 | 13 | 14 | 15 |

Not Acceptable   **Meets**   **Exceeds**
                                    Minimum Standards   **Minimum Standards**

TEST ENVIRONMENTS

L: Laboratory/Classroom Testing
C: Clinical/Field Testing
P: Practicum Testing
A: Assessment/Mock Exam Testing
S: Self-Reporting

SKILL TEST INFORMATION

Positive Finding:	Splaying of the toes
Involved Structure:	Upper motor neuron lesion
Special Considerations:	N/A
Reference(s):	Magee
Supplies Needed:	Table, pointed object

REFLEX TESTING
(RT-L-Test 4)

Skill Acquisition: _____   Practice Opportunities: _____

This problem allows you the opportunity to demonstrate a superficial reflex known as the **superficial abdominal reflex** *in order to rule out an upper motor neuron lesion. You have 2 minutes to complete this task.*

Tester places athlete and limb in appropriate position	Test 1	Test 2	Test 3
Supine	Ⓨ Ⓝ	Ⓨ Ⓝ	Ⓨ Ⓝ
Tester performs test according to accepted guidelines	**Test 1**	**Test 2**	**Test 3**
Maintains relaxation of the abdominal region	Ⓨ Ⓝ	Ⓨ Ⓝ	Ⓨ Ⓝ
Uses a pointed object to stroke each of the four quadrants of the abdomen	Ⓨ Ⓝ	Ⓨ Ⓝ	Ⓨ Ⓝ
Strokes in a triangular motion around the umbilicus	Ⓨ Ⓝ	Ⓨ Ⓝ	Ⓨ Ⓝ

The psychomotor skill was performed completely and in the appropriate order   **0 1 2 3 4 5**

The tester had control of the subject and the situation (showed confidence)   **0 1 2 3 4 5**

Method of performing the skill allowed the tester the ability to determine: severity, proper progression, and the *fit* in the overall picture (Oral)   **0 1 2 3 4 5**

In order for a grade of *minimum standard* to be given, the total must be ≥11   **TOTAL = _____**

```
 1    2    3    4    5    6    7    8    9   10   11   12   13   14   15
 |    |    |    |    |    |    |    |    |    |    |    |    |    |    |
```

Not Acceptable   **Meets**   **Exceeds**
                                   Minimum Standards   **Minimum Standards**

TEST ENVIRONMENTS

L: Laboratory/Classroom Testing
C: Clinical/Field Testing
P: Practicum Testing
A: Assessment/Mock Exam Testing
S: Self-Reporting

SKILL TEST INFORMATION

Positive Finding: No movement of the skin
Involved Structure: Upper motor neuron lesion— unilateral absence indicates a lower motor neuron lesion (T7-L2)
Special Considerations: N/A
Reference(s): Magee
Supplies Needed: Table, pointed object

REFLEX TESTING
(RT-L-Test 5)

Peer Review _____ Peer Review _____

Skill Acquisition: _____   Practice Opportunities: _____

Please demonstrate how you would perform a test to check the **deep tendon reflex of L5 (posterior tibial).** *You have 2 minutes to complete this task.*

Tester places athlete and limb in appropriate position	Test 1	Test 2	Test 3
Prone	Ⓨ Ⓝ	Ⓨ Ⓝ	Ⓨ Ⓝ
Foot hanging over the edge of the table	Ⓨ Ⓝ	Ⓨ Ⓝ	Ⓨ Ⓝ
Tester performs test according to accepted guidelines	**Test 1**	**Test 2**	**Test 3**
Applies slight stretch (plantar flexion)	Ⓨ Ⓝ	Ⓨ Ⓝ	Ⓨ Ⓝ
Maintains relaxation of the limb	Ⓨ Ⓝ	Ⓨ Ⓝ	Ⓨ Ⓝ
Strikes the posterior tibial tendon (just behind the medial malleolus)	Ⓨ Ⓝ	Ⓨ Ⓝ	Ⓨ Ⓝ
Uses the pointed end of the neurological hammer	Ⓨ Ⓝ	Ⓨ Ⓝ	Ⓨ Ⓝ
Elicits reflex	Ⓨ Ⓝ	Ⓨ Ⓝ	Ⓨ Ⓝ
Performs assessment bilaterally	Ⓨ Ⓝ	Ⓨ Ⓝ	Ⓨ Ⓝ

The psychomotor skill was performed completely and in the appropriate order   0 1 2 3 4 5

The tester had control of the subject and the situation (showed confidence)   0 1 2 3 4 5

Method of performing the skill allowed the tester the ability to determine:
severity, proper progression, and the *fit* in the overall picture (Oral)   0 1 2 3 4 5

In order for a grade of *minimum standard* to be given, the total must be ≥11   TOTAL = _____

```
  1     2     3     4     5     6     7     8     9    10    11    12    13    14    15
  |─────|─────|─────|─────|─────|─────|─────|─────|─────|─────|─────|─────|─────|─────|
```

Not Acceptable   **Meets**   **Exceeds**
                                   Minimum Standards   **Minimum Standards**

TEST ENVIRONMENTS

L: Laboratory/Classroom Testing
C: Clinical/Field Testing
P: Practicum Testing
A: Assessment/Mock Exam Testing
S: Self-Reporting

SKILL TEST INFORMATION

Positive Finding: No reflex or abnormal movement (hyper/hypo)
Involved Structure: Nerve root coming off L4/L5
Special Considerations: N/A
Reference(s): Magee
Supplies Needed: Table, reflex hammer

REFLEX TESTING
(RT-L-Test 6)

Peer Review _____ Peer Review _____

Skill Acquisition: _____   Practice Opportunities: _____

Please demonstrate how you would perform a test for the pathological reflex known as the **Oppenheim Reflex** *to rule out an upper motor neuron lesion. You have 2 minutes to complete this task.*

Tester places athlete and limb in appropriate position	Test 1	Test 2	Test 3
Supine	Ⓨ Ⓝ	Ⓨ Ⓝ	Ⓨ Ⓝ
Tester performs test according to accepted guidelines	**Test 1**	**Test 2**	**Test 3**
Maintains relaxation of the limb	Ⓨ Ⓝ	Ⓨ Ⓝ	Ⓨ Ⓝ
Uses a pointed object along the crest of the tibia:			
Anteromedial border	Ⓨ Ⓝ	Ⓨ Ⓝ	Ⓨ Ⓝ
Even/appropriate pressure	Ⓨ Ⓝ	Ⓨ Ⓝ	Ⓨ Ⓝ
Performs assessment bilaterally	Ⓨ Ⓝ	Ⓨ Ⓝ	Ⓨ Ⓝ

The psychomotor skill was performed completely and in the appropriate order   **0 1 2 3 4 5**

The tester had control of the subject and the situation (showed confidence)   **0 1 2 3 4 5**

Method of performing the skill allowed the tester the ability to determine:
severity, proper progression, and the *fit* in the overall picture (Oral)   **0 1 2 3 4 5**

In order for a grade of *minimum standard* to be given, the total must be ≥11   **TOTAL = _____**

```
 1    2    3    4    5    6    7    8    9   10   11   12   13   14   15
 |____|____|____|____|____|____|____|____|____|____|____|____|____|____|
```

Not Acceptable   **Meets**   **Exceeds**
                                    Minimum Standards   **Minimum Standards**

TEST ENVIRONMENTS	**SKILL TEST INFORMATION**	
L: Laboratory/Classroom Testing	**Positive Finding:**	Splaying of toes
C: Clinical/Field Testing	**Involved Structure:**	Upper motor neuron lesion
P: Practicum Testing	**Special Considerations:**	N/A
A: Assessment/Mock Exam Testing	**Reference(s):**	Magee
S: Self-Reporting	**Supplies Needed:**	Table, pointed object

SENSORY TESTING

SENSORY TESTING
(SST-U-Test 1)

Peer Review _____ Peer Review _____

Skill Acquisition: _____   Practice Opportunities: _____

This problem allows you the opportunity to demonstrate a **Dermatome Sensory Test** *in order to rule out damage to the nerve root* **C5***. You have 2 minutes to complete this task.*

Tester places athlete and limb in appropriate position	Test 1	Test 2	Test 3
Seated or prone	Ⓨ Ⓝ	Ⓨ Ⓝ	Ⓨ Ⓝ
Tester performs test according to accepted guidelines	**Test 1**	**Test 2**	**Test 3**
Gives appropriate directions to the athlete	Ⓨ Ⓝ	Ⓨ Ⓝ	Ⓨ Ⓝ
Explains differences in pressure	Ⓨ Ⓝ	Ⓨ Ⓝ	Ⓨ Ⓝ
Demonstration given away from the injured area	Ⓨ Ⓝ	Ⓨ Ⓝ	Ⓨ Ⓝ
Instructs athlete to close eyes	Ⓨ Ⓝ	Ⓨ Ⓝ	Ⓨ Ⓝ
Applies varied pressure with tool or common objects:			
Sharp	Ⓨ Ⓝ	Ⓨ Ⓝ	Ⓨ Ⓝ
Dull	Ⓨ Ⓝ	Ⓨ Ⓝ	Ⓨ Ⓝ
No touch	Ⓨ Ⓝ	Ⓨ Ⓝ	Ⓨ Ⓝ
Applies appropriate pressure to the lateral arm (deltoid tuberosity)	Ⓨ Ⓝ	Ⓨ Ⓝ	Ⓨ Ⓝ
Performs assessment bilaterally	Ⓨ Ⓝ	Ⓨ Ⓝ	Ⓨ Ⓝ

The psychomotor skill was performed completely and in the appropriate order   0 1 2 3 4 5

The tester had control of the subject and the situation (showed confidence)   0 1 2 3 4 5

Method of performing the skill allowed the tester the ability to determine:
severity, proper progression, and the *fit* in the overall picture (Oral)   0 1 2 3 4 5

In order for a grade of *minimum standard* to be given, the total must be ≥11   **TOTAL = _____**

```
 1     2     3     4     5     6     7     8     9    10    11    12    13    14    15
 |     |     |     |     |     |     |     |     |     |     |     |     |     |     |
```

Not Acceptable   **Meets**   **Exceeds**
                                              Minimum Standards   **Minimum Standards**

SKILL TEST INFORMATION

Positive Finding:	No feeling; difficulty in distinguishing varied pressure
Involved Structure:	Nerve root C5
Special Considerations:	N/A
Reference(s):	Hoppenfeld
Supplies Needed:	Table/chair, sharp/dull object

SENSORY TESTING
(SST-U-Test 2)

Peer Review _____ Peer Review _____

Skill Acquisition: _____   Practice Opportunities: _____

*This problem allows you the opportunity to demonstrate a **Dermatome Sensory Test** in order to rule out damage to the nerve root **C6**. You have 2 minutes to complete this task.*

Tester places athlete and limb in appropriate position	Test 1	Test 2	Test 3
Seated or prone	Ⓨ Ⓝ	Ⓨ Ⓝ	Ⓨ Ⓝ
Tester performs test according to accepted guidelines	**Test 1**	**Test 2**	**Test 3**
Gives appropriate directions to the athlete	Ⓨ Ⓝ	Ⓨ Ⓝ	Ⓨ Ⓝ
Explains differences in pressure	Ⓨ Ⓝ	Ⓨ Ⓝ	Ⓨ Ⓝ
Demonstration given away from the injured area	Ⓨ Ⓝ	Ⓨ Ⓝ	Ⓨ Ⓝ
Instructs athlete to close eyes	Ⓨ Ⓝ	Ⓨ Ⓝ	Ⓨ Ⓝ
Applies varied pressure with tool or common objects:			
Sharp	Ⓨ Ⓝ	Ⓨ Ⓝ	Ⓨ Ⓝ
Dull	Ⓨ Ⓝ	Ⓨ Ⓝ	Ⓨ Ⓝ
No touch	Ⓨ Ⓝ	Ⓨ Ⓝ	Ⓨ Ⓝ
Applies appropriate pressure to the lateral forearm (at web of the thumb)	Ⓨ Ⓝ	Ⓨ Ⓝ	Ⓨ Ⓝ
Performs assessment bilaterally	Ⓨ Ⓝ	Ⓨ Ⓝ	Ⓨ Ⓝ

The psychomotor skill was performed completely and in the appropriate order   **0 1 2 3 4 5**

The tester had control of the subject and the situation (showed confidence)   **0 1 2 3 4 5**

Method of performing the skill allowed the tester the ability to determine:
severity, proper progression, and the *fit* in the overall picture (Oral)   **0 1 2 3 4 5**

In order for a grade of *minimum standard* to be given, the total must be ≥11   **TOTAL = _____**

1	2	3	4	5	6	7	8	9	10	11	12	13	14	15

Not Acceptable   **Meets**   **Exceeds**
                                 Minimum Standards   **Minimum Standards**

TEST ENVIRONMENTS

L: Laboratory/Classroom Testing
C: Clinical/Field Testing
P: Practicum Testing
A: Assessment/Mock Exam Testing
S: Self-Reporting

SKILL TEST INFORMATION

Positive Finding:	No feeling; difficulty in distinguishing varied pressure
Involved Structure:	Nerve root C6
Special Considerations:	N/A
Reference(s):	Hoppenfeld
Supplies Needed:	Table/chair, sharp/dull object

SENSORY TESTING
(SST-U-Test 3)

Peer Review _____   Peer Review _____

Skill Acquisition: _____   Practice Opportunities: _____

This problem allows you the opportunity to demonstrate a **Dermatome Sensory Test** *in order to rule out damage to the nerve root* **C7**. *You have 2 minutes to complete this task.*

Tester places athlete and limb in appropriate position	Test 1	Test 2	Test 3
Seated or prone	Ⓨ Ⓝ	Ⓨ Ⓝ	Ⓨ Ⓝ
Tester performs test according to accepted guidelines	**Test 1**	**Test 2**	**Test 3**
Gives appropriate directions to the athlete	Ⓨ Ⓝ	Ⓨ Ⓝ	Ⓨ Ⓝ
Explains differences in pressure	Ⓨ Ⓝ	Ⓨ Ⓝ	Ⓨ Ⓝ
Demonstration given away from the injured area	Ⓨ Ⓝ	Ⓨ Ⓝ	Ⓨ Ⓝ
Instructs athlete to close eyes	Ⓨ Ⓝ	Ⓨ Ⓝ	Ⓨ Ⓝ
Applies varied pressure with tool or common objects:			
Sharp	Ⓨ Ⓝ	Ⓨ Ⓝ	Ⓨ Ⓝ
Dull	Ⓨ Ⓝ	Ⓨ Ⓝ	Ⓨ Ⓝ
No touch	Ⓨ Ⓝ	Ⓨ Ⓝ	Ⓨ Ⓝ
Applies appropriate pressure to the middle finger (palmar surface, distal)	Ⓨ Ⓝ	Ⓨ Ⓝ	Ⓨ Ⓝ
Performs assessment bilaterally	Ⓨ Ⓝ	Ⓨ Ⓝ	Ⓨ Ⓝ

The psychomotor skill was performed completely and in the appropriate order   0 1 2 3 4 5

The tester had control of the subject and the situation (showed confidence)   0 1 2 3 4 5

Method of performing the skill allowed the tester the ability to determine:
severity, proper progression, and the *fit* in the overall picture (Oral)   0 1 2 3 4 5

In order for a grade of *minimum standard* to be given, the total must be ≥11   **TOTAL = _____**

```
 1    2    3    4    5    6    7    8    9   10   11   12   13   14   15
 |____|____|____|____|____|____|____|____|____|____|____|____|____|____|
```

Not Acceptable   **Meets**   **Exceeds**
                                        Minimum Standards   **Minimum Standards**

TEST ENVIRONMENTS

L: Laboratory/Classroom Testing
C: Clinical/Field Testing
P: Practicum Testing
A: Assessment/Mock Exam Testing
S: Self-Reporting

SKILL TEST INFORMATION

Positive Finding:	No feeling; difficulty in distinguishing varied pressure
Involved Structure:	Nerve root C7
Special Considerations:	N/A
Reference(s):	Hoppenfeld
Supplies Needed:	Table/chair, sharp/dull object

SENSORY TESTING
(SST-U-Test 4)

Peer Review _____ Peer Review _____

Skill Acquisition: _____   Practice Opportunities: _____

This problem allows you the opportunity to demonstrate a **Dermatome Sensory Test** *in order to rule out damage to the nerve root* **C8**. *You have 2 minutes to complete this task.*

Tester places athlete and limb in appropriate position	Test 1	Test 2	Test 3
Seated or prone	Ⓨ Ⓝ	Ⓨ Ⓝ	Ⓨ Ⓝ
Tester performs test according to accepted guidelines	**Test 1**	**Test 2**	**Test 3**
Gives appropriate directions to the athlete	Ⓨ Ⓝ	Ⓨ Ⓝ	Ⓨ Ⓝ
Explains differences in pressure	Ⓨ Ⓝ	Ⓨ Ⓝ	Ⓨ Ⓝ
Demonstration given away from the injured area	Ⓨ Ⓝ	Ⓨ Ⓝ	Ⓨ Ⓝ
Instructs athlete to close eyes	Ⓨ Ⓝ	Ⓨ Ⓝ	Ⓨ Ⓝ
Applies varied pressure with tool or common objects:			
Sharp	Ⓨ Ⓝ	Ⓨ Ⓝ	Ⓨ Ⓝ
Dull	Ⓨ Ⓝ	Ⓨ Ⓝ	Ⓨ Ⓝ
No touch	Ⓨ Ⓝ	Ⓨ Ⓝ	Ⓨ Ⓝ
Applies appropriate pressure to the fourth and fifth fingers at the outside of little finger	Ⓨ Ⓝ	Ⓨ Ⓝ	Ⓨ Ⓝ
Performs assessment bilaterally	Ⓨ Ⓝ	Ⓨ Ⓝ	Ⓨ Ⓝ

The psychomotor skill was performed completely and in the appropriate order   **0 1 2 3 4 5**

The tester had control of the subject and the situation (showed confidence)   **0 1 2 3 4 5**

Method of performing the skill allowed the tester the ability to determine:
severity, proper progression, and the *fit* in the overall picture (Oral)   **0 1 2 3 4 5**

In order for a grade of *minimum standard* to be given, the total must be ≥11   **TOTAL = _____**

1	2	3	4	5	6	7	8	9	10	11	12	13	14	15

Not Acceptable   **Meets**   **Exceeds**
                            Minimum Standards   **Minimum Standards**

TEST ENVIRONMENTS

L: Laboratory/Classroom Testing
C: Clinical/Field Testing
P: Practicum Testing
A: Assessment/Mock Exam Testing
S: Self-Reporting

SKILL TEST INFORMATION

Positive Finding:	No feeling; difficulty in distinguishing varied pressure
Involved Structure:	Nerve root C8
Special Considerations:	N/A
Reference(s):	Hoppenfeld
Supplies Needed:	Table/chair, sharp/dull objects

SENSORY TESTING
(SST-U-Test 5)

Peer Review _____ Peer Review _____

Skill Acquisition: _____   Practice Opportunities: _____

This problem allows you the opportunity to demonstrate a **Dermatome Sensory Test** *in order to rule out damage to the nerve root* **T1.** *You have 2 minutes to complete this task.*

Tester places athlete and limb in appropriate position	Test 1	Test 2	Test 3
Seated or prone	Ⓨ Ⓝ	Ⓨ Ⓝ	Ⓨ Ⓝ
Tester performs test according to accepted guidelines	**Test 1**	**Test 2**	**Test 3**
Gives appropriate directions to the athlete	Ⓨ Ⓝ	Ⓨ Ⓝ	Ⓨ Ⓝ
Explains differences in pressure	Ⓨ Ⓝ	Ⓨ Ⓝ	Ⓨ Ⓝ
Demonstration given away from the injured area	Ⓨ Ⓝ	Ⓨ Ⓝ	Ⓨ Ⓝ
Instructs athlete to close eyes	Ⓨ Ⓝ	Ⓨ Ⓝ	Ⓨ Ⓝ
Applies varied pressure with tool or common objects:			
Sharp	Ⓨ Ⓝ	Ⓨ Ⓝ	Ⓨ Ⓝ
Dull	Ⓨ Ⓝ	Ⓨ Ⓝ	Ⓨ Ⓝ
No touch	Ⓨ Ⓝ	Ⓨ Ⓝ	Ⓨ Ⓝ
Applies appropriate pressure to the upper half of the medial forearm (medial epicondyle)	Ⓨ Ⓝ	Ⓨ Ⓝ	Ⓨ Ⓝ
Performs assessment bilaterally	Ⓨ Ⓝ	Ⓨ Ⓝ	Ⓨ Ⓝ

The psychomotor skill was performed completely and in the appropriate order   **0 1 2 3 4 5**

The tester had control of the subject and the situation (showed confidence)   **0 1 2 3 4 5**

Method of performing the skill allowed the tester the ability to determine:
severity, proper progression, and the *fit* in the overall picture (Oral)   **0 1 2 3 4 5**

In order for a grade of *minimum standard* to be given, the total must be ≥11   **TOTAL = _____**

| 1 | 2 | 3 | 4 | 5 | 6 | 7 | 8 | 9 | 10 | 11 | 12 | 13 | 14 | 15 |

Not Acceptable   **Meets Minimum Standards**   **Exceeds Minimum Standards**

TEST ENVIRONMENTS

L: Laboratory/Classroom Testing
C: Clinical/Field Testing
P: Practicum Testing
A: Assessment/Mock Exam Testing
S: Self-Reporting

SKILL TEST INFORMATION

Positive Finding: No feeling; difficulty in distinguishing varied pressure
Involved Structure: Nerve root T1
Special Considerations: N/A
Reference(s): Hoppenfeld
Supplies Needed: Table/chair, sharp/dull objects

SENSORY TESTING
(SST-U-Test 6)

Peer Review _____ Peer Review _____

Skill Acquisition: _____   Practice Opportunities: _____

*Please demonstrate how you would evaluate an athlete who is suspected of a cranial nerve injury to the **olfactory nerve (cranial nerve #1)**. You have 2 minutes to complete this task.*

Tester places athlete and limb in appropriate position	Test 1	Test 2	Test 3
Seated or standing	Ⓨ Ⓝ	Ⓨ Ⓝ	Ⓨ Ⓝ
Tester performs test according to accepted guidelines	**Test 1**	**Test 2**	**Test 3**
Gives appropriate directions to the athlete	Ⓨ Ⓝ	Ⓨ Ⓝ	Ⓨ Ⓝ
Instructs the athlete to close eyes	Ⓨ Ⓝ	Ⓨ Ⓝ	Ⓨ Ⓝ
Asks the athlete to identify a familiar odor	Ⓨ Ⓝ	Ⓨ Ⓝ	Ⓨ Ⓝ

The psychomotor skill was performed completely and in the appropriate order **0 1 2 3 4 5**

The tester had control of the subject and the situation (showed confidence) **0 1 2 3 4 5**

Method of performing the skill allowed the tester the ability to determine:
severity, proper progression, and the *fit* in the overall picture (Oral) **0 1 2 3 4 5**

In order for a grade of *minimum standard* to be given, the total must be ≥11 **TOTAL = _____**

```
 1    2    3    4    5    6    7    8    9   10   11   12   13   14   15
 |    |    |    |    |    |    |    |    |    |    |    |    |    |    |
```

Not Acceptable   **Meets**   **Exceeds**
                              Minimum Standards   **Minimum Standards**

TEST ENVIRONMENTS
L: Laboratory/Classroom Testing
C: Clinical/Field Testing
P: Practicum Testing
A: Assessment/Mock Exam Testing
S: Self-Reporting

SKILL TEST INFORMATION
Positive Finding: Inability to distinguish odor
Involved Structure: Cranial nerve #1
Special Considerations: Sensory only
Reference(s): Magee; Starkey et al
Supplies Needed: Familiar odor (eg, tape adhesive)

SENSORY TESTING
(SST-U-Test 7)

Peer Review _____ Peer Review _____

Skill Acquisition: _____   Practice Opportunities: _____

*Please demonstrate how you would evaluate an athlete who is suspected of a cranial nerve injury to the **optic nerve (cranial nerve #2)**. You have 2 minutes to complete this task.*

Tester places athlete and limb in appropriate position	Test 1	Test 2	Test 3
Seated or standing	Ⓨ Ⓝ	Ⓨ Ⓝ	Ⓨ Ⓝ
Tester performs test according to accepted guidelines	**Test 1**	**Test 2**	**Test 3**
Gives appropriate directions to the athlete	Ⓨ Ⓝ	Ⓨ Ⓝ	Ⓨ Ⓝ
Asks athlete to read from chart or scoreboard (visual field and distance acuity)	Ⓨ Ⓝ	Ⓨ Ⓝ	Ⓨ Ⓝ
Asks the athlete to tell how many fingers he or she sees (visual field and near acuity)	Ⓨ Ⓝ	Ⓨ Ⓝ	Ⓨ Ⓝ

The psychomotor skill was performed completely and in the appropriate order   **0 1 2 3 4 5**

The tester had control of the subject and the situation (showed confidence)   **0 1 2 3 4 5**

Method of performing the skill allowed the tester the ability to determine:
severity, proper progression, and the *fit* in the overall picture (Oral)   **0 1 2 3 4 5**

In order for a grade of *minimum standard* to be given, the total must be ≥11   **TOTAL = _____**

| 1 | 2 | 3 | 4 | 5 | 6 | 7 | 8 | 9 | 10 | 11 | 12 | 13 | 14 | 15 |

Not Acceptable   **Meets**   **Exceeds**
                Minimum Standards   **Minimum Standards**

<table>
<tr><td>

TEST ENVIRONMENTS

L: Laboratory/Classroom Testing
C: Clinical/Field Testing
P: Practicum Testing
A: Assessment/Mock Exam Testing
S: Self-Reporting

</td><td>

SKILL TEST INFORMATION

Positive Finding: Inability to see/read requested material
Involved Structure: Cranial nerve #2
Special Considerations: Sensory only
Reference(s): Magee; Starkey et al
Supplies Needed: Vision card, etc

</td></tr>
</table>

SENSORY TESTING
(SST-U-Test 8)

Peer Review _____   Peer Review _____

Skill Acquisition: _____   Practice Opportunities: _____

Please demonstrate how you would evaluate an athlete who is suspected of a cranial nerve injury to the **oculomotor nerve (cranial nerve #3)**. *You have 2 minutes to complete this task.*

Tester places athlete and limb in appropriate position	Test 1	Test 2	Test 3
Seated or standing	Ⓨ Ⓝ	Ⓨ Ⓝ	Ⓨ Ⓝ
Tester performs test according to accepted guidelines	**Test 1**	**Test 2**	**Test 3**
Gives appropriate directions to the athlete	Ⓨ Ⓝ	Ⓨ Ⓝ	Ⓨ Ⓝ
Checks the athlete's reaction to light (pupil reaction)	Ⓨ Ⓝ	Ⓨ Ⓝ	Ⓨ Ⓝ
Asks the athlete to raise the upper eyelid	Ⓨ Ⓝ	Ⓨ Ⓝ	Ⓨ Ⓝ
Asks the athlete to roll the eye downward, upward, and medially	Ⓨ Ⓝ	Ⓨ Ⓝ	Ⓨ Ⓝ

The psychomotor skill was performed completely and in the appropriate order   **0 1 2 3 4 5**

The tester had control of the subject and the situation (showed confidence)   **0 1 2 3 4 5**

Method of performing the skill allowed the tester the ability to determine:
severity, proper progression, and the *fit* in the overall picture (Oral)   **0 1 2 3 4 5**

In order for a grade of *minimum standard* to be given, the total must be ≥11   **TOTAL = _____**

```
  1     2     3     4     5     6     7     8     9    10    11    12    13    14    15
  |     |     |     |     |     |     |     |     |     |     |     |     |     |     |
```

Not Acceptable   **Meets**   **Exceeds**
                                          Minimum Standards   **Minimum Standards**

TEST ENVIRONMENTS

L: Laboratory/Classroom Testing
C: Clinical/Field Testing
P: Practicum Testing
A: Assessment/Mock Exam Testing
S: Self-Reporting

SKILL TEST INFORMATION

Positive Finding:	Inability to complete the above tasks
Involved Structure:	Cranial nerve #3
Special Considerations:	Motor only
Reference(s):	Magee; Starkey et al
Supplies Needed:	Pen light

SENSORY TESTING
(SST-U-Test 9)

Skill Acquisition: _____   Practice Opportunities: _____

Please demonstrate how you would evaluate an athlete who is suspected of a cranial nerve injury to the **trochlear nerve (cranial nerve #4)**. *You have 2 minutes to complete this task.*

Tester places athlete and limb in appropriate position	Test 1	Test 2	Test 3
Seated or standing	Ⓨ Ⓝ	Ⓨ Ⓝ	Ⓨ Ⓝ
Tester performs test according to accepted guidelines	**Test 1**	**Test 2**	**Test 3**
Gives appropriate directions to the athlete	Ⓨ Ⓝ	Ⓨ Ⓝ	Ⓨ Ⓝ
Asks the athlete to elevate eyes (upward rolling of the eyes)	Ⓨ Ⓝ	Ⓨ Ⓝ	Ⓨ Ⓝ

The psychomotor skill was performed completely and in the appropriate order   0 1 2 3 4 5

The tester had control of the subject and the situation (showed confidence)   0 1 2 3 4 5

Method of performing the skill allowed the tester the ability to determine:
severity, proper progression, and the *fit* in the overall picture (Oral)   0 1 2 3 4 5

In order for a grade of *minimum standard* to be given, the total must be ≥11   **TOTAL = _____**

```
  1    2    3    4    5    6    7    8    9   10   11   12   13   14   15
  |----|----|----|----|----|----|----|----|----|----|----|----|----|----|
```

Not Acceptable   **Meets**   **Exceeds**
                                          Minimum Standards   **Minimum Standards**

TEST ENVIRONMENTS
L: Laboratory/Classroom Testing
C: Clinical/Field Testing
P: Practicum Testing
A: Assessment/Mock Exam Testing
S: Self-Reporting

SKILL TEST INFORMATION

Positive Finding:	Inability to complete the above tasks
Involved Structure:	Cranial nerve #4
Special Considerations:	Motor only
Reference(s):	Starkey et al
Supplies Needed:	Penlight

SENSORY TESTING
(SST-U-Test 10)

Peer Review _____   Peer Review _____

Skill Acquisition: _____   Practice Opportunities: _____

Demonstrate how you would evaluate an athlete who is suspected of suffering a cranial nerve injury to the **trigeminal nerve**. *This problem requires you to demonstrate assessment of both the sensory and motor functions of* **cranial nerve #5**. *You have 2 minutes to complete this task.*

Tester places athlete and limb in appropriate position	Test 1	Test 2	Test 3
Seated or standing	Ⓨ Ⓝ	Ⓨ Ⓝ	Ⓨ Ⓝ
Tester performs test according to accepted guidelines	**Test 1**	**Test 2**	**Test 3**
Gives appropriate directions to the athlete	Ⓨ Ⓝ	Ⓨ Ⓝ	Ⓨ Ⓝ
Instructs the athlete to close eyes	Ⓨ Ⓝ	Ⓨ Ⓝ	Ⓨ Ⓝ
Asks the athlete to recognize a light touch to the face (sensory)	Ⓨ Ⓝ	Ⓨ Ⓝ	Ⓨ Ⓝ
Asks the athlete to clench teeth together (motor)	Ⓨ Ⓝ	Ⓨ Ⓝ	Ⓨ Ⓝ

The psychomotor skill was performed completely and in the appropriate order   **0 1 2 3 4 5**

The tester had control of the subject and the situation (showed confidence)   **0 1 2 3 4 5**

Method of performing the skill allowed the tester the ability to determine:
severity, proper progression, and the *fit* in the overall picture (Oral)   **0 1 2 3 4 5**

In order for a grade of *minimum standard* to be given, the total must be ≥11   **TOTAL = _____**

```
 1    2    3    4    5    6    7    8    9   10   11   12   13   14   15
 |____|____|____|____|____|____|____|____|____|____|____|____|____|____|
```

Not Acceptable   **Meets**   **Exceeds**
                                          Minimum Standards   **Minimum Standards**

TEST ENVIRONMENTS

L: Laboratory/Classroom Testing
C: Clinical/Field Testing
P: Practicum Testing
A: Assessment/Mock Exam Testing
S: Self-Reporting

SKILL TEST INFORMATION

Positive Finding: Inability to complete the above tasks
Involved Structure: Cranial nerve #5
Special Considerations: Motor/sensory
Reference(s): Magee; Starkey et al
Supplies Needed: N/A

SENSORY TESTING
(SST-U-Test 11)

Peer Review _____ Peer Review _____

Skill Acquisition: _____   Practice Opportunities: _____

Please demonstrate how you would evaluate an athlete who is suspected of a cranial nerve injury to the **abducens nerve (cranial nerve #6)**. *You have 2 minutes to complete this task.*

Tester places athlete and limb in appropriate position	Test 1	Test 2	Test 3
Seated or standing	Ⓨ Ⓝ	Ⓨ Ⓝ	Ⓨ Ⓝ

Tester performs test according to accepted guidelines	Test 1	Test 2	Test 3
Gives appropriate directions to the athlete	Ⓨ Ⓝ	Ⓨ Ⓝ	Ⓨ Ⓝ
Asks the athlete to move the eye laterally	Ⓨ Ⓝ	Ⓨ Ⓝ	Ⓨ Ⓝ

The psychomotor skill was performed completely and in the appropriate order   0 1 2 3 4 5

The tester had control of the subject and the situation (showed confidence)   0 1 2 3 4 5

Method of performing the skill allowed the tester the ability to determine:
severity, proper progression, and the *fit* in the overall picture (Oral)   0 1 2 3 4 5

In order for a grade of *minimum standard* to be given, the total must be ≥11   TOTAL = _____

```
  1    2    3    4    5    6    7    8    9   10   11   12   13   14   15
  |____|____|____|____|____|____|____|____|____|____|____|____|____|____|
```

Not Acceptable   **Meets**   **Exceeds**
                                   Minimum Standards   **Minimum Standards**

TEST ENVIRONMENTS

L: Laboratory/Classroom Testing
C: Clinical/Field Testing
P: Practicum Testing
A: Assessment/Mock Exam Testing
S: Self-Reporting

SKILL TEST INFORMATION

Positive Finding: Inability to complete the above tasks
Involved Structure: Cranial nerve #6
Special Considerations: Motor only
Reference(s): Magee; Starkey et al
Supplies Needed: Penlight

SENSORY TESTING
(SST-U-Test 12)

Peer Review _____ Peer Review _____

Skill Acquisition: _____   Practice Opportunities: _____

Demonstrate how you would evaluate an athlete who is suspected of suffering a cranial nerve injury to the **facial nerve**. *This problem requires you to demonstrate assessment of both the sensory and motor functions of* **cranial nerve #7**. *You have 2 minutes to complete this task.*

Tester places athlete and limb in appropriate position	Test 1	Test 2	Test 3
Seated or standing	Ⓨ Ⓝ	Ⓨ Ⓝ	Ⓨ Ⓝ
Tester performs test according to accepted guidelines	**Test 1**	**Test 2**	**Test 3**
Gives appropriate directions to the athlete	Ⓨ Ⓝ	Ⓨ Ⓝ	Ⓨ Ⓝ
Instructs the athlete to close eyes	Ⓨ Ⓝ	Ⓨ Ⓝ	Ⓨ Ⓝ
Asks the athlete to recognize a familiar taste on the anterior portion of the tongue (sensory)	Ⓨ Ⓝ	Ⓨ Ⓝ	Ⓨ Ⓝ
Asks the athlete to smile, puff cheeks, etc to show control of facial muscles (motor)	Ⓨ Ⓝ	Ⓨ Ⓝ	Ⓨ Ⓝ

The psychomotor skill was performed completely and in the appropriate order   0 1 2 3 4 5

The tester had control of the subject and the situation (showed confidence)   0 1 2 3 4 5

Method of performing the skill allowed the tester the ability to determine:
severity, proper progression, and the *fit* in the overall picture (Oral)   0 1 2 3 4 5

In order for a grade of *minimum standard* to be given, the total must be ≥11   TOTAL = _____

```
 1    2    3    4    5    6    7    8    9   10   11   12   13   14   15
 |    |    |    |    |    |    |    |    |    |    |    |    |    |    |
```

Not Acceptable   **Meets**   **Exceeds**
                                   Minimum Standards   **Minimum Standards**

TEST ENVIRONMENTS

L: Laboratory/Classroom Testing
C: Clinical/Field Testing
P: Practicum Testing
A: Assessment/Mock Exam Testing
S: Self-Reporting

SKILL TEST INFORMATION

Positive Finding:	Inability to complete the above tasks
Involved Structure:	Cranial nerve #7
Special Considerations:	Motor/sensory
Reference(s):	Magee; Starkey et al
Supplies Needed:	Sugar, etc

SENSORY TESTING
(SST-U-Test 13)

Peer Review _____ Peer Review _____

Skill Acquisition: _____   Practice Opportunities: _____

Please demonstrate how you would evaluate an athlete who is suspected of a cranial nerve injury to the **vestibulocochlear nerve (cranial nerve #8)**. *You have 2 minutes to complete this task.*

Tester places athlete and limb in appropriate position	Test 1	Test 2	Test 3
Seated or standing	Ⓨ Ⓝ	Ⓨ Ⓝ	Ⓨ Ⓝ
Tester performs test according to accepted guidelines	**Test 1**	**Test 2**	**Test 3**
Gives appropriate directions to the athlete	Ⓨ Ⓝ	Ⓨ Ⓝ	Ⓨ Ⓝ
Asks the athlete to listen for sounds (eg, watch ticking)	Ⓨ Ⓝ	Ⓨ Ⓝ	Ⓨ Ⓝ
Moves sound further away (compared bilaterally)	Ⓨ Ⓝ	Ⓨ Ⓝ	Ⓨ Ⓝ
Asks the athlete to maintain normal balance (balance/coordination test)	Ⓨ Ⓝ	Ⓨ Ⓝ	Ⓨ Ⓝ

The psychomotor skill was performed completely and in the appropriate order   0 1 2 3 4 5

The tester had control of the subject and the situation (showed confidence)   0 1 2 3 4 5

Method of performing the skill allowed the tester the ability to determine:
severity, proper progression, and the *fit* in the overall picture (Oral)   0 1 2 3 4 5

In order for a grade of *minimum standard* to be given, the total must be ≥11   TOTAL = _____

```
 1    2    3    4    5    6    7    8    9   10   11   12   13   14   15
 |    |    |    |    |    |    |    |    |    |    |    |    |    |    |
```
Not Acceptable　　　　　　　　　　　**Meets**　　　　　　**Exceeds**
　　　　　　　　　　　　　　　　Minimum Standards　　**Minimum Standards**

SKILL TEST INFORMATION

TEST ENVIRONMENTS

L: Laboratory/Classroom Testing
C: Clinical/Field Testing
P: Practicum Testing
A: Assessment/Mock Exam Testing
S: Self-Reporting

Positive Finding: Inability to complete the above tasks
Involved Structure: Cranial nerve #8
Special Considerations: Sensory only (may be called acoustic nerve)
Reference(s): Magee; Starkey et al
Supplies Needed: Some type of noise

SENSORY TESTING
(SST-U-Test 14)

Skill Acquisition: _____   Practice Opportunities: _____

Demonstrate how you would evaluate an athlete who is suspected of suffering a cranial nerve injury to the **glossopharyngeal nerve**. *This problem requires you to demonstrate assessment of both the sensory and motor functions of* **cranial nerve #9**. *You have 2 minutes to complete this task.*

Tester places athlete and limb in appropriate position	Test 1	Test 2	Test 3
Seated or standing	Ⓨ Ⓝ	Ⓨ Ⓝ	Ⓨ Ⓝ

Tester performs test according to accepted guidelines	Test 1	Test 2	Test 3
Gives appropriate directions to the athlete	Ⓨ Ⓝ	Ⓨ Ⓝ	Ⓨ Ⓝ
Instructs the athlete to close eyes	Ⓨ Ⓝ	Ⓨ Ⓝ	Ⓨ Ⓝ
Asks the athlete to recognize a familiar taste on the posterior portion of the tongue (sensory)	Ⓨ Ⓝ	Ⓨ Ⓝ	Ⓨ Ⓝ
Asks the athlete to swallow to demonstrate gag reflex (motor)	Ⓨ Ⓝ	Ⓨ Ⓝ	Ⓨ Ⓝ

The psychomotor skill was performed completely and in the appropriate order   **0 1 2 3 4 5**

The tester had control of the subject and the situation (showed confidence)   **0 1 2 3 4 5**

Method of performing the skill allowed the tester the ability to determine:
severity, proper progression, and the *fit* in the overall picture (Oral)   **0 1 2 3 4 5**

In order for a grade of *minimum standard* to be given, the total must be ≥11   **TOTAL = _____**

| 1 | 2 | 3 | 4 | 5 | 6 | 7 | 8 | 9 | 10 | 11 | 12 | 13 | 14 | 15 |

Not Acceptable   **Meets**   **Exceeds**
                                    Minimum Standards   **Minimum Standards**

TEST ENVIRONMENTS

L: Laboratory/Classroom Testing
C: Clinical/Field Testing
P: Practicum Testing
A: Assessment/Mock Exam Testing
S: Self-Reporting

SKILL TEST INFORMATION

Positive Finding:	Inability to complete the above tasks
Involved Structure:	Cranial nerve #9
Special Considerations:	Motor/sensory
Reference(s):	Magee
Supplies Needed:	Sugar, etc

SENSORY TESTING
(SST-U-Test 15)

Demonstrate how you would evaluate an athlete who is suspected of suffering a cranial nerve injury to the **vagus nerve**. *This problem requires you to demonstrate assessment of both the sensory and motor functions of* **cranial nerve #10**. *You have 2 minutes to complete this task.*

Tester places athlete and limb in appropriate position	Test 1	Test 2	Test 3
Seated or standing	Ⓨ Ⓝ	Ⓨ Ⓝ	Ⓨ Ⓝ
Tester performs test according to accepted guidelines	**Test 1**	**Test 2**	**Test 3**
Gives appropriate directions to the athlete	Ⓨ Ⓝ	Ⓨ Ⓝ	Ⓨ Ⓝ
Asks athlete to swallow (motor)	Ⓨ Ⓝ	Ⓨ Ⓝ	Ⓨ Ⓝ
Asks athlete to recognize a light touch to the pharynx, larynx (sensory)	Ⓨ Ⓝ	Ⓨ Ⓝ	Ⓨ Ⓝ

The psychomotor skill was performed completely and in the appropriate order   **0 1 2 3 4 5**

The tester had control of the subject and the situation (showed confidence)   **0 1 2 3 4 5**

Method of performing the skill allowed the tester the ability to determine:
severity, proper progression, and the *fit* in the overall picture (Oral)   **0 1 2 3 4 5**

In order for a grade of *minimum standard* to be given, the total must be ≥11   **TOTAL = _____**

```
  1     2     3     4     5     6     7     8     9    10    11    12    13    14    15
  |_____|_____|_____|_____|_____|_____|_____|_____|_____|_____|_____|_____|_____|_____|
```

Not Acceptable   **Meets**   **Exceeds**
                                          Minimum Standards   **Minimum Standards**

TEST ENVIRONMENTS

L: Laboratory/Classroom Testing
C: Clinical/Field Testing
P: Practicum Testing
A: Assessment/Mock Exam Testing
S: Self-Reporting

SKILL TEST INFORMATION

Positive Finding: Inability to complete the above tasks
Involved Structure: Cranial nerve #10
Special Considerations: Motor/sensory
Reference(s): Starkey et al
Supplies Needed: N/A

Sensory Testing
(SST-U-Test 16)

Peer Review _____ Peer Review _____

Skill Acquisition: _____   Practice Opportunities: _____

Please demonstrate how you would evaluate an athlete who is suspected of a cranial nerve injury to the **accessory nerve (cranial nerve #11)**. *You have 2 minutes to complete this task.*

Tester places athlete and limb in appropriate position	Test 1	Test 2	Test 3
Seated or standing	Ⓨ Ⓝ	Ⓨ Ⓝ	Ⓨ Ⓝ
Tester performs test according to accepted guidelines	Test 1	Test 2	Test 3
Gives appropriate directions to the athlete	Ⓨ Ⓝ	Ⓨ Ⓝ	Ⓨ Ⓝ
Asks the athlete to shrug shoulders against resistance	Ⓨ Ⓝ	Ⓨ Ⓝ	Ⓨ Ⓝ
Holds resistance for 5 seconds	Ⓨ Ⓝ	Ⓨ Ⓝ	Ⓨ Ⓝ

The psychomotor skill was performed completely and in the appropriate order   **0 1 2 3 4 5**

The tester had control of the subject and the situation (showed confidence)   **0 1 2 3 4 5**

Method of performing the skill allowed the tester the ability to determine:
severity, proper progression, and the *fit* in the overall picture (Oral)   **0 1 2 3 4 5**

In order for a grade of *minimum standard* to be given, the total must be ≥11   **TOTAL = _____**

```
  1     2     3     4     5     6     7     8     9    10    11    12    13    14    15
  |     |     |     |     |     |     |     |     |     |     |     |     |     |     |
```

Not Acceptable   **Meets**   **Exceeds**
                               Minimum Standards   **Minimum Standards**

TEST ENVIRONMENTS

L: Laboratory/Classroom Testing
C: Clinical/Field Testing
P: Practicum Testing
A: Assessment/Mock Exam Testing
S: Self-Reporting

SKILL TEST INFORMATION

Positive Finding:	Inability to complete the above tasks
Involved Structure:	Cranial nerve #11
Special Considerations:	Motor only
Reference(s):	Magee; Starkey et al
Supplies Needed:	N/A

SENSORY TESTING
(SST-U-Test 17)

Peer Review _____ Peer Review _____

Skill Acquisition: _____   Practice Opportunities: _____

Please demonstrate how you would evaluate an athlete who is suspected of a cranial nerve injury to the **hypoglossal nerve (cranial nerve #12)**. *You have 2 minutes to complete this task.*

Tester places athlete and limb in appropriate position	Test 1	Test 2	Test 3
Seated or standing	Ⓨ Ⓝ	Ⓨ Ⓝ	Ⓨ Ⓝ
Tester performs test according to accepted guidelines	**Test 1**	**Test 2**	**Test 3**
Gives appropriate directions to the athlete	Ⓨ Ⓝ	Ⓨ Ⓝ	Ⓨ Ⓝ
Asks the athlete to stick out the tongue (general tongue movements)	Ⓨ Ⓝ	Ⓨ Ⓝ	Ⓨ Ⓝ

The psychomotor skill was performed completely and in the appropriate order   **0 1 2 3 4 5**

The tester had control of the subject and the situation (showed confidence)   **0 1 2 3 4 5**

Method of performing the skill allowed the tester the ability to determine:
severity, proper progression, and the *fit* in the overall picture (Oral)   **0 1 2 3 4 5**

In order for a grade of *minimum standard* to be given, the total must be ≥11   **TOTAL = _____**

```
 1   2   3   4   5   6   7   8   9   10  11  12  13  14  15
 |   |   |   |   |   |   |   |   |   |   |   |   |   |   |
```
Not Acceptable   **Meets**   **Exceeds**
                                    Minimum Standards   **Minimum Standards**

TEST ENVIRONMENTS

L: Laboratory/Classroom Testing
C: Clinical/Field Testing
P: Practicum Testing
A: Assessment/Mock Exam Testing
S: Self-Reporting

SKILL TEST INFORMATION

Positive Finding: Inability to complete the above tasks
Involved Structure: Cranial nerve #12
Special Considerations: Motor only
Reference(s): Magee; Starkey et al
Supplies Needed: N/A

SENSORY TESTING
(SST-L-Test 1)

Skill Acquisition: _____   Practice Opportunities: _____

*This problem allows you the opportunity to demonstrate a **Dermatome Sensory Test** in order to rule out damage to the nerve root **T12**. You have 2 minutes to complete this task.*

Tester places athlete and limb in appropriate position	Test 1	Test 2	Test 3
Seated or prone	Ⓨ Ⓝ	Ⓨ Ⓝ	Ⓨ Ⓝ
Tester performs test according to accepted guidelines	**Test 1**	**Test 2**	**Test 3**
Gives appropriate directions to the athlete	Ⓨ Ⓝ	Ⓨ Ⓝ	Ⓨ Ⓝ
Explains differences in pressure	Ⓨ Ⓝ	Ⓨ Ⓝ	Ⓨ Ⓝ
Demonstration given away from the injured area	Ⓨ Ⓝ	Ⓨ Ⓝ	Ⓨ Ⓝ
Instructs athlete to close eyes	Ⓨ Ⓝ	Ⓨ Ⓝ	Ⓨ Ⓝ
Applies varied pressure with tool or common objects:			
Sharp	Ⓨ Ⓝ	Ⓨ Ⓝ	Ⓨ Ⓝ
Dull	Ⓨ Ⓝ	Ⓨ Ⓝ	Ⓨ Ⓝ
No touch	Ⓨ Ⓝ	Ⓨ Ⓝ	Ⓨ Ⓝ
Applies appropriate pressure to the area just above the inguinal ligament	Ⓨ Ⓝ	Ⓨ Ⓝ	Ⓨ Ⓝ
Performs assessment bilaterally	Ⓨ Ⓝ	Ⓨ Ⓝ	Ⓨ Ⓝ

The psychomotor skill was performed completely and in the appropriate order   **0 1 2 3 4 5**

The tester had control of the subject and the situation (showed confidence)   **0 1 2 3 4 5**

Method of performing the skill allowed the tester the ability to determine: severity, proper progression, and the *fit* in the overall picture (Oral)   **0 1 2 3 4 5**

In order for a grade of *minimum standard* to be given, the total must be ≥11   **TOTAL = _____**

1	2	3	4	5	6	7	8	9	10	11	12	13	14	15

Not Acceptable   **Meets Minimum Standards**   **Exceeds Minimum Standards**

TEST ENVIRONMENTS

L: Laboratory/Classroom Testing
C: Clinical/Field Testing
P: Practicum Testing
A: Assessment/Mock Exam Testing
S: Self-Reporting

SKILL TEST INFORMATION

Positive Finding: No feeling; difficulty distinguishing varied pressure
Involved Structure: Nerve root T12
Special Considerations: N/A
Reference(s): Magee
Supplies Needed: Table/chair, sharp/dull objects

SENSORY TESTING
(SST-L-Test 2)

Peer Review _____ Peer Review _____

Skill Acquisition: _____ Practice Opportunities: _____

*This problem allows you the opportunity to demonstrate a **Dermatome Sensory Test** in order to rule out damage to the nerve root **L1**. You have 2 minutes to complete this task.*

Tester places athlete and limb in appropriate position	Test 1	Test 2	Test 3
Seated or prone	Ⓨ Ⓝ	Ⓨ Ⓝ	Ⓨ Ⓝ
Tester performs test according to accepted guidelines	**Test 1**	**Test 2**	**Test 3**
Gives appropriate directions to the athlete	Ⓨ Ⓝ	Ⓨ Ⓝ	Ⓨ Ⓝ
Explains differences in pressure	Ⓨ Ⓝ	Ⓨ Ⓝ	Ⓨ Ⓝ
Demonstration given away from the injured area	Ⓨ Ⓝ	Ⓨ Ⓝ	Ⓨ Ⓝ
Instructs athlete to close eyes	Ⓨ Ⓝ	Ⓨ Ⓝ	Ⓨ Ⓝ
Applies varied pressure with tool or common objects:			
Sharp	Ⓨ Ⓝ	Ⓨ Ⓝ	Ⓨ Ⓝ
Dull	Ⓨ Ⓝ	Ⓨ Ⓝ	Ⓨ Ⓝ
No touch	Ⓨ Ⓝ	Ⓨ Ⓝ	Ⓨ Ⓝ
Applies appropriate pressure to the area just below the inguinal ligament (upper anterior thigh)	Ⓨ Ⓝ	Ⓨ Ⓝ	Ⓨ Ⓝ
Performs assessment bilaterally	Ⓨ Ⓝ	Ⓨ Ⓝ	Ⓨ Ⓝ

The psychomotor skill was performed completely and in the appropriate order   0 1 2 3 4 5

The tester had control of the subject and the situation (showed confidence)   0 1 2 3 4 5

Method of performing the skill allowed the tester the ability to determine: severity, proper progression, and the *fit* in the overall picture (Oral)   0 1 2 3 4 5

In order for a grade of *minimum standard* to be given, the total must be ≥11   TOTAL = _____

1   2   3   4   5   6   7   8   9   10   11   12   13   14   15

Not Acceptable   **Meets Minimum Standards**   **Exceeds Minimum Standards**

TEST ENVIRONMENTS

L: Laboratory/Classroom Testing
C: Clinical/Field Testing
P: Practicum Testing
A: Assessment/Mock Exam Testing
S: Self-Reporting

SKILL TEST INFORMATION

Positive Finding: No feeling; difficulty distinguishing varied pressure
Involved Structure: Nerve root L1
Special Considerations: N/A
Reference(s): Hoppenfeld
Supplies Needed: Table/chair, sharp/dull objects

SENSORY TESTING
(SST-L-Test 3)

Peer Review _____ Peer Review _____

Skill Acquisition: _____   Practice Opportunities: _____

*This problem allows you the opportunity to demonstrate a **Dermatome Sensory Test** in order to rule out damage to the nerve root **L2**. You have 2 minutes to complete this task.*

Tester places athlete and limb in appropriate position	Test 1	Test 2	Test 3
Seated or prone	Ⓨ Ⓝ	Ⓨ Ⓝ	Ⓨ Ⓝ
Tester performs test according to accepted guidelines	**Test 1**	**Test 2**	**Test 3**
Gives appropriate directions to the athlete	Ⓨ Ⓝ	Ⓨ Ⓝ	Ⓨ Ⓝ
Explains differences in pressure	Ⓨ Ⓝ	Ⓨ Ⓝ	Ⓨ Ⓝ
Demonstration given away from the injured area	Ⓨ Ⓝ	Ⓨ Ⓝ	Ⓨ Ⓝ
Instructs athlete to close eyes	Ⓨ Ⓝ	Ⓨ Ⓝ	Ⓨ Ⓝ
Applies varied pressure with tool or common objects:			
Sharp	Ⓨ Ⓝ	Ⓨ Ⓝ	Ⓨ Ⓝ
Dull	Ⓨ Ⓝ	Ⓨ Ⓝ	Ⓨ Ⓝ
No touch	Ⓨ Ⓝ	Ⓨ Ⓝ	Ⓨ Ⓝ
Applies appropriate pressure to the area of the midthigh (middle quadriceps)	Ⓨ Ⓝ	Ⓨ Ⓝ	Ⓨ Ⓝ
Performs assessment bilaterally	Ⓨ Ⓝ	Ⓨ Ⓝ	Ⓨ Ⓝ

The psychomotor skill was performed completely and in the appropriate order   **0 1 2 3 4 5**

The tester had control of the subject and the situation (showed confidence)   **0 1 2 3 4 5**

Method of performing the skill allowed the tester the ability to determine:
severity, proper progression, and the *fit* in the overall picture (Oral)   **0 1 2 3 4 5**

In order for a grade of *minimum standard* to be given, the total must be ≥11   **TOTAL = _____**

```
  1    2    3    4    5    6    7    8    9   10   11   12   13   14   15
  |    |    |    |    |    |    |    |    |    |    |    |    |    |    |
```

Not Acceptable   **Meets**   **Exceeds**
                                    Minimum Standards   **Minimum Standards**

TEST ENVIRONMENTS

L: Laboratory/Classroom Testing
C: Clinical/Field Testing
P: Practicum Testing
A: Assessment/Mock Exam Testing
S: Self-Reporting

SKILL TEST INFORMATION

Positive Finding:	No feeling; difficulty distinguishing varied pressure
Involved Structure:	Nerve root L2
Special Considerations:	N/A
Reference(s):	Magee
Supplies Needed:	Table/chair, sharp/dull objects

SENSORY TESTING
(SST-L-Test 4)

Peer Review _____ Peer Review _____

Skill Acquisition: _____   Practice Opportunities: _____

This problem allows you the opportunity to demonstrate a **Dermatome Sensory Test** *in order to rule out damage to the nerve root* **L3**. *You have 2 minutes to complete this task.*

Tester places athlete and limb in appropriate position	Test 1	Test 2	Test 3
Seated or prone	Ⓨ Ⓝ	Ⓨ Ⓝ	Ⓨ Ⓝ
Tester performs test according to accepted guidelines	**Test 1**	**Test 2**	**Test 3**
Gives appropriate directions to the athlete	Ⓨ Ⓝ	Ⓨ Ⓝ	Ⓨ Ⓝ
Explains differences in pressure	Ⓨ Ⓝ	Ⓨ Ⓝ	Ⓨ Ⓝ
Demonstration given away from the injured area	Ⓨ Ⓝ	Ⓨ Ⓝ	Ⓨ Ⓝ
Instructs athlete to close eyes	Ⓨ Ⓝ	Ⓨ Ⓝ	Ⓨ Ⓝ
Applies varied pressure with tool or common objects:			
Sharp	Ⓨ Ⓝ	Ⓨ Ⓝ	Ⓨ Ⓝ
Dull	Ⓨ Ⓝ	Ⓨ Ⓝ	Ⓨ Ⓝ
No touch	Ⓨ Ⓝ	Ⓨ Ⓝ	Ⓨ Ⓝ
Applies appropriate pressure to the area just above the superior pole of the patella	Ⓨ Ⓝ	Ⓨ Ⓝ	Ⓨ Ⓝ
Performs assessment bilaterally	Ⓨ Ⓝ	Ⓨ Ⓝ	Ⓨ Ⓝ

The psychomotor skill was performed completely and in the appropriate order   **0 1 2 3 4 5**

The tester had control of the subject and the situation (showed confidence)   **0 1 2 3 4 5**

Method of performing the skill allowed the tester the ability to determine:
severity, proper progression, and the *fit* in the overall picture (Oral)   **0 1 2 3 4 5**

In order for a grade of *minimum standard* to be given, the total must be ≥11   **TOTAL = _____**

1	2	3	4	5	6	7	8	9	10	11	12	13	14	15

Not Acceptable   **Meets**   **Exceeds**
                              Minimum Standards   **Minimum Standards**

TEST ENVIRONMENTS

L: Laboratory/Classroom Testing
C: Clinical/Field Testing
P: Practicum Testing
A: Assessment/Mock Exam Testing
S: Self-Reporting

SKILL TEST INFORMATION

Positive Finding: No feeling; difficulty in distinguishing varied pressure
Involved Structure: Nerve root L3
Special Considerations: N/A
Reference(s): Magee
Supplies Needed: Table/chair, sharp/dull objects

SENSORY TESTING
(SST-L-Test 5)

Peer Review _____ Peer Review _____

Skill Acquisition: _____   Practice Opportunities: _____

*This problem allows you the opportunity to demonstrate a **Dermatome Sensory Test** in order to rule out damage to the nerve root **L4**. You have 2 minutes to complete this task.*

Tester places athlete and limb in appropriate position	Test 1	Test 2	Test 3
Seated or prone	Ⓨ Ⓝ	Ⓨ Ⓝ	Ⓨ Ⓝ
Shoes and socks off	Ⓨ Ⓝ	Ⓨ Ⓝ	Ⓨ Ⓝ
Tester performs test according to accepted guidelines	**Test 1**	**Test 2**	**Test 3**
Gives appropriate directions to the athlete	Ⓨ Ⓝ	Ⓨ Ⓝ	Ⓨ Ⓝ
Explain differences in pressure	Ⓨ Ⓝ	Ⓨ Ⓝ	Ⓨ Ⓝ
Demonstration given away from the injured area	Ⓨ Ⓝ	Ⓨ Ⓝ	Ⓨ Ⓝ
Instructs athlete to close eyes	Ⓨ Ⓝ	Ⓨ Ⓝ	Ⓨ Ⓝ
Applies varied pressure with tool or common objects:			
Sharp	Ⓨ Ⓝ	Ⓨ Ⓝ	Ⓨ Ⓝ
Dull	Ⓨ Ⓝ	Ⓨ Ⓝ	Ⓨ Ⓝ
No touch	Ⓨ Ⓝ	Ⓨ Ⓝ	Ⓨ Ⓝ
Applies appropriate pressure to the medial side of the lower leg	Ⓨ Ⓝ	Ⓨ Ⓝ	Ⓨ Ⓝ
Performs assessment bilaterally	Ⓨ Ⓝ	Ⓨ Ⓝ	Ⓨ Ⓝ

The psychomotor skill was performed completely and in the appropriate order   **0 1 2 3 4 5**

The tester had control of the subject and the situation (showed confidence)   **0 1 2 3 4 5**

Method of performing the skill allowed the tester the ability to determine:
severity, proper progression, and the *fit* in the overall picture (Oral)   **0 1 2 3 4 5**

In order for a grade of *minimum standard* to be given, the total must be ≥11   **TOTAL = _____**

```
  1    2    3    4    5    6    7    8    9    10   11   12   13   14   15
  |    |    |    |    |    |    |    |    |    |    |    |    |    |    |
```

Not Acceptable   **Meets**   **Exceeds**
                             Minimum Standards   **Minimum Standards**

TEST ENVIRONMENTS

L: Laboratory/Classroom Testing
C: Clinical/Field Testing
P: Practicum Testing
A: Assessment/Mock Exam Testing
S: Self-Reporting

SKILL TEST INFORMATION

Positive Finding:	No feeling; difficulty distinguishing varied pressure
Involved Structure:	Nerve root L4
Special Considerations:	N/A
Reference(s):	Hoppenfeld
Supplies Needed:	Table/chair, sharp/dull objects

SENSORY TESTING
(SST-L-Test 6)

Peer Review _____ Peer Review _____

Skill Acquisition: _____   Practice Opportunities: _____

This problem allows you the opportunity to demonstrate a **Dermatome Sensory Test** *in order to rule out damage to the nerve root* **L5.** *You have 2 minutes to complete this task.*

Tester places athlete and limb in appropriate position	Test 1	Test 2	Test 3
Seated or prone	Ⓨ Ⓝ	Ⓨ Ⓝ	Ⓨ Ⓝ
Shoes and socks off	Ⓨ Ⓝ	Ⓨ Ⓝ	Ⓨ Ⓝ
Tester performs test according to accepted guidelines	**Test 1**	**Test 2**	**Test 3**
Gives appropriate directions to the athlete	Ⓨ Ⓝ	Ⓨ Ⓝ	Ⓨ Ⓝ
Explains differences in pressure	Ⓨ Ⓝ	Ⓨ Ⓝ	Ⓨ Ⓝ
Demonstration given away from the injured area	Ⓨ Ⓝ	Ⓨ Ⓝ	Ⓨ Ⓝ
Instructs athlete to close eyes	Ⓨ Ⓝ	Ⓨ Ⓝ	Ⓨ Ⓝ
Applies varied pressure with tool or common objects:			
Sharp	Ⓨ Ⓝ	Ⓨ Ⓝ	Ⓨ Ⓝ
Dull	Ⓨ Ⓝ	Ⓨ Ⓝ	Ⓨ Ⓝ
No touch	Ⓨ Ⓝ	Ⓨ Ⓝ	Ⓨ Ⓝ
Applies appropriate pressure to the top of the foot (and/or below the head of fibula)	Ⓨ Ⓝ	Ⓨ Ⓝ	Ⓨ Ⓝ
Performs assessment bilaterally	Ⓨ Ⓝ	Ⓨ Ⓝ	Ⓨ Ⓝ

The psychomotor skill was performed completely and in the appropriate order   0   1   2   3   4   5

The tester had control of the subject and the situation (showed confidence)   0   1   2   3   4   5

Method of performing the skill allowed the tester the ability to determine:
severity, proper progression, and the *fit* in the overall picture (Oral)   0   1   2   3   4   5

In order for a grade of *minimum standard* to be given, the total must be ≥11   **TOTAL = _____**

| 1 | 2 | 3 | 4 | 5 | 6 | 7 | 8 | 9 | 10 | 11 | 12 | 13 | 14 | 15 |

Not Acceptable   **Meets**   **Exceeds**
                                  Minimum Standards   **Minimum Standards**

TEST ENVIRONMENTS

L: Laboratory/Classroom Testing
C: Clinical/Field Testing
P: Practicum Testing
A: Assessment/Mock Exam Testing
S: Self-Reporting

SKILL TEST INFORMATION

Positive Finding: No feeling; difficulty distinguishing varied pressure
Involved Structure: Nerve root L5
Special Considerations: N/A
Reference(s): Hoppenfeld
Supplies Needed: Table/chair, sharp/dull objects

SENSORY TESTING
(SST-L-Test 7)

Peer Review _____ Peer Review _____

Skill Acquisition: _____   Practice Opportunities: _____

*This problem allows you the opportunity to demonstrate a **Dermatome Sensory Test** in order to rule out damage to the nerve root **S1**. You have 2 minutes to complete this task.*

Tester places athlete and limb in appropriate position	Test 1	Test 2	Test 3
Seated or prone	Ⓨ Ⓝ	Ⓨ Ⓝ	Ⓨ Ⓝ
Shoes and socks off	Ⓨ Ⓝ	Ⓨ Ⓝ	Ⓨ Ⓝ
Tester performs test according to accepted guidelines	**Test 1**	**Test 2**	**Test 3**
Gives appropriate directions to the athlete	Ⓨ Ⓝ	Ⓨ Ⓝ	Ⓨ Ⓝ
Explains differences in pressure	Ⓨ Ⓝ	Ⓨ Ⓝ	Ⓨ Ⓝ
Demonstration given away from the injured area	Ⓨ Ⓝ	Ⓨ Ⓝ	Ⓨ Ⓝ
Instructs athlete to close eyes	Ⓨ Ⓝ	Ⓨ Ⓝ	Ⓨ Ⓝ
Applies varied pressure with tool or common objects:			
Sharp	Ⓨ Ⓝ	Ⓨ Ⓝ	Ⓨ Ⓝ
Dull	Ⓨ Ⓝ	Ⓨ Ⓝ	Ⓨ Ⓝ
No touch	Ⓨ Ⓝ	Ⓨ Ⓝ	Ⓨ Ⓝ
Applies appropriate pressure to the lateral malleolus and/or fifth metatarsal	Ⓨ Ⓝ	Ⓨ Ⓝ	Ⓨ Ⓝ
Performs assessment bilaterally	Ⓨ Ⓝ	Ⓨ Ⓝ	Ⓨ Ⓝ

The psychomotor skill was performed completely and in the appropriate order   **0 1 2 3 4 5**

The tester had control of the subject and the situation (showed confidence)   **0 1 2 3 4 5**

Method of performing the skill allowed the tester the ability to determine:
severity, proper progression, and the *fit* in the overall picture (Oral)   **0 1 2 3 4 5**

In order for a grade of *minimum standard* to be given, the total must be ≥11   **TOTAL = _____**

| 1 | 2 | 3 | 4 | 5 | 6 | 7 | 8 | 9 | 10 | 11 | 12 | 13 | 14 | 15 |

Not Acceptable   **Meets**   **Exceeds**
                          Minimum Standards   **Minimum Standards**

TEST ENVIRONMENTS

L: Laboratory/Classroom Testing
C: Clinical/Field Testing
P: Practicum Testing
A: Assessment/Mock Exam Testing
S: Self-Reporting

SKILL TEST INFORMATION

Positive Finding: No feeling; difficulty distinguishing varied pressure
Involved Structure: Nerve root S1
Special Considerations: N/A
Reference(s): Hoppenfeld
Supplies Needed: Table/chair, sharp/dull objects

SENSORY TESTING
(SST-L-Test 8)

Peer Review _____ Peer Review _____

Skill Acquisition: _____   Practice Opportunities: _____

*This problem allows you the opportunity to demonstrate a **Dermatome Sensory Test** in order to rule out damage to the nerve root **S2**. You have 2 minutes to complete this task.*

Tester places athlete and limb in appropriate position	Test 1	Test 2	Test 3
Seated or prone	Ⓨ Ⓝ	Ⓨ Ⓝ	Ⓨ Ⓝ
Tester performs test according to accepted guidelines	**Test 1**	**Test 2**	**Test 3**
Gives appropriate directions to the athlete	Ⓨ Ⓝ	Ⓨ Ⓝ	Ⓨ Ⓝ
Explains differences in pressure	Ⓨ Ⓝ	Ⓨ Ⓝ	Ⓨ Ⓝ
Demonstration given away from the injured area	Ⓨ Ⓝ	Ⓨ Ⓝ	Ⓨ Ⓝ
Instructs athlete to close eyes	Ⓨ Ⓝ	Ⓨ Ⓝ	Ⓨ Ⓝ
Applies varied pressure with tool or common objects:			
Sharp	Ⓨ Ⓝ	Ⓨ Ⓝ	Ⓨ Ⓝ
Dull	Ⓨ Ⓝ	Ⓨ Ⓝ	Ⓨ Ⓝ
No touch	Ⓨ Ⓝ	Ⓨ Ⓝ	Ⓨ Ⓝ
Applies appropriate pressure to the area in and around the popliteal fossa (posterior knee)	Ⓨ Ⓝ	Ⓨ Ⓝ	Ⓨ Ⓝ
Performs assessment bilaterally	Ⓨ Ⓝ	Ⓨ Ⓝ	Ⓨ Ⓝ

The psychomotor skill was performed completely and in the appropriate order   0 1 2 3 4 5

The tester had control of the subject and the situation (showed confidence)   0 1 2 3 4 5

Method of performing the skill allowed the tester the ability to determine: severity, proper progression, and the *fit* in the overall picture (Oral)   0 1 2 3 4 5

In order for a grade of *minimum standard* to be given, the total must be ≥11   **TOTAL = _____**

  1   2   3   4   5   6   7   8   9   10   11   12   13   14   15

Not Acceptable   **Meets Minimum Standards**   **Exceeds Minimum Standards**

TEST ENVIRONMENTS

L: Laboratory/Classroom Testing
C: Clinical/Field Testing
P: Practicum Testing
A: Assessment/Mock Exam Testing
S: Self-Reporting

SKILL TEST INFORMATION

Positive Finding:	No feeling; difficulty distinguishing varied pressure
Involved Structure:	Nerve root S2
Special Considerations:	N/A
Reference(s):	Magee
Supplies Needed:	Table/chair, sharp/dull objects

Chapter

Special Tests

SPECIAL TESTS
(ST-U-Test 1)

Peer Review _____ Peer Review _____

Skill Acquisition: _____   Practice Opportunities: _____

*Please demonstrate how you would perform the orthopedic test known as the **Adson's Maneuver** to help rule out the condition known as thoracic outlet syndrome. You have 2 minutes to complete this task.*

Tester places athlete and limb in appropriate position	Test 1	Test 2	Test 3
Seated or standing	Ⓨ Ⓝ	Ⓨ Ⓝ	Ⓨ Ⓝ
Arm at the side (approximately 30 degrees abduction)	Ⓨ Ⓝ	Ⓨ Ⓝ	Ⓨ Ⓝ
Externally rotate the shoulder (thumb pointing upward)	Ⓨ Ⓝ	Ⓨ Ⓝ	Ⓨ Ⓝ
Extend the shoulder and elbow	Ⓨ Ⓝ	Ⓨ Ⓝ	Ⓨ Ⓝ
Tester placed in proper position	**Test 1**	**Test 2**	**Test 3**
Stands behind and to the side of the athlete	Ⓨ Ⓝ	Ⓨ Ⓝ	Ⓨ Ⓝ
Places two fingers over the radial pulse	Ⓨ Ⓝ	Ⓨ Ⓝ	Ⓨ Ⓝ
Tester performs test according to accepted guidelines	Ⓨ Ⓝ	Ⓨ Ⓝ	Ⓨ Ⓝ
Asks the athlete to extend and laterally rotate the head to the involved side	Ⓨ Ⓝ	Ⓨ Ⓝ	Ⓨ Ⓝ
Asks the athlete to take a deep breath	Ⓨ Ⓝ	Ⓨ Ⓝ	Ⓨ Ⓝ
Asks the athlete to hold it	Ⓨ Ⓝ	Ⓨ Ⓝ	Ⓨ Ⓝ
Performs assessment bilaterally	Ⓨ Ⓝ	Ⓨ Ⓝ	Ⓨ Ⓝ

The psychomotor skill was performed completely and in the appropriate order   0 1 2 3 4 5

The tester had control of the subject and the situation (showed confidence)   0 1 2 3 4 5

Method of performing the skill allowed the tester the ability to determine:
severity, proper progression, and the *fit* in the overall picture (Oral)   0 1 2 3 4 5

In order for a grade of *minimum standard* to be given, the total must be ≥11   **TOTAL = _____**

| 1 | 2 | 3 | 4 | 5 | 6 | 7 | 8 | 9 | 10 | 11 | 12 | 13 | 14 | 15 |

Not Acceptable   **Meets**   **Exceeds**
                                   Minimum Standards   **Minimum Standards**

TEST ENVIRONMENTS

L: Laboratory/Classroom Testing
C: Clinical/Field Testing
P: Practicum Testing
A: Assessment/Mock Exam Testing
S: Self-Reporting

SKILL TEST INFORMATION

Positive Finding: Disappearance of the radial pulse

Involved Structure: Subclavian artery (indicative of thoracic outlet syndrome)

Special Considerations: N/A

Reference(s): Konin et al (2002); Magee; Starkey et al (2002)

Supplies Needed: N/A

Special Tests
(ST-U-Test 2)

Peer Review _____ Peer Review _____

Skill Acquisition: _____   Practice Opportunities: _____

Please demonstrate how you would perform the orthopedic test known as the **Empty Can Test (Supraspinatus Test)** *for the shoulder. You have 2 minutes to complete this task.*

Tester places athlete and limb in appropriate position	Test 1	Test 2	Test 3
Standing or seated	Y N	Y N	Y N
Shoulder abducted to 90 degrees	Y N	Y N	Y N
Horizontally flex shoulder to approximately 30 degrees	Y N	Y N	Y N
Internally rotate shoulder thumb pointing toward the floor (ending position is similar to draining a can)	Y N	Y N	Y N
Tester placed in proper position	**Test 1**	**Test 2**	**Test 3**
Stands, facing the athlete	Y N	Y N	Y N
Places hand on the distal portion of the forearm	Y N	Y N	Y N
Tester performs test according to accepted guidelines	**Test 1**	**Test 2**	**Test 3**
Directs athlete to hold arms in this position	Y N	Y N	Y N
Applies downward pressure (resist abduction)	Y N	Y N	Y N

The psychomotor skill was performed completely and in the appropriate order   **0 1 2 3 4 5**

The tester had control of the subject and the situation (showed confidence)   **0 1 2 3 4 5**

Method of performing the skill allowed the tester the ability to determine:
severity, proper progression, and the *fit* in the overall picture (Oral)   **0 1 2 3 4 5**

In order for a grade of *minimum standard* to be given, the total must be ≥11   **TOTAL = _____**

```
   1    2    3    4    5    6    7    8    9    10   11   12   13   14   15
   |    |    |    |    |    |    |    |    |    |    |    |    |    |    |
```

Not Acceptable   **Meets**   **Exceeds**
                                   Minimum Standards   **Minimum Standards**

TEST ENVIRONMENTS

L: Laboratory/Classroom Testing
C: Clinical/Field Testing
P: Practicum Testing
A: Assessment/Mock Exam Testing
S: Self-Reporting

SKILL TEST INFORMATION

Positive Finding: Pain and/or weakness
Involved Structure: Supraspinatus, suprascapular nerve
Special Considerations: N/A
Reference(s): Konin et al (2002); Magee; Starkey et al (2002)
Supplies Needed: N/A

SPECIAL TESTS
(ST-U-Test 3)

Peer Review _____ Peer Review _____

Skill Acquisition: _____   Practice Opportunities: _____

Please demonstrate how you would perform the orthopedic test known as **Ludington's Test** *for the shoulder. You have 2 minutes to complete this task.*

Tester places athlete and limb in appropriate position	Test 1	Test 2	Test 3
Standing or seated	Ⓨ Ⓝ	Ⓨ Ⓝ	Ⓨ Ⓝ
Athlete clasps both hands (with fingers interlocked) behind or on top of the head	Ⓨ Ⓝ	Ⓨ Ⓝ	Ⓨ Ⓝ
Tester placed in proper position	**Test 1**	**Test 2**	**Test 3**
Stands directly behind the athlete	Ⓨ Ⓝ	Ⓨ Ⓝ	Ⓨ Ⓝ
Places fingers over the biceps tendon long head (bicipital groove)	Ⓨ Ⓝ	Ⓨ Ⓝ	Ⓨ Ⓝ
Tester performs test according to accepted guidelines	**Test 1**	**Test 2**	**Test 3**
Asks the athlete to alternately contract biceps (contract/relax)	Ⓨ Ⓝ	Ⓨ Ⓝ	Ⓨ Ⓝ
Palpation of the biceps tendon occurs during the contraction phase	Ⓨ Ⓝ	Ⓨ Ⓝ	Ⓨ Ⓝ

The psychomotor skill was performed completely and in the appropriate order   **0 1 2 3 4 5**

The tester had control of the subject and the situation (showed confidence)   **0 1 2 3 4 5**

Method of performing the skill allowed the tester the ability to determine:
severity, proper progression, and the *fit* in the overall picture (Oral)   **0 1 2 3 4 5**

In order for a grade of *minimum standard* to be given, the total must be ≥11   **TOTAL = _____**

```
 1    2    3    4    5    6    7    8    9   10   11   12   13   14   15
 |____|____|____|____|____|____|____|____|____|____|____|____|____|____|
```

Not Acceptable   **Meets**   **Exceeds**
                                   Minimum Standards   **Minimum Standards**

TEST ENVIRONMENTS

L: Laboratory/Classroom Testing
C: Clinical/Field Testing
P: Practicum Testing
A: Assessment/Mock Exam Testing
S: Self-Reporting

SKILL TEST INFORMATION

Positive Finding: Pain and/or inability to feel the biceps tendon during contraction

Involved Structure: Biceps

Special Considerations: N/A

Reference(s): Magee; Starkey et al (2002)

Supplies Needed: N/A

SPECIAL TESTS
(ST-U-Test 4)

Peer Review _____ Peer Review _____

Skill Acquisition: _____   Practice Opportunities: _____

Please demonstrate how you would perform the orthopedic test known as the **Military Brace Position (Costoclavicular Syndrome Test)** *for the shoulder. You have 2 minutes to complete this task.*

Tester places athlete and limb in appropriate position	Test 1	Test 2	Test 3
Seated or standing	Ⓨ Ⓝ	Ⓨ Ⓝ	Ⓨ Ⓝ
Arms to the side (relaxed posture)	Ⓨ Ⓝ	Ⓨ Ⓝ	Ⓨ Ⓝ
Tester placed in proper position	**Test 1**	**Test 2**	**Test 3**
Stands directly behind the athlete	Ⓨ Ⓝ	Ⓨ Ⓝ	Ⓨ Ⓝ
Palpates the radial pulse	Ⓨ Ⓝ	Ⓨ Ⓝ	Ⓨ Ⓝ
Tester performs test according to accepted guidelines	**Test 1**	**Test 2**	**Test 3**
Depresses and retracts the scapula	Ⓨ Ⓝ	Ⓨ Ⓝ	Ⓨ Ⓝ
Extends and abducts the shoulder approximately 30 degrees	Ⓨ Ⓝ	Ⓨ Ⓝ	Ⓨ Ⓝ
Hyperextends the head	Ⓨ Ⓝ	Ⓨ Ⓝ	Ⓨ Ⓝ
Performs assessment bilaterally	Ⓨ Ⓝ	Ⓨ Ⓝ	Ⓨ Ⓝ

The psychomotor skill was performed completely and in the appropriate order   **0 1 2 3 4 5**

The tester had control of the subject and the situation (showed confidence)   **0 1 2 3 4 5**

Method of performing the skill allowed the tester the ability to determine:
severity, proper progression, and the *fit* in the overall picture (Oral)   **0 1 2 3 4 5**

In order for a grade of *minimum standard* to be given, the total must be ≥11   **TOTAL = _____**

| 1 | 2 | 3 | 4 | 5 | 6 | 7 | 8 | 9 | 10 | 11 | 12 | 13 | 14 | 15 |

Not Acceptable   **Meets**   **Exceeds**
                              Minimum Standards   **Minimum Standards**

TEST ENVIRONMENTS

L: Laboratory/Classroom Testing
C: Clinical/Field Testing
P: Practicum Testing
A: Assessment/Mock Exam Testing
S: Self-Reporting

SKILL TEST INFORMATION

Positive Finding: Absence of a radial pulse
Involved Structure: Subclavian artery, thoracic outlet syndrome
Special Considerations: N/A
Reference(s): Magee; Starkey et al (2002)
Supplies Needed: N/A

SPECIAL TESTS
(ST-U-Test 5)

Peer Review _____ Peer Review _____

Skill Acquisition: _____   Practice Opportunities: _____

Please demonstrate how you would perform the orthopedic test known as the **Roos Test (Elevated Arm Stress Test)**. *You have 4 minutes to complete this task.*

Tester places athlete and limb in appropriate position	Test 1	Test 2	Test 3
Standing	Ⓨ Ⓝ	Ⓨ Ⓝ	Ⓨ Ⓝ
Shoulder abducted to 90 degrees	Ⓨ Ⓝ	Ⓨ Ⓝ	Ⓨ Ⓝ
Shoulder externally rotated to 90 degrees	Ⓨ Ⓝ	Ⓨ Ⓝ	Ⓨ Ⓝ
Elbow flexed to 45 degrees	Ⓨ Ⓝ	Ⓨ Ⓝ	Ⓨ Ⓝ
Tester placed in proper position	**Test 1**	**Test 2**	**Test 3**
Facing the athlete (observing only)	Ⓨ Ⓝ	Ⓨ Ⓝ	Ⓨ Ⓝ
Tester performs test according to accepted guidelines	**Test 1**	**Test 2**	**Test 3**
Instructs the athlete to continually open and close hand (make fist, then release)	Ⓨ Ⓝ	Ⓨ Ⓝ	Ⓨ Ⓝ
Instructs the athlete to maintain this position for 3 minutes	Ⓨ Ⓝ	Ⓨ Ⓝ	Ⓨ Ⓝ

The psychomotor skill was performed completely and in the appropriate order   **0 1 2 3 4 5**

The tester had control of the subject and the situation (showed confidence)   **0 1 2 3 4 5**

Method of performing the skill allowed the tester the ability to determine: severity, proper progression, and the *fit* in the overall picture (Oral)   **0 1 2 3 4 5**

In order for a grade of *minimum standard* to be given, the total must be ≥11   **TOTAL = _____**

```
 1    2    3    4    5    6    7    8    9   10   11   12   13   14   15
 |    |    |    |    |    |    |    |    |    |    |    |    |    |    |
```

Not Acceptable   **Meets**   **Exceeds**
                                    Minimum Standards   **Minimum Standards**

TEST ENVIRONMENTS

L: Laboratory/Classroom Testing
C: Clinical/Field Testing
P: Practicum Testing
A: Assessment/Mock Exam Testing
S: Self-Reporting

SKILL TEST INFORMATION

Positive Finding: Ischemic pain; heaviness and/or weakness
Involved Structure: Subclavian artery (indicative of thoracic outlet syndrome)
Special Considerations: N/A
Reference(s): Konin et al (2002); Magee
Supplies Needed: N/A

SPECIAL TESTS
(ST-U-Test 6)

Peer Review _____   Peer Review _____

Skill Acquisition: _____   Practice Opportunities: _____

This problem allows you the opportunity to demonstrate the special test known as the **Valsalva's Maneuver**. *You have 2 minutes to complete this task. Please inform the "room captain" when you have completed the task.*

Tester places athlete and limb in appropriate position	Test 1	Test 2	Test 3
Seated	Ⓨ Ⓝ	Ⓨ Ⓝ	Ⓨ Ⓝ
Tester placed in proper position	**Test 1**	**Test 2**	**Test 3**
Facing the athlete (observing only)	Ⓨ Ⓝ	Ⓨ Ⓝ	Ⓨ Ⓝ
Tester performs test according to accepted guidelines	**Test 1**	**Test 2**	**Test 3**
Instructs the athlete to take a deep breath and hold throughout	Ⓨ Ⓝ	Ⓨ Ⓝ	Ⓨ Ⓝ
Instructs the athlete to bear down (as if having a bowel movement)	Ⓨ Ⓝ	Ⓨ Ⓝ	Ⓨ Ⓝ

The psychomotor skill was performed completely and in the appropriate order   **0 1 2 3 4 5**

The tester had control of the subject and the situation (showed confidence)   **0 1 2 3 4 5**

Method of performing the skill allowed the tester the ability to determine: severity, proper progression, and the *fit* in the overall picture (Oral)   **0 1 2 3 4 5**

In order for a grade of *minimum standard* to be given, the total must be ≥11   **TOTAL = _____**

```
 1    2    3    4    5    6    7    8    9   10   11   12   13   14   15
 |----|----|----|----|----|----|----|----|----|----|----|----|----|----|
```

Not Acceptable   **Meets**   **Exceeds**
                                    Minimum Standards   **Minimum Standards**

TEST ENVIRONMENTS

L: Laboratory/Classroom Testing
C: Clinical/Field Testing
P: Practicum Testing
A: Assessment/Mock Exam Testing
S: Self-Reporting

SKILL TEST INFORMATION

Positive Finding: Increased pain
Involved Structure: Possible disc, tumor (space-occupying lesion)
Special Considerations: Results are subjective
Reference(s):   Konin et al (2002); Magee; Starkey et al (2002)
Supplies Needed: Chair

SPECIAL TESTS
(ST-U-Test 7)

Peer Review _____   Peer Review _____

Skill Acquisition: _____   Practice Opportunities: _____

Please demonstrate how you would perform the orthopedic test known as the **Speed's Test (Biceps or Straight-Arm Test)** *for the shoulder. You have 2 minutes to complete this task.*

Tester places athlete and limb in appropriate position	Test 1	Test 2	Test 3
Seated or standing	Ⓨ Ⓝ	Ⓨ Ⓝ	Ⓨ Ⓝ
Shoulder/elbow placed in anatomical position	Ⓨ Ⓝ	Ⓨ Ⓝ	Ⓨ Ⓝ
Tester placed in proper position	**Test 1**	**Test 2**	**Test 3**
Stands to the side, facing the athlete	Ⓨ Ⓝ	Ⓨ Ⓝ	Ⓨ Ⓝ
Places one finger on the bicipital groove	Ⓨ Ⓝ	Ⓨ Ⓝ	Ⓨ Ⓝ
Places the other hand on the distal portion of the wrist	Ⓨ Ⓝ	Ⓨ Ⓝ	Ⓨ Ⓝ
Tester performs test according to accepted guidelines	**Test 1**	**Test 2**	**Test 3**
Resists flexion of the shoulder to 90 degrees	Ⓨ Ⓝ	Ⓨ Ⓝ	Ⓨ Ⓝ
Palpates the biceps tendon (bicipital groove)	Ⓨ Ⓝ	Ⓨ Ⓝ	Ⓨ Ⓝ
Performs break test (90 degrees of shoulder flexion)	Ⓨ Ⓝ	Ⓨ Ⓝ	Ⓨ Ⓝ
Performs assessment bilaterally	Ⓨ Ⓝ	Ⓨ Ⓝ	Ⓨ Ⓝ

The psychomotor skill was performed completely and in the appropriate order   0 1 2 3 4 5

The tester had control of the subject and the situation (showed confidence)   0 1 2 3 4 5

Method of performing the skill allowed the tester the ability to determine:
severity, proper progression, and the *fit* in the overall picture (Oral)   0 1 2 3 4 5

In order for a grade of *minimum standard* to be given, the total must be ≥11   TOTAL = _____

```
  1    2    3    4    5    6    7    8    9   10   11   12   13   14   15
  |____|____|____|____|____|____|____|____|____|____|____|____|____|____|
```

Not Acceptable   **Meets**   **Exceeds**
                          Minimum Standards   **Minimum Standards**

TEST ENVIRONMENTS

L: Laboratory/Classroom Testing
C: Clinical/Field Testing
P: Practicum Testing
A: Assessment/Mock Exam Testing
S: Self-Reporting

SKILL TEST INFORMATION

Positive Finding: Pain/tenderness (bicipital groove)
Involved Structure: Long head of the biceps brachii
Special Considerations: N/A
Reference(s): Konin et al (2002); Magee; Starkey et al (2002)
Supplies Needed: N/A

SPECIAL TESTS
(ST-U-Test 8)

Peer Review _____   Peer Review _____

Skill Acquisition: _____   Practice Opportunities: _____

*Please demonstrate how you would perform the orthopedic test known as the **Yergason's Test** for the shoulder. You have 2 minutes to complete this task.*

Tester places athlete and limb in appropriate position	Test 1	Test 2	Test 3
Seated or standing	Ⓨ Ⓝ	Ⓨ Ⓝ	Ⓨ Ⓝ
Elbow flexed to 90 degrees (stabilized against the side of the body)	Ⓨ Ⓝ	Ⓨ Ⓝ	Ⓨ Ⓝ
Forearm fully pronated	Ⓨ Ⓝ	Ⓨ Ⓝ	Ⓨ Ⓝ
Tester placed in proper position	**Test 1**	**Test 2**	**Test 3**
Stands to the side, facing the athlete	Ⓨ Ⓝ	Ⓨ Ⓝ	Ⓨ Ⓝ
Places one finger over the bicipital groove	Ⓨ Ⓝ	Ⓨ Ⓝ	Ⓨ Ⓝ
Places the other hand around the distal portion of the wrist	Ⓨ Ⓝ	Ⓨ Ⓝ	Ⓨ Ⓝ
Tester performs test according to accepted guidelines	**Test 1**	**Test 2**	**Test 3**
Resists supination of the forearm through full range of motion	Ⓨ Ⓝ	Ⓨ Ⓝ	Ⓨ Ⓝ
Resists external rotation of the shoulder through full range of motion	Ⓨ Ⓝ	Ⓨ Ⓝ	Ⓨ Ⓝ
Palpates the biceps tendon bicipital groove (gently)	Ⓨ Ⓝ	Ⓨ Ⓝ	Ⓨ Ⓝ
Performs assessment bilaterally	Ⓨ Ⓝ	Ⓨ Ⓝ	Ⓨ Ⓝ

The psychomotor skill was performed completely and in the appropriate order   **0 1 2 3 4 5**

The tester had control of the subject and the situation (showed confidence)   **0 1 2 3 4 5**

Method of performing the skill allowed the tester the ability to determine:
severity, proper progression, and the *fit* in the overall picture (Oral)   **0 1 2 3 4 5**

In order for a grade of *minimum standard* to be given, the total must be ≥11   **TOTAL = _____**

| 1 | 2 | 3 | 4 | 5 | 6 | 7 | 8 | 9 | 10 | 11 | 12 | 13 | 14 | 15 |

Not Acceptable   **Meets**   **Exceeds**
                                     Minimum Standards   **Minimum Standards**

TEST ENVIRONMENTS

L: Laboratory/Classroom Testing
C: Clinical/Field Testing
P: Practicum Testing
A: Assessment/Mock Exam Testing
S: Self-Reporting

SKILL TEST INFORMATION

Positive Finding: Pain and/or snapping; biceps tendon popping out of the bicipital groove

Involved Structure: Biceps tendon, transverse humeral ligament

Special Considerations: N/A

Reference(s): Hoppenfeld; Konin et al (2002); Magee; Starkey et al (2002)

Supplies Needed: Chair

SPECIAL TESTS
(ST-U-Test 9)

Peer Review _____ Peer Review _____

Skill Acquisition: _____   Practice Opportunities: _____

*This problem allows you the opportunity to demonstrate the **Hawkins-Kennedy Test for Impingement** of the shoulder. You have 2 minutes to complete this task.*

Tester places athlete and limb in appropriate position	Test 1	Test 2	Test 3
Seated or standing	Ⓨ Ⓝ	Ⓨ Ⓝ	Ⓨ Ⓝ
Shoulder horizontally flexed to 90 degrees (forward flexion)	Ⓨ Ⓝ	Ⓨ Ⓝ	Ⓨ Ⓝ
Elbow flexed to 90 degrees	Ⓨ Ⓝ	Ⓨ Ⓝ	Ⓨ Ⓝ
Forearm fully pronated (palm facing the floor)	Ⓨ Ⓝ	Ⓨ Ⓝ	Ⓨ Ⓝ
Tester placed in proper position	**Test 1**	**Test 2**	**Test 3**
Stands in front, facing the athlete	Ⓨ Ⓝ	Ⓨ Ⓝ	Ⓨ Ⓝ
Places one hand under the elbow	Ⓨ Ⓝ	Ⓨ Ⓝ	Ⓨ Ⓝ
Places the other hand over the distal portion of the wrist	Ⓨ Ⓝ	Ⓨ Ⓝ	Ⓨ Ⓝ
Tester performs test according to accepted guidelines	**Test 1**	**Test 2**	**Test 3**
Maintains relaxation of the limb	Ⓨ Ⓝ	Ⓨ Ⓝ	Ⓨ Ⓝ
Maintains horizontally flexed position (may move into a greater forward flexed position)	Ⓨ Ⓝ	Ⓨ Ⓝ	Ⓨ Ⓝ
Passively, internally rotates the shoulder	Ⓨ Ⓝ	Ⓨ Ⓝ	Ⓨ Ⓝ
Performs assessment bilaterally	Ⓨ Ⓝ	Ⓨ Ⓝ	Ⓨ Ⓝ

The psychomotor skill was performed completely and in the appropriate order   0 1 2 3 4 5

The tester had control of the subject and the situation (showed confidence)   0 1 2 3 4 5

Method of performing the skill allowed the tester the ability to determine:
severity, proper progression, and the *fit* in the overall picture (Oral)   0 1 2 3 4 5

In order for a grade of *minimum standard* to be given, the total must be ≥11   TOTAL = _____

```
 1    2    3    4    5    6    7    8    9   10   11   12   13   14   15
 |    |    |    |    |    |    |    |    |    |    |    |    |    |    |
```

Not Acceptable   **Meets**   **Exceeds**
                          Minimum Standards   **Minimum Standards**

TEST ENVIRONMENTS

L: Laboratory/Classroom Testing
C: Clinical/Field Testing
P: Practicum Testing
A: Assessment/Mock Exam Testing
S: Self-Reporting

SKILL TEST INFORMATION

Positive Finding: Pain
Involved Structure: Supraspinatus tendon
Special Considerations: N/A
Reference(s): Konin et al (2002); Magee; Starkey et al (2002)
Supplies Needed: N/A

SPECIAL TESTS
(ST-U-Test 10)

Peer Review _____ Peer Review _____

Skill Acquisition: _____   Practice Opportunities: _____

This problem allows you the opportunity to demonstrate the **Neer Impingement Test (Shoulder Impingement Test)** *of the shoulder. You have 2 minutes to complete this task.'*

Tester places athlete and limb in appropriate position	Test 1	Test 2	Test 3
Standing or seated	Ⓨ Ⓝ	Ⓨ Ⓝ	Ⓨ Ⓝ
Arms placed at athlete's side	Ⓨ Ⓝ	Ⓨ Ⓝ	Ⓨ Ⓝ
Shoulder internally rotated, elbow pronated	Ⓨ Ⓝ	Ⓨ Ⓝ	Ⓨ Ⓝ
Tester placed in proper position	**Test 1**	**Test 2**	**Test 3**
Stands to the side, facing the athlete	Ⓨ Ⓝ	Ⓨ Ⓝ	Ⓨ Ⓝ
Places one hand against the scapula	Ⓨ Ⓝ	Ⓨ Ⓝ	Ⓨ Ⓝ
Places the other hand under the elbow (supporting the arm)	Ⓨ Ⓝ	Ⓨ Ⓝ	Ⓨ Ⓝ
Tester performs test according to accepted guidelines	**Test 1**	**Test 2**	**Test 3**
Maintains relaxation of the limb	Ⓨ Ⓝ	Ⓨ Ⓝ	Ⓨ Ⓝ
Pushes/jams the greater tuberosity into the border of the acromion	Ⓨ Ⓝ	Ⓨ Ⓝ	Ⓨ Ⓝ
Passively flexes the shoulder through a full range of motion	Ⓨ Ⓝ	Ⓨ Ⓝ	Ⓨ Ⓝ
Performs assessment bilaterally	Ⓨ Ⓝ	Ⓨ Ⓝ	Ⓨ Ⓝ

The psychomotor skill was performed completely and in the appropriate order   **0 1 2 3 4 5**

The tester had control of the subject and the situation (showed confidence)   **0 1 2 3 4 5**

Method of performing the skill allowed the tester the ability to determine:
severity, proper progression, and the *fit* in the overall picture (Oral)   **0 1 2 3 4 5**

In order for a grade of *minimum standard* to be given, the total must be ≥11   **TOTAL = _____**

```
  1     2     3     4     5     6     7     8     9    10    11    12    13    14    15
  |     |     |     |     |     |     |     |     |     |     |     |     |     |     |
```
Not Acceptable   **Meets**   **Exceeds**
                                          Minimum Standards   **Minimum Standards**

TEST ENVIRONMENTS

L: Laboratory/Classroom Testing
C: Clinical/Field Testing
P: Practicum Testing
A: Assessment/Mock Exam Testing
S: Self-Reporting

SKILL TEST INFORMATION

Positive Finding:	Pain with movement
Involved Structure:	Supraspinatus; biceps long head tendon
Special Considerations:	N/A
Reference(s):	Konin et al (2002); Magee; Starkey et al (2002)
Supplies Needed:	N/A

SPECIAL TESTS
(ST-U-Test 11)

Peer Review _____ Peer Review _____

Skill Acquisition: _____   Practice Opportunities: _____

This problem allows you the opportunity to demonstrate the **Drop Arm Test (Codman's Test)** *to help rule out rotator cuff pathology. You have 2 minutes to complete this task.*

Tester places athlete and limb in appropriate position	Test 1	Test 2	Test 3
Seated or standing	Ⓨ Ⓝ	Ⓨ Ⓝ	Ⓨ Ⓝ
Arms placed at athlete's side	Ⓨ Ⓝ	Ⓨ Ⓝ	Ⓨ Ⓝ
Shoulder internally rotated, elbow pronated	Ⓨ Ⓝ	Ⓨ Ⓝ	Ⓨ Ⓝ

Tester placed in proper position	Test 1	Test 2	Test 3
Stands in front, facing the athlete (may stand behind the athlete)	Ⓨ Ⓝ	Ⓨ Ⓝ	Ⓨ Ⓝ
Places one hand under the wrist	Ⓨ Ⓝ	Ⓨ Ⓝ	Ⓨ Ⓝ

Tester performs test according to accepted guidelines	Test 1	Test 2	Test 3
Passively abducts the shoulder to 90 degrees, then releases arm	Ⓨ Ⓝ	Ⓨ Ⓝ	Ⓨ Ⓝ
Asks athlete to slowly lower the arm to the side (adduction)	Ⓨ Ⓝ	Ⓨ Ⓝ	Ⓨ Ⓝ
Performs assessment bilaterally	Ⓨ Ⓝ	Ⓨ Ⓝ	Ⓨ Ⓝ

The psychomotor skill was performed completely and in the appropriate order   **0 1 2 3 4 5**

The tester had control of the subject and the situation (showed confidence)   **0 1 2 3 4 5**

Method of performing the skill allowed the tester the ability to determine:
severity, proper progression, and the *fit* in the overall picture (Oral)   **0 1 2 3 4 5**

In order for a grade of *minimum standard* to be given, the total must be ≥11   **TOTAL = _____**

```
 1    2    3    4    5    6    7    8    9   10   11   12   13   14   15
 |    |    |    |    |    |    |    |    |    |    |    |    |    |    |
```
Not Acceptable   **Meets**   **Exceeds**
                                    Minimum Standards   **Minimum Standards**

TEST ENVIRONMENTS

L: Laboratory/Classroom Testing
C: Clinical/Field Testing
P: Practicum Testing
A: Assessment/Mock Exam Testing
S: Self-Reporting

SKILL TEST INFORMATION

Positive Finding:	Inability to slowly return the arm to the side
Involved Structure:	Rotator cuff
Special Considerations:	N/A
Reference(s):	Konin et al (2002); Magee; Starkey et al (2002)
Supplies Needed:	N/A

Special Tests
(ST-U-Test 12)

Peer Review _____ Peer Review _____

Skill Acquisition: _____   Practice Opportunities: _____

This problem allows you the opportunity to demonstrate the **Pectoralis Major Contracture Test** *in order to determine muscle flexibility. You have 2 minutes to complete this task.*

Tester places athlete and limb in appropriate position	Test 1	Test 2	Test 3
Supine	Ⓨ Ⓝ	Ⓨ Ⓝ	Ⓨ Ⓝ
Athletes clasps both hands behind the head fingers interlocked	Ⓨ Ⓝ	Ⓨ Ⓝ	Ⓨ Ⓝ
Tester placed in proper position	**Test 1**	**Test 2**	**Test 3**
Stands behind the athlete's head	Ⓨ Ⓝ	Ⓨ Ⓝ	Ⓨ Ⓝ
Tester performs test according to accepted guidelines	**Test 1**	**Test 2**	**Test 3**
Asks the athlete to relax arms	Ⓨ Ⓝ	Ⓨ Ⓝ	Ⓨ Ⓝ
Passively forces the elbows to the table (hyperextension of the shoulder)	Ⓨ Ⓝ	Ⓨ Ⓝ	Ⓨ Ⓝ

The psychomotor skill was performed completely and in the appropriate order   **0 1 2 3 4 5**

The tester had control of the subject and the situation (showed confidence)   **0 1 2 3 4 5**

Method of performing the skill allowed the tester the ability to determine:
severity, proper progression, and the *fit* in the overall picture (Oral)   **0 1 2 3 4 5**

In order for a grade of *minimum standard* to be given, the total must be ≥11   **TOTAL = _____**

| 1 | 2 | 3 | 4 | 5 | 6 | 7 | 8 | 9 | 10 | 11 | 12 | 13 | 14 | 15 |

Not Acceptable   **Meets**   **Exceeds**
                      Minimum Standards   **Minimum Standards**

TEST ENVIRONMENTS

L: Laboratory/Classroom Testing
C: Clinical/Field Testing
P: Practicum Testing
A: Assessment/Mock Exam Testing
S: Self-Reporting

SKILL TEST INFORMATION

Positive Finding:	Elbows unable to touch the table
Involved Structure:	Pectoralis major
Special Considerations:	N/A
Reference(s):	Magee
Supplies Needed:	Table

SPECIAL TESTS
(ST-U-Test 13)

Peer Review _____ Peer Review _____

Skill Acquisition: _____   Practice Opportunities: _____

This problem allows you the opportunity to demonstrate **Apley's Scratch Tests** *in order to determine general shoulder flexibility. You have 2 minutes to complete this task.*

Tester places athlete and limb in appropriate position	Test 1	Test 2	Test 3
Seated or standing	Y N	Y N	Y N
Arms placed at athlete's side	Y N	Y N	Y N

Tester placed in proper position	Test 1	Test 2	Test 3
Facing the athlete (observing only)	Y N	Y N	Y N

Tester performs test according to accepted guidelines	Test 1	Test 2	Test 3
Instructs athlete to actively take one hand and touch opposite shoulder (front)	Y N	Y N	Y N
Instructs athlete to actively take one hand and touch opposite shoulder (behind head)	Y N	Y N	Y N
Instructs athlete to actively take one hand and reach behind and touch opposite scapula	Y N	Y N	Y N
Performs assessment bilaterally	Y N	Y N	Y N

The psychomotor skill was performed completely and in the appropriate order   **0 1 2 3 4 5**

The tester had control of the subject and the situation (showed confidence)   **0 1 2 3 4 5**

Method of performing the skill allowed the tester the ability to determine:
severity, proper progression, and the *fit* in the overall picture (Oral)   **0 1 2 3 4 5**

In order for a grade of *minimum standard* to be given, the total must be ≥11   **TOTAL = _____**

```
  1    2    3    4    5    6    7    8    9    10   11   12   13   14   15
  |    |    |    |    |    |    |    |    |    |    |    |    |    |    |
```

Not Acceptable   **Meets**   **Exceeds**
                                    Minimum Standards   **Minimum Standards**

TEST ENVIRONMENTS

L: Laboratory/Classroom Testing
C: Clinical/Field Testing
P: Practicum Testing
A: Assessment/Mock Exam Testing
S: Self-Reporting

SKILL TEST INFORMATION

Positive Finding:	Inability to touch opposite shoulder
Involved Structure:	Structures in and around the glenohumeral joint
Special Considerations:	N/A
Reference(s):	Konin; Starkey et al (2002)
Supplies Needed:	N/A

SPECIAL TESTS
(ST-U-Test 14)

Peer Review _____ Peer Review _____

Skill Acquisition: _____   Practice Opportunities: _____

This problem allows you the opportunity to demonstrate **Allen's Test** *in order to rule out thoracic outlet syndrome. You have 2 minutes to complete this task.*

Tester places athlete and limb in appropriate position	Test 1	Test 2	Test 3
Seated or standing	Y N	Y N	Y N
Shoulder abducted to 90 degrees	Y N	Y N	Y N
Shoulder externally rotated to 90 degrees	Y N	Y N	Y N
Elbow flexed to 90 degrees	Y N	Y N	Y N
Tester placed in proper position	**Test 1**	**Test 2**	**Test 3**
Stands behind the athlete	Y N	Y N	Y N
Places fingers over the radial pulse (palpate pulse)	Y N	Y N	Y N
Places the other hand under the elbow (supporting the arm)	Y N	Y N	Y N
Tester performs test according to accepted guidelines	**Test 1**	**Test 2**	**Test 3**
Instructs athlete to look away (laterally rotates toward opposite side)	Y N	Y N	Y N
Passively horizontally extends the shoulder (horizontal abduction)	Y N	Y N	Y N
Performs assessment bilaterally	Y N	Y N	Y N

The psychomotor skill was performed completely and in the appropriate order   **0 1 2 3 4 5**

The tester had control of the subject and the situation (showed confidence)   **0 1 2 3 4 5**

Method of performing the skill allowed the tester the ability to determine:
severity, proper progression, and the *fit* in the overall picture (Oral)   **0 1 2 3 4 5**

In order for a grade of *minimum standard* to be given, the total must be ≥11   **TOTAL = _____**

```
  1    2    3    4    5    6    7    8    9   10   11   12   13   14   15
  |----|----|----|----|----|----|----|----|----|----|----|----|----|----|
```

Not Acceptable   **Meets**   **Exceeds**
                              Minimum Standards   **Minimum Standards**

TEST ENVIRONMENTS

L: Laboratory/Classroom Testing
C: Clinical/Field Testing
P: Practicum Testing
A: Assessment/Mock Exam Testing
S: Self-Reporting

SKILL TEST INFORMATION

Positive Finding: Diminished or absent pulse
Involved Structure: Vascular structures, thoracic outlet syndrome
Special Considerations: N/A
Reference(s): Konin et al (2002); Magee; Starkey et al (2002)
Supplies Needed: N/A

SPECIAL TESTS
(ST-U-Test 15)

Peer Review _____ Peer Review _____

Skill Acquisition: _____ Practice Opportunities: _____

This problem allows you the opportunity to demonstrate the **Cozen's Test (Test for Lateral Epicondylitis/Tennis Elbow, Method 1/Resistive Tennis Elbow Test)** *in order to help rule out lateral epicondylitis. You have 2 minutes to complete this task.*

Tester places athlete and limb in appropriate position	Test 1	Test 2	Test 3
Seated or standing	Ⓨ Ⓝ	Ⓨ Ⓝ	Ⓨ Ⓝ
Elbow flexed to 90 degrees	Ⓨ Ⓝ	Ⓨ Ⓝ	Ⓨ Ⓝ
Forearm/elbow placed in full pronation	Ⓨ Ⓝ	Ⓨ Ⓝ	Ⓨ Ⓝ
Fingers flexed (make into a fist)	Ⓨ Ⓝ	Ⓨ Ⓝ	Ⓨ Ⓝ
Tester placed in proper position	**Test 1**	**Test 2**	**Test 3**
Stands in front, facing the athlete	Ⓨ Ⓝ	Ⓨ Ⓝ	Ⓨ Ⓝ
Places hand around the wrist	Ⓨ Ⓝ	Ⓨ Ⓝ	Ⓨ Ⓝ
Places the other hand under the elbow supporting the arm (palpating lateral epicondyle)	Ⓨ Ⓝ	Ⓨ Ⓝ	Ⓨ Ⓝ
Tester performs test according to accepted guidelines	**Test 1**	**Test 2**	**Test 3**
Resists wrist extension through a full range of motion	Ⓨ Ⓝ	Ⓨ Ⓝ	Ⓨ Ⓝ
Resists radial deviation through a full range of motion	Ⓨ Ⓝ	Ⓨ Ⓝ	Ⓨ Ⓝ
Performs assessment bilaterally	Ⓨ Ⓝ	Ⓨ Ⓝ	Ⓨ Ⓝ

The psychomotor skill was performed completely and in the appropriate order   **0 1 2 3 4 5**

The tester had control of the subject and the situation (showed confidence)   **0 1 2 3 4 5**

Method of performing the skill allowed the tester the ability to determine:
severity, proper progression, and the *fit* in the overall picture (Oral)   **0 1 2 3 4 5**

In order for a grade of *minimum standard* to be given, the total must be ≥11   **TOTAL = _____**

```
 1    2    3    4    5    6    7    8    9   10   11   12   13   14   15
 |    |    |    |    |    |    |    |    |    |    |    |    |    |    |
```
Not Acceptable   **Meets**   **Exceeds**
                                    Minimum Standards   **Minimum Standards**

TEST ENVIRONMENTS

L: Laboratory/Classroom Testing
C: Clinical/Field Testing
P: Practicum Testing
A: Assessment/Mock Exam Testing
S: Self-Reporting

SKILL TEST INFORMATION

Positive Finding: Pain (sudden)
Involved Structure: Lateral epicondyle (epicondylitis)
Special Considerations: May also resist pronation
Reference(s): Konin et al (2002); Magee; Starkey et al (2002)
Supplies Needed: N/A

SPECIAL TESTS
(ST-U-Test 16)

Peer Review _____ Peer Review _____

Skill Acquisition: _____   Practice Opportunities: _____

This problem allows you the opportunity to demonstrate the **Golfer's Elbow Test (Test for Medial Epicondylitis)** *in order to help rule out medial epicondylitis. You have 2 minutes to complete this task.*

Tester places athlete and limb in appropriate position	Test 1	Test 2	Test 3
Seated or standing	Y N	Y N	Y N
Elbow flexed to 90 degrees	Y N	Y N	Y N
Forearm/elbow placed in full pronation	Y N	Y N	Y N
Fingers flexed (make into a fist)	Y N	Y N	Y N
Tester placed in proper position	**Test 1**	**Test 2**	**Test 3**
Stands in front, facing the athlete	Y N	Y N	Y N
Places hand around the wrist	Y N	Y N	Y N
Places the other hand under the elbow supporting the arm (palpating medial epicondyle)	Y N	Y N	Y N
Tester performs test according to accepted guidelines	**Test 1**	**Test 2**	**Test 3**
Passively supinates the forearm through a full range of motion	Y N	Y N	Y N
Passively extend the elbow through a full range of motion	Y N	Y N	Y N
Passively extend the wrist through a full range of motion	Y N	Y N	Y N
Performs assessment bilaterally	Y N	Y N	Y N

The psychomotor skill was performed completely and in the appropriate order   **0 1 2 3 4 5**

The tester had control of the subject and the situation (showed confidence)   **0 1 2 3 4 5**

Method of performing the skill allowed the tester the ability to determine:
severity, proper progression, and the *fit* in the overall picture (Oral)   **0 1 2 3 4 5**

In order for a grade of *minimum standard* to be given, the total must be ≥11   **TOTAL = _____**

```
  1    2    3    4    5    6    7    8    9   10   11   12   13   14   15
  |    |    |    |    |    |    |    |    |    |    |    |    |    |    |
```

Not Acceptable   **Meets**   **Exceeds**
                              Minimum Standards   **Minimum Standards**

TEST ENVIRONMENTS

L: Laboratory/Classroom Testing
C: Clinical/Field Testing
P: Practicum Testing
A: Assessment/Mock Exam Testing
S: Self-Reporting

SKILL TEST INFORMATION

Positive Finding:	Pain
Involved Structure:	Medial epicondyle (epicondylitis)
Special Considerations:	N/A
Reference(s):	Magee
Supplies Needed:	N/A

SPECIAL TESTS
(ST-U-Test 17)

Peer Review _____ Peer Review _____

Skill Acquisition: _____   Practice Opportunities: _____

Please demonstrate the **Tinel's Sign** *in order to rule out a possible injury to the* **ulnar nerve (elbow)**. *You have 2 minutes to complete this task.*

Tester places athlete and limb in appropriate position	Test 1	Test 2	Test 3
Standing or seated	Y N	Y N	Y N
Elbow placed in slight flexion	Y N	Y N	Y N
Tester placed in proper position	**Test 1**	**Test 2**	**Test 3**
Stands in front, facing the athlete	Y N	Y N	Y N
Places hand around the wrist supporting the arm	Y N	Y N	Y N
Places the other hand against the medial aspect of the elbow	Y N	Y N	Y N
Tester performs test according to accepted guidelines	**Test 1**	**Test 2**	**Test 3**
Applies pressure (tapping motion) over the ulnar nerve (between the olecranon process and medial epicondyle)	Y N	Y N	Y N
Performs assessment bilaterally	Y N	Y N	Y N

The psychomotor skill was performed completely and in the appropriate order   **0 1 2 3 4 5**

The tester had control of the subject and the situation (showed confidence)   **0 1 2 3 4 5**

Method of performing the skill allowed the tester the ability to determine:
severity, proper progression, and the *fit* in the overall picture (Oral)   **0 1 2 3 4 5**

In order for a grade of *minimum standard* to be given, the total must be ≥11   **TOTAL = _____**

```
 1    2    3    4    5    6    7    8    9   10   11   12   13   14   15
 |----|----|----|----|----|----|----|----|----|----|----|----|----|----|
```

Not Acceptable   **Meets**   **Exceeds**
                                    Minimum Standards   **Minimum Standards**

TEST ENVIRONMENTS

L: Laboratory/Classroom Testing
C: Clinical/Field Testing
P: Practicum Testing
A: Assessment/Mock Exam Testing
S: Self-Reporting

SKILL TEST INFORMATION

Positive Finding: Tingling/pain
Involved Structure: Ulnar nerve
Special Considerations: N/A
Reference(s): Konin et al (2002); Magee
Supplies Needed: N/A

Special Tests
(ST-U-Test 18)

Peer Review _____ Peer Review _____

Skill Acquisition: _____   Practice Opportunities: _____

This problem allows you the opportunity to demonstrate the **Pinch Grip Test** *in order to help rule out injury to the anterior interosseous nerve. You have 2 minutes to complete this task.*

Tester places athlete and limb in appropriate position	Test 1	Test 2	Test 3
Seated or standing	Ⓨ Ⓝ	Ⓨ Ⓝ	Ⓨ Ⓝ
Tester placed in proper position	**Test 1**	**Test 2**	**Test 3**
Facing the athlete (observing only)	Ⓨ Ⓝ	Ⓨ Ⓝ	Ⓨ Ⓝ
Tester performs test according to accepted guidelines	**Test 1**	**Test 2**	**Test 3**
Instructs the athlete to pinch the tips of the thumb and index finger together (tip-to-tip pinch)	Ⓨ Ⓝ	Ⓨ Ⓝ	Ⓨ Ⓝ
Performs assessment bilaterally	Ⓨ Ⓝ	Ⓨ Ⓝ	Ⓨ Ⓝ

The psychomotor skill was performed completely and in the appropriate order   **0 1 2 3 4 5**

The tester had control of the subject and the situation (showed confidence)   **0 1 2 3 4 5**

Method of performing the skill allowed the tester the ability to determine:
severity, proper progression, and the *fit* in the overall picture (Oral)   **0 1 2 3 4 5**

In order for a grade of *minimum standard* to be given, the total must be ≥11   **TOTAL = _____**

| 1 | 2 | 3 | 4 | 5 | 6 | 7 | 8 | 9 | 10 | 11 | 12 | 13 | 14 | 15 |

Not Acceptable   **Meets**   **Exceeds**
                         Minimum Standards   **Minimum Standards**

TEST ENVIRONMENTS

L: Laboratory/Classroom Testing
C: Clinical/Field Testing
P: Practicum Testing
A: Assessment/Mock Exam Testing
S: Self-Reporting

SKILL TEST INFORMATION

Positive Finding: Inability to touch tips together
Involved Structure: Anterior interosseous nerve (branch of the median nerve)
Special Considerations: N/A
Reference(s): Konin et al (2002); Magee
Supplies Needed: N/A

Special Tests
(ST-U-Test 19)

Peer Review _____ Peer Review _____

Skill Acquisition: _____   Practice Opportunities: _____

This problem allows you the opportunity to demonstrate **Finkelstein's Test** *in order to help rule out de Quervain's disease or Hoffmann's disease. You have 2 minutes to complete this task.*

Tester places athlete and limb in appropriate position	Test 1	Test 2	Test 3
Standing or seated	Y N	Y N	Y N
Athlete is asked to form a fist around the thumb (fist with thumb inside)	Y N	Y N	Y N
Tester placed in proper position	**Test 1**	**Test 2**	**Test 3**
Stands in front, facing the athlete	Y N	Y N	Y N
Places hand under the forearm supporting the arm	Y N	Y N	Y N
Places the other hand around the fist	Y N	Y N	Y N
Tester performs test according to accepted guidelines	**Test 1**	**Test 2**	**Test 3**
Maintains relaxation of the involved limb	Y N	Y N	Y N
Passively deviates the wrist toward the ulna (ulnar deviation)	Y N	Y N	Y N
Performs assessment bilaterally	Y N	Y N	Y N

The psychomotor skill was performed completely and in the appropriate order   0 1 2 3 4 5

The tester had control of the subject and the situation (showed confidence)   0 1 2 3 4 5

Method of performing the skill allowed the tester the ability to determine:
severity, proper progression, and the *fit* in the overall picture (Oral)   0 1 2 3 4 5

In order for a grade of *minimum standard* to be given, the total must be ≥11   **TOTAL = _____**

```
   1    2    3    4    5    6    7    8    9    10   11   12   13   14   15
   |    |    |    |    |    |    |    |    |    |    |    |    |    |    |
```
Not Acceptable   **Meets**   **Exceeds**
                                            Minimum Standards   **Minimum Standards**

TEST ENVIRONMENTS
L: Laboratory/Classroom Testing
C: Clinical/Field Testing
P: Practicum Testing
A: Assessment/Mock Exam Testing
S: Self-Reporting

SKILL TEST INFORMATION
Positive Finding: Pain
Involved Structure: Abductor pollicis longus, extensor pollicis brevis
Special Considerations: N/A
Reference(s): Konin et al (2002); Magee; Starkey et al (2002)
Supplies Needed: N/A

SPECIAL TESTS
(ST-U-Test 20)

Peer Review _____ Peer Review _____

Skill Acquisition: _____   Practice Opportunities: _____

Please demonstrate the **Tinel's Sign** *in order to rule out a possible injury to the* **median nerve (wrist)** *such as carpal tunnel syndrome). You have 2 minutes to complete this task.*

Tester places athlete and limb in appropriate position	Test 1	Test 2	Test 3
Seated	Y N	Y N	Y N
Elbow flexed to approximately 90 degrees	Y N	Y N	Y N
Forearm placed in full supination (palm up)	Y N	Y N	Y N
Forearm resting on the table (supporting surface)	Y N	Y N	Y N
Tester placed in proper position	**Test 1**	**Test 2**	**Test 3**
Sits to the involved side, facing the athlete	Y N	Y N	Y N
Places one hand over the middle portion of the forearm	Y N	Y N	Y N
Places the other hand over the carpal tunnel area	Y N	Y N	Y N
Tester performs test according to accepted guidelines	**Test 1**	**Test 2**	**Test 3**
Applies pressure (tapping motion) over the carpal tunnel area (distal forearm)	Y N	Y N	Y N
Performs assessment bilaterally	Y N	Y N	Y N

The psychomotor skill was performed completely and in the appropriate order   0 1 2 3 4 5

The tester had control of the subject and the situation (showed confidence)   0 1 2 3 4 5

Method of performing the skill allowed the tester the ability to determine:
severity, proper progression, and the *fit* in the overall picture (Oral)   0 1 2 3 4 5

In order for a grade of *minimum standard* to be given, the total must be ≥11   TOTAL = _____

```
  1     2     3     4     5     6     7     8     9    10    11    12    13    14    15
  |     |     |     |     |     |     |     |     |     |     |     |     |     |     |
```
  Not Acceptable   **Meets**   **Exceeds**
                                       Minimum Standards   **Minimum Standards**

TEST ENVIRONMENTS	**SKILL TEST INFORMATION**

TEST ENVIRONMENTS

L: Laboratory/Classroom Testing
C: Clinical/Field Testing
P: Practicum Testing
A: Assessment/Mock Exam Testing
S: Self-Reporting

SKILL TEST INFORMATION

Positive Finding: Tingling and pain
Involved Structure: Median nerve
Special Considerations: N/A
Reference(s): Konin et al (2002); Magee
Supplies Needed: Chair/table

Special Tests
(ST-U-Test 21)

Peer Review _____ Peer Review _____

Skill Acquisition: _____   Practice Opportunities: _____

This problem allows you the opportunity to demonstrate **Phalen's Test (Wrist Flexion Test)** *for the wrist. You have 3 minutes to perform this task.*

Tester places athlete and limb in appropriate position	Test 1	Test 2	Test 3
Standing or seated	Ⓨ Ⓝ	Ⓨ Ⓝ	Ⓨ Ⓝ
Shoulders, elbows, and wrists flexed to 90 degrees	Ⓨ Ⓝ	Ⓨ Ⓝ	Ⓨ Ⓝ
Dorsal aspect of both hands are in complete contact	Ⓨ Ⓝ	Ⓨ Ⓝ	Ⓨ Ⓝ
Tester placed in proper position	**Test 1**	**Test 2**	**Test 3**
Stands in front, facing the athlete	Ⓨ Ⓝ	Ⓨ Ⓝ	Ⓨ Ⓝ
Places hand around one wrist	Ⓨ Ⓝ	Ⓨ Ⓝ	Ⓨ Ⓝ
Places the other hand around the other wrist	Ⓨ Ⓝ	Ⓨ Ⓝ	Ⓨ Ⓝ
Tester performs test according to accepted guidelines	**Test 1**	**Test 2**	**Test 3**
Applies steady compressive force inward (pushes wrist together)	Ⓨ Ⓝ	Ⓨ Ⓝ	Ⓨ Ⓝ
Holds compression for 1 minute	Ⓨ Ⓝ	Ⓨ Ⓝ	Ⓨ Ⓝ

The psychomotor skill was performed completely and in the appropriate order   **0 1 2 3 4 5**

The tester had control of the subject and the situation (showed confidence)   **0 1 2 3 4 5**

Method of performing the skill allowed the tester the ability to determine:
severity, proper progression, and the *fit* in the overall picture (Oral)   **0 1 2 3 4 5**

In order for a grade of *minimum standard* to be given, the total must be ≥11   **TOTAL = _____**

```
  1    2    3    4    5    6    7    8    9   10   11   12   13   14   15
  |    |    |    |    |    |    |    |    |    |    |    |    |    |    |
```

Not Acceptable   **Meets**   **Exceeds**
                            Minimum Standards   **Minimum Standards**

TEST ENVIRONMENTS

L: Laboratory/Classroom Testing
C: Clinical/Field Testing
P: Practicum Testing
A: Assessment/Mock Exam Testing
S: Self-Reporting

SKILL TEST INFORMATION

Positive Finding: Tingling and/or numbness
Involved Structure: Median nerve, carpal tunnel syndrome
Special Considerations: N/A
Reference(s): Konin et al (2002); Magee; Starkey et al (2002)
Supplies Needed: N/A

Special Tests
(ST-U-Test 22)

Peer Review _____ Peer Review _____

Skill Acquisition: _____   Practice Opportunities: _____

This problem allows you the opportunity to demonstrate the **Foraminal Compression Test (Spurling's Test/ Cervical Compression Test)** *in order to confirm pressure on a nerve root. You have 3 minutes to perform this task. Please inform the examiner when you have completed the task.*

Tester places athlete and limb in appropriate position	Test 1	Test 2	Test 3
Seated	Ⓨ Ⓝ	Ⓨ Ⓝ	Ⓨ Ⓝ
Stage 1: Head is placed in a neutral position (cervical compression test)	Ⓨ Ⓝ	Ⓨ Ⓝ	Ⓨ Ⓝ
Stage 2: Head is placed in a slightly extended position	Ⓨ Ⓝ	Ⓨ Ⓝ	Ⓨ Ⓝ
Stage 3: Head is placed in a slightly extended position and laterally flexes to the involved side (Spurling's test)	Ⓨ Ⓝ	Ⓨ Ⓝ	Ⓨ Ⓝ
Tester placed in proper position	**Test 1**	**Test 2**	**Test 3**
Stands behind the athlete	Ⓨ Ⓝ	Ⓨ Ⓝ	Ⓨ Ⓝ
Places both hands on top of the head (fingers interlocked)	Ⓨ Ⓝ	Ⓨ Ⓝ	Ⓨ Ⓝ
Tester performs test according to accepted guidelines	**Test 1**	**Test 2**	**Test 3**
Maintains relaxation of the head	Ⓨ Ⓝ	Ⓨ Ⓝ	Ⓨ Ⓝ
Applies a compressive force downward: Stage 1, Stage 2, Stage 3	Ⓨ Ⓝ	Ⓨ Ⓝ	Ⓨ Ⓝ

The psychomotor skill was performed completely and in the appropriate order   **0 1 2 3 4 5**

The tester had control of the subject and the situation (showed confidence)   **0 1 2 3 4 5**

Method of performing the skill allowed the tester the ability to determine:
severity, proper progression, and the *fit* in the overall picture (Oral)   **0 1 2 3 4 5**

In order for a grade of *minimum standard* to be given, the total must be ≥11   **TOTAL = _____**

1	2	3	4	5	6	7	8	9	10	11	12	13	14	15

Not Acceptable   **Meets**   **Exceeds**
                      Minimum Standards   **Minimum Standards**

TEST ENVIRONMENTS

L: Laboratory/Classroom Testing
C: Clinical/Field Testing
P: Practicum Testing
A: Assessment/Mock Exam Testing
S: Self-Reporting

SKILL TEST INFORMATION

Positive Finding: Radiating pain
Involved Structure: Nerve root(s)
Special Considerations: Several medical conditions warrant precautions when applying pressure
Reference(s): Konin et al (2002); Magee; Starkey et al (2002)
Supplies Needed: Chair

SPECIAL TESTS
(ST-U-Test 23)

Peer Review _____   Peer Review _____

Skill Acquisition: _____   Practice Opportunities: _____

This problem allows you the opportunity to demonstrate the **Foraminal Distraction Test (Cervical Distraction Test)** *in order to confirm pressure on a nerve root. You have 2 minutes to perform this task. Please inform the examiner when you have completed the task.*

Tester places athlete and limb in appropriate position	Test 1	Test 2	Test 3
Seated or supine	Ⓨ Ⓝ	Ⓨ Ⓝ	Ⓨ Ⓝ
Tester placed in proper position	**Test 1**	**Test 2**	**Test 3**
Stands behind the athlete	Ⓨ Ⓝ	Ⓨ Ⓝ	Ⓨ Ⓝ
Places one hand under the athlete's chin	Ⓨ Ⓝ	Ⓨ Ⓝ	Ⓨ Ⓝ
Places the other hand against the base of the occiput	Ⓨ Ⓝ	Ⓨ Ⓝ	Ⓨ Ⓝ
Tester performs test according to accepted guidelines	**Test 1**	**Test 2**	**Test 3**
Maintains relaxation of the head	Ⓨ Ⓝ	Ⓨ Ⓝ	Ⓨ Ⓝ
Applies a distractive force upward (slowly lifts or pulls the head)	Ⓨ Ⓝ	Ⓨ Ⓝ	Ⓨ Ⓝ

The psychomotor skill was performed completely and in the appropriate order   **0 1 2 3 4 5**

The tester had control of the subject and the situation (showed confidence)   **0 1 2 3 4 5**

Method of performing the skill allowed the tester the ability to determine:
severity, proper progression, and the *fit* in the overall picture (Oral)   **0 1 2 3 4 5**

In order for a grade of *minimum standard* to be given, the total must be ≥11   **TOTAL = _____**

1	2	3	4	5	6	7	8	9	10	11	12	13	14	15

Not Acceptable   **Meets**   **Exceeds**
                                      Minimum Standards   **Minimum Standards**

TEST ENVIRONMENTS

L: Laboratory/Classroom Testing
C: Clinical/Field Testing
P: Practicum Testing
A: Assessment/Mock Exam Testing
S: Self-Reporting

SKILL TEST INFORMATION

Positive Finding: Pain decreases
Involved Structure: Nerve root
Special Considerations: Distraction should not be performed if there are any signs of instability
Reference(s): Konin et al (2002); Magee; Starkey et al (2002)
Supplies Needed: Chair and/or table

Special Tests
(ST-U-Test 24)

Peer Review _____   Peer Review _____

Skill Acquisition: _____.   Practice Opportunities: _____

This problem allows you the opportunity to demonstrate the **Shoulder Abduction Test** *in order to help rule out a herniated disc or nerve root compression. You have 2 minutes to complete this task. Please inform the examiner when you have completed the task.*

Tester places athlete and limb in appropriate position	Test 1	Test 2	Test 3
Seated or standing	Ⓨ Ⓝ	Ⓨ Ⓝ	Ⓨ Ⓝ
Tester placed in proper position	**Test 1**	**Test 2**	**Test 3**
Facing the athlete (observing only)	Ⓨ Ⓝ	Ⓨ Ⓝ	Ⓨ Ⓝ
Tester performs test according to accepted guidelines	**Test 1**	**Test 2**	**Test 3**
Instructs the athlete to actively abduct the shoulder	Ⓨ Ⓝ	Ⓨ Ⓝ	Ⓨ Ⓝ
Instructs the athlete to flex elbow by placing the palm of the hand on top of the head	Ⓨ Ⓝ	Ⓨ Ⓝ	Ⓨ Ⓝ
Performs assessment bilaterally	Ⓨ Ⓝ	Ⓨ Ⓝ	Ⓨ Ⓝ

The psychomotor skill was performed completely and in the appropriate order   0 1 2 3 4 5

The tester had control of the subject and the situation (showed confidence)   0 1 2 3 4 5

Method of performing the skill allowed the tester the ability to determine:
severity, proper progression, and the *fit* in the overall picture (Oral)   0 1 2 3 4 5

In order for a grade of *minimum standard* to be given, the total must be ≥11   TOTAL = _____

| 1   2   3   4   5   6   7   8   9   10   11   12   13   14   15 |

Not Acceptable   **Meets**   **Exceeds**
                              Minimum Standards   **Minimum Standards**

TEST ENVIRONMENTS

L: Laboratory/Classroom Testing
C: Clinical/Field Testing
P: Practicum Testing
A: Assessment/Mock Exam Testing
S: Self-Reporting

SKILL TEST INFORMATION

Positive Finding: Decreased symptoms (pain)
Involved Structure: Nerve root/herniated disc
Special Considerations: N/A
Reference(s): Starkey et al (2002)
Supplies Needed: N/A

SPECIAL TESTS
(ST-U-Test 25)

Peer Review _____ Peer Review _____

Skill Acquisition: _____   Practice Opportunities: _____

This problem allows you the opportunity to demonstrate the **Brachial Plexus Tension Test (Brachial Plexus Traction Test/Shoulder Depression Test/Brachial Plexus Stretch Test)**. *You have 2 minutes to complete this task. Please inform the examiner when you have completed the task.*

Tester places athlete and limb in appropriate position	Test 1	Test 2	Test 3
Standing or seated	Ⓨ Ⓝ	Ⓨ Ⓝ	Ⓨ Ⓝ

Tester placed in proper position	Test 1	Test 2	Test 3
Stands behind the athlete	Ⓨ Ⓝ	Ⓨ Ⓝ	Ⓨ Ⓝ
Places one hand on the side of the athlete's head (involved side)	Ⓨ Ⓝ	Ⓨ Ⓝ	Ⓨ Ⓝ
Places the other hand on top of the acromioclavicular joint (involved side)	Ⓨ Ⓝ	Ⓨ Ⓝ	Ⓨ Ⓝ

Tester performs test according to accepted guidelines	Test 1	Test 2	Test 3
Maintains relaxation of the head, neck, and shoulder area	Ⓨ Ⓝ	Ⓨ Ⓝ	Ⓨ Ⓝ
Passively laterally flexes the head (away from the shoulder)	Ⓨ Ⓝ	Ⓨ Ⓝ	Ⓨ Ⓝ
Depresses the shoulder (away from the head)	Ⓨ Ⓝ	Ⓨ Ⓝ	Ⓨ Ⓝ

The psychomotor skill was performed completely and in the appropriate order   0 1 2 3 4 5

The tester had control of the subject and the situation (showed confidence)   0 1 2 3 4 5

Method of performing the skill allowed the tester the ability to determine:
severity, proper progression, and the *fit* in the overall picture (Oral)   0 1 2 3 4 5

In order for a grade of *minimum standard* to be given, the total must be ≥11   **TOTAL = _____**

```
 1    2    3    4    5    6    7    8    9    10   11   12   13   14   15
 |____|____|____|____|____|____|____|____|____|____|____|____|____|____|
```
Not Acceptable   **Meets**   **Exceeds**
                                   Minimum Standards   **Minimum Standards**

TEST ENVIRONMENTS
L: Laboratory/Classroom Testing
C: Clinical/Field Testing
P: Practicum Testing
A: Assessment/Mock Exam Testing
S: Self-Reporting

SKILL TEST INFORMATION
Positive Finding: Pain (radiating)
Involved Structure: Brachial plexus/nerve root
Special Considerations: N/A
Reference(s): Konin et al (2002); Shultz et al; Starkey et al (2002)
Supplies Needed: N/A

SPECIAL TESTS
(ST-U-Test 26)

Peer Review _____ Peer Review _____

Skill Acquisition: _____   Practice Opportunities: _____

This problem allows you the opportunity to demonstrate **Tinel's Sign for the Cervical Spine** *to help rule out problems to the brachial plexus. You have 2 minutes to complete this task. Please inform the examiner when you have completed the task.*

Tester places athlete and limb in appropriate position	Test 1	Test 2	Test 3
Seated	Ⓨ Ⓝ	Ⓨ Ⓝ	Ⓨ Ⓝ
Head slightly flexed	Ⓨ Ⓝ	Ⓨ Ⓝ	Ⓨ Ⓝ
Tester placed in proper position	**Test 1**	**Test 2**	**Test 3**
Stands behind the athlete	Ⓨ Ⓝ	Ⓨ Ⓝ	Ⓨ Ⓝ
Places one hand over the transverse processes (each of the cervical vertebra)	Ⓨ Ⓝ	Ⓨ Ⓝ	Ⓨ Ⓝ
Tester performs test according to accepted guidelines	**Test 1**	**Test 2**	**Test 3**
Applies pressure (tapping motion) over each transverse process	Ⓨ Ⓝ	Ⓨ Ⓝ	Ⓨ Ⓝ
Taps multiple vertebrae	Ⓨ Ⓝ	Ⓨ Ⓝ	Ⓨ Ⓝ
Performs assessment on both sides of the vertebrae	Ⓨ Ⓝ	Ⓨ Ⓝ	Ⓨ Ⓝ

The psychomotor skill was performed completely and in the appropriate order   0 1 2 3 4 5

The tester had control of the subject and the situation (showed confidence)   0 1 2 3 4 5

Method of performing the skill allowed the tester the ability to determine:
severity, proper progression, and the *fit* in the overall picture (Oral)   0 1 2 3 4 5

In order for a grade of *minimum standard* to be given, the total must be ≥11   TOTAL = _____

```
  1     2     3     4     5     6     7     8     9    10    11    12    13    14    15
  |     |     |     |     |     |     |     |     |     |     |     |     |     |     |
```
Not Acceptable   **Meets**   **Exceeds**
                                          Minimum Standards   **Minimum Standards**

TEST ENVIRONMENTS

L: Laboratory/Classroom Testing
C: Clinical/Field Testing
P: Practicum Testing
A: Assessment/Mock Exam Testing
S: Self-Reporting

SKILL TEST INFORMATION

Positive Finding: Pain (radiating)
Involved Structure: Brachial plexus
Special Considerations: N/A
Reference(s): Shultz et al
Supplies Needed: Chair

SPECIAL TESTS
(ST-U-Test 27)

Peer Review _____ Peer Review _____

Skill Acquisition: _____   Practice Opportunities: _____

*This problem allows you the opportunity to demonstrate the **Vertebral Artery Test**. You have 2 minutes to complete this task. Please inform the examiner when you have completed the task.*

Tester places athlete and limb in appropriate position	Test 1	Test 2	Test 3
Supine	Ⓨ Ⓝ	Ⓨ Ⓝ	Ⓨ Ⓝ
Head positioned off the table	Ⓨ Ⓝ	Ⓨ Ⓝ	Ⓨ Ⓝ
Tester placed in proper position	**Test 1**	**Test 2**	**Test 3**
Standing or seated behind the athlete (at the head)	Ⓨ Ⓝ	Ⓨ Ⓝ	Ⓨ Ⓝ
Places both hands under the occiput (holding the head)	Ⓨ Ⓝ	Ⓨ Ⓝ	Ⓨ Ⓝ
Tester performs test according to accepted guidelines	**Test 1**	**Test 2**	**Test 3**
Maintains relaxation of the head, neck, and shoulder area	Ⓨ Ⓝ	Ⓨ Ⓝ	Ⓨ Ⓝ
Passively extends and laterally flexes the head	Ⓨ Ⓝ	Ⓨ Ⓝ	Ⓨ Ⓝ
Passively laterally rotates the head	Ⓨ Ⓝ	Ⓨ Ⓝ	Ⓨ Ⓝ
Maintains the position for 30 seconds	Ⓨ Ⓝ	Ⓨ Ⓝ	Ⓨ Ⓝ
Performs assessment to the opposite side	Ⓨ Ⓝ	Ⓨ Ⓝ	Ⓨ Ⓝ

The psychomotor skill was performed completely and in the appropriate order   0 1 2 3 4 5

The tester had control of the subject and the situation (showed confidence)   0 1 2 3 4 5

Method of performing the skill allowed the tester the ability to determine:
severity, proper progression, and the *fit* in the overall picture (Oral)   0 1 2 3 4 5

In order for a grade of *minimum standard* to be given, the total must be ≥11   **TOTAL =** _____

```
 1    2    3    4    5    6    7    8    9   10   11   12   13   14   15
 |    |    |    |    |    |    |    |    |    |    |    |    |    |    |
```
Not Acceptable   **Meets**   **Exceeds**
                                         Minimum Standards   **Minimum Standards**

TEST ENVIRONMENTS

L: Laboratory/Classroom Testing
C: Clinical/Field Testing
P: Practicum Testing
A: Assessment/Mock Exam Testing
S: Self-Reporting

SKILL TEST INFORMATION

Positive Finding:	Dizziness, confusion, pupil changes
Involved Structure:	Vertebral artery
Special Considerations:	Positive test-refer to a physician
Reference(s):	Starkey et al (2002)
Supplies Needed:	Table

SPECIAL TESTS
(ST-U-Test 28)

Peer Review _____ Peer Review _____

Skill Acquisition: _____   Practice Opportunities: _____

This problem allows you the opportunity to demonstrate the **Loading Test** *in order to rule out or confirm problems at the temporo-mandibular joint. You have 2 minutes to complete this task.*

Tester places athlete and limb in appropriate position	Test 1	Test 2	Test 3
Seated	Ⓨ Ⓝ	Ⓨ Ⓝ	Ⓨ Ⓝ
Tester placed in proper position	**Test 1**	**Test 2**	**Test 3**
Places cotton roll between the molars on the uninvolved side	Ⓨ Ⓝ	Ⓨ Ⓝ	Ⓨ Ⓝ
Tester performs test according to accepted guidelines	**Test 1**	**Test 2**	**Test 3**
Instructs the athlete to bite down forcefully and/or	Ⓨ Ⓝ	Ⓨ Ⓝ	Ⓨ Ⓝ
Instructs the athlete to chew on the cotton roll	Ⓨ Ⓝ	Ⓨ Ⓝ	Ⓨ Ⓝ

The psychomotor skill was performed completely and in the appropriate order   **0 1 2 3 4 5**

The tester had control of the subject and the situation (showed confidence)   **0 1 2 3 4 5**

Method of performing the skill allowed the tester the ability to determine:
severity, proper progression, and the *fit* in the overall picture (Oral)   **0 1 2 3 4 5**

In order for a grade of *minimum standard* to be given, the total must be ≥11   **TOTAL = _____**

```
  1    2    3    4    5    6    7    8    9    10    11    12    13    14    15
  |    |    |    |    |    |    |    |    |    |    |    |    |    |    |
```
Not Acceptable   **Meets**   **Exceeds**
                                          Minimum Standards   **Minimum Standards**

<table>
<tr><td>

TEST ENVIRONMENTS

L: Laboratory/Classroom Testing
C: Clinical/Field Testing
P: Practicum Testing
A: Assessment/Mock Exam Testing
S: Self-Reporting

</td><td>

SKILL TEST INFORMATION

Positive Finding: Pain on the involved side
Involved Structure: Temporo-mandibular joint
Special Considerations: N/A
Reference(s): Konin (2002)
Supplies Needed: Chair, cotton roll

</td></tr>
</table>

SPECIAL TESTS
(ST-L-Test 1)

Peer Review _____ Peer Review _____

Skill Acquisition: _____   Practice Opportunities: _____

*This problem allows you the opportunity to demonstrate **Thompson's Test (Simmonds' Test)**. You have 2 minutes to complete this task.*

Tester places athlete and limb in appropriate position	Test 1	Test 2	Test 3
Prone with feet over the edge of the table	Ⓨ Ⓝ	Ⓨ Ⓝ	Ⓨ Ⓝ
Tester placed in proper position	**Test 1**	**Test 2**	**Test 3**
Stands to the side of the athlete	Ⓨ Ⓝ	Ⓨ Ⓝ	Ⓨ Ⓝ
Tester performs test according to accepted guidelines	**Test 1**	**Test 2**	**Test 3**
Squeezes belly of the calf muscle (gastrocnemius/soleus)	Ⓨ Ⓝ	Ⓨ Ⓝ	Ⓨ Ⓝ
Maintains relaxation of the limb	Ⓨ Ⓝ	Ⓨ Ⓝ	Ⓨ Ⓝ
Performs assessment bilaterally	Ⓨ Ⓝ	Ⓨ Ⓝ	Ⓨ Ⓝ

The psychomotor skill was performed completely and in the appropriate order   0 1 2 3 4 5

The tester had control of the subject and the situation (showed confidence)   0 1 2 3 4 5

Method of performing the skill allowed the tester the ability to determine:
severity, proper progression, and the *fit* in the overall picture (Oral)   0 1 2 3 4 5

In order for a grade of *minimum standard* to be given, the total must be ≥11   **TOTAL = _____**

```
  1    2    3    4    5    6    7    8    9    10   11   12   13   14   15
  |    |    |    |    |    |    |    |    |    |    |    |    |    |    |
```

Not Acceptable   **Meets**   **Exceeds**
                                    Minimum Standards   **Minimum Standards**

TEST ENVIRONMENTS

L: Laboratory/Classroom Testing
C: Clinical/Field Testing
P: Practicum Testing
A: Assessment/Mock Exam Testing
S: Self-Reporting

SKILL TEST INFORMATION

Positive Finding:	Foot does not plantar flex
Involved Structure:	Achilles' tendon (rupture)
Special Considerations:	N/A
Reference(s):	Konin et al (2002); Magee; Starkey et al (2002)
Supplies Needed:	Table

SPECIAL TESTS
(ST-L-Test 2)

Peer Review _____ Peer Review _____

Skill Acquisition: _____   Practice Opportunities: _____

This problem allows you the opportunity to demonstrate the **Percussion (Tap) Test** *to rule out a fracture to the* **ankle**. *You have 2 minutes to complete this task.*

Tester places athlete and limb in appropriate position	Test 1	Test 2	Test 3
Supine with foot off the table	Ⓨ Ⓝ	Ⓨ Ⓝ	Ⓨ Ⓝ
Knee placed in full extension	Ⓨ Ⓝ	Ⓨ Ⓝ	Ⓨ Ⓝ
Tester placed in proper position	**Test 1**	**Test 2**	**Test 3**
Stands to the side of the athlete	Ⓨ Ⓝ	Ⓨ Ⓝ	Ⓨ Ⓝ
Places one hand on the foot	Ⓨ Ⓝ	Ⓨ Ⓝ	Ⓨ Ⓝ
Places the other hand in position to tap the heel	Ⓨ Ⓝ	Ⓨ Ⓝ	Ⓨ Ⓝ
Tester performs test according to accepted guidelines	**Test 1**	**Test 2**	**Test 3**
Passively dorsiflexes the foot	Ⓨ Ⓝ	Ⓨ Ⓝ	Ⓨ Ⓝ
Taps firmly on the bottom of the heel (calcaneus)	Ⓨ Ⓝ	Ⓨ Ⓝ	Ⓨ Ⓝ

The psychomotor skill was performed completely and in the appropriate order   **0 1 2 3 4 5**

The tester had control of the subject and the situation (showed confidence)   **0 1 2 3 4 5**

Method of performing the skill allowed the tester the ability to determine:
severity, proper progression, and the *fit* in the overall picture (Oral)   **0 1 2 3 4 5**

In order for a grade of *minimum standard* to be given, the total must be ≥11   **TOTAL = _____**

1	2	3	4	5	6	7	8	9	10	11	12	13	14	15

Not Acceptable   **Meets**   **Exceeds**
                               Minimum Standards   **Minimum Standards**

TEST ENVIRONMENTS

L: Laboratory/Classroom Testing
C: Clinical/Field Testing
P: Practicum Testing
A: Assessment/Mock Exam Testing
S: Self-Reporting

SKILL TEST INFORMATION

Positive Finding:	Pain at the site of the injury
Involved Structure:	Bone (fracture)
Special Considerations:	Do not attempt if obvious deformity exists
Reference(s):	Konin et al (2002)
Supplies Needed:	Table

SPECIAL TESTS
(ST-L-Test 3)

Peer Review _____ Peer Review _____

Skill Acquisition: _____   Practice Opportunities: _____

*This problem allows you the opportunity to demonstrate the **Compression Test** to rule out a fracture to the **tibia**. You have 2 minutes to complete this task.*

Tester places athlete and limb in appropriate position	Test 1	Test 2	Test 3
Supine with foot off the table	Ⓨ Ⓝ	Ⓨ Ⓝ	Ⓨ Ⓝ
Knee placed in full extension	Ⓨ Ⓝ	Ⓨ Ⓝ	Ⓨ Ⓝ
Tester placed in proper position	**Test 1**	**Test 2**	**Test 3**
Stands to the side of the athlete	Ⓨ Ⓝ	Ⓨ Ⓝ	Ⓨ Ⓝ
Places both hands around the lower leg (tibia/fibula)	Ⓨ Ⓝ	Ⓨ Ⓝ	Ⓨ Ⓝ
Tester performs test according to accepted guidelines	**Test 1**	**Test 2**	**Test 3**
Squeezes the tibia and fibula together (proximal to the injury site)	Ⓨ Ⓝ	Ⓨ Ⓝ	Ⓨ Ⓝ
Squeezes the tibia and fibula together (distal to the injury site	Ⓨ Ⓝ	Ⓨ Ⓝ	Ⓨ Ⓝ

The psychomotor skill was performed completely and in the appropriate order   **0 1 2 3 4 5**

The tester had control of the subject and the situation (showed confidence)   **0 1 2 3 4 5**

Method of performing the skill allowed the tester the ability to determine:
severity, proper progression, and the *fit* in the overall picture (Oral)   **0 1 2 3 4 5**

In order for a grade of *minimum standard* to be given, the total must be ≥11   **TOTAL = _____**

```
  1    2    3    4    5    6    7    8    9   10   11   12   13   14   15
  |    |    |    |    |    |    |    |    |    |    |    |    |    |    |
```
Not Acceptable   **Meets**   **Exceeds**
                                    Minimum Standards   **Minimum Standards**

TEST ENVIRONMENTS

L: Laboratory/Classroom Testing
C: Clinical/Field Testing
P: Practicum Testing
A: Assessment/Mock Exam Testing
S: Self-Reporting

SKILL TEST INFORMATION

Positive Finding: Pain at the site of the injury
Involved Structure: Bone (fracture)
Special Considerations: Do not attempt if obvious deformity exists
Reference(s): Konin et al (2002)
Supplies Needed: Table

Special Tests
(ST-L-Test 4)

Peer Review _____ Peer Review _____

Skill Acquisition: _____   Practice Opportunities: _____

This problem allows you the opportunity to demonstrate **Homan's Sign**. *You have 2 minutes to complete this task.*

Tester places athlete and limb in appropriate position	Test 1	Test 2	Test 3
Supine	Ⓨ Ⓝ	Ⓨ Ⓝ	Ⓨ Ⓝ
Knee placed in full extension	Ⓨ Ⓝ	Ⓨ Ⓝ	Ⓨ Ⓝ
Tester placed in proper position	**Test 1**	**Test 2**	**Test 3**
Stands to the side of the athlete	Ⓨ Ⓝ	Ⓨ Ⓝ	Ⓨ Ⓝ
Places one hand over the lower leg (supporting the limb)	Ⓨ Ⓝ	Ⓨ Ⓝ	Ⓨ Ⓝ
Places the other hand on the plantar surface of the foot	Ⓨ Ⓝ	Ⓨ Ⓝ	Ⓨ Ⓝ
Tester performs test according to accepted guidelines	**Test 1**	**Test 2**	**Test 3**
Passively dorsiflexes the foot	Ⓨ Ⓝ	Ⓨ Ⓝ	Ⓨ Ⓝ
Maintains relaxation of the limb	Ⓨ Ⓝ	Ⓨ Ⓝ	Ⓨ Ⓝ
Performs assessment bilaterally	Ⓨ Ⓝ	Ⓨ Ⓝ	Ⓨ Ⓝ

The psychomotor skill was performed completely and in the appropriate order   **0 1 2 3 4 5**

The tester had control of the subject and the situation (showed confidence)   **0 1 2 3 4 5**

Method of performing the skill allowed the tester the ability to determine:
severity, proper progression, and the *fit* in the overall picture (Oral)   **0 1 2 3 4 5**

In order for a grade of *minimum standard* to be given, the total must be ≥11   **TOTAL = _____**

```
 1    2    3    4    5    6    7    8    9   10   11   12   13   14   15
 |    |    |    |    |    |    |    |    |    |    |    |    |    |    |
```

Not Acceptable   **Meets**   **Exceeds**
                                          Minimum Standards   **Minimum Standards**

TEST ENVIRONMENTS

L: Laboratory/Classroom Testing
C: Clinical/Field Testing
P: Practicum Testing
A: Assessment/Mock Exam Testing
S: Self-Reporting

SKILL TEST INFORMATION

Positive Finding: Pain in the calf area (gastrocnemius/soleus complex)
Involved Structure: Thrombophlebitis (possible)
Special Considerations: Rule out muscle injury; check dorsalis pedis pulse
Reference(s): Konin et al (2002); Magee; Starkey
Supplies Needed: Table

SPECIAL TESTS
(ST-L-Test 5)

Peer Review _____ Peer Review _____

Skill Acquisition: _____   Practice Opportunities: _____

This problem allows you the opportunity to demonstrate the **Tinel's Sign** *at the* **Ankle (Percussion Sign).** *You have 2 minutes to complete this task.*

Tester places athlete and limb in appropriate position	Test 1	Test 2	Test 3
Foot placed in a stable position (seated, prone, etc)	Ⓨ Ⓝ	Ⓨ Ⓝ	Ⓨ Ⓝ
Tester placed in proper position	**Test 1**	**Test 2**	**Test 3**
Stands to the side of the limb	Ⓨ Ⓝ	Ⓨ Ⓝ	Ⓨ Ⓝ
Places one hand on the lower leg	Ⓨ Ⓝ	Ⓨ Ⓝ	Ⓨ Ⓝ
Places the other hand in position to tap the area around the medial malleolus	Ⓨ Ⓝ	Ⓨ Ⓝ	Ⓨ Ⓝ
Tester performs test according to accepted guidelines	**Test 1**	**Test 2**	**Test 3**
Taps firmly on the dorsum of the ankle (anterior tibial branch of the deep peroneal nerve)	Ⓨ Ⓝ	Ⓨ Ⓝ	Ⓨ Ⓝ
Taps firmly behind the medial malleolus (posterior tibial nerve)	Ⓨ Ⓝ	Ⓨ Ⓝ	Ⓨ Ⓝ
Performs assessment bilaterally	Ⓨ Ⓝ	Ⓨ Ⓝ	Ⓨ Ⓝ

The psychomotor skill was performed completely and in the appropriate order   **0 1 2 3 4 5**

The tester had control of the subject and the situation (showed confidence)   **0 1 2 3 4 5**

Method of performing the skill allowed the tester the ability to determine:
severity, proper progression, and the *fit* in the overall picture (Oral)   **0 1 2 3 4 5**

In order for a grade of *minimum standard* to be given, the total must be ≥11   **TOTAL = _____**

```
 1    2    3    4    5    6    7    8    9   10   11   12   13   14   15
 |____|____|____|____|____|____|____|____|____|____|____|____|____|____|
```

Not Acceptable   **Meets**   **Exceeds**
                            Minimum Standards   **Minimum Standards**

TEST ENVIRONMENTS

L: Laboratory/Classroom Testing
C: Clinical/Field Testing
P: Practicum Testing
A: Assessment/Mock Exam Testing
S: Self-Reporting

SKILL TEST INFORMATION

Positive Finding: Tingling and/or paresthesia
Involved Structure: Anterior tibial branch of the deep peroneal nerve, posterior tibial nerve
Special Considerations: N/A
Reference(s): Magee
Supplies Needed: Supporting surface (table, floor)

Special Tests
(ST-L-Test 6)

Peer Review _____ Peer Review _____

Skill Acquisition: _____   Practice Opportunities: _____

This problem allows you the opportunity to demonstrate **McMurray's Test for the Knee.** *You have 2 minutes to complete this task.*

Tester places athlete and limb in appropriate position	Test 1	Test 2	Test 3
Supine	Ⓨ Ⓝ	Ⓨ Ⓝ	Ⓨ Ⓝ
Knee flexed to 90 degrees or knee extended to 0 degrees (starting with either knee)	Ⓨ Ⓝ	Ⓨ Ⓝ	Ⓨ Ⓝ
Tester placed in proper position	**Test 1**	**Test 2**	**Test 3**
Stands to the side of the athlete	Ⓨ Ⓝ	Ⓨ Ⓝ	Ⓨ Ⓝ
Grasps the involved foot (heel) with one hand	Ⓨ Ⓝ	Ⓨ Ⓝ	Ⓨ Ⓝ
Places the other hand in the position to palpate and support the knee	Ⓨ Ⓝ	Ⓨ Ⓝ	Ⓨ Ⓝ
Tester performs test according to accepted guidelines	**Test 1**	**Test 2**	**Test 3**
Passively medially rotates the knee while palpating the lateral joint line	Ⓨ Ⓝ	Ⓨ Ⓝ	Ⓨ Ⓝ
Applies valgus stress to the knee	Ⓨ Ⓝ	Ⓨ Ⓝ	Ⓨ Ⓝ
Passively moves the knee through a figure-8 motion (extension and flexion)	Ⓨ Ⓝ	Ⓨ Ⓝ	Ⓨ Ⓝ
Passively laterally rotates the knee while palpating the medial joint line	Ⓨ Ⓝ	Ⓨ Ⓝ	Ⓨ Ⓝ
Applies a varus stress to the knee	Ⓨ Ⓝ	Ⓨ Ⓝ	Ⓨ Ⓝ
Passively moves the knee through a figure-8 motion (extension and flexion)	Ⓨ Ⓝ	Ⓨ Ⓝ	Ⓨ Ⓝ
Maintains relaxation of the limb	Ⓨ Ⓝ	Ⓨ Ⓝ	Ⓨ Ⓝ
Performs assessment bilaterally	Ⓨ Ⓝ	Ⓨ Ⓝ	Ⓨ Ⓝ

The psychomotor skill was performed completely and in the appropriate order   **0 1 2 3 4 5**

The tester had control of the subject and the situation (showed confidence)   **0 1 2 3 4 5**

Method of performing the skill allowed the tester the ability to determine:
severity, proper progression, and the *fit* in the overall picture (Oral)   **0 1 2 3 4 5**

In order for a grade of *minimum standard* to be given, the total must be ≥11   **TOTAL = _____**

```
  1     2     3     4     5     6     7     8     9    10    11    12    13    14    15
  |     |     |     |     |     |     |     |     |     |     |     |     |     |     |
```
Not Acceptable   **Meets**   **Exceeds**
                                          Minimum Standards   **Minimum Standards**

TEST ENVIRONMENTS

L: Laboratory/Classroom Testing
C: Clinical/Field Testing
P: Practicum Testing
A: Assessment/Mock Exam Testing
S: Self-Reporting

SKILL TEST INFORMATION

Positive Finding:	Clicking or locking within knee joint
Involved Structure:	Meniscus (medial/lateral)
Special Considerations:	Rule out patella femoral problems
Reference(s):	Konin et al (2002); Magee; Starkey et al (2002)
Supplies Needed:	Table

Special Tests
(ST-L-Test 7)

Skill Acquisition: _____   Practice Opportunities: _____

This problem allows you the opportunity to demonstrate **Steinman's Tenderness Displacement Test (First Steinman's Sign)**. *You have 2 minutes to complete this task.*

Tester places athlete and limb in appropriate position	Test 1	Test 2	Test 3
Supine	Ⓨ Ⓝ	Ⓨ Ⓝ	Ⓨ Ⓝ
Knee placed in full extension (0 degrees)	Ⓨ Ⓝ	Ⓨ Ⓝ	Ⓨ Ⓝ
Tester placed in proper position	**Test 1**	**Test 2**	**Test 3**
Stands to the side of the athlete	Ⓨ Ⓝ	Ⓨ Ⓝ	Ⓨ Ⓝ
Grasps the involved foot (heel) with one hand	Ⓨ Ⓝ	Ⓨ Ⓝ	Ⓨ Ⓝ
Places the other hand in the position to support the knee	Ⓨ Ⓝ	Ⓨ Ⓝ	Ⓨ Ⓝ
Tester performs test according to accepted guidelines	**Test 1**	**Test 2**	**Test 3**
Passively moves the knee into full flexion	Ⓨ Ⓝ	Ⓨ Ⓝ	Ⓨ Ⓝ
Passively rotates the knee medially	Ⓨ Ⓝ	Ⓨ Ⓝ	Ⓨ Ⓝ
Passively rotates the knee laterally	Ⓨ Ⓝ	Ⓨ Ⓝ	Ⓨ Ⓝ
Repeats medial and lateral rotation	Ⓨ Ⓝ	Ⓨ Ⓝ	Ⓨ Ⓝ
Maintains relaxation of the limb	Ⓨ Ⓝ	Ⓨ Ⓝ	Ⓨ Ⓝ
Performs assessment bilaterally	Ⓨ Ⓝ	Ⓨ Ⓝ	Ⓨ Ⓝ

The psychomotor skill was performed completely and in the appropriate order   **0 1 2 3 4 5**

The tester had control of the subject and the situation (showed confidence)   **0 1 2 3 4 5**

Method of performing the skill allowed the tester the ability to determine:
severity, proper progression, and the *fit* in the overall picture (Oral)   **0 1 2 3 4 5**

In order for a grade of *minimum standard* to be given, the total must be ≥11   **TOTAL = _____**

```
 1    2    3    4    5    6    7    8    9   10   11   12   13   14   15
 |    |    |    |    |    |    |    |    |    |    |    |    |    |    |
```

Not Acceptable   **Meets**   **Exceeds**
                              Minimum Standards   **Minimum Standards**

TEST ENVIRONMENTS

L: Laboratory/Classroom Testing
C: Clinical/Field Testing
P: Practicum Testing
A: Assessment/Mock Exam Testing
S: Self-Reporting

SKILL TEST INFORMATION

Positive Finding:	Pain during rotation, lacks full flexion
Involved Structure:	Meniscus (medial/lateral)
Special Considerations:	N/A
Reference(s):	Magee
Supplies Needed:	Table

SPECIAL TESTS
(ST-L-Test 8)

Peer Review _____   Peer Review _____

Skill Acquisition: _____   Practice Opportunities: _____

This problem allows you the opportunity to demonstrate the **Patellofemoral Grind Test (Clarke's Test/Patella Hold/Zohler's Sign)** *for the knee. You have 2 minutes to complete this task.*

Tester places athlete and limb in appropriate position	Test 1	Test 2	Test 3
Supine	Ⓨ Ⓝ	Ⓨ Ⓝ	Ⓨ Ⓝ
Knee placed in full extension (heels on the table)	Ⓨ Ⓝ	Ⓨ Ⓝ	Ⓨ Ⓝ
Tester placed in proper position	**Test 1**	**Test 2**	**Test 3**
Stands to the side of the athlete	Ⓨ Ⓝ	Ⓨ Ⓝ	Ⓨ Ⓝ
Places hand over the superior pole of the patella (web of the hand)	Ⓨ Ⓝ	Ⓨ Ⓝ	Ⓨ Ⓝ
Tester performs test according to accepted guidelines	**Test 1**	**Test 2**	**Test 3**
Applies downward-inferior pressure on the patella	Ⓨ Ⓝ	Ⓨ Ⓝ	Ⓨ Ⓝ
Instructs the athlete to actively contract the quadriceps	Ⓨ Ⓝ	Ⓨ Ⓝ	Ⓨ Ⓝ
Performs the assessment bilaterally	Ⓨ Ⓝ	Ⓨ Ⓝ	Ⓨ Ⓝ

The psychomotor skill was performed completely and in the appropriate order   0 1 2 3 4 5

The tester had control of the subject and the situation (showed confidence)   0 1 2 3 4 5

Method of performing the skill allowed the tester the ability to determine:
severity, proper progression, and the *fit* in the overall picture (Oral)   0 1 2 3 4 5

In order for a grade of *minimum standard* to be given, the total must be ≥11   **TOTAL = _____**

```
  1    2    3    4    5    6    7    8    9    10   11   12   13   14   15
  |    |    |    |    |    |    |    |    |    |    |    |    |    |    |
```

Not Acceptable   **Meets**   **Exceeds**
                              Minimum Standards   **Minimum Standards**

TEST ENVIRONMENTS

L: Laboratory/Classroom Testing
C: Clinical/Field Testing
P: Practicum Testing
A: Assessment/Mock Exam Testing
S: Self-Reporting

SKILL TEST INFORMATION

Positive Finding: Pain/crepitation
Involved Structure: Patella
Special Considerations: N/A
Reference(s): Konin et al (2002); Magee
Supplies Needed: N/A

SPECIAL TESTS
(ST-L-Test 9)

Peer Review _____ Peer Review _____

Skill Acquisition: _____   Practice Opportunities: _____

This problem allows you the opportunity to demonstrate the **Patellar Apprehension Test (Fairbank's Apprehension Test)***. You have 2 minutes to complete this task.*

Tester places athlete and limb in appropriate position	Test 1	Test 2	Test 3
Supine	Ⓨ Ⓝ	Ⓨ Ⓝ	Ⓨ Ⓝ
Knee placed in full extension (heels on the table)	Ⓨ Ⓝ	Ⓨ Ⓝ	Ⓨ Ⓝ
Tester placed in proper position	**Test 1**	**Test 2**	**Test 3**
Stands to the side of the athlete	Ⓨ Ⓝ	Ⓨ Ⓝ	Ⓨ Ⓝ
Places thumbs over the medial border of the patella	Ⓨ Ⓝ	Ⓨ Ⓝ	Ⓨ Ⓝ
Tester performs test according to accepted guidelines	**Test 1**	**Test 2**	**Test 3**
Passively moves the patella in a lateral direction	Ⓨ Ⓝ	Ⓨ Ⓝ	Ⓨ Ⓝ
Performs assessment bilaterally	Ⓨ Ⓝ	Ⓨ Ⓝ	Ⓨ Ⓝ

The psychomotor skill was performed completely and in the appropriate order   **0 1 2 3 4 5**

The tester had control of the subject and the situation (showed confidence)   **0 1 2 3 4 5**

Method of performing the skill allowed the tester the ability to determine:
severity, proper progression, and the *fit* in the overall picture (Oral)   **0 1 2 3 4 5**

In order for a grade of *minimum standard* to be given, the total must be ≥11   **TOTAL = _____**

```
  1    2    3    4    5    6    7    8    9   10   11   12   13   14   15
  |____|____|____|____|____|____|____|____|____|____|____|____|____|____|
```

Not Acceptable   **Meets**   **Exceeds**
                            Minimum Standards   **Minimum Standards**

TEST ENVIRONMENTS
L: Laboratory/Classroom Testing
C: Clinical/Field Testing
P: Practicum Testing
A: Assessment/Mock Exam Testing
S: Self-Reporting

SKILL TEST INFORMATION
Positive Finding: Pain, apprehension, tightening of the quads
Involved Structure: Patella
Special Considerations: N/A
Reference(s): Konin et al (2002); Magee
Supplies Needed: Table

SPECIAL TESTS
(ST-L-Test 10)

Peer Review _____ Peer Review _____

Skill Acquisition: _____   Practice Opportunities: _____

This problem allows you the opportunity to demonstrate the **Ballottable Patella (Patella Tap Test)**. *You have 2 minutes to complete this task.*

Tester places athlete and limb in appropriate position	Test 1	Test 2	Test 3
Supine	Ⓨ Ⓝ	Ⓨ Ⓝ	Ⓨ Ⓝ
Knee placed in full extension (heels on the table)	Ⓨ Ⓝ	Ⓨ Ⓝ	Ⓨ Ⓝ
Tester placed in proper position	**Test 1**	**Test 2**	**Test 3**
Stands to the side of the athlete	Ⓨ Ⓝ	Ⓨ Ⓝ	Ⓨ Ⓝ
Places one hand over the suprapatellar pouch (just above the superior pole of the patella)	Ⓨ Ⓝ	Ⓨ Ⓝ	Ⓨ Ⓝ
Places the other hand over the central portion of the patella	Ⓨ Ⓝ	Ⓨ Ⓝ	Ⓨ Ⓝ
Tester performs test according to accepted guidelines	**Test 1**	**Test 2**	**Test 3**
Applies downward pressure on the patella	Ⓨ Ⓝ	Ⓨ Ⓝ	Ⓨ Ⓝ
Maintains relaxation of the limb	Ⓨ Ⓝ	Ⓨ Ⓝ	Ⓨ Ⓝ
Performs assessment bilaterally	Ⓨ Ⓝ	Ⓨ Ⓝ	Ⓨ Ⓝ

The psychomotor skill was performed completely and in the appropriate order   **0 1 2 3 4 5**

The tester had control of the subject and the situation (showed confidence)   **0 1 2 3 4 5**

Method of performing the skill allowed the tester the ability to determine:
severity, proper progression, and the *fit* in the overall picture (Oral)   **0 1 2 3 4 5**

In order for a grade of *minimum standard* to be given, the total must be ≥11   **TOTAL = _____**

```
 1    2    3    4    5    6    7    8    9   10   11   12   13   14   15
 |    |    |    |    |    |    |    |    |    |    |    |    |    |    |
```

Not Acceptable   Meets   Exceeds
                                        Minimum Standards   Minimum Standards

TEST ENVIRONMENTS

L: Laboratory/Classroom Testing
C: Clinical/Field Testing
P: Practicum Testing
A: Assessment/Mock Exam Testing
S: Self-Reporting

SKILL TEST INFORMATION

Positive Finding: Rebound of the patella
Involved Structure: Joint (effusion)
Special Considerations: Measure thigh girth
Reference(s): Konin et al (2002); Starkey et al (2002)
Supplies Needed: Table

SPECIAL TESTS
(ST-L-Test 11)

Peer Review _____ Peer Review _____

Skill Acquisition: _____   Practice Opportunities: _____

This problem allows you the opportunity to demonstrate the **Sweep Test.** *You have 2 minutes to complete this task.*

Tester places athlete and limb in appropriate position	Test 1	Test 2	Test 3
Supine	Ⓨ Ⓝ	Ⓨ Ⓝ	Ⓨ Ⓝ
Knee placed in full extension (heels on the table)	Ⓨ Ⓝ	Ⓨ Ⓝ	Ⓨ Ⓝ
Tester placed in proper position	**Test 1**	**Test 2**	**Test 3**
Stands to the side of the athlete	Ⓨ Ⓝ	Ⓨ Ⓝ	Ⓨ Ⓝ
Places hands on the medial side of the patella	Ⓨ Ⓝ	Ⓨ Ⓝ	Ⓨ Ⓝ
Tester performs test according to accepted guidelines	**Test 1**	**Test 2**	**Test 3**
Pushes edema/swelling proximally and/or laterally ("milking")	Ⓨ Ⓝ	Ⓨ Ⓝ	Ⓨ Ⓝ
Applies pressure to the lateral aspect of the knee	Ⓨ Ⓝ	Ⓨ Ⓝ	Ⓨ Ⓝ
Maintains relaxation of the limb	Ⓨ Ⓝ	Ⓨ Ⓝ	Ⓨ Ⓝ
Performs assessment bilaterally	Ⓨ Ⓝ	Ⓨ Ⓝ	Ⓨ Ⓝ

The psychomotor skill was performed completely and in the appropriate order   **0 1 2 3 4 5**

The tester had control of the subject and the situation (showed confidence)   **0 1 2 3 4 5**

Method of performing the skill allowed the tester the ability to determine:
severity, proper progression, and the *fit* in the overall picture (Oral)   **0 1 2 3 4 5**

In order for a grade of *minimum standard* to be given, the total must be ≥11   **TOTAL = _____**

```
 1    2    3    4    5    6    7    8    9   10   11   12   13   14   15
 |____|____|____|____|____|____|____|____|____|____|____|____|____|____|
```
Not Acceptable   **Meets**   **Exceeds**
                                    Minimum Standards   **Minimum Standards**

TEST ENVIRONMENTS

L: Laboratory/Classroom Testing
C: Clinical/Field Testing
P: Practicum Testing
A: Assessment/Mock Exam Testing
S: Self-Reporting

SKILL TEST INFORMATION

Positive Finding:	Fluid reforms on the medial side
Involved Structure:	Intracapsular swelling
Special Considerations:	N/A
Reference(s):	Starkey et al (2002)
Supplies Needed:	Table

SPECIAL TESTS
(ST-L-Test 12)

*This problem allows you the opportunity to demonstrate the **Bounce Home Test** for the knee. You have 2 minutes to complete this task.*

Tester places athlete and limb in appropriate position	Test 1	Test 2	Test 3
Supine	Y N	Y N	Y N
Knee placed into slight flexion	Y N	Y N	Y N
Tester placed in proper position	**Test 1**	**Test 2**	**Test 3**
Stands to the side of the athlete	Y N	Y N	Y N
Places one hand under the heel of the involved limb	Y N	Y N	Y N
Places other hand under the knee joint	Y N	Y N	Y N
Tester performs test according to accepted guidelines	**Test 1**	**Test 2**	**Test 3**
Passively flexes the knee (approximately 30 degrees)	Y N	Y N	Y N
Allows the knee to fall to neutral (gravity)	Y N	Y N	Y N
Maintains relaxation of the limb	Y N	Y N	Y N
Performs assessment bilaterally	Y N	Y N	Y N

The psychomotor skill was performed completely and in the appropriate order   **0 1 2 3 4 5**

The tester had control of the subject and the situation (showed confidence)   **0 1 2 3 4 5**

Method of performing the skill allowed the tester the ability to determine:
severity, proper progression, and the *fit* in the overall picture (Oral)   **0 1 2 3 4 5**

In order for a grade of *minimum standard* to be given, the total must be ≥11   **TOTAL = _____**

1 2 3 4 5 6 7 8 9 10 11 12 13 14 15

Not Acceptable   **Meets Minimum Standards**   **Exceeds Minimum Standards**

TEST ENVIRONMENTS
L: Laboratory/Classroom Testing
C: Clinical/Field Testing
P: Practicum Testing
A: Assessment/Mock Exam Testing
S: Self-Reporting

SKILL TEST INFORMATION
Positive Finding: Rubbery end-feel, springy block, lacks full extension
Involved Structure: Structural block; meniscus
Special Considerations: N/A
Reference(s): Konin et al (2002); Magee
Supplies Needed: Table

SPECIAL TESTS
(ST-L-Test 13)

Peer Review _____ Peer Review _____

Skill Acquisition: _____   Practice Opportunities: _____

This problem allows you the opportunity to demonstrate **Apley's Compression Test** *for the knee. You have 2 minutes to complete this task.*

Tester places athlete and limb in appropriate position	Test 1	Test 2	Test 3
Prone	Y N	Y N	Y N
Knee flexed to 90 degrees	Y N	Y N	Y N
Tester placed in proper position	**Test 1**	**Test 2**	**Test 3**
Stands to the side of the athlete	Y N	Y N	Y N
Places one hand over the posterior femur (may stabilize with knee)	Y N	Y N	Y N
Grasps other hand around the distal portion of the tibia/fibula	Y N	Y N	Y N
Tester performs test according to accepted guidelines	**Test 1**	**Test 2**	**Test 3**
Applies downward pressure of the tibia/fibula (compressing the knee joint)	Y N	Y N	Y N
Simultaneously medially/laterally rotates the tibia	Y N	Y N	Y N
Maintains relaxation of the limb	Y N	Y N	Y N
Performs assessment bilaterally	Y N	Y N	Y N

The psychomotor skill was performed completely and in the appropriate order   0 1 2 3 4 5

The tester had control of the subject and the situation (showed confidence)   0 1 2 3 4 5

Method of performing the skill allowed the tester the ability to determine:
severity, proper progression, and the *fit* in the overall picture (Oral)   0 1 2 3 4 5

In order for a grade of *minimum standard* to be given, the total must be ≥11   TOTAL = _____

```
  1    2    3    4    5    6    7    8    9   10   11   12   13   14   15
  |----|----|----|----|----|----|----|----|----|----|----|----|----|----|
```

Not Acceptable   **Meets**   **Exceeds**
                                    Minimum Standards   **Minimum Standards**

TEST ENVIRONMENTS

L: Laboratory/Classroom Testing
C: Clinical/Field Testing
P: Practicum Testing
A: Assessment/Mock Exam Testing
S: Self-Reporting

SKILL TEST INFORMATION

Positive Finding: Pain, clicking, restriction
Involved Structure: Meniscus
Special Considerations: Combine with Apley's distraction test
Reference(s): Konin et al (2002); Magee; Starkey et al (2002)
Supplies Needed: Table

SPECIAL TESTS
(ST-L-Test 14)

Peer Review _____ Peer Review _____

Skill Acquisition: _____   Practice Opportunities: _____

*This problem allows you the opportunity to demonstrate **Apley's Distraction Test** for the knee. You have 2 minutes to complete this task.*

Tester places athlete and limb in appropriate position	Test 1	Test 2	Test 3
Prone	Ⓨ Ⓝ	Ⓨ Ⓝ	Ⓨ Ⓝ
Knee flexed to 90 degrees	Ⓨ Ⓝ	Ⓨ Ⓝ	Ⓨ Ⓝ
Tester placed in proper position	**Test 1**	**Test 2**	**Test 3**
Stands to the side of the athlete	Ⓨ Ⓝ	Ⓨ Ⓝ	Ⓨ Ⓝ
Places one hand over posterior femur (may stabilize with knee)	Ⓨ Ⓝ	Ⓨ Ⓝ	Ⓨ Ⓝ
Grasp other hand around the distal portion of the tibia/fibula	Ⓨ Ⓝ	Ⓨ Ⓝ	Ⓨ Ⓝ
Tester performs test according to accepted guidelines	**Test 1**	**Test 2**	**Test 3**
Applies upward pressure of the tibia/fibula (distracting the knee)	Ⓨ Ⓝ	Ⓨ Ⓝ	Ⓨ Ⓝ
Simultaneously medially/laterally rotates the tibia	Ⓨ Ⓝ	Ⓨ Ⓝ	Ⓨ Ⓝ
Maintains relaxation of the limb	Ⓨ Ⓝ	Ⓨ Ⓝ	Ⓨ Ⓝ
Performs assessment bilaterally	Ⓨ Ⓝ	Ⓨ Ⓝ	Ⓨ Ⓝ

The psychomotor skill was performed completely and in the appropriate order   **0 1 2 3 4 5**

The tester had control of the subject and the situation (showed confidence)   **0 1 2 3 4 5**

Method of performing the skill allowed the tester the ability to determine:
severity, proper progression, and the *fit* in the overall picture (Oral)   **0 1 2 3 4 5**

In order for a grade of *minimum standard* to be given, the total must be ≥11   **TOTAL = _____**

```
 1    2    3    4    5    6    7    8    9    10   11   12   13   14   15
 |----|----|----|----|----|----|----|----|----|----|----|----|----|----|
```
Not Acceptable   Meets   Exceeds
                                  Minimum Standards   Minimum Standards

TEST ENVIRONMENTS
L: Laboratory/Classroom Testing
C: Clinical/Field Testing
P: Practicum Testing
A: Assessment/Mock Exam Testing
S: Self-Reporting

SKILL TEST INFORMATION
Positive Finding:	Pain
Involved Structure:	General ligamentous meniscus (pain goes away)
Special Considerations:	Combine with Apley's compression test
Reference(s):	Konin et al (2002); Magee; Starkey et al (2002)
Supplies Needed:	Table

Special Tests
(ST-L-Test 15)

Peer Review _____ Peer Review _____

Skill Acquisition: _____   Practice Opportunities: _____

This problem allows you the opportunity to demonstrate the **FABER Test (Figure-Four Test/Patrick's Test/Jansen's Test)**. *You have 2 minutes to complete this task.*

Tester places athlete and limb in appropriate position	Test 1	Test 2	Test 3
Supine	Ⓨ Ⓝ	Ⓨ Ⓝ	Ⓨ Ⓝ
Hip flexed, abducted, and externally rotated (FABER) figure-4 position	Ⓨ Ⓝ	Ⓨ Ⓝ	Ⓨ Ⓝ
Foot placed on opposite knee (above the superior pole of the patella)	Ⓨ Ⓝ	Ⓨ Ⓝ	Ⓨ Ⓝ
Tester placed in proper position	**Test 1**	**Test 2**	**Test 3**
Stands to the side of the athlete	Ⓨ Ⓝ	Ⓨ Ⓝ	Ⓨ Ⓝ
Places one hand on the ASIS (opposite the involved side)	Ⓨ Ⓝ	Ⓨ Ⓝ	Ⓨ Ⓝ
Places the other hand on the involved knee	Ⓨ Ⓝ	Ⓨ Ⓝ	Ⓨ Ⓝ
Tester performs test according to accepted guidelines	**Test 1**	**Test 2**	**Test 3**
Slowly press the knee toward the table	Ⓨ Ⓝ	Ⓨ Ⓝ	Ⓨ Ⓝ
Maintains relaxation of the limb	Ⓨ Ⓝ	Ⓨ Ⓝ	Ⓨ Ⓝ
Performs assessment bilaterally	Ⓨ Ⓝ	Ⓨ Ⓝ	Ⓨ Ⓝ

The psychomotor skill was performed completely and in the appropriate order   0 1 2 3 4 5

The tester had control of the subject and the situation (showed confidence)   0 1 2 3 4 5

Method of performing the skill allowed the tester the ability to determine: severity, proper progression, and the *fit* in the overall picture (Oral)   0 1 2 3 4 5

In order for a grade of *minimum standard* to be given, the total must be ≥11   **TOTAL =** _____

```
 1    2    3    4    5    6    7    8    9   10   11   12   13   14   15
 |    |    |    |    |    |    |    |    |    |    |    |    |    |    |
```

Not Acceptable   **Meets**   **Exceeds**
                                   Minimum Standards   **Minimum Standards**

TEST ENVIRONMENTS

L: Laboratory/Classroom Testing
C: Clinical/Field Testing
P: Practicum Testing
A: Assessment/Mock Exam Testing
S: Self-Reporting

SKILL TEST INFORMATION

Positive Finding:	Knee does not move to the table (ideal parallel to the table)
Involved Structure:	Iliopsoas, sacroiliac joint
Special Considerations:	N/A
Reference(s):	Konin et al (2002); Magee; Starkey et al (2002)
Supplies Needed:	Table

SPECIAL TESTS
(ST-L-Test 16)

Peer Review _____ Peer Review _____

Skill Acquisition: _____   Practice Opportunities: _____

This problem allows you the opportunity to demonstrate the **Gaenslen's Test**. *You have 2 minutes to complete this task.*

Tester places athlete and limb in appropriate position	Test 1	Test 2	Test 3
Side lying	Ⓨ Ⓝ	Ⓨ Ⓝ	Ⓨ Ⓝ
Hip hyperextended (upper limb)	Ⓨ Ⓝ	Ⓨ Ⓝ	Ⓨ Ⓝ
Hip/knee flexed (lower limb) with leg held against chest	Ⓨ Ⓝ	Ⓨ Ⓝ	Ⓨ Ⓝ
Tester placed in proper position	**Test 1**	**Test 2**	**Test 3**
Stands behind the athlete	Ⓨ Ⓝ	Ⓨ Ⓝ	Ⓨ Ⓝ
Places one hand on the pelvis (stabilize)	Ⓨ Ⓝ	Ⓨ Ⓝ	Ⓨ Ⓝ
Places other hand against the anterior knee	Ⓨ Ⓝ	Ⓨ Ⓝ	Ⓨ Ⓝ
Tester performs test according to accepted guidelines	**Test 1**	**Test 2**	**Test 3**
Passively extends the hip (over pressure)	Ⓨ Ⓝ	Ⓨ Ⓝ	Ⓨ Ⓝ
Maintains relaxation of the limb	Ⓨ Ⓝ	Ⓨ Ⓝ	Ⓨ Ⓝ
Performs assessment bilaterally	Ⓨ Ⓝ	Ⓨ Ⓝ	Ⓨ Ⓝ

The psychomotor skill was performed completely and in the appropriate order   **0 1 2 3 4 5**

The tester had control of the subject and the situation (showed confidence)   **0 1 2 3 4 5**

Method of performing the skill allowed the tester the ability to determine:
severity, proper progression, and the *fit* in the overall picture (Oral)   **0 1 2 3 4 5**

In order for a grade of *minimum standard* to be given, the total must be ≥11   **TOTAL = _____**

```
1    2    3    4    5    6    7    8    9    10    11    12    13    14    15
|    |    |    |    |    |    |    |    |    |     |     |     |     |     |
```

Not Acceptable   **Meets**   **Exceeds**
                                        Minimum Standards   **Minimum Standards**

TEST ENVIRONMENTS

L: Laboratory/Classroom Testing
C: Clinical/Field Testing
P: Practicum Testing
A: Assessment/Mock Exam Testing
S: Self-Reporting

SKILL TEST INFORMATION

Positive Finding:	Pain
Involved Structure:	Sacroiliac joint, hip
Special Considerations:	May be done supine (leg hanging off the table)
Reference(s):	Magee
Supplies Needed:	Table

SPECIAL TESTS
(ST-L-Test 17)

Peer Review _____ Peer Review _____

Skill Acquisition: _____   Practice Opportunities: _____

This problem allows you the opportunity to demonstrate the **Sacroiliac Compression Test (Gapping Test/ Transverse Anterior Stress Test)**. *You have 2 minutes to complete this task.*

Tester places athlete and limb in appropriate position	Test 1	Test 2	Test 3
Supine	Ⓨ Ⓝ	Ⓨ Ⓝ	Ⓨ Ⓝ
Tester placed in proper position	**Test 1**	**Test 2**	**Test 3**
Stands behind the athlete	Ⓨ Ⓝ	Ⓨ Ⓝ	Ⓨ Ⓝ
Places hands over the ASIS (X pattern/cross-arm pattern)	Ⓨ Ⓝ	Ⓨ Ⓝ	Ⓨ Ⓝ
Tester performs test according to accepted guidelines	**Test 1**	**Test 2**	**Test 3**
Applies downward and outward pressure (attempting to spread the ASIS)	Ⓨ Ⓝ	Ⓨ Ⓝ	Ⓨ Ⓝ
Asks the athlete to relax	Ⓨ Ⓝ	Ⓨ Ⓝ	Ⓨ Ⓝ
Performs assessment bilaterally	Ⓨ Ⓝ	Ⓨ Ⓝ	Ⓨ Ⓝ

The psychomotor skill was performed completely and in the appropriate order   0 1 2 3 4 5

The tester had control of the subject and the situation (showed confidence)   0 1 2 3 4 5

Method of performing the skill allowed the tester the ability to determine:
severity, proper progression, and the *fit* in the overall picture (Oral)   0 1 2 3 4 5

In order for a grade of *minimum standard* to be given, the total must be ≥11   TOTAL = _____

```
 1    2    3    4    5    6    7    8    9   10   11   12   13   14   15
 |    |    |    |    |    |    |    |    |    |    |    |    |    |    |
```

Not Acceptable   **Meets**   **Exceeds**
                          Minimum Standards   **Minimum Standards**

TEST ENVIRONMENTS

L: Laboratory/Classroom Testing
C: Clinical/Field Testing
P: Practicum Testing
A: Assessment/Mock Exam Testing
S: Self-Reporting

SKILL TEST INFORMATION

Positive Finding: Pain (sacroiliac area)
Involved Structure: Sacroiliac joint
Special Considerations: N/A
Reference(s): Magee; Starkey et al (2002)
Supplies Needed: Table

SPECIAL TESTS
(ST-L-Test 18)

Peer Review _____ Peer Review _____

Skill Acquisition: _____ Practice Opportunities: _____

This problem allows you the opportunity to demonstrate the **Sacroiliac Distraction Test (Approximation Test/ Transverse Posterior Stress Test)**. *You have 2 minutes to complete this task.*

Tester places athlete and limb in appropriate position	Test 1	Test 2	Test 3
Side lying	Ⓨ Ⓝ	Ⓨ Ⓝ	Ⓨ Ⓝ
Tester placed in proper position	**Test 1**	**Test 2**	**Test 3**
Stands behind the athlete	Ⓨ Ⓝ	Ⓨ Ⓝ	Ⓨ Ⓝ
Places both hands over the lateral aspect of the pelvis (iliac crest)	Ⓨ Ⓝ	Ⓨ Ⓝ	Ⓨ Ⓝ
Tester performs test according to accepted guidelines	**Test 1**	**Test 2**	**Test 3**
Applies downward pressure (pushing toward the table)	Ⓨ Ⓝ	Ⓨ Ⓝ	Ⓨ Ⓝ
Asks the athlete to relax	Ⓨ Ⓝ	Ⓨ Ⓝ	Ⓨ Ⓝ
Performs assessment bilaterally	Ⓨ Ⓝ	Ⓨ Ⓝ	Ⓨ Ⓝ

The psychomotor skill was performed completely and in the appropriate order   **0 1 2 3 4 5**

The tester had control of the subject and the situation (showed confidence)   **0 1 2 3 4 5**

Method of performing the skill allowed the tester the ability to determine:
severity, proper progression, and the *fit* in the overall picture (Oral)   **0 1 2 3 4 5**

In order for a grade of *minimum standard* to be given, the total must be ≥11   **TOTAL = _____**

```
 1    2    3    4    5    6    7    8    9   10   11   12   13   14   15
 |    |    |    |    |    |    |    |    |    |    |    |    |    |    |
```
Not Acceptable   **Meets**   **Exceeds**
                                            Minimum Standards   **Minimum Standards**

TEST ENVIRONMENTS

L: Laboratory/Classroom Testing
C: Clinical/Field Testing
P: Practicum Testing
A: Assessment/Mock Exam Testing
S: Self-Reporting

SKILL TEST INFORMATION

Positive Finding: Pain (sacroiliac area)
Involved Structure: Sacroiliac joint
Special Considerations: N/A
Reference(s): Magee; Starkey et al (2002)
Supplies Needed: Table

SPECIAL TESTS
(ST-L-Test 19)

Skill Acquisition: _____   Practice Opportunities: _____

This problem allows you the opportunity to demonstrate the **Tripod Sign (Hamstrings Contracture, Method 2)** *for hamstring flexibility. You have 2 minutes to complete this task.*

Tester places athlete and limb in appropriate position	Test 1	Test 2	Test 3
Seated	Ⓨ Ⓝ	Ⓨ Ⓝ	Ⓨ Ⓝ
Knees flexed to 90 degrees (hanging over the edge of the table)	Ⓨ Ⓝ	Ⓨ Ⓝ	Ⓨ Ⓝ
Tester placed in proper position	**Test 1**	**Test 2**	**Test 3**
Stands to the side of the athlete	Ⓨ Ⓝ	Ⓨ Ⓝ	Ⓨ Ⓝ
Places hand around the distal aspect of the lower leg	Ⓨ Ⓝ	Ⓨ Ⓝ	Ⓨ Ⓝ
Places the other hand over the distal aspect of the femur (above the knee)	Ⓨ Ⓝ	Ⓨ Ⓝ	Ⓨ Ⓝ
Tester performs test according to accepted guidelines	**Test 1**	**Test 2**	**Test 3**
Passively extends the knee	Ⓨ Ⓝ	Ⓨ Ⓝ	Ⓨ Ⓝ
Maintains relaxation of the limb	Ⓨ Ⓝ	Ⓨ Ⓝ	Ⓨ Ⓝ
Performs assessment bilaterally	Ⓨ Ⓝ	Ⓨ Ⓝ	Ⓨ Ⓝ

The psychomotor skill was performed completely and in the appropriate order   **0 1 2 3 4 5**

The tester had control of the subject and the situation (showed confidence)   **0 1 2 3 4 5**

Method of performing the skill allowed the tester the ability to determine:
severity, proper progression, and the *fit* in the overall picture (Oral)   **0 1 2 3 4 5**

In order for a grade of *minimum standard* to be given, the total must be ≥11   **TOTAL = _____**

```
 1    2    3    4    5    6    7    8    9    10   11   12   13   14   15
 |    |    |    |    |    |    |    |    |    |    |    |    |    |    |
```
Not Acceptable   **Meets**   **Exceeds**
                                          Minimum Standards   **Minimum Standards**

TEST ENVIRONMENTS	**SKILL TEST INFORMATION**	
L: Laboratory/Classroom Testing	**Positive Finding:**	Hyperextends the trunk
C: Clinical/Field Testing	**Involved Structure:**	Hamstrings
P: Practicum Testing	**Special Considerations:**	N/A
A: Assessment/Mock Exam Testing	**Reference(s):**	Magee
S: Self-Reporting	**Supplies Needed:**	Table

SPECIAL TESTS
(ST-L-Test 20)

Peer Review _____ Peer Review _____

Skill Acquisition: _____   Practice Opportunities: _____

This problem allows you the opportunity to demonstrate the **Ely's Test (Tight Rectus Femoris, Method 2).** *You have 2 minutes to complete this task.*

Tester places athlete and limb in appropriate position	Test 1	Test 2	Test 3
Prone	Ⓨ Ⓝ	Ⓨ Ⓝ	Ⓨ Ⓝ
Knees extended	Ⓨ Ⓝ	Ⓨ Ⓝ	Ⓨ Ⓝ
Tester placed in proper position	**Test 1**	**Test 2**	**Test 3**
Stands to the side of the athlete	Ⓨ Ⓝ	Ⓨ Ⓝ	Ⓨ Ⓝ
Places hand around distal aspect of the lower leg	Ⓨ Ⓝ	Ⓨ Ⓝ	Ⓨ Ⓝ
Places the other over the distal aspect of the femur (above the knee)	Ⓨ Ⓝ	Ⓨ Ⓝ	Ⓨ Ⓝ
Tester performs test according to accepted guidelines	**Test 1**	**Test 2**	**Test 3**
Passively flexes the knee (overpressure)	Ⓨ Ⓝ	Ⓨ Ⓝ	Ⓨ Ⓝ
Maintains relaxation of the limb	Ⓨ Ⓝ	Ⓨ Ⓝ	Ⓨ Ⓝ
Performs assessment bilaterally	Ⓨ Ⓝ	Ⓨ Ⓝ	Ⓨ Ⓝ

The psychomotor skill was performed completely and in the appropriate order   **0 1 2 3 4 5**

The tester had control of the subject and the situation (showed confidence)   **0 1 2 3 4 5**

Method of performing the skill allowed the tester the ability to determine:
severity, proper progression, and the *fit* in the overall picture (Oral)   **0 1 2 3 4 5**

In order for a grade of *minimum standard* to be given, the total must be ≥11   **TOTAL = _____**

| 1 | 2 | 3 | 4 | 5 | 6 | 7 | 8 | 9 | 10 | 11 | 12 | 13 | 14 | 15 |

Not Acceptable   **Meets**   **Exceeds**
                                         Minimum Standards   **Minimum Standards**

TEST ENVIRONMENTS

L: Laboratory/Classroom Testing
C: Clinical/Field Testing
P: Practicum Testing
A: Assessment/Mock Exam Testing
S: Self-Reporting

SKILL TEST INFORMATION

Positive Finding: Hip moves off the table on the involved side
Involved Structure: Rectus femoris
Special Considerations: N/A
Reference(s): Konin et al (2002); Magee
Supplies Needed: Table

SPECIAL TESTS
(ST-L-Test 21)

Peer Review _____ Peer Review _____

Skill Acquisition: _____   Practice Opportunities: _____

This problem allows you the opportunity to demonstrate the **Femoral Nerve Traction Test.** *You have 2 minutes to complete this task.*

Tester places athlete and limb in appropriate position	Test 1	Test 2	Test 3
Side lying	Y N	Y N	Y N
Torso, hip, and leg in straight alignment	Y N	Y N	Y N
Hip/knee slightly flexed (bottom leg uninvolved limb)	Y N	Y N	Y N
Head slightly flexed	Y N	Y N	Y N
Tester placed in proper position	**Test 1**	**Test 2**	**Test 3**
Stands behind the athlete	Y N	Y N	Y N
Places hand under the knee (supporting the lower leg)	Y N	Y N	Y N
Places the other hand over the lateral aspect of the pelvis (iliac crest)	Y N	Y N	Y N
Tester performs test according to accepted guidelines	**Test 1**	**Test 2**	**Test 3**
Passively extends the hip	Y N	Y N	Y N
Passively flexes the knee	Y N	Y N	Y N
Maintains relaxation of the limb	Y N	Y N	Y N
Performs assessment bilaterally	Y N	Y N	Y N

The psychomotor skill was performed completely and in the appropriate order   **0 1 2 3 4 5**

The tester had control of the subject and the situation (showed confidence)   **0 1 2 3 4 5**

Method of performing the skill allowed the tester the ability to determine:
severity, proper progression, and the *fit* in the overall picture (Oral)   **0 1 2 3 4 5**

In order for a grade of *minimum standard* to be given, the total must be ≥11   **TOTAL = _____**

```
 1    2    3    4    5    6    7    8    9   10   11   12   13   14   15
 |----|----|----|----|----|----|----|----|----|----|----|----|----|----|
```
Not Acceptable   **Meets**   **Exceeds**
                                    Minimum Standards   **Minimum Standards**

TEST ENVIRONMENTS

L: Laboratory/Classroom Testing
C: Clinical/Field Testing
P: Practicum Testing
A: Assessment/Mock Exam Testing
S: Self-Reporting

SKILL TEST INFORMATION

Positive Finding:	Pain shooting down the anterior thigh
Involved Structure:	Femoral nerve
Special Considerations:	May also serve as a traction test for L2 to L4
Reference(s):	Magee
Supplies Needed:	N/A

SPECIAL TESTS
(ST-L-Test 22)

Peer Review _____ Peer Review _____

Skill Acquisition: _____ Practice Opportunities: _____

*This problem allows you the opportunity to demonstrate the **Trendelenburg Test (Trendelenburg Sign)**. You have 2 minutes to complete this task.*

Tester places athlete and limb in appropriate position	Test 1	Test 2	Test 3
Standing	Ⓨ Ⓝ	Ⓨ Ⓝ	Ⓨ Ⓝ
Tester placed in proper position	**Test 1**	**Test 2**	**Test 3**
Stands behind the athlete (observing only movement of the pelvis)	Ⓨ Ⓝ	Ⓨ Ⓝ	Ⓨ Ⓝ
Tester performs test according to accepted guidelines	**Test 1**	**Test 2**	**Test 3**
Instructs the athlete to balance on one leg (10 seconds)	Ⓨ Ⓝ	Ⓨ Ⓝ	Ⓨ Ⓝ
Performs assessment bilaterally	Ⓨ Ⓝ	Ⓨ Ⓝ	Ⓨ Ⓝ

The psychomotor skill was performed completely and in the appropriate order   0 1 2 3 4 5

The tester had control of the subject and the situation (showed confidence)   0 1 2 3 4 5

Method of performing the skill allowed the tester the ability to determine:
severity, proper progression, and the *fit* in the overall picture (Oral)   0 1 2 3 4 5

In order for a grade of *minimum standard* to be given, the total must be ≥11   TOTAL = _____

1 2 3 4 5 6 7 8 9 10 11 12 13 14 15

Not Acceptable   **Meets Minimum Standards**   **Exceeds Minimum Standards**

TEST ENVIRONMENTS

L: Laboratory/Classroom Testing
C: Clinical/Field Testing
P: Practicum Testing
A: Assessment/Mock Exam Testing
S: Self-Reporting

SKILL TEST INFORMATION

Positive Finding: Pelvis on the unsupported side/nonstance leg drops
Involved Structure: Gluteus medius (weakness)
Special Considerations: May view from the front
Reference(s): Konin et al (2002); Magee; Starkey et al (2002)
Supplies Needed: N/A

SPECIAL TESTS
(ST-L-Test 23)

Skill Acquisition: _____   Practice Opportunities: _____

This problem allows you the opportunity to demonstrate the **Thomas Test.** *You have 2 minutes to complete this task.*

Tester places athlete and limb in appropriate position	Test 1	Test 2	Test 3
Supine	Y N	Y N	Y N
Hips/knees in full extension	Y N	Y N	Y N
Tester placed in proper position	**Test 1**	**Test 2**	**Test 3**
Stands to the side of the athlete	Y N	Y N	Y N
Places one hand over the pelvis (monitors lumbar lordosis and/or pelvic tilt)	Y N	Y N	Y N
Places the other hand around the knee	Y N	Y N	Y N
Tester performs test according to accepted guidelines	**Test 1**	**Test 2**	**Test 3**
Passively flexes the hip and knee—overpressure (opposite limb is the involved hip)	Y N	Y N	Y N
Maintains relaxation of the limb	Y N	Y N	Y N
Performs assessment bilaterally	Y N	Y N	Y N

The psychomotor skill was performed completely and in the appropriate order   **0 1 2 3 4 5**

The tester had control of the subject and the situation (showed confidence)   **0 1 2 3 4 5**

Method of performing the skill allowed the tester the ability to determine: severity, proper progression, and the *fit* in the overall picture (Oral)   **0 1 2 3 4 5**

In order for a grade of *minimum standard* to be given, the total must be ≥11   **TOTAL = _____**

```
1    2    3    4    5    6    7    8    9   10   11   12   13   14   15
|____|____|____|____|____|____|____|____|____|____|____|____|____|____|
```
Not Acceptable   **Meets**   **Exceeds**
                                    Minimum Standards   **Minimum Standards**

TEST ENVIRONMENTS

L: Laboratory/Classroom Testing
C: Clinical/Field Testing
P: Practicum Testing
A: Assessment/Mock Exam Testing
S: Self-Reporting

SKILL TEST INFORMATION

Positive Finding: Opposite leg comes off the table

Involved Structure: Iliopsoas, rectus femoris

Special Considerations: Starting position may be full flexion, move to extension

Reference(s): Konin et al (2002); Magee; Starkey et al (2002)

Supplies Needed: Table

SPECIAL TESTS
(ST-L-Test 24)

Peer Review _____ Peer Review _____

Skill Acquisition: _____   Practice Opportunities: _____

This problem allows you the opportunity to demonstrate the **Rectus Femoris Contracture Test, Method 1.** *You have 2 minutes to complete this task.*

Tester places athlete and limb in appropriate position	Test 1	Test 2	Test 3
Supine	Ⓨ Ⓝ	Ⓨ Ⓝ	Ⓨ Ⓝ
Knees flexed to 90 degrees (legs off the edge of the table)	Ⓨ Ⓝ	Ⓨ Ⓝ	Ⓨ Ⓝ
Tester placed in proper position	**Test 1**	**Test 2**	**Test 3**
Stands to the side of the athlete (observing only)	Ⓨ Ⓝ	Ⓨ Ⓝ	Ⓨ Ⓝ
Tester performs test according to accepted guidelines	**Test 1**	**Test 2**	**Test 3**
Instructs the athlete to actively flex the hip and knee of the opposite side (may be done passively by the tester)	Ⓨ Ⓝ	Ⓨ Ⓝ	Ⓨ Ⓝ
Performs assessment bilaterally	Ⓨ Ⓝ	Ⓨ Ⓝ	Ⓨ Ⓝ

The psychomotor skill was performed completely and in the appropriate order   **0 1 2 3 4 5**

The tester had control of the subject and the situation (showed confidence)   **0 1 2 3 4 5**

Method of performing the skill allowed the tester the ability to determine:
severity, proper progression, and the *fit* in the overall picture (Oral)   **0 1 2 3 4 5**

In order for a grade of *minimum standard* to be given, the total must be ≥11   **TOTAL = _____**

```
1   2   3   4   5   6   7   8   9   10   11   12   13   14   15
```
Not Acceptable   **Meets**   **Exceeds**
                          Minimum Standards   **Minimum Standards**

TEST ENVIRONMENTS
L: Laboratory/Classroom Testing
C: Clinical/Field Testing
P: Practicum Testing
A: Assessment/Mock Exam Testing
S: Self-Reporting

SKILL TEST INFORMATION
Positive Finding: Opposite leg moves into an extended position (flexion and extension)
Involved Structure: Iliopsoas, rectus femoris
Special Considerations: N/A
Reference(s): Konin et al (2002); Magee
Supplies Needed: Table

SPECIAL TESTS
(ST-L-Test 25)

Peer Review _____ Peer Review _____

Skill Acquisition: _____   Practice Opportunities: _____

This problem allows you the opportunity to demonstrate **Ober's Test**. *You have 2 minutes to complete this task.*

Tester places athlete and limb in appropriate position	Test 1	Test 2	Test 3
Side lying (involved limb on top)	Ⓨ Ⓝ	Ⓨ Ⓝ	Ⓨ Ⓝ
Hip/knee of the opposite limb is flexed	Ⓨ Ⓝ	Ⓨ Ⓝ	Ⓨ Ⓝ
Tester placed in proper position	**Test 1**	**Test 2**	**Test 3**
Stands behind the athlete	Ⓨ Ⓝ	Ⓨ Ⓝ	Ⓨ Ⓝ
Places hand over the lateral aspect of the pelvis (prevent rolling/stabilize)	Ⓨ Ⓝ	Ⓨ Ⓝ	Ⓨ Ⓝ
Places the other hand under the lower leg (support)	Ⓨ Ⓝ	Ⓨ Ⓝ	Ⓨ Ⓝ
Tester performs test according to accepted guidelines	**Test 1**	**Test 2**	**Test 3**
Passively abducts and extends the hip	Ⓨ Ⓝ	Ⓨ Ⓝ	Ⓨ Ⓝ
Instructs the athlete to slowly lower the hip (adduction)	Ⓨ Ⓝ	Ⓨ Ⓝ	Ⓨ Ⓝ
Performs assessment bilaterally	Ⓨ Ⓝ	Ⓨ Ⓝ	Ⓨ Ⓝ

The psychomotor skill was performed completely and in the appropriate order   **0 1 2 3 4 5**

The tester had control of the subject and the situation (showed confidence)   **0 1 2 3 4 5**

Method of performing the skill allowed the tester the ability to determine:
severity, proper progression, and the *fit* in the overall picture (Oral)   **0 1 2 3 4 5**

In order for a grade of *minimum standard* to be given, the total must be ≥11   **TOTAL = _____**

```
 1    2    3    4    5    6    7    8    9   10   11   12   13   14   15
 |    |    |    |    |    |    |    |    |    |    |    |    |    |    |
```

Not Acceptable   **Meets**   **Exceeds**
                            Minimum Standards   **Minimum Standards**

TEST ENVIRONMENTS

L: Laboratory/Classroom Testing
C: Clinical/Field Testing
P: Practicum Testing
A: Assessment/Mock Exam Testing
S: Self-Reporting

SKILL TEST INFORMATION

Positive Finding: Unable to adduct the hip
Involved Structure: Iliotibial band, tensor fasciae-latae
Special Considerations: N/A
Reference(s): Konin et al (2002); Magee; Starkey et al (2002)
Supplies Needed: Table

SPECIAL TESTS
(ST-L-Test 26)

Peer Review _____ Peer Review _____

Skill Acquisition: _____   Practice Opportunities: _____

This problem allows you the opportunity to demonstrate **Noble's Compression Test (Noble's Test)** *in order to help rule out iliotibial band friction syndrome. You have 2 minutes to complete this task.*

Tester places athlete and limb in appropriate position	Test 1	Test 2	Test 3
Supine	Ⓨ Ⓝ	Ⓨ Ⓝ	Ⓨ Ⓝ
Knee flexed to 90 degrees	Ⓨ Ⓝ	Ⓨ Ⓝ	Ⓨ Ⓝ
Tester placed in proper position	**Test 1**	**Test 2**	**Test 3**
Stands to the side of the athlete	Ⓨ Ⓝ	Ⓨ Ⓝ	Ⓨ Ⓝ
Places thumb and/or fingers over the lateral femoral epicondyle	Ⓨ Ⓝ	Ⓨ Ⓝ	Ⓨ Ⓝ
Places other hand under the knee for support	Ⓨ Ⓝ	Ⓨ Ⓝ	Ⓨ Ⓝ
Tester performs test according to accepted guidelines	**Test 1**	**Test 2**	**Test 3**
Applies pressure over the lateral femoral epicondyle	Ⓨ Ⓝ	Ⓨ Ⓝ	Ⓨ Ⓝ
Instructs the athlete to actively extend the knee at slow pace (may be performed passively)	Ⓨ Ⓝ	Ⓨ Ⓝ	Ⓨ Ⓝ
Performs assessment bilaterally	Ⓨ Ⓝ	Ⓨ Ⓝ	Ⓨ Ⓝ

The psychomotor skill was performed completely and in the appropriate order   0 1 2 3 4 5

The tester had control of the subject and the situation (showed confidence)   0 1 2 3 4 5

Method of performing the skill allowed the tester the ability to determine:
severity, proper progression, and the *fit* in the overall picture (Oral)   0 1 2 3 4 5

In order for a grade of *minimum standard* to be given, the total must be ≥11   **TOTAL = _____**

```
  1     2     3     4     5     6     7     8     9     10    11    12    13    14    15
  |     |     |     |     |     |     |     |     |     |     |     |     |     |     |
```

Not Acceptable   **Meets**   **Exceeds**
                                      Minimum Standards   **Minimum Standards**

TEST ENVIRONMENTS

L: Laboratory/Classroom Testing
C: Clinical/Field Testing
P: Practicum Testing
A: Assessment/Mock Exam Testing
S: Self-Reporting

SKILL TEST INFORMATION

Positive Finding:	Increased pain around 30 degrees of extension
Involved Structure:	Iliotibial band
Special Considerations:	N/A
Reference(s):	Magee; Starkey et al (2002)
Supplies Needed:	Table

SPECIAL TESTS
(ST-L-Test 27)

Skill Acquisition: _____   Practice Opportunities: _____

This problem allows you the opportunity to demonstrate the **Piriformis Test**. *You have 2 minutes to complete this task.*

Tester places athlete and limb in appropriate position	Test 1	Test 2	Test 3
Side lying near the edge to the table (involved side on top)	Ⓨ Ⓝ	Ⓨ Ⓝ	Ⓨ Ⓝ
Hip flexed to 60 degrees	Ⓨ Ⓝ	Ⓨ Ⓝ	Ⓨ Ⓝ
Knee in slight flexion	Ⓨ Ⓝ	Ⓨ Ⓝ	Ⓨ Ⓝ
Tester placed in proper position	**Test 1**	**Test 2**	**Test 3**
Stands behind the athlete	Ⓨ Ⓝ	Ⓨ Ⓝ	Ⓨ Ⓝ
Places hand over the lateral aspect of the pelvis (prevent rolling/stabilize)	Ⓨ Ⓝ	Ⓨ Ⓝ	Ⓨ Ⓝ
Places the other hand over the knee	Ⓨ Ⓝ	Ⓨ Ⓝ	Ⓨ Ⓝ
Tester performs test according to accepted guidelines	**Test 1**	**Test 2**	**Test 3**
Applies a downward pressure on the knee	Ⓨ Ⓝ	Ⓨ Ⓝ	Ⓨ Ⓝ
Maintains relaxation of the limb	Ⓨ Ⓝ	Ⓨ Ⓝ	Ⓨ Ⓝ
Performs assessment bilaterally	Ⓨ Ⓝ	Ⓨ Ⓝ	Ⓨ Ⓝ

The psychomotor skill was performed completely and in the appropriate order   0 1 2 3 4 5

The tester had control of the subject and the situation (showed confidence)   0 1 2 3 4 5

Method of performing the skill allowed the tester the ability to determine:
severity, proper progression, and the *fit* in the overall picture (Oral)   0 1 2 3 4 5

In order for a grade of *minimum standard* to be given, the total must be ≥11   **TOTAL = _____**

```
    1    2    3    4    5    6    7    8    9   10   11   12   13   14   15
    |    |    |    |    |    |    |    |    |    |    |    |    |    |    |
 Not Acceptable                           Meets                  Exceeds
                                     Minimum Standards      Minimum Standards
```

TEST ENVIRONMENTS	**SKILL TEST INFORMATION**	
L: Laboratory/Classroom Testing	**Positive Finding:**	Tightness and/or pain
C: Clinical/Field Testing	**Involved Structure:**	Piriformis/sciatic nerve
P: Practicum Testing	**Special Considerations:**	N/A
A: Assessment/Mock Exam Testing	**Reference(s):**	Konin et al (2002); Magee
S: Self-Reporting	**Supplies Needed:**	Table

SPECIAL TESTS
(ST-L-Test 28)

Skill Acquisition: _____   Practice Opportunities: _____

This problem allows you the opportunity to demonstrate the **90/90 Straight Leg Raise Test (Hamstrings Contracture, Method 3)**. *You have 2 minutes to complete this task.*

Tester places athlete and limb in appropriate position	Test 1	Test 2	Test 3
Supine	Ⓨ Ⓝ	Ⓨ Ⓝ	Ⓨ Ⓝ
Hips flexed to 90 degrees (supported by the athlete)	Ⓨ Ⓝ	Ⓨ Ⓝ	Ⓨ Ⓝ
Knees flexed to 90 degrees	Ⓨ Ⓝ	Ⓨ Ⓝ	Ⓨ Ⓝ
Tester placed in proper position	**Test 1**	**Test 2**	**Test 3**
Standing to the side of the athlete (observing only)	Ⓨ Ⓝ	Ⓨ Ⓝ	Ⓨ Ⓝ
Tester performs test according to accepted guidelines	**Test 1**	**Test 2**	**Test 3**
Instructs athlete to actively extend knee	Ⓨ Ⓝ	Ⓨ Ⓝ	Ⓨ Ⓝ
Performs assessment bilaterally	Ⓨ Ⓝ	Ⓨ Ⓝ	Ⓨ Ⓝ

The psychomotor skill was performed completely and in the appropriate order   **0 1 2 3 4 5**

The tester had control of the subject and the situation (showed confidence)   **0 1 2 3 4 5**

Method of performing the skill allowed the tester the ability to determine:
severity, proper progression, and the *fit* in the overall picture (Oral)   **0 1 2 3 4 5**

In order for a grade of *minimum standard* to be given, the total must be ≥11   **TOTAL = _____**

1	2	3	4	5	6	7	8	9	10	11	12	13	14	15

Not Acceptable   **Meets**   **Exceeds**
                          Minimum Standards   **Minimum Standards**

TEST ENVIRONMENTS

L: Laboratory/Classroom Testing
C: Clinical/Field Testing
P: Practicum Testing
A: Assessment/Mock Exam Testing
S: Self-Reporting

SKILL TEST INFORMATION

Positive Finding:	Not able to extend to 20 degrees
Involved Structure:	Hamstrings
Special Considerations:	N/A
Reference(s):	Konin et al (2002); Magee
Supplies Needed:	Table

SPECIAL TESTS
(ST-L-Test 29)

Peer Review _____ Peer Review _____

Skill Acquisition: _____   Practice Opportunities: _____

This problem allows you the opportunity to demonstrate the special test known as the **Gillet's Test (Sacral Fixation Test)**. *You have 2 minutes to complete this task.*

Tester places athlete and limb in appropriate position	Test 1	Test 2	Test 3
Standing	Ⓨ Ⓝ	Ⓨ Ⓝ	Ⓨ Ⓝ

Tester placed in proper position	Test 1	Test 2	Test 3
Standing behind the athlete	Ⓨ Ⓝ	Ⓨ Ⓝ	Ⓨ Ⓝ
Hands palpating the PSIS (monitor movement of the PSIS)	Ⓨ Ⓝ	Ⓨ Ⓝ	Ⓨ Ⓝ

Tester performs test according to accepted guidelines	Test 1	Test 2	Test 3
Instructs the athlete to actively flex the knee and hip while balancing on one leg (pulling toward the chest)	Ⓨ Ⓝ	Ⓨ Ⓝ	Ⓨ Ⓝ
Performs assessment bilaterally	Ⓨ Ⓝ	Ⓨ Ⓝ	Ⓨ Ⓝ

The psychomotor skill was performed completely and in the appropriate order   0 1 2 3 4 5

The tester had control of the subject and the situation (showed confidence)   0 1 2 3 4 5

Method of performing the skill allowed the tester the ability to determine: severity, proper progression, and the *fit* in the overall picture (Oral)   0 1 2 3 4 5

In order for a grade of *minimum standard* to be given, the total must be ≥11   TOTAL = _____

```
 1   2   3   4   5   6   7   8   9   10   11   12   13   14   15
 |   |   |   |   |   |   |   |   |   |    |    |    |    |    |
```
Not Acceptable   **Meets**   **Exceeds**
                          Minimum Standards   **Minimum Standards**

TEST ENVIRONMENTS
L: Laboratory/Classroom Testing
C: Clinical/Field Testing
P: Practicum Testing
A: Assessment/Mock Exam Testing
S: Self-Reporting

SKILL TEST INFORMATION
Positive Finding: Flexed side moves upward hypomobility
Involved Structure: Sacroiliac
Special Considerations: Normal movement should be downward (inferiorly)
Reference(s): Magee
Supplies Needed: N/A

SPECIAL TESTS
(ST-L-Test 30)

Peer Review _____ Peer Review _____

Skill Acquisition: _____   Practice Opportunities: _____

This problem allows you the opportunity to demonstrate the special test known as the **Squish Test.** *You have 2 minutes to complete this task.*

Tester places athlete and limb in appropriate position	Test 1	Test 2	Test 3
Supine	Ⓨ Ⓝ	Ⓨ Ⓝ	Ⓨ Ⓝ
Tester placed in proper position	**Test 1**	**Test 2**	**Test 3**
Stands behind the athlete	Ⓨ Ⓝ	Ⓨ Ⓝ	Ⓨ Ⓝ
Places hands over the ASIS/iliac crest	Ⓨ Ⓝ	Ⓨ Ⓝ	Ⓨ Ⓝ
Tester performs test according to accepted guidelines	**Test 1**	**Test 2**	**Test 3**
Passively push down and in (45 degree angle)	Ⓨ Ⓝ	Ⓨ Ⓝ	Ⓨ Ⓝ
Maintains relaxation of the limb	Ⓨ Ⓝ	Ⓨ Ⓝ	Ⓨ Ⓝ

The psychomotor skill was performed completely and in the appropriate order   0 1 2 3 4 5

The tester had control of the subject and the situation (showed confidence)   0 1 2 3 4 5

Method of performing the skill allowed the tester the ability to determine:
severity, proper progression, and the *fit* in the overall picture (Oral)   0 1 2 3 4 5

In order for a grade of *minimum standard* to be given, the total must be ≥11   TOTAL = _____

```
 1    2    3    4    5    6    7    8    9   10   11   12   13   14   15
 |    |    |    |    |    |    |    |    |    |    |    |    |    |    |
```

Not Acceptable   **Meets**   **Exceeds**
                                     Minimum Standards   **Minimum Standards**

TEST ENVIRONMENTS

L: Laboratory/Classroom Testing
C: Clinical/Field Testing
P: Practicum Testing
A: Assessment/Mock Exam Testing
S: Self-Reporting

SKILL TEST INFORMATION

Positive Finding: Pain
Involved Structure: Posterior sacroiliac ligament
Special Considerations: N/A
Reference(s): Magee
Supplies Needed: Table

SPECIAL TESTS
(ST-L-Test 31)

Peer Review _____ Peer Review _____

Skill Acquisition: _____   Practice Opportunities: _____

This problem allows you the opportunity to demonstrate the special test known as the **Long Sit Test (Supine-to-Sit Test)**. *You have 2 minutes to perform this task.*

Tester places athlete and limb in appropriate position	Test 1	Test 2	Test 3
Supine	Ⓨ Ⓝ	Ⓨ Ⓝ	Ⓨ Ⓝ
Heels off the table (both medial malleoli should be even with each other)	Ⓨ Ⓝ	Ⓨ Ⓝ	Ⓨ Ⓝ
Tester placed in proper position	**Test 1**	**Test 2**	**Test 3**
Stands at the athlete's feet	Ⓨ Ⓝ	Ⓨ Ⓝ	Ⓨ Ⓝ
Places hands/thumbs over the medial malleoli	Ⓨ Ⓝ	Ⓨ Ⓝ	Ⓨ Ⓝ
Tester performs test according to accepted guidelines	**Test 1**	**Test 2**	**Test 3**
Instructs the athlete to actively sit up (supine to sitting)	Ⓨ Ⓝ	Ⓨ Ⓝ	Ⓨ Ⓝ
Repeat (confirm the results)	Ⓨ Ⓝ	Ⓨ Ⓝ	Ⓨ Ⓝ

The psychomotor skill was performed completely and in the appropriate order   0 1 2 3 4 5

The tester had control of the subject and the situation (showed confidence)   0 1 2 3 4 5

Method of performing the skill allowed the tester the ability to determine:
severity, proper progression, and the *fit* in the overall picture (Oral)   0 1 2 3 4 5

In order for a grade of *minimum standard* to be given, the total must be ≥11   TOTAL = _____

```
 1   2   3   4   5   6   7   8   9   10  11  12  13  14  15
 |   |   |   |   |   |   |   |   |   |   |   |   |   |   |
Not Acceptable                    Meets              Exceeds
                             Minimum Standards   Minimum Standards
```

TEST ENVIRONMENTS
L: Laboratory/Classroom Testing
C: Clinical/Field Testing
P: Practicum Testing
A: Assessment/Mock Exam Testing
S: Self-Reporting

SKILL TEST INFORMATION
Positive Finding: One leg moves further than the other (medial malleoli)
Involved Structure: Ilium (rotation/functional)
Special Considerations: N/A
Reference(s): Magee; Starkey et al (2002)
Supplies Needed: Table

SPECIAL TESTS
(ST-L-Test 32)

Peer Review _____ Peer Review _____

Skill Acquisition: _____ Practice Opportunities: _____

*This problem allows you the opportunity to demonstrate the **Slump Test**. You have 2 minutes to complete this task.*

Tester places athlete and limb in appropriate position	Test 1	Test 2	Test 3
Seated (knees off the edge of the table at 90 degrees)	Y N	Y N	Y N
Hands positioned behind the back	Y N	Y N	Y N
Tester placed in proper position	**Test 1**	**Test 2**	**Test 3**
Stands to the side of the athlete	Y N	Y N	Y N
Hand position changes throughout the assessment	Y N	Y N	Y N
Tester performs test according to accepted guidelines	**Test 1**	**Test 2**	**Test 3**
Instructs the athlete to actively flex the thoracic and lumbar area (head remains neutral)	Y N	Y N	Y N
Passively applies overpressure to maintain flexion of the thoracic and lumbar areas	Y N	Y N	Y N
Instructs the athlete to actively flex the head (chin to chest)	Y N	Y N	Y N
Passively applies overpressure to maintain flexion of the head	Y N	Y N	Y N
Passively dorsiflexes the foot (maintains)	Y N	Y N	Y N
Instructs the athlete to actively extend the knee	Y N	Y N	Y N
Performs assessment bilaterally	Y N	Y N	Y N

The psychomotor skill was performed completely and in the appropriate order   0 1 2 3 4 5

The tester had control of the subject and the situation (showed confidence)   0 1 2 3 4 5

Method of performing the skill allowed the tester the ability to determine:
severity, proper progression, and the *fit* in the overall picture (Oral)   0 1 2 3 4 5

In order for a grade of *minimum standard* to be given, the total must be ≥11   TOTAL = _____

```
  1    2    3    4    5    6    7    8    9    10   11   12   13   14   15
  |    |    |    |    |    |    |    |    |    |    |    |    |    |    |
```

Not Acceptable   **Meets**   **Exceeds**
                          Minimum Standards   **Minimum Standards**

TEST ENVIRONMENTS

L: Laboratory/Classroom Testing
C: Clinical/Field Testing
P: Practicum Testing
A: Assessment/Mock Exam Testing
S: Self-Reporting

SKILL TEST INFORMATION

Positive Finding: Pain/neurological symptoms
Involved Structure: Nerve root; neurological structures
Special Considerations: Do not continue to next stage if pain occurs
Reference(s): Konin et al (2002); Magee; Starkey et al (2002)
Supplies Needed: Table

SPECIAL TESTS
(ST-L-Test 33)

Peer Review _____ Peer Review _____

Skill Acquisition: _____   Practice Opportunities: _____

This problem allows you the opportunity to demonstrate the special test known as the **Straight Leg Raise Test (Unilateral Straight Leg Raise/Lasegue Test)***. You have 2 minutes to complete this task..*

Tester places athlete and limb in appropriate position	Test 1	Test 2	Test 3
Supine	Ⓨ Ⓝ	Ⓨ Ⓝ	Ⓨ Ⓝ
Hip slightly adducted and medially rotated	Ⓨ Ⓝ	Ⓨ Ⓝ	Ⓨ Ⓝ
Tester placed in proper position	**Test 1**	**Test 2**	**Test 3**
Stands to the side of the athlete (may kneel on the table)	Ⓨ Ⓝ	Ⓨ Ⓝ	Ⓨ Ⓝ
Places one hand on the anterior thigh (maintains knee extension)	Ⓨ Ⓝ	Ⓨ Ⓝ	Ⓨ Ⓝ
Places the other hand around the foot	Ⓨ Ⓝ	Ⓨ Ⓝ	Ⓨ Ⓝ
Tester performs test according to accepted guidelines	**Test 1**	**Test 2**	**Test 3**
Passively flexes the hip (until painful)	Ⓨ Ⓝ	Ⓨ Ⓝ	Ⓨ Ⓝ
Slowly lowers the limb until pain dissipates	Ⓨ Ⓝ	Ⓨ Ⓝ	Ⓨ Ⓝ
Passively dorsiflexes the foot	Ⓨ Ⓝ	Ⓨ Ⓝ	Ⓨ Ⓝ
Instructs the athlete to actively flex the head (chin to chest)	Ⓨ Ⓝ	Ⓨ Ⓝ	Ⓨ Ⓝ
Maintains relaxation of the limb	Ⓨ Ⓝ	Ⓨ Ⓝ	Ⓨ Ⓝ
Performs assessment bilaterally	Ⓨ Ⓝ	Ⓨ Ⓝ	Ⓨ Ⓝ

The psychomotor skill was performed completely and in the appropriate order   0 1 2 3 4 5

The tester had control of the subject and the situation (showed confidence)   0 1 2 3 4 5

Method of performing the skill allowed the tester the ability to determine:
severity, proper progression, and the *fit* in the overall picture (Oral)   0 1 2 3 4 5

In order for a grade of *minimum standard* to be given, the total must be ≥11   **TOTAL = _____**

| 1 | 2 | 3 | 4 | 5 | 6 | 7 | 8 | 9 | 10 | 11 | 12 | 13 | 14 | 15 |

Not Acceptable   **Meets**   **Exceeds**
                              Minimum Standards   **Minimum Standards**

TEST ENVIRONMENTS

L: Laboratory/Classroom Testing
C: Clinical/Field Testing
P: Practicum Testing
A: Assessment/Mock Exam Testing
S: Self-Reporting

SKILL TEST INFORMATION

Positive Finding: Increased pain with dorsiflexion and/or flexion of the head
Involved Structure: Dural involvement
Special Considerations: Must rule out hamstrings
Reference(s): Konin et al (2002); Magee; Starkey et al (2002)
Supplies Needed: Table

Special Tests
(ST-L-Test 34)

Peer Review _____ Peer Review _____

Skill Acquisition: _____   Practice Opportunities: _____

This problem allows you the opportunity to demonstrate the special test known as the **Well Straight Leg Raise Test (Well Straight Leg Raise Test of Fajersztajn/Lhermitt's Test/Crossover Sign)**. *You have 2 minutes to complete this task.*

Tester places athlete and limb in appropriate position	Test 1	Test 2	Test 3
Supine	Ⓨ Ⓝ	Ⓨ Ⓝ	Ⓨ Ⓝ
Tester placed in proper position	**Test 1**	**Test 2**	**Test 3**
Stands to the side of the athlete (may kneel on the table)	Ⓨ Ⓝ	Ⓨ Ⓝ	Ⓨ Ⓝ
Places one hand on anterior thigh (maintain knee extension)	Ⓨ Ⓝ	Ⓨ Ⓝ	Ⓨ Ⓝ
Place the other hand around the foot	Ⓨ Ⓝ	Ⓨ Ⓝ	Ⓨ Ⓝ
Tester performs test according to accepted guidelines	**Test 1**	**Test 2**	**Test 3**
Passively flexes the hip (until painful at opposite side)	Ⓨ Ⓝ	Ⓨ Ⓝ	Ⓨ Ⓝ
Maintains relaxation of the limb	Ⓨ Ⓝ	Ⓨ Ⓝ	Ⓨ Ⓝ
Performs assessment bilaterally	Ⓨ Ⓝ	Ⓨ Ⓝ	Ⓨ Ⓝ

The psychomotor skill was performed completely and in the appropriate order   **0 1 2 3 4 5**

The tester had control of the subject and the situation (showed confidence)   **0 1 2 3 4 5**

Method of performing the skill allowed the tester the ability to determine:
severity, proper progression, and the *fit* in the overall picture (Oral)   **0 1 2 3 4 5**

In order for a grade of *minimum standard* to be given, the total must be ≥11   **TOTAL = _____**

```
  1    2    3    4    5    6    7    8    9    10   11   12   13   14   15
  |    |    |    |    |    |    |    |    |    |    |    |    |    |    |
```

Not Acceptable   Meets   Exceeds
                                          Minimum Standards   Minimum Standards

TEST ENVIRONMENTS

L: Laboratory/Classroom Testing
C: Clinical/Field Testing
P: Practicum Testing
A: Assessment/Mock Exam Testing
S: Self-Reporting

SKILL TEST INFORMATION

Positive Finding:	Pain on opposite side
Involved Structure:	Space-occupying lesion
Special Considerations:	N/A
Reference(s):	Konin et al (2002); Magee; Starkey et al (2002)
Supplies Needed:	Table

SPECIAL TESTS
(ST-L-Test 35)

Peer Review _____ Peer Review _____

Skill Acquisition: _____   Practice Opportunities: _____

*This problem allows you the opportunity to demonstrate the special test known as the **Kernig's Sign***. *You have 2 minutes to complete this task.*

Tester places athlete and limb in appropriate position	Test 1	Test 2	Test 3
Supine	Ⓨ Ⓝ	Ⓨ Ⓝ	Ⓨ Ⓝ
Tester placed in proper position	**Test 1**	**Test 2**	**Test 3**
Stands to the side of the athlete (observes only)	Ⓨ Ⓝ	Ⓨ Ⓝ	Ⓨ Ⓝ
Tester performs test according to accepted guidelines	**Test 1**	**Test 2**	**Test 3**
Instructs the athlete to actively flex the hip until painful (maintain knee extension)	Ⓨ Ⓝ	Ⓨ Ⓝ	Ⓨ Ⓝ
Instructs the athlete to slowly flex the knee until pain dissipates	Ⓨ Ⓝ	Ⓨ Ⓝ	Ⓨ Ⓝ
Performs assessment bilaterally	Ⓨ Ⓝ	Ⓨ Ⓝ	Ⓨ Ⓝ

Adding head flexion: Kernig-Brudzinski Test

The psychomotor skill was performed completely and in the appropriate order   0 1 2 3 4 5

The tester had control of the subject and the situation (showed confidence)   0 1 2 3 4 5

Method of performing the skill allowed the tester the ability to determine:
severity, proper progression, and the *fit* in the overall picture (Oral)   0 1 2 3 4 5

In order for a grade of *minimum standard* to be given, the total must be ≥11   TOTAL = _____

```
  1    2    3    4    5    6    7    8    9   10   11   12   13   14   15
  |    |    |    |    |    |    |    |    |    |    |    |    |    |    |
```

Not Acceptable   **Meets**   **Exceeds**
                                        Minimum Standards   **Minimum Standards**

TEST ENVIRONMENTS

L: Laboratory/Classroom Testing
C: Clinical/Field Testing
P: Practicum Testing
A: Assessment/Mock Exam Testing
S: Self-Reporting

SKILL TEST INFORMATION

Positive Finding:	Pain is relieved with flexion of the knee
Involved Structure:	Nerve root (impingement)
Special Considerations:	N/A
Reference(s):	Konin et al (2002); Starkey et al (2002)
Supplies Needed:	Table

SPECIAL TESTS
(ST-L-Test 36)

Peer Review _____ Peer Review _____

Skill Acquisition: _____   Practice Opportunities: _____

This problem allows you the opportunity to demonstrate the special test known as the **Brudzinski's Sign***. You have 2 minutes to complete this task.*

Tester places athlete and limb in appropriate position	Test 1	Test 2	Test 3
Supine	Ⓨ Ⓝ	Ⓨ Ⓝ	Ⓨ Ⓝ
Cupped hands behind the neck	Ⓨ Ⓝ	Ⓨ Ⓝ	Ⓨ Ⓝ
Tester placed in proper position	**Test 1**	**Test 2**	**Test 3**
Stands to the side of the athlete	Ⓨ Ⓝ	Ⓨ Ⓝ	Ⓨ Ⓝ
Tester performs test according to accepted guidelines	**Test 1**	**Test 2**	**Test 3**
Instructs the athlete to actively flex the head (chin to chest)	Ⓨ Ⓝ	Ⓨ Ⓝ	Ⓨ Ⓝ
May flex the head passively (overpressure)	Ⓨ Ⓝ	Ⓨ Ⓝ	Ⓨ Ⓝ

The psychomotor skill was performed completely and in the appropriate order   **0 1 2 3 4 5**

The tester had control of the subject and the situation (showed confidence)   **0 1 2 3 4 5**

Method of performing the skill allowed the tester the ability to determine:
severity, proper progression, and the *fit* in the overall picture (Oral)   **0 1 2 3 4 5**

In order for a grade of *minimum standard* to be given, the total must be ≥11   **TOTAL = _____**

```
  1    2    3    4    5    6    7    8    9    10   11   12   13   14   15
  |    |    |    |    |    |    |    |    |    |    |    |    |    |    |
```

Not Acceptable   **Meets**   **Exceeds**
                                   Minimum Standards   **Minimum Standards**

TEST ENVIRONMENTS

L: Laboratory/Classroom Testing
C: Clinical/Field Testing
P: Practicum Testing
A: Assessment/Mock Exam Testing
S: Self-Reporting

SKILL TEST INFORMATION

Positive Finding: Pain; involuntarily flexes knee(s)
Involved Structure: Nerve root
Special Considerations: N/A
Reference(s): Konin et al (2002); Magee; Starkey et al (2002)
Supplies Needed: Table

SPECIAL TESTS
(ST-L-Test 37)

Peer Review _____ Peer Review _____

Skill Acquisition: _____   Practice Opportunities: _____

This problem allows you the opportunity to demonstrate the **Bowstring Test (Cram Test/Popliteal Pressure Sign)** *in order to help rule out pressure on the sciatic nerve. You have 2 minutes to complete this task.*

Tester places athlete and limb in appropriate position	Test 1	Test 2	Test 3
Supine	Ⓨ Ⓝ	Ⓨ Ⓝ	Ⓨ Ⓝ
Hip slightly adducted and medially rotated	Ⓨ Ⓝ	Ⓨ Ⓝ	Ⓨ Ⓝ
Tester placed in proper position	**Test 1**	**Test 2**	**Test 3**
Stands to the side of the athlete (may kneel on the table)	Ⓨ Ⓝ	Ⓨ Ⓝ	Ⓨ Ⓝ
Places one hand on the anterior thigh (maintains knee extension)	Ⓨ Ⓝ	Ⓨ Ⓝ	Ⓨ Ⓝ
Places the other hand around the foot	Ⓨ Ⓝ	Ⓨ Ⓝ	Ⓨ Ⓝ
Tester performs test according to accepted guidelines	**Test 1**	**Test 2**	**Test 3**
Passively flexes the hip (until painful)	Ⓨ Ⓝ	Ⓨ Ⓝ	Ⓨ Ⓝ
Slowly flexes the knee about 20 degrees	Ⓨ Ⓝ	Ⓨ Ⓝ	Ⓨ Ⓝ
Applies pressure into the popliteal space	Ⓨ Ⓝ	Ⓨ Ⓝ	Ⓨ Ⓝ
Maintains relaxation of the limb	Ⓨ Ⓝ	Ⓨ Ⓝ	Ⓨ Ⓝ
Performs assessment bilaterally	Ⓨ Ⓝ	Ⓨ Ⓝ	Ⓨ Ⓝ

The psychomotor skill was performed completely and in the appropriate order   0 1 2 3 4 5

The tester had control of the subject and the situation (showed confidence)   0 1 2 3 4 5

Method of performing the skill allowed the tester the ability to determine:
severity, proper progression, and the *fit* in the overall picture (Oral)   0 1 2 3 4 5

In order for a grade of *minimum standard* to be given, the total must be ≥11   TOTAL = _____

```
  1     2     3     4     5     6     7     8     9    10    11    12    13    14    15
  |     |     |     |     |     |     |     |     |     |     |     |     |     |     |
```

Not Acceptable   **Meets**   **Exceeds**
                                    Minimum Standards   **Minimum Standards**

TEST ENVIRONMENTS	**SKILL TEST INFORMATION**	
L: Laboratory/Classroom Testing	**Positive Finding:**	Pain (with pressure)
C: Clinical/Field Testing	**Involved Structure:**	Sciatic nerve
P: Practicum Testing	**Special Considerations:**	N/A
A: Assessment/Mock Exam Testing	**Reference(s):**	Konin et al (2002); Magee
S: Self-Reporting	**Supplies Needed:**	Table

SPECIAL TESTS
(ST-L-Test 38)

Peer Review _____   Peer Review _____

Skill Acquisition: _____   Practice Opportunities: _____

This problem allows you the opportunity to demonstrate the special test known as the **Hoover's Sign**. *You have 2 minutes to complete this task.*

Tester places athlete and limb in appropriate position	Test 1	Test 2	Test 3
Supine (heels completely on the table)	Ⓨ Ⓝ	Ⓨ Ⓝ	Ⓨ Ⓝ
Tester placed in proper position	**Test 1**	**Test 2**	**Test 3**
Stands at the athlete's feet	Ⓨ Ⓝ	Ⓨ Ⓝ	Ⓨ Ⓝ
Places the palms of the hands under the heels (calcaneus)	Ⓨ Ⓝ	Ⓨ Ⓝ	Ⓨ Ⓝ
Tester performs test according to accepted guidelines	**Test 1**	**Test 2**	**Test 3**
Instructs the athlete to actively flex the hip	Ⓨ Ⓝ	Ⓨ Ⓝ	Ⓨ Ⓝ
Instructs the athlete to actively flex the other hip	Ⓨ Ⓝ	Ⓨ Ⓝ	Ⓨ Ⓝ

The psychomotor skill was performed completely and in the appropriate order   0 1 2 3 4 5

The tester had control of the subject and the situation (showed confidence)   0 1 2 3 4 5

Method of performing the skill allowed the tester the ability to determine:
severity, proper progression, and the *fit* in the overall picture (Oral)   0 1 2 3 4 5

In order for a grade of *minimum standard* to be given, the total must be ≥11   **TOTAL = _____**

```
  1     2     3     4     5     6     7     8     9    10    11    12    13    14    15
  |     |     |     |     |     |     |     |     |     |     |     |     |     |     |
```

Not Acceptable   **Meets**   **Exceeds**
                                           Minimum Standards   **Minimum Standards**

TEST ENVIRONMENTS

L: Laboratory/Classroom Testing
C: Clinical/Field Testing
P: Practicum Testing
A: Assessment/Mock Exam Testing
S: Self-Reporting

SKILL TEST INFORMATION

Positive Finding: No downward pressure by the opposite leg
Involved Structure: Neuromuscular weakness or lack of effort by the subject
Special Considerations: N/A
Reference(s): Konin et al (2002); Magee
Supplies Needed: Table

SPECIAL TESTS
(ST-L-Test 39)

Peer Review _____ Peer Review _____

Skill Acquisition: _____   Practice Opportunities: _____

This problem allows you the opportunity to demonstrate the special test known as the **Stork Standing Test (One Leg Standing Lumbar Extension Test)**. *You have 2 minutes to complete this task.*

Tester places athlete and limb in appropriate position	Test 1	Test 2	Test 3
Standing	Ⓨ Ⓝ	Ⓨ Ⓝ	Ⓨ Ⓝ
Tester placed in proper position	**Test 1**	**Test 2**	**Test 3**
Stands behind the athlete (observe only)	Ⓨ Ⓝ	Ⓨ Ⓝ	Ⓨ Ⓝ
Tester performs test according to accepted guidelines	**Test 1**	**Test 2**	**Test 3**
Instructs the athlete to balance on one leg	Ⓨ Ⓝ	Ⓨ Ⓝ	Ⓨ Ⓝ
Instructs the athlete to hyperextend the trunk (maintain balance)	Ⓨ Ⓝ	Ⓨ Ⓝ	Ⓨ Ⓝ
Repeat test on opposite leg	Ⓨ Ⓝ	Ⓨ Ⓝ	Ⓨ Ⓝ

The psychomotor skill was performed completely and in the appropriate order   0 1 2 3 4 5

The tester had control of the subject and the situation (showed confidence)   0 1 2 3 4 5

Method of performing the skill allowed the tester the ability to determine:
severity, proper progression, and the *fit* in the overall picture (Oral)   0 1 2 3 4 5

In order for a grade of *minimum standard* to be given, the total must be ≥11   **TOTAL = _____**

```
 1    2    3    4    5    6    7    8    9   10   11   12   13   14   15
 |    |    |    |    |    |    |    |    |    |    |    |    |    |    |
```

Not Acceptable   **Meets**   **Exceeds**
                                      Minimum Standards   **Minimum Standards**

TEST ENVIRONMENTS	**SKILL TEST INFORMATION**	
L: Laboratory/Classroom Testing	**Positive Finding:**	Pain
C: Clinical/Field Testing	**Involved Structure:**	Pars interarticularis (lumbar area)
P: Practicum Testing	**Special Considerations:**	N/A
A: Assessment/Mock Exam Testing	**Reference(s):**	Magee
S: Self-Reporting	**Supplies Needed:**	N/A

SPECIAL TESTS
(ST-L-Test 40)

Peer Review _____ Peer Review _____

Skill Acquisition: _____   Practice Opportunities: _____

*This problem allows you the opportunity to demonstrate the **Spring Test** to help rule out problems with hypomobility of the vertebrae. You have 2 minutes to complete this task.*

Tester places athlete and limb in appropriate position	Test 1	Test 2	Test 3
Prone	Ⓨ Ⓝ	Ⓨ Ⓝ	Ⓨ Ⓝ
Tester placed in proper position	**Test 1**	**Test 2**	**Test 3**
Stands to the side of the athlete	Ⓨ Ⓝ	Ⓨ Ⓝ	Ⓨ Ⓝ
Places thumbs (or hypothenar eminence) over the spinous process	Ⓨ Ⓝ	Ⓨ Ⓝ	Ⓨ Ⓝ
Tester performs test according to accepted guidelines	**Test 1**	**Test 2**	**Test 3**
Applies pressure downward (P-A motion through the spinous process toward the table)	Ⓨ Ⓝ	Ⓨ Ⓝ	Ⓨ Ⓝ
Repeats downward pressure (each lumbar vertebra)	Ⓨ Ⓝ	Ⓨ Ⓝ	Ⓨ Ⓝ

The psychomotor skill was performed completely and in the appropriate order   0 1 2 3 4 5

The tester had control of the subject and the situation (showed confidence)   0 1 2 3 4 5

Method of performing the skill allowed the tester the ability to determine:
severity, proper progression, and the *fit* in the overall picture (Oral)   0 1 2 3 4 5

In order for a grade of *minimum standard* to be given, the total must be ≥11   **TOTAL =** _____

```
   1     2     3     4     5     6     7     8     9    10    11    12    13    14    15
   |     |     |     |     |     |     |     |     |     |     |     |     |     |     |
```

Not Acceptable   **Meets**   **Exceeds**
                                          Minimum Standards   **Minimum Standards**

TEST ENVIRONMENTS

L: Laboratory/Classroom Testing
C: Clinical/Field Testing
P: Practicum Testing
A: Assessment/Mock Exam Testing
S: Self-Reporting

SKILL TEST INFORMATION

Positive Finding:	Lack of movement; pain
Involved Structure:	Facet joints (lumbar)
Special Considerations:	N/A
Reference(s):	Konin et al (2002); Starkey et al (2002)
Supplies Needed:	Table

Special Tests
(ST-L-Test 41)

Peer Review _____ Peer Review _____

Skill Acquisition: _____   Practice Opportunities: _____

This problem allows you the opportunity to demonstrate the special test known as the **Yeoman's Test**. *You have 2 minutes to complete this task.*

Tester places athlete and limb in appropriate position	Test 1	Test 2	Test 3
Prone	Ⓨ Ⓝ	Ⓨ Ⓝ	Ⓨ Ⓝ
Knee flexed to 90 degrees	Ⓨ Ⓝ	Ⓨ Ⓝ	Ⓨ Ⓝ
Tester placed in proper position	**Test 1**	**Test 2**	**Test 3**
Stands to the side of the athlete	Ⓨ Ⓝ	Ⓨ Ⓝ	Ⓨ Ⓝ
Places one hand under the knee (anterior thigh)	Ⓨ Ⓝ	Ⓨ Ⓝ	Ⓨ Ⓝ
Places the other hand at the pelvis (stabilizes)	Ⓨ Ⓝ	Ⓨ Ⓝ	Ⓨ Ⓝ
Tester performs test according to accepted guidelines	**Test 1**	**Test 2**	**Test 3**
Maintains knee flexion	Ⓨ Ⓝ	Ⓨ Ⓝ	Ⓨ Ⓝ
Passively hyperextends the hip	Ⓨ Ⓝ	Ⓨ Ⓝ	Ⓨ Ⓝ
Maintains relaxation of the limb	Ⓨ Ⓝ	Ⓨ Ⓝ	Ⓨ Ⓝ
Performs assessment bilaterally	Ⓨ Ⓝ	Ⓨ Ⓝ	Ⓨ Ⓝ

The psychomotor skill was performed completely and in the appropriate order   0 1 2 3 4 5

The tester had control of the subject and the situation (showed confidence)   0 1 2 3 4 5

Method of performing the skill allowed the tester the ability to determine:
severity, proper progression, and the *fit* in the overall picture (Oral)   0 1 2 3 4 5

In order for a grade of *minimum standard* to be given, the total must be ≥11   TOTAL = _____

```
1    2    3    4    5    6    7    8    9    10   11   12   13   14   15
|----|----|----|----|----|----|----|----|----|----|----|----|----|----|
```

Not Acceptable   **Meets**   **Exceeds**
                               Minimum Standards   **Minimum Standards**

TEST ENVIRONMENTS

L: Laboratory/Classroom Testing
C: Clinical/Field Testing
P: Practicum Testing
A: Assessment/Mock Exam Testing
S: Self-Reporting

SKILL TEST INFORMATION

Positive Finding:	Pain
Involved Structure:	Sacroiliac joint, lumbar joints, femoral nerve
Special Considerations:	N/A
Reference(s):	Magee
Supplies Needed:	Table

Chapter

9

TAPING/WRAPPING

Taping/Wrapping
(TW-U-Test 1)

Peer Review _____ Peer Review _____

Skill Acquisition: _____   Practice Opportunities: _____

This problem allows you the opportunity to demonstrate a **taping technique to prevent hyperextension of the elbow**. *You have 3 minutes to complete this task.*

Tester places athlete and limb in appropriate position	Test 1	Test 2	Test 3
Seated or standing	Ⓨ Ⓝ	Ⓨ Ⓝ	Ⓨ Ⓝ
Extends elbow to the point of pain (backs off approximately 10 to 20 degrees)	Ⓨ Ⓝ	Ⓨ Ⓝ	Ⓨ Ⓝ
Contracts biceps and forearm	Ⓨ Ⓝ	Ⓨ Ⓝ	Ⓨ Ⓝ
Taping technique	**Test 1**	**Test 2**	**Test 3**
Applies tape adhesive/applies underwrap (optional)	Ⓨ Ⓝ	Ⓨ Ⓝ	Ⓨ Ⓝ
Applies anchor(s) to skin, mid-to-upper humerus	Ⓨ Ⓝ	Ⓨ Ⓝ	Ⓨ Ⓝ
Applies anchor(s) to skin, mid-to-lower forearm	Ⓨ Ⓝ	Ⓨ Ⓝ	Ⓨ Ⓝ
Applies longitudinal fan to anterior surface of the elbow (approximately 5 strips)	Ⓨ Ⓝ	Ⓨ Ⓝ	Ⓨ Ⓝ
Reinforces the center of the fan	Ⓨ Ⓝ	Ⓨ Ⓝ	Ⓨ Ⓝ
Secures fan at proximal and distal ends	Ⓨ Ⓝ	Ⓨ Ⓝ	Ⓨ Ⓝ
Applies closures to secure holes and loose ends	Ⓨ Ⓝ	Ⓨ Ⓝ	Ⓨ Ⓝ
Closes with stretch tape or elastic compression wrap	Ⓨ Ⓝ	Ⓨ Ⓝ	Ⓨ Ⓝ
Support and neatness	**Test 1**	**Test 2**	**Test 3**
Prevents elbow from moving into full extension	Ⓨ Ⓝ	Ⓨ Ⓝ	Ⓨ Ⓝ
Maintains good circulation to the hand	Ⓨ Ⓝ	Ⓨ Ⓝ	Ⓨ Ⓝ
No holes and/or loose ends	Ⓨ Ⓝ	Ⓨ Ⓝ	Ⓨ Ⓝ

The psychomotor skill was performed completely and in the appropriate order   0 1 2 3 4 5

The tester had control of the subject and the situation (showed confidence)   0 1 2 3 4 5

Method of performing the skill allowed the tester the ability to determine:
severity, proper progression, and the *fit* in the overall picture (Oral)   0 1 2 3 4 5

In order for a grade of *minimum standard* to be given, the total must be ≥11   **TOTAL = _____**

```
  1    2    3    4    5    6    7    8    9   10   11   12   13   14   15
  |    |    |    |    |    |    |    |    |    |    |    |    |    |    |
```

Not Acceptable   **Meets**   **Exceeds**
                                     Minimum Standards   **Minimum Standards**

TEST ENVIRONMENTS

L: Laboratory/Classroom Testing
C: Clinical/Field Testing
P: Practicum Testing
A: Assessment/Mock Exam Testing
S: Self-Reporting

SKILL TEST INFORMATION

Positive Finding: Prevent hyperextension
Involved Structure: Elbow
Special Considerations: N/A
Reference(s): Perrin; Wright et al
Supplies Needed: 1.5-inch white tape, stretch tape or elastic wrap, prewrap

Taping/Wrapping
(TW-U-Test 2)

Peer Review_____   Peer Review _____

Skill Acquisition: _____   Practice Opportunities: _____

*Please demonstrate how you would perform a **shoulder spica taping** of the **glenohumeral joint** to help prevent external rotation. You have 3 minutes to complete this task.*

Tester places athlete and limb in appropriate position	Test 1	Test 2	Test 3
Standing	Ⓨ Ⓝ	Ⓨ Ⓝ	Ⓨ Ⓝ
Shoulder abducted with the hand resting on the low back (elbow flexed)	Ⓨ Ⓝ	Ⓨ Ⓝ	Ⓨ Ⓝ
Contracts biceps			
For a male athlete, cover both nipples with either gauze or band-aids	Ⓨ Ⓝ	Ⓨ Ⓝ	Ⓨ Ⓝ
For a female athlete, tape over a sports bra	Ⓨ Ⓝ	Ⓨ Ⓝ	Ⓨ Ⓝ
Taping technique	**Test 1**	**Test 2**	**Test 3**
Taping begins at the distal portion of the affected upper arm and moves anteriorly, encircling the affected arm	Ⓨ Ⓝ	Ⓨ Ⓝ	Ⓨ Ⓝ
Continues the tape across the anterior portion of the chest, under the opposite arm, and across the back	Ⓨ Ⓝ	Ⓨ Ⓝ	Ⓨ Ⓝ
Repeats the above procedure a second time, ending by encircling the affected upper arm	Ⓨ Ⓝ	Ⓨ Ⓝ	Ⓨ Ⓝ
Places a check rein between the upper arm and the torso (optional)	Ⓨ Ⓝ	Ⓨ Ⓝ	Ⓨ Ⓝ
Support and neatness	**Test 1**	**Test 2**	**Test 3**
Prevents abduction and external rotation of the shoulder	Ⓨ Ⓝ	Ⓨ Ⓝ	Ⓨ Ⓝ
Maintains good circulation to the hands and finger	Ⓨ Ⓝ	Ⓨ Ⓝ	Ⓨ Ⓝ
No holes and/or loose ends	Ⓨ Ⓝ	Ⓨ Ⓝ	Ⓨ Ⓝ

The psychomotor skill was performed completely and in the appropriate order   **0 1 2 3 4 5**

The tester had control of the subject and the situation (showed confidence)   **0 1 2 3 4 5**

Method of performing the skill allowed the tester the ability to determine:
severity, proper progression, and the *fit* in the overall picture (Oral)   **0 1 2 3 4 5**

In order for a grade of *minimum standard* to be given, the total must be ≥11   **TOTAL = _____**

```
   1    2    3    4    5    6    7    8    9   10   11   12   13   14   15
   |    |    |    |    |    |    |    |    |    |    |    |    |    |    |
```
Not Acceptable   **Meets**   **Exceeds**
                                   Minimum Standards   **Minimum Standards**

TEST ENVIRONMENTS

L: Laboratory/Classroom Testing
C: Clinical/Field Testing
P: Practicum Testing
A: Assessment/Mock Exam Testing
S: Self-Reporting

SKILL TEST INFORMATION

Positive Finding:	Restrict abduction/external rotation
Involved Structure:	Glenohumeral joint
Special Considerations:	May practice with ACE wrap
Reference(s):	Wright et al
Supplies Needed:	Elastic tape, 1.5-inch white tape, gauze/band-aids, prewrap

TAPING/WRAPPING
(TW-U-Test 3)

Peer Review _____ Peer Review _____

Skill Acquisition: _____ Practice Opportunities: _____

*Please demonstrate how you would perform a **shoulder spica elastic wrap** in order to help support the* **glenohumeral joint***. You have 3 minutes to complete this task.*

Tester places athlete and limb in appropriate position	Test 1	Test 2	Test 3
Standing	Ⓨ Ⓝ	Ⓨ Ⓝ	Ⓨ Ⓝ
Shoulder abducted with hand resting on low back (elbow flexed)	Ⓨ Ⓝ	Ⓨ Ⓝ	Ⓨ Ⓝ
Contracts biceps	Ⓨ Ⓝ	Ⓨ Ⓝ	Ⓨ Ⓝ
Instructs the athlete to breathe deeply (expand the chest)	Ⓨ Ⓝ	Ⓨ Ⓝ	Ⓨ Ⓝ
Taping technique	**Test 1**	**Test 2**	**Test 3**
Using 6-inch elastic (double) wrap, begins at the distal aspect of the biceps muscle and encircles the arm, pulling the wrap from posterior to anterior	Ⓨ Ⓝ	Ⓨ Ⓝ	Ⓨ Ⓝ
Continues the wrap across the chest, beneath the opposite arm, around the back, and encircles the upper arm	Ⓨ Ⓝ	Ⓨ Ⓝ	Ⓨ Ⓝ
Repeats the above steps until the wrap runs out	Ⓨ Ⓝ	Ⓨ Ⓝ	Ⓨ Ⓝ
Secures the wrap with elastic tape and adhesive tape	Ⓨ Ⓝ	Ⓨ Ⓝ	Ⓨ Ⓝ
Support and neatness	**Test 1**	**Test 2**	**Test 3**
Provides support to the glenohumeral joint	Ⓨ Ⓝ	Ⓨ Ⓝ	Ⓨ Ⓝ
Maintains good circulation to the hand and fingers	Ⓨ Ⓝ	Ⓨ Ⓝ	Ⓨ Ⓝ
No gaps and/or loose ends	Ⓨ Ⓝ	Ⓨ Ⓝ	Ⓨ Ⓝ

The psychomotor skill was performed completely and in the appropriate order   0 1 2 3 4 5

The tester had control of the subject and the situation (showed confidence)   0 1 2 3 4 5

Method of performing the skill allowed the tester the ability to determine:
severity, proper progression, and the *fit* in the overall picture (Oral)   0 1 2 3 4 5

In order for a grade of *minimum standard* to be given, the total must be ≥11   TOTAL = _____

1	2	3	4	5	6	7	8	9	10	11	12	13	14	15

Not Acceptable   **Meets**   **Exceeds**
         Minimum Standards   **Minimum Standards**

TEST ENVIRONMENTS

L: Laboratory/Classroom Testing
C: Clinical/Field Testing
P: Practicum Testing
A: Assessment/Mock Exam Testing
S: Self-Reporting

SKILL TEST INFORMATION

Positive Finding:	Support/stabilize
Involved Structure:	Glenohumeral joint
Special Considerations:	N/A
Reference(s):	Wright et al; Perrin
Supplies Needed:	1.5-inch white tape, 6- to 4-inch reusable elastic wrap

Taping/Wrapping
(TW-U-Test 4)

Peer Review _____ Peer Review _____

Skill Acquisition: _____   Practice Opportunities: _____

Please demonstrate how you would perform a **shoulder spica taping** *for injury to the* **acromioclavicular joint.**
You have 3 minutes to complete this task.

Tester places athlete and limb in appropriate position	Test 1	Test 2	Test 3
Standing	Ⓨ Ⓝ	Ⓨ Ⓝ	Ⓨ Ⓝ
Shoulder abducted with hand resting on low back (elbow flexed)	Ⓨ Ⓝ	Ⓨ Ⓝ	Ⓨ Ⓝ
Contracts biceps			
For a male athlete, cover both nipples with either gauze or band-aids	Ⓨ Ⓝ	Ⓨ Ⓝ	Ⓨ Ⓝ
For a female athlete, tape over a sports bra	Ⓨ Ⓝ	Ⓨ Ⓝ	Ⓨ Ⓝ
Taping technique	**Test 1**	**Test 2**	**Test 3**
Places a horizontal anchor from the anterior to posterior midline of the body, covering the mid-to-lower portion of the ribs (note: on a female athlete, all strips should end above the breast)	Ⓨ Ⓝ	Ⓨ Ⓝ	Ⓨ Ⓝ
Applies strips of tape over the AC joint by placing the middle of the strip over the AC joint and applying equal tension toward both the anterior and posterior ends, attaching the tape to the midline anchor	Ⓨ Ⓝ	Ⓨ Ⓝ	Ⓨ Ⓝ
Repeats the above step three more times (overlap)	Ⓨ Ⓝ	Ⓨ Ⓝ	Ⓨ Ⓝ
Applies another anchor that encircles the entire torso, securing the strips	Ⓨ Ⓝ	Ⓨ Ⓝ	Ⓨ Ⓝ
Support and neatness	**Test 1**	**Test 2**	**Test 3**
Provides proper support to the AC joint	Ⓨ Ⓝ	Ⓨ Ⓝ	Ⓨ Ⓝ
Maintains good circulation to hands and fingers	Ⓨ Ⓝ	Ⓨ Ⓝ	Ⓨ Ⓝ
Should not hinder movement or breathing	Ⓨ Ⓝ	Ⓨ Ⓝ	Ⓨ Ⓝ
No holes and/or loose ends	Ⓨ Ⓝ	Ⓨ Ⓝ	Ⓨ Ⓝ

The psychomotor skill was performed completely and in the appropriate order   **0 1 2 3 4 5**

The tester had control of the subject and the situation (showed confidence)   **0 1 2 3 4 5**

Method of performing the skill allowed the tester the ability to determine:
severity, proper progression, and the *fit* in the overall picture (Oral)   **0 1 2 3 4 5**

In order for a grade of *minimum standard* to be given, the total must be ≥11   **TOTAL = _____**

1	2	3	4	5	6	7	8	9	10	11	12	13	14	15

Not Acceptable   **Meets
Minimum Standards**   **Exceeds
Minimum Standards**

TEST ENVIRONMENTS

L: Laboratory/Classroom Testing
C: Clinical/Field Testing
P: Practicum Testing
A: Assessment/Mock Exam Testing
S: Self-Reporting

SKILL TEST INFORMATION

Positive Finding:	Support
Involved Structure:	AC joint
Special Considerations:	N/A
Reference(s):	Perrin; Wright et al
Supplies Needed:	2-inch elastic tape, 1.5-inch white tape, gauze/band-aids

TAPING/WRAPPING
(TW-U-Test 5)

Peer Review _____ Peer Review _____

Skill Acquisition: _____   Practice Opportunities: _____

Please demonstrate how you would perform a **shoulder spica elastic wrap** *to secure a doughnut pad over the* **acromioclavicular joint***. You have 3 minutes to complete this task.*

Tester places athlete and limb in appropriate position	Test 1	Test 2	Test 3
Standing	Ⓨ Ⓝ	Ⓨ Ⓝ	Ⓨ Ⓝ
Shoulder abducted with hand resting on low back (elbow flexed)	Ⓨ Ⓝ	Ⓨ Ⓝ	Ⓨ Ⓝ
Contracts biceps	Ⓨ Ⓝ	Ⓨ Ⓝ	Ⓨ Ⓝ
Instructs the athlete to breathe deeply (expand the chest)	Ⓨ Ⓝ	Ⓨ Ⓝ	Ⓨ Ⓝ
Taping technique	**Test 1**	**Test 2**	**Test 3**
Places the doughnut pad over the AC joint	Ⓨ Ⓝ	Ⓨ Ⓝ	Ⓨ Ⓝ
Using 6-inch elastic wrap, begins at the distal aspect of the biceps muscle and encircles the arm, pulling the wrap from posterior to anterior	Ⓨ Ⓝ	Ⓨ Ⓝ	Ⓨ Ⓝ
Continues the wrap across the chest, beneath the opposite arm, around the back, and encircle the upper arm	Ⓨ Ⓝ	Ⓨ Ⓝ	Ⓨ Ⓝ
Repeats the above steps until you run out of wrap	Ⓨ Ⓝ	Ⓨ Ⓝ	Ⓨ Ⓝ
Secures the wrap with elastic tape and adhesive tape	Ⓨ Ⓝ	Ⓨ Ⓝ	Ⓨ Ⓝ
Support and neatness	**Test 1**	**Test 2**	**Test 3**
Holds pad over the AC joint	Ⓨ Ⓝ	Ⓨ Ⓝ	Ⓨ Ⓝ
Maintains good circulation to hand and fingers	Ⓨ Ⓝ	Ⓨ Ⓝ	Ⓨ Ⓝ
No gaps and/or loose ends	Ⓨ Ⓝ	Ⓨ Ⓝ	Ⓨ Ⓝ

The psychomotor skill was performed completely and in the appropriate order   0 1 2 3 4 5

The tester had control of the subject and the situation (showed confidence)   0 1 2 3 4 5

Method of performing the skill allowed the tester the ability to determine:
severity, proper progression, and the *fit* in the overall picture (Oral)   0 1 2 3 4 5

In order for a grade of *minimum standard* to be given, the total must be ≥11   TOTAL = _____

```
   1     2     3     4     5     6     7     8     9    10    11    12    13    14    15
   |     |     |     |     |     |     |     |     |     |     |     |     |     |     |
```

Not Acceptable   **Meets**   **Exceeds**
                                    Minimum Standards   **Minimum Standards**

TEST ENVIRONMENTS

L: Laboratory/Classroom Testing
C: Clinical/Field Testing
P: Practicum Testing
A: Assessment/Mock Exam Testing
S: Self-Reporting

SKILL TEST INFORMATION

Positive Finding:	Secure pad
Involved Structure:	AC joint
Special Considerations:	N/A
Reference(s):	Perrin
Supplies Needed:	1.5-inch white tape, AC pad, 6- to 4-inch double elastic wrap

TAPING/WRAPPING
(TW-U-Test 6)

Peer Review _____   Peer Review _____

Skill Acquisition: _____   Practice Opportunities: _____

Please demonstrate how you would perform **wrist taping neutralization** *to prevent flexion and extension. You have 3 minutes to complete this task.*

Tester places athlete and limb in appropriate position	Test 1	Test 2	Test 3
Seated or standing	Y N	Y N	Y N
Wrist position into neutral (0 degrees)	Y N	Y N	Y N
Taping technique	**Test 1**	**Test 2**	**Test 3**
Applies a 2-inch anchor around the distal forearm	Y N	Y N	Y N
Applies a smaller anchor around the hand (second to fifth metacarpal heads)	Y N	Y N	Y N
Constructs a fan of tape ("X-shaped"), extending from proximal to distal anchors (fan placed on dorsal side to prevent hyperflexion and on palmar side to prevent hyperextension)	Y N	Y N	Y N
Applies a second set of anchors (holding the fan down)	Y N	Y N	Y N
Applies tape in a figure-8 pattern, encircling the wrist	Y N	Y N	Y N
Closes with a spiral taping from proximal anchor to distal anchor	Y N	Y N	Y N
Support and neatness	**Test 1**	**Test 2**	**Test 3**
Prevents hyperextension and flexion of the wrist (good support)	Y N	Y N	Y N
Maintains good circulation to hand and fingers	Y N	Y N	Y N
No holes and/or loose ends	Y N	Y N	Y N

The psychomotor skill was performed completely and in the appropriate order   0 1 2 3 4 5

The tester had control of the subject and the situation (showed confidence)   0 1 2 3 4 5

Method of performing the skill allowed the tester the ability to determine:
severity, proper progression, and the *fit* in the overall picture (Oral)   0 1 2 3 4 5

In order for a grade of *minimum standard* to be given, the total must be ≥11   TOTAL = _____

```
 1    2    3    4    5    6    7    8    9   10   11   12   13   14   15
 |    |    |    |    |    |    |    |    |    |    |    |    |    |    |
```

Not Acceptable   **Meets**   **Exceeds**
                                              Minimum Standards   **Minimum Standards**

TEST ENVIRONMENTS

L: Laboratory/Classroom Testing
C: Clinical/Field Testing
P: Practicum Testing
A: Assessment/Mock Exam Testing
S: Self-Reporting

SKILL TEST INFORMATION

Positive Finding:	Neutralize the wrist (flexion/extension)
Involved Structure:	Wrist
Special Considerations:	N/A
Reference(s):	Perrin; Wright et al
Supplies Needed:	1.5-inch white tape/prewrap

TAPING/WRAPPING
(TW-U-Test 7)

Peer Review _____ Peer Review _____

Skill Acquisition: _____   Practice Opportunities: _____

Please demonstrate how you would perform a **thumb spica taping** *in order to support the first metacarpophalangeal joint of the hand. You have 3 minutes to complete this task.*

Tester places athlete and limb in appropriate position	Test 1	Test 2	Test 3
Standing or seated	Ⓨ Ⓝ	Ⓨ Ⓝ	Ⓨ Ⓝ
Hand pronated and slightly extended	Ⓨ Ⓝ	Ⓨ Ⓝ	Ⓨ Ⓝ
Thumb slightly flexed/fingers abducted	Ⓨ Ⓝ	Ⓨ Ⓝ	Ⓨ Ⓝ
Taping technique	**Test 1**	**Test 2**	**Test 3**
Applies an anchor around the distal forearm just above the ulnar condyle	Ⓨ Ⓝ	Ⓨ Ⓝ	Ⓨ Ⓝ
Applies a figure-eight around the thumb, starting at the ulnar condyle, across the dorsal aspect of the hand, around the thumb, across the palmar aspect of the hand, and back to the ulnar condyle	Ⓨ Ⓝ	Ⓨ Ⓝ	Ⓨ Ⓝ
Repeats the above step one to two more times	Ⓨ Ⓝ	Ⓨ Ⓝ	Ⓨ Ⓝ
Secures tape with a second anchor around the wrist	Ⓨ Ⓝ	Ⓨ Ⓝ	Ⓨ Ⓝ
Support and neatness	**Test 1**	**Test 2**	**Test 3**
Provides support and stability to the MP joint	Ⓨ Ⓝ	Ⓨ Ⓝ	Ⓨ Ⓝ
Maintains good circulation to the hand and thumb (check capillary refill)	Ⓨ Ⓝ	Ⓨ Ⓝ	Ⓨ Ⓝ
No holes and/or loose ends	Ⓨ Ⓝ	Ⓨ Ⓝ	Ⓨ Ⓝ

The psychomotor skill was performed completely and in the appropriate order   **0 1 2 3 4 5**

The tester had control of the subject and the situation (showed confidence)   **0 1 2 3 4 5**

Method of performing the skill allowed the tester the ability to determine:
severity, proper progression, and the *fit* in the overall picture (Oral)   **0 1 2 3 4 5**

In order for a grade of *minimum standard* to be given, the total must be ≥11   **TOTAL = _____**

```
  1    2    3    4    5    6    7    8    9   10   11   12   13   14   15
  |____|____|____|____|____|____|____|____|____|____|____|____|____|____|
```

Not Acceptable   **Meets**   **Exceeds**
                                    Minimum Standards   **Minimum Standards**

TEST ENVIRONMENTS

L: Laboratory/Classroom Testing
C: Clinical/Field Testing
P: Practicum Testing
A: Assessment/Mock Exam Testing
S: Self-Reporting

SKILL TEST INFORMATION

Positive Finding: Support and stabilize
Involved Structure: MP joint (thumb) and wrist
Special Considerations: N/A
Reference(s): Perrin; Wright et al
Supplies Needed: 1.5-inch white tape/prewrap

TAPING/WRAPPING
(TW-U-Test 8)

Peer Review _____ Peer Review _____

Skill Acquisition: _____   Practice Opportunities: _____

Please demonstrate how you would perform a **collateral interphalangeal joint taping** *of the fourth finger. You have 2 minutes to complete this task.*

Tester places athlete and limb in appropriate position	Test 1	Test 2	Test 3
Standing or seated	Ⓨ Ⓝ	Ⓨ Ⓝ	Ⓨ Ⓝ
Finger slightly flexed (PIP joint)	Ⓨ Ⓝ	Ⓨ Ⓝ	Ⓨ Ⓝ
Fingers abducted (spread apart)	Ⓨ Ⓝ	Ⓨ Ⓝ	Ⓨ Ⓝ
Taping technique	**Test 1**	**Test 2**	**Test 3**
Applies anchor strips around the proximal and distal aspects of the finger	Ⓨ Ⓝ	Ⓨ Ⓝ	Ⓨ Ⓝ
Applies a strip of tape, beginning on the anterior proximal anchor, crossing the medial joint line, under the finger, and ending on the posterior distal anchor			
Applies a strip of tape from the anterior distal anchor, across the medial joint line, under the finger, and ending on the posterior proximal anchor	Ⓨ Ⓝ	Ⓨ Ⓝ	Ⓨ Ⓝ
Repeats the above two steps, crossing on the lateral joint line	Ⓨ Ⓝ	Ⓨ Ⓝ	Ⓨ Ⓝ
Secures the tape with a second set of proximal and distal anchors	Ⓨ Ⓝ	Ⓨ Ⓝ	Ⓨ Ⓝ
Support and neatness	**Test 1**	**Test 2**	**Test 3**
Prevents valgus and varus stress on the PIP joint	Ⓨ Ⓝ	Ⓨ Ⓝ	Ⓨ Ⓝ
Maintains good circulation to the finger (check capillary refill)	Ⓨ Ⓝ	Ⓨ Ⓝ	Ⓨ Ⓝ
No holes and/or loose ends	Ⓨ Ⓝ	Ⓨ Ⓝ	Ⓨ Ⓝ

The psychomotor skill was performed completely and in the appropriate order   **0 1 2 3 4 5**

The tester had control of the subject and the situation (showed confidence)   **0 1 2 3 4 5**

Method of performing the skill allowed the tester the ability to determine:
severity, proper progression, and the *fit* in the overall picture (Oral)   **0 1 2 3 4 5**

In order for a grade of *minimum standard* to be given, the total must be ≥11   **TOTAL = _____**

1	2	3	4	5	6	7	8	9	10	11	12	13	14	15

Not Acceptable   **Meets**   **Exceeds**
                                    Minimum Standards   **Minimum Standards**

TEST ENVIRONMENTS
L: Laboratory/Classroom Testing
C: Clinical/Field Testing
P: Practicum Testing
A: Assessment/Mock Exam Testing
S: Self-Reporting

SKILL TEST INFORMATION
Positive Finding: Supports/prevents motion
Involved Structure: PIP joint
Special Considerations: N/A
Reference(s): Perrin; Wright et al
Supplies Needed: 1.5-inch white tape/prewrap

TAPING/WRAPPING
(TW-L-Test 1)

Peer Review _____ Peer Review _____

Skill Acquisition: _____   Practice Opportunities: _____

*Please demonstrate how you would perform a **hip spica wrap (hip flexor wrap)** for an injury to the hip flexors. You have 3 minutes to complete this task.*

Tester places athlete and limb in appropriate position	Test 1	Test 2	Test 3
Standing	Ⓨ Ⓝ	Ⓨ Ⓝ	Ⓨ Ⓝ
Hip in slight flexion (heel may be propped up on a small block)	Ⓨ Ⓝ	Ⓨ Ⓝ	Ⓨ Ⓝ
Foot/lower leg in a neutral position (quadriceps contracted)	Ⓨ Ⓝ	Ⓨ Ⓝ	Ⓨ Ⓝ
Taping technique	**Test 1**	**Test 2**	**Test 3**
Beginning at the proximal end of the thigh, wraps a 6-inch elastic wrap down to the distal lateral aspect of the quadriceps (pulls down and out)	Ⓨ Ⓝ	Ⓨ Ⓝ	Ⓨ Ⓝ
Spirals back up the thigh (pulls up and out), overlapping each layer by half the wrap's width	Ⓨ Ⓝ	Ⓨ Ⓝ	Ⓨ Ⓝ
At the proximal end up the thigh, continues the wrap around the waist, across the back, around the torso, and back to the proximal hip	Ⓨ Ⓝ	Ⓨ Ⓝ	Ⓨ Ⓝ
Repeats the above steps until the wrap in gone (start and finish on the thigh)	Ⓨ Ⓝ	Ⓨ Ⓝ	Ⓨ Ⓝ
Secures the wrap with elastic and white adhesive tape	Ⓨ Ⓝ	Ⓨ Ⓝ	Ⓨ Ⓝ
Support and neatness	**Test 1**	**Test 2**	**Test 3**
Provides support and stability	Ⓨ Ⓝ	Ⓨ Ⓝ	Ⓨ Ⓝ
Good circulation to the lower leg and foot	Ⓨ Ⓝ	Ⓨ Ⓝ	Ⓨ Ⓝ
No gaps and/or loose ends	Ⓨ Ⓝ	Ⓨ Ⓝ	Ⓨ Ⓝ

The psychomotor skill was performed completely and in the appropriate order   **0 1 2 3 4 5**

The tester had control of the subject and the situation (showed confidence)   **0 1 2 3 4 5**

Method of performing the skill allowed the tester the ability to determine: severity, proper progression, and the *fit* in the overall picture (Oral)   **0 1 2 3 4 5**

In order for a grade of *minimum standard* to be given, the total must be ≥11   **TOTAL = _____**

```
  1    2    3    4    5    6    7    8    9   10   11   12   13   14   15
  |    |    |    |    |    |    |    |    |    |    |    |    |    |    |
```
Not Acceptable   **Meets**   **Exceeds**
                                    Minimum Standards   **Minimum Standards**

TEST ENVIRONMENTS

L: Laboratory/Classroom Testing
C: Clinical/Field Testing
P: Practicum Testing
A: Assessment/Mock Exam Testing
S: Self-Reporting

SKILL TEST INFORMATION

Positive Finding: Support
Involved Structure: Hip flexors
Special Considerations: Adductors (pull inward)
Reference(s): Perrin; Wright et al
Supplies Needed: 6-inch double elastic wrap; elastic tape; 1.5-inch white adhesive tape

TAPING/WRAPPING
(TW-L-Test 2)

Peer Review _____   Peer Review _____

Skill Acquisition: _____   Practice Opportunities: _____

Please demonstrate how you would perform a **hip spica wrap (hip adductor wrap)** *for an injury to the groin area. You have 3 minutes to complete this task.*

Tester places athlete and limb in appropriate position	Test 1	Test 2	Test 3
Standing	Ⓨ Ⓝ	Ⓨ Ⓝ	Ⓨ Ⓝ
Hip in slight flexion (heel may be propped up on a small block)	Ⓨ Ⓝ	Ⓨ Ⓝ	Ⓨ Ⓝ
Foot/lower leg in slight internal rotation (quadriceps contracted)	Ⓨ Ⓝ	Ⓨ Ⓝ	Ⓨ Ⓝ
Taping technique	**Test 1**	**Test 2**	**Test 3**
Beginning at the proximal end of the thigh, wrap a 6-inch (double) elastic wrap down to the distal medial aspect of the quadriceps, pulling the wrap down and in	Ⓨ Ⓝ	Ⓨ Ⓝ	Ⓨ Ⓝ
Spirals back up, overlapping each layer by half the wrap's width	Ⓨ Ⓝ	Ⓨ Ⓝ	Ⓨ Ⓝ
At the proximal end of the thigh, continue the wrap around the waist, pulling across the abdomen, around the torso, and back to the proximal hip	Ⓨ Ⓝ	Ⓨ Ⓝ	Ⓨ Ⓝ
Repeats the above steps until the wrap is gone (start and finish on the thigh)	Ⓨ Ⓝ	Ⓨ Ⓝ	Ⓨ Ⓝ
Secures the ends with elastic and white adhesive tape	Ⓨ Ⓝ	Ⓨ Ⓝ	Ⓨ Ⓝ
Support and neatness	**Test 1**	**Test 2**	**Test 3**
Provides support and stability	Ⓨ Ⓝ	Ⓨ Ⓝ	Ⓨ Ⓝ
Good circulation to the lower leg and foot	Ⓨ Ⓝ	Ⓨ Ⓝ	Ⓨ Ⓝ
No gaps and/or loose ends	Ⓨ Ⓝ	Ⓨ Ⓝ	Ⓨ Ⓝ

The psychomotor skill was performed completely and in the appropriate order   **0 1 2 3 4 5**

The tester had control of the subject and the situation (showed confidence)   **0 1 2 3 4 5**

Method of performing the skill allowed the tester the ability to determine: severity, proper progression, and the *fit* in the overall picture (Oral)   **0 1 2 3 4 5**

In order for a grade of *minimum standard* to be given, the total must be ≥11   **TOTAL = _____**

```
  1    2    3    4    5    6    7    8    9   10   11   12   13   14   15
  |    |    |    |    |    |    |    |    |    |    |    |    |    |    |
```
Not Acceptable   **Meets**   **Exceeds**
                                    Minimum Standards   **Minimum Standards**

TEST ENVIRONMENTS

L: Laboratory/Classroom Testing
C: Clinical/Field Testing
P: Practicum Testing
A: Assessment/Mock Exam Testing
S: Self-Reporting

SKILL TEST INFORMATION

Positive Finding:	Support
Involved Structure:	Adductors
Special Considerations:	Hip flexors (pull outward)
Reference(s):	Perrin; Wright et al
Supplies Needed:	6-inch double elastic wrap; elastic tape; 1.5-inch white adhesive tape

TAPING/WRAPPING
(TW-L-Test 3)

Peer Review _____ Peer Review _____

Skill Acquisition: _____   Practice Opportunities: _____

*Please demonstrate how you would perform a **knee compression wrap** to secure an ice bag over the medial pole of the patella. You have 2 minutes to complete this task.*

Tester places athlete and limb in appropriate position	Test 1	Test 2	Test 3
Supine	Ⓨ Ⓝ	Ⓨ Ⓝ	Ⓨ Ⓝ
Knee slightly flexed	Ⓨ Ⓝ	Ⓨ Ⓝ	Ⓨ Ⓝ
Place ice bag in appropriate area	Ⓨ Ⓝ	Ⓨ Ⓝ	Ⓨ Ⓝ
Taping technique	**Test 1**	**Test 2**	**Test 3**
Begin wrapping the leg with a 6-inch elastic wrap, beginning about 6 inches below the knee	Ⓨ Ⓝ	Ⓨ Ⓝ	Ⓨ Ⓝ
Spirals up the leg, overlapping each layer by half the wrap's width	Ⓨ Ⓝ	Ⓨ Ⓝ	Ⓨ Ⓝ
Wraps should end above the knee at approximately mid-quadriceps	Ⓨ Ⓝ	Ⓨ Ⓝ	Ⓨ Ⓝ
Secures the wrap with white adhesive tape	Ⓨ Ⓝ	Ⓨ Ⓝ	Ⓨ Ⓝ
Support and neatness	**Test 1**	**Test 2**	**Test 3**
Provides compression to the knee (holds ice bag in place)	Ⓨ Ⓝ	Ⓨ Ⓝ	Ⓨ Ⓝ
Maintains good circulation to the foot	Ⓨ Ⓝ	Ⓨ Ⓝ	Ⓨ Ⓝ
No gaps and/or loose ends	Ⓨ Ⓝ	Ⓨ Ⓝ	Ⓨ Ⓝ

The psychomotor skill was performed completely and in the appropriate order   0 1 2 3 4 5

The tester had control of the subject and the situation (showed confidence)   0 1 2 3 4 5

Method of performing the skill allowed the tester the ability to determine:
severity, proper progression, and the *fit* in the overall picture (Oral)   0 1 2 3 4 5

In order for a grade of *minimum standard* to be given, the total must be ≥11   **TOTAL = _____**

```
 1    2    3    4    5    6    7    8    9   10   11   12   13   14   15
 |    |    |    |    |    |    |    |    |    |    |    |    |    |    |
```

Not Acceptable   **Meets**   **Exceeds**
                                        Minimum Standards   **Minimum Standards**

TEST ENVIRONMENTS

L: Laboratory/Classroom Testing
C: Clinical/Field Testing
P: Practicum Testing
A: Assessment/Mock Exam Testing
S: Self-Reporting

SKILL TEST INFORMATION

Positive Finding: Compression/holds bag in place
Involved Structure: Knee
Special Considerations: N/A
Reference(s): Wright et al
Supplies Needed: 6-inch elastic wrap, white adhesive tape, ice bag

Taping/Wrapping
(TW-L-Test 4)

Peer Review _____ Peer Review _____

Skill Acquisition: _____   Practice Opportunities: _____

*Please demonstrate how you would perform a **patellar check strap** in order help reduce symptoms of patella tendonitis. You have 2 minutes to complete this task.*

Tester places athlete and limb in appropriate position	Test 1	Test 2	Test 3
Standing	Ⓨ Ⓝ	Ⓨ Ⓝ	Ⓨ Ⓝ
Knee slightly flexed (lower leg muscles relaxed)	Ⓨ Ⓝ	Ⓨ Ⓝ	Ⓨ Ⓝ
Taping technique	Test 1	Test 2	Test 3
Applies a strip of tape between the distal patella and superior tibial tuberosity, applying direct pressure on the patellar tendon	Ⓨ Ⓝ	Ⓨ Ⓝ	Ⓨ Ⓝ
Applies tape in a circling motion from lateral to medial across the tendon	Ⓨ Ⓝ	Ⓨ Ⓝ	Ⓨ Ⓝ
Repeats above steps (two to three times)	Ⓨ Ⓝ	Ⓨ Ⓝ	Ⓨ Ⓝ
Support and neatness	Test 1	Test 2	Test 3
Reduces stress on the patellar tendon	Ⓨ Ⓝ	Ⓨ Ⓝ	Ⓨ Ⓝ
Good circulation to the lower leg, no numbness or tingling	Ⓨ Ⓝ	Ⓨ Ⓝ	Ⓨ Ⓝ
No holes and/or loose ends	Ⓨ Ⓝ	Ⓨ Ⓝ	Ⓨ Ⓝ

The psychomotor skill was performed completely and in the appropriate order   0 1 2 3 4 5

The tester had control of the subject and the situation (showed confidence)   0 1 2 3 4 5

Method of performing the skill allowed the tester the ability to determine:
severity, proper progression, and the *fit* in the overall picture (Oral)   0 1 2 3 4 5

In order for a grade of *minimum standard* to be given, the total must be ≥11   TOTAL = _____

```
  1   2   3   4   5   6   7   8   9   10  11  12  13  14  15
  |   |   |   |   |   |   |   |   |   |   |   |   |   |   |
```
Not Acceptable   **Meets**   **Exceeds**
                                    Minimum Standards   **Minimum Standards**

TEST ENVIRONMENTS
L: Laboratory/Classroom Testing
C: Clinical/Field Testing
P: Practicum Testing
A: Assessment/Mock Exam Testing
S: Self-Reporting

SKILL TEST INFORMATION
Positive Finding: Apply pressure
Involved Structure: Patella tendon
Special Considerations: N/A
Reference(s): Wright et al
Supplies Needed: Prewrap, white adhesive tape

TAPING/WRAPPING
(TW-L-Test 5)

Peer Review _____ Peer Review _____

Skill Acquisition: _____   Practice Opportunities: _____

Please demonstrate how you would perform a **closed basketweave taping** *to prevent excessive inversion of the* **ankle**. *You have 2 minutes to complete this task.*

Tester places athlete and limb in appropriate position	Test 1	Test 2	Test 3
Seated (leg supported in full extension)	Ⓨ Ⓝ	Ⓨ Ⓝ	Ⓨ Ⓝ
Ankle/foot dorsiflexed to 0 degrees (maintained throughout)	Ⓨ Ⓝ	Ⓨ Ⓝ	Ⓨ Ⓝ
Taping technique	**Test 1**	**Test 2**	**Test 3**
Places heel/lace pads to dorsal ankle joint line (distal Achilles' tendon [optional])	Ⓨ Ⓝ	Ⓨ Ⓝ	Ⓨ Ⓝ
Secures pads with a layer of prewrap	Ⓨ Ⓝ	Ⓨ Ⓝ	Ⓨ Ⓝ
Places two anchors around the lower leg at the base of the gastrocnemius muscle	Ⓨ Ⓝ	Ⓨ Ⓝ	Ⓨ Ⓝ
Places a second anchor around the instep, proximal to the base of the fifth metatarsal	Ⓨ Ⓝ	Ⓨ Ⓝ	Ⓨ Ⓝ
Applies a stirrup (medial to lateral)	Ⓨ Ⓝ	Ⓨ Ⓝ	Ⓨ Ⓝ
Places a horseshoe around the foot just below the malleoli	Ⓨ Ⓝ	Ⓨ Ⓝ	Ⓨ Ⓝ
Repeats the above two steps two additional times	Ⓨ Ⓝ	Ⓨ Ⓝ	Ⓨ Ⓝ
Applies a figure-8, starting at the dorsal aspect of the ankle, followed by heel-locks (repeat)	Ⓨ Ⓝ	Ⓨ Ⓝ	Ⓨ Ⓝ
Closes taping with horseshoes, overlapping by half the tape width, from distal to proximal	Ⓨ Ⓝ	Ⓨ Ⓝ	Ⓨ Ⓝ
Places a final anchor around the instep, proximal to the base of the fifth metatarsal	Ⓨ Ⓝ	Ⓨ Ⓝ	Ⓨ Ⓝ
Support and neatness	**Test 1**	**Test 2**	**Test 3**
Limits excessive inversion	Ⓨ Ⓝ	Ⓨ Ⓝ	Ⓨ Ⓝ
Maintains good circulation to the foot and toes	Ⓨ Ⓝ	Ⓨ Ⓝ	Ⓨ Ⓝ
No holes and/or loose ends	Ⓨ Ⓝ	Ⓨ Ⓝ	Ⓨ Ⓝ

The psychomotor skill was performed completely and in the appropriate order   0 1 2 3 4 5

The tester had control of the subject and the situation (showed confidence)   0 1 2 3 4 5

Method of performing the skill allowed the tester the ability to determine:
severity, proper progression, and the *fit* in the overall picture (Oral)   0 1 2 3 4 5

In order for a grade of *minimum standard* to be given, the total must be ≥11   **TOTAL =** _____

```
 1    2    3    4    5    6    7    8    9   10   11   12   13   14   15
 |----|----|----|----|----|----|----|----|----|----|----|----|----|----|
```

Not Acceptable   **Meets**   **Exceeds**
                                   Minimum Standards   **Minimum Standards**

TEST ENVIRONMENTS

L: Laboratory/Classroom Testing
C: Clinical/Field Testing
P: Practicum Testing
A: Assessment/Mock Exam Testing
S: Self-Reporting

SKILL TEST INFORMATION

Positive Finding:	Prevent excessive inversion
Involved Structure:	Subtalar joint (ankle)
Special Considerations:	N/A
Reference(s):	Perrin; Wright et al
Supplies Needed:	1.5-inch white adhesive tape, prewrap

TAPING/WRAPPING
(TW-L-Test 6)

Peer Review _____   Peer Review _____

Skill Acquisition: _____   Practice Opportunities: _____

Please demonstrate how you would perform an **Achilles' tendon taping** *in order to prevent dorsiflexion of the* **ankle**. *You have 3 minutes to complete this task.*

Tester places athlete and limb in appropriate position	Test 1	Test 2	Test 3
Seated (leg supported in full extension)	Ⓨ Ⓝ	Ⓨ Ⓝ	Ⓨ Ⓝ
Ankle/foot plantar flexed (approximately 25 degrees)	Ⓨ Ⓝ	Ⓨ Ⓝ	Ⓨ Ⓝ
Taping technique	**Test 1**	**Test 2**	**Test 3**
Places heel/lace pad over the dorsal ankle joint (distal Achilles' tendon)	Ⓨ Ⓝ	Ⓨ Ⓝ	Ⓨ Ⓝ
Places anchor around the proximal gastrocnemius and around the instep of the foot	Ⓨ Ⓝ	Ⓨ Ⓝ	Ⓨ Ⓝ
Measures a strip of elastic tape slightly longer than the distance between the two anchors and cuts both ends of the strip about 1 inch longitudinally	Ⓨ Ⓝ	Ⓨ Ⓝ	Ⓨ Ⓝ
With one end of the strip, wraps the split under the plantar side of the foot to anchor the strip to the foot	Ⓨ Ⓝ	Ⓨ Ⓝ	Ⓨ Ⓝ
Pulls the strip up, pulling the foot into plantar flexion and attaches it to the proximal anchor by wrapping the split ends of the strip around the gastrocnemius (*Note*: the above three steps may be repeated for added support)	Ⓨ Ⓝ	Ⓨ Ⓝ	Ⓨ Ⓝ
Secures both ends of the elastic strip with adhesive tape anchors	Ⓨ Ⓝ	Ⓨ Ⓝ	Ⓨ Ⓝ
Closes the tape job with either elastic or adhesive tape from distal to proximal	Ⓨ Ⓝ	Ⓨ Ⓝ	Ⓨ Ⓝ
Support and neatness	**Test 1**	**Test 2**	**Test 3**
Limits excessive dorsiflexion	Ⓨ Ⓝ	Ⓨ Ⓝ	Ⓨ Ⓝ
Good circulation to the foot	Ⓨ Ⓝ	Ⓨ Ⓝ	Ⓨ Ⓝ
No holes and/or loose ends	Ⓨ Ⓝ	Ⓨ Ⓝ	Ⓨ Ⓝ

The psychomotor skill was performed completely and in the appropriate order   0 1 2 3 4 5

The tester had control of the subject and the situation (showed confidence)   0 1 2 3 4 5

Method of performing the skill allowed the tester the ability to determine:
severity, proper progression, and the *fit* in the overall picture (Oral)   0 1 2 3 4 5

In order for a grade of *minimum standard* to be given, the total must be ≥11   **TOTAL = _____**

```
  1     2     3     4     5     6     7     8     9    10    11    12    13    14    15
  |     |     |     |     |     |     |     |     |     |     |     |     |     |     |
```
Not Acceptable   **Meets**   **Exceeds**
                                              Minimum Standards   **Minimum Standards**

SKILL TEST INFORMATION

TEST ENVIRONMENTS

L: Laboratory/Classroom Testing
C: Clinical/Field Testing
P: Practicum Testing
A: Assessment/Mock Exam Testing
S: Self-Reporting

Positive Finding:	Reduce stress to tendon; prevent dorsiflexion
Involved Structure:	Achilles' tendon, talocrural joint
Special Considerations:	N/A
Reference(s):	Wright et al
Supplies Needed:	Elastic tape, white adhesive tape, heel/lace pads

TAPING/WRAPPING
(TW-L-Test 7)

Peer Review _____ Peer Review _____

Skill Acquisition: _____   Practice Opportunities: _____

Please demonstrate how you would perform **longitudinal arch taping** *to give added support to the involved bones, ligaments, and muscles. You have 3 minutes to complete this task.*

Tester places athlete and limb in appropriate position	Test 1	Test 2	Test 3
Seated (leg supported in full extension)	Ⓨ Ⓝ	Ⓨ Ⓝ	Ⓨ Ⓝ
Ankle/foot slightly plantar flexed	Ⓨ Ⓝ	Ⓨ Ⓝ	Ⓨ Ⓝ
Taping technique	**Test 1**	**Test 2**	**Test 3**
Place an anchor at the head of the metatarsals	Ⓨ Ⓝ	Ⓨ Ⓝ	Ⓨ Ⓝ
Begins at the medial head (first metatarsal); attaches a strip of tape, bringing the tape along the medial foot from anterior-posterior, around the heel, and diagonally along the plantar side of the foot, back to the medial head of the first metatarsal	Ⓨ Ⓝ	Ⓨ Ⓝ	Ⓨ Ⓝ
Repeats above step	Ⓨ Ⓝ	Ⓨ Ⓝ	Ⓨ Ⓝ
Makes a teardrop beginning on the plantar side of the third metatarsal head, back around the heel, and returns to the starting point	Ⓨ Ⓝ	Ⓨ Ⓝ	Ⓨ Ⓝ
Repeats above step	Ⓨ Ⓝ	Ⓨ Ⓝ	Ⓨ Ⓝ
Places the tape on the plantar side of the fifth metatarsal head and draws the tape diagonally across the foot to the medial side of the heel, around the heel, and back to the lateral head of the fifth metatarsal	Ⓨ Ⓝ	Ⓨ Ⓝ	Ⓨ Ⓝ
Repeats above step	Ⓨ Ⓝ	Ⓨ Ⓝ	Ⓨ Ⓝ
Places tape strips along the plantar surface of the foot, pulling the tape from lateral to medial, beginning distally and moving proximally; each strip should overlap by half the width of the tape	Ⓨ Ⓝ	Ⓨ Ⓝ	Ⓨ Ⓝ
Places tape around the heads of the metatarsals to anchor	Ⓨ Ⓝ	Ⓨ Ⓝ	Ⓨ Ⓝ
Support and neatness	**Test 1**	**Test 2**	**Test 3**
Provides support to the longitudinal arch	Ⓨ Ⓝ	Ⓨ Ⓝ	Ⓨ Ⓝ
Maintains good circulation throughout the foot	Ⓨ Ⓝ	Ⓨ Ⓝ	Ⓨ Ⓝ
No holes and/or loose ends	Ⓨ Ⓝ	Ⓨ Ⓝ	Ⓨ Ⓝ

The psychomotor skill was performed completely and in the appropriate order   **0 1 2 3 4 5**

The tester had control of the subject and the situation (showed confidence)   **0 1 2 3 4 5**

Method of performing the skill allowed the tester the ability to determine:
severity, proper progression, and the *fit* in the overall picture (Oral)   **0 1 2 3 4 5**

In order for a grade of *minimum standard* to be given, the total must be ≥11   **TOTAL = _____**

```
 1    2    3    4    5    6    7    8    9   10   11   12   13   14   15
 |    |    |    |    |    |    |    |    |    |    |    |    |    |    |
```

Not Acceptable	Meets Minimum Standards	Exceeds Minimum Standards

TEST ENVIRONMENTS

L: Laboratory/Classroom Testing
C: Clinical/Field Testing
P: Practicum Testing
A: Assessment/Mock Exam Testing
S: Self-Reporting

SKILL TEST INFORMATION

Positive Finding: Support longitudinal arch
Involved Structure: Plantar surface of the foot
Special Considerations: N/A
Reference(s): Perrin; Wright et al
Supplies Needed: White adhesive tape

Taping/Wrapping
(TW-L-Test 8)

Peer Review _____ Peer Review _____

Skill Acquisition: _____   Practice Opportunities: _____

Please demonstrate **great toe taping** *in order to neutralize the first metatarsophalangeal joint. You have 3 minutes to complete this task.*

Tester places athlete and limb in appropriate position	Test 1	Test 2	Test 3
Seated (leg supported in full extension)	Ⓨ Ⓝ	Ⓨ Ⓝ	Ⓨ Ⓝ
First metatarsal placed in a neutral position	Ⓨ Ⓝ	Ⓨ Ⓝ	Ⓨ Ⓝ
Taping technique	**Test 1**	**Test 2**	**Test 3**
Places 2 inches elastic anchor around midfoot (lateral to medial), 1-inch adhesive tape anchor around the distal great toe	Ⓨ Ⓝ	Ⓨ Ⓝ	Ⓨ Ⓝ
A fan of four to six strips of adhesive tape should be placed on the dorsal side of the foot, beginning on the distal anchor and attaching on the proximal anchor	Ⓨ Ⓝ	Ⓨ Ⓝ	Ⓨ Ⓝ
A fan of four to six strips of adhesive tape should be placed on the planter side of the foot, beginning on the distal anchor and attaching on the proximal anchor	Ⓨ Ⓝ	Ⓨ Ⓝ	Ⓨ Ⓝ
Using a continuous strip of elastic tape, make a figure-eight around the great toe and midfoot, aiding the abduction of the first metatarsal joint	Ⓨ Ⓝ	Ⓨ Ⓝ	Ⓨ Ⓝ
Secure the figure-8 with adhesive tape	Ⓨ Ⓝ	Ⓨ Ⓝ	Ⓨ Ⓝ
Support and neatness	**Test 1**	**Test 2**	**Test 3**
Limits excessive motion of the first MP joint (flexion/extension)	Ⓨ Ⓝ	Ⓨ Ⓝ	Ⓨ Ⓝ
Maintains good circulation to the great toe (check capillary refill)	Ⓨ Ⓝ	Ⓨ Ⓝ	Ⓨ Ⓝ
No holes and/or loose ends	Ⓨ Ⓝ	Ⓨ Ⓝ	Ⓨ Ⓝ

The psychomotor skill was performed completely and in the appropriate order   **0 1 2 3 4 5**

The tester had control of the subject and the situation (showed confidence)   **0 1 2 3 4 5**

Method of performing the skill allowed the tester the ability to determine:
severity, proper progression, and the *fit* in the overall picture (Oral)   **0 1 2 3 4 5**

In order for a grade of *minimum standard* to be given, the total must be ≥11   **TOTAL = _____**

```
 1     2     3     4     5     6     7     8     9     10    11    12    13    14    15
 |__|__|__|__|__|__|__|__|__|__|__|__|__|__|__|
```

Not Acceptable   **Meets**   **Exceeds**
                                   Minimum Standards   **Minimum Standards**

TEST ENVIRONMENTS

L: Laboratory/Classroom Testing
C: Clinical/Field Testing
P: Practicum Testing
A: Assessment/Mock Exam Testing
S: Self-Reporting

SKILL TEST INFORMATION

Positive Finding:	Limits flexion and extension
Involved Structure:	First MP joint
Special Considerations:	N/A
Reference(s):	Perrin; Wright et al
Supplies Needed:	Elastic tape; white adhesive tape

TAPING/WRAPPING
(TW-L-Test 9)

Peer Review _____ Peer Review _____

Skill Acquisition: _____   Practice Opportunities: _____

Please demonstrate a **taping technique for patellofemoral stabilization** *in order to help realign the patella. You have 3 minutes to complete this task response.*

Tester places athlete and limb in appropriate position	Test 1	Test 2	Test 3
Supine or seated	Ⓨ Ⓝ	Ⓨ Ⓝ	Ⓨ Ⓝ
Knee fully extended	Ⓨ Ⓝ	Ⓨ Ⓝ	Ⓨ Ⓝ
Taping technique	**Test 1**	**Test 2**	**Test 3**
Assesses the patella for tilt and rotation	Ⓨ Ⓝ	Ⓨ Ⓝ	Ⓨ Ⓝ
Applies cover roll tape to protect affected area	Ⓨ Ⓝ	Ⓨ Ⓝ	Ⓨ Ⓝ
Correct tilt of the patella by applying Leukotape from middle of the patella to the medial femoral condyle	Ⓨ Ⓝ	Ⓨ Ⓝ	Ⓨ Ⓝ
Correct glide of the patella by applying Leukotape from the lateral border of the patella and pulling medially to the medial femoral condyle	Ⓨ Ⓝ	Ⓨ Ⓝ	Ⓨ Ⓝ
Correct external rotation of the patella by applying Leukotape from the inferior pole of the patella and pulling upward at a 45 degree angle	Ⓨ Ⓝ	Ⓨ Ⓝ	Ⓨ Ⓝ
Support and neatness	**Test 1**	**Test 2**	**Test 3**
Provides proper support to patellofemoral joint	Ⓨ Ⓝ	Ⓨ Ⓝ	Ⓨ Ⓝ
No holes and/loose ends	Ⓨ Ⓝ	Ⓨ Ⓝ	Ⓨ Ⓝ
Assesses the athlete for pain while performing functional activities	Ⓨ Ⓝ	Ⓨ Ⓝ	Ⓨ Ⓝ

The psychomotor skill was performed completely and in the appropriate order   0 1 2 3 4 5

The tester had control of the subject and the situation (showed confidence)   0 1 2 3 4 5

Method of performing the skill allowed the tester the ability to determine:
severity, proper progression, and the *fit* in the overall picture (Oral)   0 1 2 3 4 5

In order for a grade of *minimum standard* to be given, the total must be ≥11   TOTAL = _____

```
 1    2    3    4    5    6    7    8    9   10   11   12   13   14   15
 |    |    |    |    |    |    |    |    |    |    |    |    |    |    |
```

Not Acceptable   **Meets**   **Exceeds**
                                    Minimum Standards   **Minimum Standards**

TEST ENVIRONMENTS	**SKILL TEST INFORMATION**

TEST ENVIRONMENTS

L: Laboratory/Classroom Testing
C: Clinical/Field Testing
P: Practicum Testing
A: Assessment/Mock Exam Testing
S: Self-Reporting

SKILL TEST INFORMATION

Involved Structure: Patellofemoral joint
Special Considerations: N/A
Reference(s): Perrin
Supplies Needed: Leukotape tape and cover roll tape

TAPING/WRAPPING
(TW-L-Test 10)

Peer Review _____ Peer Review _____

Skill Acquisition: _____   Practice Opportunities: _____

Please demonstrate how you would perform an **open basketweave taping technique** *to contain swelling of the* **ankle**. *You have 3 minutes to complete this task response.*

Tester places athlete and limb in appropriate position	Test 1	Test 2	Test 3
Supine or seated	Ⓨ Ⓝ	Ⓨ Ⓝ	Ⓨ Ⓝ
Ankle in neutral position	Ⓨ Ⓝ	Ⓨ Ⓝ	Ⓨ Ⓝ
Taping technique	**Test 1**	**Test 2**	**Test 3**
Places one anchor distal to the base of the fifth metatarsal, leaving approximately an inch open on the dorsum of the foot	Ⓨ Ⓝ	Ⓨ Ⓝ	Ⓨ Ⓝ
Places one anchor distal to the base of the gastrocnemius muscle, leaving approximately an inch open on the anterior tibia	Ⓨ Ⓝ	Ⓨ Ⓝ	Ⓨ Ⓝ
Applies a stirrup (medial to lateral)	Ⓨ Ⓝ	Ⓨ Ⓝ	Ⓨ Ⓝ
Applies a horseshoe around the foot alternating with the stirrups	Ⓨ Ⓝ	Ⓨ Ⓝ	Ⓨ Ⓝ
Repeats above steps to complete three to four alternating stirrups/horseshoes	Ⓨ Ⓝ	Ⓨ Ⓝ	Ⓨ Ⓝ
Closes plantar surface of foot with c-strips from distal to proximal	Ⓨ Ⓝ	Ⓨ Ⓝ	Ⓨ Ⓝ
Applies single heel locks both medially and laterally (leaving approximately an inch open on the anterior tibia)	Ⓨ Ⓝ	Ⓨ Ⓝ	Ⓨ Ⓝ
Repeats above steps to complete two to three noncontinuous heel locks (medially and laterally)	Ⓨ Ⓝ	Ⓨ Ⓝ	Ⓨ Ⓝ
Applies three stabilizer straps (distally, proximally, and midway)	Ⓨ Ⓝ	Ⓨ Ⓝ	Ⓨ Ⓝ
Applies elastic wrap over taping technique (distal to proximal)	Ⓨ Ⓝ	Ⓨ Ⓝ	Ⓨ Ⓝ
Instructs athlete to remove elastic wrap before bedtime and remove stabilizer straps if swelling becomes uncomfortable	Ⓨ Ⓝ	Ⓨ Ⓝ	Ⓨ Ⓝ
Support and neatness	**Test 1**	**Test 2**	**Test 3**
Maintains circulation to the foot and toes while limiting swelling	Ⓨ Ⓝ	Ⓨ Ⓝ	Ⓨ Ⓝ
No holes or loose ends	Ⓨ Ⓝ	Ⓨ Ⓝ	Ⓨ Ⓝ

The psychomotor skill was performed completely and in the appropriate order   0 1 2 3 4 5

The tester had control of the subject and the situation (showed confidence)   0 1 2 3 4 5

Method of performing the skill allowed the tester the ability to determine:
severity, proper progression, and the *fit* in the overall picture (Oral)   0 1 2 3 4 5

In order for a grade of *minimum standard* to be given, the total must be ≥11   TOTAL = _____

```
 1    2    3    4    5    6    7    8    9   10   11   12   13   14   15
 |    |    |    |    |    |    |    |    |    |    |    |    |    |    |
```

Not Acceptable   **Meets**   **Exceeds**
                                          Minimum Standards   **Minimum Standards**

TEST ENVIRONMENTS

L: Laboratory/Classroom Testing
C: Clinical/Field Testing
P: Practicum Testing
A: Assessment/Mock Exam Testing
S: Self-Reporting

SKILL TEST INFORMATION

Positive Finding:	Prevent additional swelling
Involved Structure:	Subtalar joint (ankle)
Special Considerations:	N/A
Reference(s):	Perrin
Supplies Needed:	1.5-inch white adhesive tape, elastic wrap

TAPING/WRAPPING
(TW-L-Test 11)

Peer Review _____ Peer Review _____

Skill Acquisition: _____   Practice Opportunities: _____

Please demonstrate how you would perform a **closed basketweave taping technique** *to prevent excessive eversion of the* **ankle**. *You have 3 minutes to complete this task response.*

Tester places athlete and limb in appropriate position	Test 1	Test 2	Test 3
Seated (leg supported in full extension)	Ⓨ Ⓝ	Ⓨ Ⓝ	Ⓨ Ⓝ
Ankle/foot dorsiflexed to 0 degrees (maintained throughout)	Ⓨ Ⓝ	Ⓨ Ⓝ	Ⓨ Ⓝ
Taping technique	**Test 1**	**Test 2**	**Test 3**
Places heel/lace pads on dorsal ankle joint line	Ⓨ Ⓝ	Ⓨ Ⓝ	Ⓨ Ⓝ
Secures pads with a layer of prewrap	Ⓨ Ⓝ	Ⓨ Ⓝ	Ⓨ Ⓝ
Places two anchors around the lower leg at the base of the gastrocnemius	Ⓨ Ⓝ	Ⓨ Ⓝ	Ⓨ Ⓝ
Places a second anchor proximal to the base of the fifth metatarsal	Ⓨ Ⓝ	Ⓨ Ⓝ	Ⓨ Ⓝ
Applies a stirrup (even upward pressure to both sides or slight lateral to medial pressure)	Ⓨ Ⓝ	Ⓨ Ⓝ	Ⓨ Ⓝ
Places a horseshoe around the foot just below the malleoli	Ⓨ Ⓝ	Ⓨ Ⓝ	Ⓨ Ⓝ
Repeats the above two steps three additional times (alternating lateral-medial and medial-lateral)	Ⓨ Ⓝ	Ⓨ Ⓝ	Ⓨ Ⓝ
Applies a figure-8 starting at the dorsal aspect of the ankle, followed by heel-locks (repeat)	Ⓨ Ⓝ	Ⓨ Ⓝ	Ⓨ Ⓝ
Closes taping with horseshoes from distal to proximal (overlap half width)	Ⓨ Ⓝ	Ⓨ Ⓝ	Ⓨ Ⓝ
Places a final anchor proximal to the base of the fifth metatarsal	Ⓨ Ⓝ	Ⓨ Ⓝ	Ⓨ Ⓝ
Support and neatness	**Test 1**	**Test 2**	**Test 3**
Limits excessive eversion	Ⓨ Ⓝ	Ⓨ Ⓝ	Ⓨ Ⓝ
Maintains good circulation of the foot and toes	Ⓨ Ⓝ	Ⓨ Ⓝ	Ⓨ Ⓝ
No holes or loose ends	Ⓨ Ⓝ	Ⓨ Ⓝ	Ⓨ Ⓝ

The psychomotor skill was performed completely and in the appropriate order   **0 1 2 3 4 5**

The tester had control of the subject and the situation (showed confidence)   **0 1 2 3 4 5**

Method of performing the skill allowed the tester the ability to determine:
severity, proper progression, and the *fit* in the overall picture (Oral)   **0 1 2 3 4 5**

In order for a grade of *minimum standard* to be given, the total must be ≥11   **TOTAL = _____**

1	2	3	4	5	6	7	8	9	10	11	12	13	14	15

Not Acceptable   **Meets**   **Exceeds**
                              Minimum Standards   **Minimum Standards**

TEST ENVIRONMENTS

L: Laboratory/Classroom Testing
C: Clinical/Field Testing
P: Practicum Testing
A: Assessment/Mock Exam Testing
S: Self-Reporting

SKILL TEST INFORMATION

Positive Finding:	Prevent excessive eversion
Involved Structure:	Subtalar joint (ankle)
Special Considerations:	N/A
Reference(s):	Perrin
Supplies Needed:	1.5-inch white adhesive tape, prewrap

10

PROTECTIVE DEVICE CONSTRUCTION/EQUIPMENT FITTING

PROTECTIVE DEVICE CONSTRUCTION/EQUIPMENT FITTING
(PDC-U-Test 1)

Peer Review _____   Peer Review _____

Skill Acquisition: _____   Practice Opportunities: _____

This situation allows you to demonstrate your proficiency in properly **fitting a football helmet**. *You have 3 minutes to complete this task.*

Tester places athlete and limb in appropriate position	Test 1	Test 2	Test 3
Standing	Ⓨ Ⓝ	Ⓨ Ⓝ	Ⓨ Ⓝ
Head looking forward (neutral position)	Ⓨ Ⓝ	Ⓨ Ⓝ	Ⓨ Ⓝ
Tester placed in proper position	**Test 1**	**Test 2**	**Test 3**
Standing (facing the athlete)	Ⓨ Ⓝ	Ⓨ Ⓝ	Ⓨ Ⓝ
Tester performs test according to accepted guidelines	**Test 1**	**Test 2**	**Test 3**
Inspects the helmet (no visual damage and NOCSAE [National Operating Committee on Standards for Athletic Equipment] sticker is in place)	Ⓨ Ⓝ	Ⓨ Ⓝ	Ⓨ Ⓝ
Helmet pads cover the base of the skull (occipital)	Ⓨ Ⓝ	Ⓨ Ⓝ	Ⓨ Ⓝ
Space between helmet pad and eyebrows should be .75 inch (two fingers' width)	Ⓨ Ⓝ	Ⓨ Ⓝ	Ⓨ Ⓝ
Ear holes of the athlete should match the helmet ear holes	Ⓨ Ⓝ	Ⓨ Ⓝ	Ⓨ Ⓝ
Space between the facemask and nose should be 2 inches (three fingers' width)	Ⓨ Ⓝ	Ⓨ Ⓝ	Ⓨ Ⓝ
Chin strap should be centered (4-point attachment)	Ⓨ Ⓝ	Ⓨ Ⓝ	Ⓨ Ⓝ
Helmet should fit snugly around all parts of the athlete's head grabs facemask (manual pressure), asks athlete to look upward and downward	Ⓨ Ⓝ	Ⓨ Ⓝ	Ⓨ Ⓝ
Helmet should fit snugly around all parts of the athlete's head grabs facemask (manual pressure), asks athlete to rotate head left and right	Ⓨ Ⓝ	Ⓨ Ⓝ	Ⓨ Ⓝ

The psychomotor skill was performed completely and in the appropriate order   0 1 2 3 4 5

The tester had control of the subject and the situation (showed confidence)   0 1 2 3 4 5

Method of performing the skill allowed the tester the ability to determine:
severity, proper progression, and the *fit* in the overall picture (Oral)   0 1 2 3 4 5

In order for a grade of *minimum standard* to be given, the total must be ≥11   **TOTAL = _____**

```
  1   2   3   4   5   6   7   8   9   10  11  12  13  14  15
  |   |   |   |   |   |   |   |   |   |   |   |   |   |   |
```
Not Acceptable   **Meets**   **Exceeds**
                          Minimum Standards   **Minimum Standards**

TEST ENVIRONMENTS
L: Laboratory/Classroom Testing
C: Clinical/Field Testing
P: Practicum Testing
A: Assessment/Mock Exam Testing
S: Self-Reporting

SKILL TEST INFORMATION
Special Considerations: May want to wet the hair first
Reference(s): Prentice (2003)
Supplies Needed: Football helmet, chin strap, cheek pads, air pump for helmet

PROTECTIVE DEVICE CONSTRUCTION/EQUIPMENT FITTING
(PDC-U-Test 2)

Peer Review _____ Peer Review _____

Skill Acquisition: _____   Practice Opportunities: _____

*This problem allows you the opportunity to demonstrate the application of a cervical arm **sling and swath** to immobilize the upper extremity. You have 3 minutes to complete this task.*

Tester places athlete and limb in appropriate position	Test 1	Test 2	Test 3
Standing	Ⓨ Ⓝ	Ⓨ Ⓝ	Ⓨ Ⓝ
Elbow flexed to approximately 70 degrees	Ⓨ Ⓝ	Ⓨ Ⓝ	Ⓨ Ⓝ
Tester applies protective device to injured area	**Test 1**	**Test 2**	**Test 3**
Slides sling underneath injured extremity with apex facing the elbow	Ⓨ Ⓝ	Ⓨ Ⓝ	Ⓨ Ⓝ
Drapes end of bandage closest to body over the injured shoulder	Ⓨ Ⓝ	Ⓨ Ⓝ	Ⓨ Ⓝ
Pulls other end of bandage over the opposite shoulder	Ⓨ Ⓝ	Ⓨ Ⓝ	Ⓨ Ⓝ
Secures sling with square knot behind the neck	Ⓨ Ⓝ	Ⓨ Ⓝ	Ⓨ Ⓝ
Fastens apex of the bandage at elbow with a safety pin	Ⓨ Ⓝ	Ⓨ Ⓝ	Ⓨ Ⓝ
Secures sling to body by applying swath around the trunk	Ⓨ Ⓝ	Ⓨ Ⓝ	Ⓨ Ⓝ
Tester evaluates injured area after device application	**Test 1**	**Test 2**	**Test 3**
Checks distal pulse	Ⓨ Ⓝ	Ⓨ Ⓝ	Ⓨ Ⓝ
Checks distal sensation and capillary refill	Ⓨ Ⓝ	Ⓨ Ⓝ	Ⓨ Ⓝ

The psychomotor skill was performed completely and in the appropriate order   0 1 2 3 4 5

The tester had control of the subject and the situation (showed confidence)   0 1 2 3 4 5

Method of performing the skill allowed the tester the ability to determine:
severity, proper progression, and the *fit* in the overall picture (Oral)   0 1 2 3 4 5

In order for a grade of *minimum standard* to be given, the total must be ≥11   **TOTAL =** _____

```
  1     2     3     4     5     6     7     8     9    10    11    12    13    14    15
  |     |     |     |     |     |     |     |     |     |     |     |     |     |     |
```
Not Acceptable   **Meets**   **Exceeds**
                                          Minimum Standards   **Minimum Standards**

TEST ENVIRONMENTS
L: Laboratory/Classroom Testing
C: Clinical/Field Testing
P: Practicum Testing
A: Assessment/Mock Exam Testing
S: Self-Reporting

SKILL TEST INFORMATION
Special Considerations: N/A
Reference(s): Prentice (2003)
Supplies Needed: Triangular bandage, swath, safety pin

PROTECTIVE DEVICE CONSTRUCTION/EQUIPMENT FITTING
(PDC-U-Test 3)

Peer Review _____ Peer Review _____

Skill Acquisition: _____   Practice Opportunities: _____

This problem allows you the opportunity to demonstrate the application of a **finger splint** *to immobilize the* **PIP joint** *of the middle finger. You have 2 minutes to complete this task.*

Tester places athlete and limb in appropriate position	Test 1	Test 2	Test 3
Seated	Ⓨ Ⓝ	Ⓨ Ⓝ	Ⓨ Ⓝ
Places hand in position of function	Ⓨ Ⓝ	Ⓨ Ⓝ	Ⓨ Ⓝ
Moves injured area as little as possible	Ⓨ Ⓝ	Ⓨ Ⓝ	Ⓨ Ⓝ
Tester applies protective device to injured area	**Test 1**	**Test 2**	**Test 3**
Slides splint under the affected finger	Ⓨ Ⓝ	Ⓨ Ⓝ	Ⓨ Ⓝ
Adjusts splint to cover one joint above and below the fracture site	Ⓨ Ⓝ	Ⓨ Ⓝ	Ⓨ Ⓝ
Secures splint to affected finger with white tape	Ⓨ Ⓝ	Ⓨ Ⓝ	Ⓨ Ⓝ
Tester evaluates injured area after device application	**Test 1**	**Test 2**	**Test 3**
Checks distal pulse	Ⓨ Ⓝ	Ⓨ Ⓝ	Ⓨ Ⓝ
Checks distal sensation and capillary refill	Ⓨ Ⓝ	Ⓨ Ⓝ	Ⓨ Ⓝ

The psychomotor skill was performed completely and in the appropriate order   **0 1 2 3 4 5**

The tester had control of the subject and the situation (showed confidence)   **0 1 2 3 4 5**

Method of performing the skill allowed the tester the ability to determine:
severity, proper progression, and the *fit* in the overall picture (Oral)   **0 1 2 3 4 5**

In order for a grade of *minimum standard* to be given, the total must be ≥11   **TOTAL = _____**

| 1 | 2 | 3 | 4 | 5 | 6 | 7 | 8 | 9 | 10 | 11 | 12 | 13 | 14 | 15 |

Not Acceptable   **Meets**   **Exceeds**
                                         Minimum Standards   **Minimum Standards**

TEST ENVIRONMENTS
L: Laboratory/Classroom Testing
C: Clinical/Field Testing
P: Practicum Testing
A: Assessment/Mock Exam Testing
S: Self-Reporting

SKILL TEST INFORMATION
Special Considerations: Do not reduce deformity
Reference(s): Street
Supplies Needed: Finger splint, white tape

PROTECTIVE DEVICE CONSTRUCTION/EQUIPMENT FITTING
(PDC-U-Test 4)

Peer Review _____ Peer Review _____

Skill Acquisition: _____ Practice Opportunities: _____

This problem allows you the opportunity to demonstrate the construction of a **hardshell doughnut pad** *to protect the* **acromioclavicular joint**. *You have 4 minutes to complete this task.*

Tester places athlete and limb in appropriate position	Test 1	Test 2	Test 3
Cuts foam to create doughnut pad	Ⓨ Ⓝ	Ⓨ Ⓝ	Ⓨ Ⓝ
Cuts hole in pad to fit around AC joint	Ⓨ Ⓝ	Ⓨ Ⓝ	Ⓨ Ⓝ
Cuts thermomoldable material to same size as doughnut pad	Ⓨ Ⓝ	Ⓨ Ⓝ	Ⓨ Ⓝ
Heats thermomoldable material until pliable	Ⓨ Ⓝ	Ⓨ Ⓝ	Ⓨ Ⓝ
Molds a convex dome in thermomoldable material	Ⓨ Ⓝ	Ⓨ Ⓝ	Ⓨ Ⓝ
Secures thermomoldable to doughnut pad with elastic tape	Ⓨ Ⓝ	Ⓨ Ⓝ	Ⓨ Ⓝ
Tester applies protective device to injured area	**Test 1**	**Test 2**	**Test 3**
Secures finished pad over the AC joint (optional)	Ⓨ Ⓝ	Ⓨ Ⓝ	Ⓨ Ⓝ

The psychomotor skill was performed completely and in the appropriate order   **0 1 2 3 4 5**

The tester had control of the subject and the situation (showed confidence)   **0 1 2 3 4 5**

Method of performing the skill allowed the tester the ability to determine:
severity, proper progression, and the *fit* in the overall picture (Oral)   **0 1 2 3 4 5**

In order for a grade of *minimum standard* to be given, the total must be ≥11   **TOTAL = _____**

```
  1    2    3    4    5    6    7    8    9    10   11   12   13   14   15
  |    |    |    |    |    |    |    |    |    |    |    |    |    |    |
```
Not Acceptable   **Meets**   **Exceeds**
                               Minimum Standards   **Minimum Standards**

TEST ENVIRONMENTS

L: Laboratory/Classroom Testing
C: Clinical/Field Testing
P: Practicum Testing
A: Assessment/Mock Exam Testing
S: Self-Reporting

SKILL TEST INFORMATION

Special Considerations: N/A
Reference(s): Perrin; Prentice (2003)
Supplies Needed: Thermomoldable material, heating source, foam/felt, elastic tape, white tape, scissors

PROTECTIVE DEVICE CONSTRUCTION/EQUIPMENT FITTING
(PDC-U-Test 5)

Peer Review _____ Peer Review _____

Skill Acquisition: _____   Practice Opportunities: _____

The athlete is suspected of having a neck injury and is having difficulty breathing. Demonstrate your ability to **remove a facemask from a standard football helmet** *using any equipment on the supply table. Assume that a second member of the medical team is stabilizing the head. For this scenario, your only concern is the removal of the facemask. You have 2 minutes to complete this task.*

Tester places athlete and limb in appropriate position	Test 1	Test 2	Test 3
Supine on the floor	Ⓨ Ⓝ	Ⓨ Ⓝ	Ⓨ Ⓝ
Tester placed in proper position	**Test 1**	**Test 2**	**Test 3**
Kneeling on the side of the athlete	Ⓨ Ⓝ	Ⓨ Ⓝ	Ⓨ Ⓝ
Tester performs task according to accepted guidelines	**Test 1**	**Test 2**	**Test 3**
Selects the proper cutting tool	Ⓨ Ⓝ	Ⓨ Ⓝ	Ⓨ Ⓝ
Removes the two side (lower) brackets first	Ⓨ Ⓝ	Ⓨ Ⓝ	Ⓨ Ⓝ
Removes the two top (upper) brackets	Ⓨ Ⓝ	Ⓨ Ⓝ	Ⓨ Ⓝ

The psychomotor skill was performed completely and in the appropriate order   0 1 2 3 4 5

The tester had control of the subject and the situation (showed confidence)   0 1 2 3 4 5

Method of performing the skill allowed the tester the ability to determine:
severity, proper progression, and the *fit* in the overall picture (Oral)   0 1 2 3 4 5

In order for a grade of *minimum standard* to be given, the total must be ≥11   TOTAL = _____

```
 1    2    3    4    5    6    7    8    9   10   11   12   13   14   15
 |    |    |    |    |    |    |    |    |    |    |    |    |    |    |
```
Not Acceptable   **Meets**   **Exceeds**
                                   Minimum Standards   **Minimum Standards**

TEST ENVIRONMENTS	SKILL TEST INFORMATION	
L: Laboratory/Classroom Testing	**Positive Finding:**	Remove facemask
C: Clinical/Field Testing	**Involved Structure:**	N/A
P: Practicum Testing	**Special Considerations:**	N/A
A: Assessment/Mock Exam Testing	**Reference(s):**	Starkey et al
S: Self-Reporting	**Supplies Needed:**	Football helmet; proper cutters

PROTECTIVE DEVICE CONSTRUCTION/EQUIPMENT FITTING
(PDC-U-Test 6)

Peer Review _____ Peer Review _____

Skill Acquisition: _____ Practice Opportunities: _____

This situation allows you the opportunity to demonstrate your proficiency in properly **fitting shoulder pads** *for a football player. You have 3 minutes to complete this task response.*

Tester places athlete in appropriate position	Test 1	Test 2	Test 3
Standing	Ⓨ Ⓝ	Ⓨ Ⓝ	Ⓨ Ⓝ
Tester applies protective device	**Test 1**	**Test 2**	**Test 3**
Measures chest size at the level of the nipples	Ⓨ Ⓝ	Ⓨ Ⓝ	Ⓨ Ⓝ
Checks the following	Ⓨ Ⓝ	Ⓨ Ⓝ	Ⓨ Ⓝ
Shoulder pads should completely cover scapula	Ⓨ Ⓝ	Ⓨ Ⓝ	Ⓨ Ⓝ
Shoulder pads should completely cover clavicle	Ⓨ Ⓝ	Ⓨ Ⓝ	Ⓨ Ⓝ
Shoulder pads should completely cover deltoids and AC joint	Ⓨ Ⓝ	Ⓨ Ⓝ	Ⓨ Ⓝ
Pads should be no more than two finger widths from body	Ⓨ Ⓝ	Ⓨ Ⓝ	Ⓨ Ⓝ
Tester evaluates protective device after application	**Test 1**	**Test 2**	**Test 3**
Checks for pinching of the neck when arms are raised above head	Ⓨ Ⓝ	Ⓨ Ⓝ	Ⓨ Ⓝ
Checks for any damage to shoulder pads	Ⓨ Ⓝ	Ⓨ Ⓝ	Ⓨ Ⓝ
Checks to see that all parts are in place	Ⓨ Ⓝ	Ⓨ Ⓝ	Ⓨ Ⓝ

The psychomotor skill was performed completely and in the appropriate order   **0 1 2 3 4 5**

The tester had control of the subject and the situation (showed confidence)   **0 1 2 3 4 5**

Method of performing the skill allowed the tester the ability to determine: severity, proper progression, and the *fit* in the overall picture (Oral)   **0 1 2 3 4 5**

In order for a grade of *minimum standard* to be given, the total must be ≥11   **TOTAL = _____**

```
 1    2    3    4    5    6    7    8    9   10   11   12   13   14   15
 |____|____|____|____|____|____|____|____|____|____|____|____|____|____|

  Not Acceptable                        Meets                    Exceeds
                                   Minimum Standards        Minimum Standards
```

TEST ENVIRONMENTS

L: Laboratory/Classroom Testing
C: Clinical/Field Testing
P: Practicum Testing
A: Assessment/Mock Exam Testing
S: Self-Reporting

SKILL TEST INFORMATION

Purpose: Help to prevent injuries to the shoulder
Special Considerations: N/A
Reference(s): Prentice (2003)
Supplies Needed: Shoulder pads

PROTECTIVE DEVICE CONSTRUCTION/EQUIPMENT FITTING
(PDC-U-Test 7)

Peer Review _____ Peer Review _____

Skill Acquisition: _____   Practice Opportunities: _____

This situation allows you to demonstrate your proficiency in properly **fitting a mouth guard**. *You have 2 minutes to complete this task response.*

Tester applies protective device	Test 1	Test 2	Test 3
Places mouth guard in hot water until pliable (about 3 seconds)	Y N	Y N	Y N
Removes mouth guard and shakes off excess water	Y N	Y N	Y N
Asks athlete to bite down on back of mouth guard	Y N	Y N	Y N
Asks athlete to apply suction to remove excess air	Y N	Y N	Y N
Asks athlete to remove mouth guard once molded	Y N	Y N	Y N
Asks athlete to run mouth guard under cold water for a few seconds	Y N	Y N	Y N

The psychomotor skill was performed completely and in the appropriate order   0 1 2 3 4 5

The tester had control of the subject and the situation (showed confidence)   0 1 2 3 4 5

Method of performing the skill allowed the tester the ability to determine:
severity, proper progression, and the *fit* in the overall picture (Oral)   0 1 2 3 4 5

In order for a grade of *minimum standard* to be given, the total must be ≥11   TOTAL = _____

```
  1    2    3    4    5    6    7    8    9    10   11   12   13   14   15
  |----|----|----|----|----|----|----|----|----|----|----|----|----|----|
Not Acceptable                          Meets                 Exceeds
                                  Minimum Standards      Minimum Standards
```

TEST ENVIRONMENTS

L: Laboratory/Classroom Testing
C: Clinical/Field Testing
P: Practicum Testing
A: Assessment/Mock Exam Testing
S: Self-Reporting

SKILL TEST INFORMATION

Purpose: Help to prevent injuries to the area of the month and teeth; absorbs external forces

Special Considerations: N/A

Reference(s): Prentice (2003)

Supplies Needed: Mouth guard, source of hot water

Protective Device Construction/Equipment Fitting
(PDC-L-Test 1)

Peer Review _____ Peer Review _____

Skill Acquisition: _____   Practice Opportunities: _____

*This problem allows you the opportunity to demonstrate the application of an **adjustable SAM splint (ladder splint)** to immobilize the ankle joint. You have 4 minutes to complete this task.*

Tester places athlete and limb in appropriate position	Test 1	Test 2	Test 3
Maintains injured body part in position it was found	Ⓨ Ⓝ	Ⓨ Ⓝ	Ⓨ Ⓝ
Limits movement of injured area as much as possible	Ⓨ Ⓝ	Ⓨ Ⓝ	Ⓨ Ⓝ
Tester selects appropriate device and applies to injured area	**Test 1**	**Test 2**	**Test 3**
Positions splint in horseshoe shape around the foot and ankle (forms around deformity and does not relocate)	Ⓨ Ⓝ	Ⓨ Ⓝ	Ⓨ Ⓝ
Applies compression wrap distal to proximal	Ⓨ Ⓝ	Ⓨ Ⓝ	Ⓨ Ⓝ
Secures splint, stabilizing the bones above and below the ankle joint	Ⓨ Ⓝ	Ⓨ Ⓝ	Ⓨ Ⓝ
Tester evaluates injured area after device application	**Test 1**	**Test 2**	**Test 3**
Checks distal pulse	Ⓨ Ⓝ	Ⓨ Ⓝ	Ⓨ Ⓝ
Checks distal sensation and capillary refill	Ⓨ Ⓝ	Ⓨ Ⓝ	Ⓨ Ⓝ

The psychomotor skill was performed completely and in the appropriate order   **0 1 2 3 4 5**

The tester had control of the subject and the situation (showed confidence)   **0 1 2 3 4 5**

Method of performing the skill allowed the tester the ability to determine:
severity, proper progression, and the *fit* in the overall picture (Oral)   **0 1 2 3 4 5**

In order for a grade of *minimum standard* to be given, the total must be ≥11   **TOTAL = _____**

```
1   2   3   4   5   6   7   8   9   10  11  12  13  14  15
```

Not Acceptable   **Meets Minimum Standards**   **Exceeds Minimum Standards**

TEST ENVIRONMENTS
L: Laboratory/Classroom Testing
C: Clinical/Field Testing
P: Practicum Testing
A: Assessment/Mock Exam Testing
S: Self-Reporting

SKILL TEST INFORMATION
Special Considerations: N/A
Reference(s): Manufacturer's recommendations
Supplies Needed: SAM splint/ladder splint, white tape, compression wrap, neuro pinwheel

PROTECTIVE DEVICE CONSTRUCTION/EQUIPMENT FITTING
(PDC-L-Test 2)

Peer Review _____ Peer Review _____

Skill Acquisition: _____   Practice Opportunities: _____

This problem allows you the opportunity to demonstrate the application of a **knee immobilizer**. *You have 2 minutes to complete this task.*

Tester places athlete and limb in appropriate position	Test 1	Test 2	Test 3
Knee extended	Ⓨ Ⓝ	Ⓨ Ⓝ	Ⓨ Ⓝ
Limits movement of injured area as much as possible	Ⓨ Ⓝ	Ⓨ Ⓝ	Ⓨ Ⓝ
Tester selects appropriate device and applies to injured area	**Test 1**	**Test 2**	**Test 3**
Obtains appropriate size immobilizer	Ⓨ Ⓝ	Ⓨ Ⓝ	Ⓨ Ⓝ
Slides immobilizer under affected limb	Ⓨ Ⓝ	Ⓨ Ⓝ	Ⓨ Ⓝ
Secures straps near joint first	Ⓨ Ⓝ	Ⓨ Ⓝ	Ⓨ Ⓝ
Follows by securing proximal and distal straps	Ⓨ Ⓝ	Ⓨ Ⓝ	Ⓨ Ⓝ
Verifies that device is snug but comfortable	Ⓨ Ⓝ	Ⓨ Ⓝ	Ⓨ Ⓝ
Tester evaluates injured area after device application	**Test 1**	**Test 2**	**Test 3**
Checks distal pulse	Ⓨ Ⓝ	Ⓨ Ⓝ	Ⓨ Ⓝ
Checks distal sensation and capillary refill	Ⓨ Ⓝ	Ⓨ Ⓝ	Ⓨ Ⓝ

The psychomotor skill was performed completely and in the appropriate order   **0 1 2 3 4 5**

The tester had control of the subject and the situation (showed confidence)   **0 1 2 3 4 5**

Method of performing the skill allowed the tester the ability to determine:
severity, proper progression, and the *fit* in the overall picture (Oral)   **0 1 2 3 4 5**

In order for a grade of *minimum standard* to be given, the total must be ≥11   **TOTAL = _____**

```
  1     2     3     4     5     6     7     8     9    10    11    12    13    14    15
  |     |     |     |     |     |     |     |     |     |     |     |     |     |     |
```

Not Acceptable   **Meets**   **Exceeds**
                                   Minimum Standards   **Minimum Standards**

TEST ENVIRONMENTS

L: Laboratory/Classroom Testing
C: Clinical/Field Testing
P: Practicum Testing
A: Assessment/Mock Exam Testing
S: Self-Reporting

SKILL TEST INFORMATION

Special Considerations: N/A
Reference(s): Perrin
Supplies Needed: Various-sized knee immobilizers, neuro pinwheel

PROTECTIVE DEVICE CONSTRUCTION/EQUIPMENT FITTING
(PDC-L-Test 3)

Peer Review _____   Peer Review _____

Skill Acquisition: _____   Practice Opportunities: _____

*This problem allows you the opportunity to demonstrate the application of a **ankle horseshoe pad and compression wrap** to prevent swelling. You have 3 minutes to complete this task.*

Tester places athlete and limb in appropriate position	Test 1	Test 2	Test 3
Seated with foot extended over the table	Ⓨ Ⓝ	Ⓨ Ⓝ	Ⓨ Ⓝ
Ankle dorsiflexed at 90 degrees (if possible)	Ⓨ Ⓝ	Ⓨ Ⓝ	Ⓨ Ⓝ
Tester selects appropriate device and applies to injured area	**Test 1**	**Test 2**	**Test 3**
Applies horseshoe pad to lateral malleolus	Ⓨ Ⓝ	Ⓨ Ⓝ	Ⓨ Ⓝ
Applies compression wrap just proximal to toes	Ⓨ Ⓝ	Ⓨ Ⓝ	Ⓨ Ⓝ
Applies compression wrap proximally to lower third of the calf	Ⓨ Ⓝ	Ⓨ Ⓝ	Ⓨ Ⓝ
Secures compression wrap with tape	Ⓨ Ⓝ	Ⓨ Ⓝ	Ⓨ Ⓝ
Tester evaluates injured area after device application	**Test 1**	**Test 2**	**Test 3**
Checks distal pulse	Ⓨ Ⓝ	Ⓨ Ⓝ	Ⓨ Ⓝ
Checks distal sensation and capillary refill	Ⓨ Ⓝ	Ⓨ Ⓝ	Ⓨ Ⓝ

The psychomotor skill was performed completely and in the appropriate order   **0 1 2 3 4 5**

The tester had control of the subject and the situation (showed confidence)   **0 1 2 3 4 5**

Method of performing the skill allowed the tester the ability to determine:
severity, proper progression, and the *fit* in the overall picture (Oral)   **0 1 2 3 4 5**

In order for a grade of *minimum standard* to be given, the total must be ≥11   **TOTAL = _____**

```
  1    2    3    4    5    6    7    8    9   10   11   12   13   14   15
  |    |    |    |    |    |    |    |    |    |    |    |    |    |    |
```

Not Acceptable   **Meets**   **Exceeds**
                                        Minimum Standards   **Minimum Standards**

TEST ENVIRONMENTS

L: Laboratory/Classroom Testing
C: Clinical/Field Testing
P: Practicum Testing
A: Assessment/Mock Exam Testing
S: Self-Reporting

SKILL TEST INFORMATION

Special Considerations: N/A
Reference(s): Prentice (2003)
Supplies Needed: Horseshoe pad, white tape, compression wrap, neuro pinwheel

PROTECTIVE DEVICE CONSTRUCTION/EQUIPMENT FITTING
(PDC-L-Test 4)

Peer Review _____ Peer Review _____

Skill Acquisition: _____   Practice Opportunities: _____

This problem allows you the opportunity to demonstrate the application of a **vacuum splint for a tibia fracture**. *You have 3 minutes to complete this task.*

Tester places athlete and limb in appropriate position	Test 1	Test 2	Test 3
Seated or supine	Ⓨ Ⓝ	Ⓨ Ⓝ	Ⓨ Ⓝ
Maintains injured body part in position it was found	Ⓨ Ⓝ	Ⓨ Ⓝ	Ⓨ Ⓝ
Tester selects appropriate device and applies to injured area	**Test 1**	**Test 2**	**Test 3**
Slides splint under affected limb	Ⓨ Ⓝ	Ⓨ Ⓝ	Ⓨ Ⓝ
Adjusts splint to cover one joint above and below fracture site	Ⓨ Ⓝ	Ⓨ Ⓝ	Ⓨ Ⓝ
Secures splint to affected limb	Ⓨ Ⓝ	Ⓨ Ⓝ	Ⓨ Ⓝ
Removes residual air from splint	Ⓨ Ⓝ	Ⓨ Ⓝ	Ⓨ Ⓝ
Tester evaluates injured area after device application	**Test 1**	**Test 2**	**Test 3**
Checks distal pulse	Ⓨ Ⓝ	Ⓨ Ⓝ	Ⓨ Ⓝ
Checks distal sensation and capillary refill	Ⓨ Ⓝ	Ⓨ Ⓝ	Ⓨ Ⓝ

The psychomotor skill was performed completely and in the appropriate order   **0 1 2 3 4 5**

The tester had control of the subject and the situation (showed confidence)   **0 1 2 3 4 5**

Method of performing the skill allowed the tester the ability to determine:
severity, proper progression, and the *fit* in the overall picture (Oral)   **0 1 2 3 4 5**

In order for a grade of *minimum standard* to be given, the total must be ≥11   **TOTAL = _____**

```
  1     2     3     4     5     6     7     8     9    10    11    12    13    14    15
  |     |     |     |     |     |     |     |     |     |     |     |     |     |     |
```
Not Acceptable   **Meets**   **Exceeds**
                                        Minimum Standards   **Minimum Standards**

TEST ENVIRONMENTS

L: Laboratory/Classroom Testing
C: Clinical/Field Testing
P: Practicum Testing
A: Assessment/Mock Exam Testing
S: Self-Reporting

SKILL TEST INFORMATION

Special Considerations: N/A
Reference(s): Manufacturer's recommendations
Supplies Needed: Vacuum splint, neuro pinwheel

PROTECTIVE DEVICE CONSTRUCTION/EQUIPMENT FITTING
(PDC-L-Test 5)

Peer Review _____ Peer Review _____

Skill Acquisition: _____   Practice Opportunities: _____

This situation allows you the opportunity to demonstrate your proficiency in **properly fitting running shoes.** *You have 3 minutes to complete this task response.*

Tester places athlete and limb in appropriate position	Test 1	Test 2	Test 3
Wears socks that will be worn during activity	Ⓨ Ⓝ	Ⓨ Ⓝ	Ⓨ Ⓝ
Fits shoes late in the day when feet have enlarged from weight-bearing	Ⓨ Ⓝ	Ⓨ Ⓝ	Ⓨ Ⓝ
Tester applies protective device	**Test 1**	**Test 2**	**Test 3**
Measures foot length	Ⓨ Ⓝ	Ⓨ Ⓝ	Ⓨ Ⓝ
Requests narrow or wide model (if applicable based on foot shape)	Ⓨ Ⓝ	Ⓨ Ⓝ	Ⓨ Ⓝ
Allows 0.5 to 0.75 inch from end of great toe to end of shoe	Ⓨ Ⓝ	Ⓨ Ⓝ	Ⓨ Ⓝ
Tester evaluates protective device after application	**Test 1**	**Test 2**	**Test 3**
Assures that 0.5 to 0.75 inches exists between great toe and end of shoe	Ⓨ Ⓝ	Ⓨ Ⓝ	Ⓨ Ⓝ
Assures that shoes bends in the places where the foot bends	Ⓨ Ⓝ	Ⓨ Ⓝ	Ⓨ Ⓝ
Assures that the show is not slipping on the heel	Ⓨ Ⓝ	Ⓨ Ⓝ	Ⓨ Ⓝ
Assures appropriate support in sole and heel	Ⓨ Ⓝ	Ⓨ Ⓝ	Ⓨ Ⓝ
Assures upper of breathable material (nylon and leather combo)	Ⓨ Ⓝ	Ⓨ Ⓝ	Ⓨ Ⓝ
Applies additional support as needed for specific biomechanical conditions (heel cup, wedges, etc)	Ⓨ Ⓝ	Ⓨ Ⓝ	Ⓨ Ⓝ
Performs assessment bilaterally	Ⓨ Ⓝ	Ⓨ Ⓝ	Ⓨ Ⓝ

The psychomotor skill was performed completely and in the appropriate order   0 1 2 3 4 5

The tester had control of the subject and the situation (showed confidence)   0 1 2 3 4 5

Method of performing the skill allowed the tester the ability to determine:
severity, proper progression, and the *fit* in the overall picture (Oral)   0 1 2 3 4 5

In order for a grade of *minimum standard* to be given, the total must be ≥11   TOTAL = _____

```
 1    2    3    4    5    6    7    8    9   10   11   12   13   14   15
 |____|____|____|____|____|____|____|____|____|____|____|____|____|____|
```

Not Acceptable   **Meets**   **Exceeds**
                              Minimum Standards   **Minimum Standards**

TEST ENVIRONMENTS

L: Laboratory/Classroom Testing
C: Clinical/Field Testing
P: Practicum Testing
A: Assessment/Mock Exam Testing
S: Self-Reporting

SKILL TEST INFORMATION

Purpose: Help prevent foot and lower leg injuries
Special Considerations: N/A
Reference(s) Prentice (2003)
Supplies Needed: Running shoes, measuring tape, socks

PROTECTIVE DEVICE CONSTRUCTION/EQUIPMENT FITTING
(PDC-L-Test 6)

Peer Review _____ Peer Review _____

Skill Acquisition: _____   Practice Opportunities: _____

This situation allows you the opportunity to demonstrate your proficiency in properly **fitting a prophylactic knee brace**. *You have 2 minutes to complete this task response.*

Tester places athlete and limb in appropriate position	Test 1	Test 2	Test 3
Standing with knee flexed at 15 to 30 degrees	Ⓨ Ⓝ	Ⓨ Ⓝ	Ⓨ Ⓝ
Tester applies protective device to injured area	**Test 1**	**Test 2**	**Test 3**
Selects appropriate sized prophylactic brace	Ⓨ Ⓝ	Ⓨ Ⓝ	Ⓨ Ⓝ
Applies sleeve over knee joint	Ⓨ Ⓝ	Ⓨ Ⓝ	Ⓨ Ⓝ
Tester evaluates protective device after application	**Test 1**	**Test 2**	**Test 3**
Has athlete actively flex the knee joint	Ⓨ Ⓝ	Ⓨ Ⓝ	Ⓨ Ⓝ
Assures snug fit above and below the knee joint	Ⓨ Ⓝ	Ⓨ Ⓝ	Ⓨ Ⓝ
Assures alignment of brace elements with joint line	Ⓨ Ⓝ	Ⓨ Ⓝ	Ⓨ Ⓝ
Confirms comfort and functionality of brace	Ⓨ Ⓝ	Ⓨ Ⓝ	Ⓨ Ⓝ

The psychomotor skill was performed completely and in the appropriate order   **0 1 2 3 4 5**

The tester had control of the subject and the situation (showed confidence)   **0 1 2 3 4 5**

Method of performing the skill allowed the tester the ability to determine: severity, proper progression, and the *fit* in the overall picture (Oral)   **0 1 2 3 4 5**

In order for a grade of *minimum standard* to be given, the total must be ≥11   **TOTAL = _____**

```
  1    2    3    4    5    6    7    8    9   10   11   12   13   14   15
  |____|____|____|____|____|____|____|____|____|____|____|____|____|____|
```

Not Acceptable   **Meets**   **Exceeds**
                                    Minimum Standards   **Minimum Standards**

TEST ENVIRONMENTS
L: Laboratory/Classroom Testing
C: Clinical/Field Testing
P: Practicum Testing
A: Assessment/Mock Exam Testing
S: Self-Reporting

SKILL TEST INFORMATION
Special Considerations: N/A
Reference(s): Perrin; Prentice (2003)
Supplies Needed: Knee brace

PROTECTIVE DEVICE CONSTRUCTION/EQUIPMENT FITTING
(PDC-L-Test 7)

Peer Review _____ Peer Review _____

Skill Acquisition: _____   Practice Opportunities: _____

This situation allows you the opportunity to demonstrate your proficiency in properly **fitting a prophylactic ankle brace**. *You have 2 minutes to complete this task response.*

Tester places athlete and limb in appropriate position	Test 1	Test 2	Test 3
Seated or supine	Ⓨ Ⓝ	Ⓨ Ⓝ	Ⓨ Ⓝ
Ankle in neutral position	Ⓨ Ⓝ	Ⓨ Ⓝ	Ⓨ Ⓝ
Tester applies protective device to injured area	**Test 1**	**Test 2**	**Test 3**
Selects appropriate sized prophylactic brace	Ⓨ Ⓝ	Ⓨ Ⓝ	Ⓨ Ⓝ
Applies sleeve over ankle joint	Ⓨ Ⓝ	Ⓨ Ⓝ	Ⓨ Ⓝ
Laces brace and tightens to comfort of athlete	Ⓨ Ⓝ	Ⓨ Ⓝ	Ⓨ Ⓝ
Tester evaluates protective device after application	**Test 1**	**Test 2**	**Test 3**
Assures snug fit above and below the ankle joint	Ⓨ Ⓝ	Ⓨ Ⓝ	Ⓨ Ⓝ
Confirms comfort and functionality of brace	Ⓨ Ⓝ	Ⓨ Ⓝ	Ⓨ Ⓝ
Has athlete actively dorsiflex and plantarflex the ankle joint	Ⓨ Ⓝ	Ⓨ Ⓝ	Ⓨ Ⓝ
Has athlete actively invert and evert the ankle joint	Ⓨ Ⓝ	Ⓨ Ⓝ	Ⓨ Ⓝ
Confirms that inversion is limited by brace	Ⓨ Ⓝ	Ⓨ Ⓝ	Ⓨ Ⓝ
Performs assessment bilaterally (if needed)	Ⓨ Ⓝ	Ⓨ Ⓝ	Ⓨ Ⓝ

The psychomotor skill was performed completely and in the appropriate order   0 1 2 3 4 5

The tester had control of the subject and the situation (showed confidence)   0 1 2 3 4 5

Method of performing the skill allowed the tester the ability to determine:
severity, proper progression, and the *fit* in the overall picture (Oral)   0 1 2 3 4 5

In order for a grade of *minimum standard* to be given, the total must be ≥11   TOTAL = _____

```
  1     2     3     4     5     6     7     8     9    10    11    12    13    14    15
  |     |     |     |     |     |     |     |     |     |     |     |     |     |     |
```
Not Acceptable   **Meets**   **Exceeds**
                                    Minimum Standards   **Minimum Standards**

TEST ENVIRONMENTS

L: Laboratory/Classroom Testing
C: Clinical/Field Testing
P: Practicum Testing
A: Assessment/Mock Exam Testing
S: Self-Reporting

SKILL TEST INFORMATION

Special Considerations: N/A
Reference(s): Perrin; Prentice (2003)
Supplies Needed: Ankle brace

Chapter

11

GENERAL MEDICAL

GENERAL MEDICAL
(GMED-Test 1)

Peer Review _____ Peer Review _____

Skill Acquisition: _____   Practice Opportunities: _____

This problem allows you the opportunity to demonstrate assessment of the **radial pulse** *for an athlete. You have 2 minutes to complete this task.*

Tester places athlete and limb in appropriate position	Test 1	Test 2	Test 3
Supine	Ⓨ Ⓝ	Ⓨ Ⓝ	Ⓨ Ⓝ
Tester placed in proper position	**Test 1**	**Test 2**	**Test 3**
Stands to the side to the athlete	Ⓨ Ⓝ	Ⓨ Ⓝ	Ⓨ Ⓝ
Locates the radial pulse using the index and middle fingers	Ⓨ Ⓝ	Ⓨ Ⓝ	Ⓨ Ⓝ
Tester performs test according to accepted guidelines	**Test 1**	**Test 2**	**Test 3**
Counts the number of beats/minute (Note: 10 seconds x 6 or 15 seconds x 4)	Ⓨ Ⓝ	Ⓨ Ⓝ	Ⓨ Ⓝ
Assesses rhythm (good, irregular, etc)	Ⓨ Ⓝ	Ⓨ Ⓝ	Ⓨ Ⓝ
Assesses strength (strong, weak)	Ⓨ Ⓝ	Ⓨ Ⓝ	Ⓨ Ⓝ
Records and rechecks at regular intervals	Ⓨ Ⓝ	Ⓨ Ⓝ	Ⓨ Ⓝ

The psychomotor skill was performed completely and in the appropriate order   0 1 2 3 4 5

The tester had control of the subject and the situation (showed confidence)   0 1 2 3 4 5

Method of performing the skill allowed the tester the ability to determine:
severity, proper progression, and the *fit* in the overall picture (Oral)   0 1 2 3 4 5

In order for a grade of *minimum standard* to be given, the total must be ≥11   TOTAL = _____

```
  1     2     3     4     5     6     7     8     9    10    11    12    13    14    15
  |     |     |     |     |     |     |     |     |     |     |     |     |     |     |
```

Not Acceptable   **Meets**   **Exceeds**
                                           Minimum Standards   **Minimum Standards**

TEST ENVIRONMENTS

L: Laboratory/Classroom Testing
C: Clinical/Field Testing
P: Practicum Testing
A: Assessment/Mock Exam Testing
S: Self-Reporting

SKILL TEST INFORMATION

Positive Finding:	Improper rate, rhythm, strength
Involved Structure:	Cardiovascular system
Special Considerations:	N/A
Reference(s):	Bickley et al; Starkey et al (2002)
Supplies Needed:	Watch (with a second hand), pencil/paper

GENERAL MEDICAL
(GMED-Test 2)

Peer Review _____ Peer Review _____

Skill Acquisition: _____   Practice Opportunities: _____

*This problem allows you the opportunity to demonstrate assessment of the **carotid pulse** of an athlete. You have 2 minutes to complete this task.*

Tester places athlete and limb in appropriate position	Test 1	Test 2	Test 3
Seated or supine	Ⓨ Ⓝ	Ⓨ Ⓝ	Ⓨ Ⓝ
Tester placed in proper position	**Test 1**	**Test 2**	**Test 3**
Stands to the side of the athlete	Ⓨ Ⓝ	Ⓨ Ⓝ	Ⓨ Ⓝ
Locates the carotid pulse (using index and middle fingers)	Ⓨ Ⓝ	Ⓨ Ⓝ	Ⓨ Ⓝ
Tester performs test according to accepted guidelines	**Test 1**	**Test 2**	**Test 3**
Counts the number beats/minute (Note: 10 seconds x 6 or 15 seconds x 4)	Ⓨ Ⓝ	Ⓨ Ⓝ	Ⓨ Ⓝ
Assesses rhythm (good, irregular, etc)	Ⓨ Ⓝ	Ⓨ Ⓝ	Ⓨ Ⓝ
Assesses strength (strong, weak)	Ⓨ Ⓝ	Ⓨ Ⓝ	Ⓨ Ⓝ
Records and rechecks at regular intervals	Ⓨ Ⓝ	Ⓨ Ⓝ	Ⓨ Ⓝ

The psychomotor skill was performed completely and in the appropriate order   **0 1 2 3 4 5**

The tester had control of the subject and the situation (showed confidence)   **0 1 2 3 4 5**

Method of performing the skill allowed the tester the ability to determine:
severity, proper progression, and the *fit* in the overall picture (Oral)   **0 1 2 3 4 5**

In order for a grade of *minimum standard* to be given, the total must be ≥11   **TOTAL = _____**

```
 1    2    3    4    5    6    7    8    9   10   11   12   13   14   15
 |    |    |    |    |    |    |    |    |    |    |    |    |    |    |
```
Not Acceptable   **Meets**   **Exceeds**
                              Minimum Standards   **Minimum Standards**

TEST ENVIRONMENTS

L: Laboratory/Classroom Testing
C: Clinical/Field Testing
P: Practicum Testing
A: Assessment/Mock Exam Testing
S: Self-Reporting

SKILL TEST INFORMATION

Positive Finding: Improper rate, rhythm, and/or strength
Involved Structure: Cardiovascular system
Special Considerations: N/A
Reference(s): Bickley et al; Starkey et al (2002)
Supplies Needed: Watch (with a second hand), pencil/paper

GENERAL MEDICAL
(GMED-Test 3)

Peer Review _____ Peer Review _____

Skill Acquisition: _____   Practice Opportunities: _____

This problem allows you the opportunity to demonstrate **blood pressure assessment** *for an athlete. You have 2 minutes to complete this task.*

Tester places athlete and limb in appropriate position	Test 1	Test 2	Test 3
Supine or seated	Ⓨ Ⓝ	Ⓨ Ⓝ	Ⓨ Ⓝ

Tester placed in proper position	Test 1	Test 2	Test 3
Stands to the side of the athlete (in position to read BP cuff)	Ⓨ Ⓝ	Ⓨ Ⓝ	Ⓨ Ⓝ

Tester performs test according to accepted guidelines	Test 1	Test 2	Test 3
Determines the appropriate size BP cuff	Ⓨ Ⓝ	Ⓨ Ⓝ	Ⓨ Ⓝ
Positions the brachial artery at approximately heart level	Ⓨ Ⓝ	Ⓨ Ⓝ	Ⓨ Ⓝ
Centers BP cuff (inflatable bladder) over the upper arm (secures the cuff snugly)	Ⓨ Ⓝ	Ⓨ Ⓝ	Ⓨ Ⓝ
Positions the diaphragm of the stethoscope over the brachial artery	Ⓨ Ⓝ	Ⓨ Ⓝ	Ⓨ Ⓝ
Inflates the cuff to about 200 mmHg of pressure or about 30 mmHg over the predicted systolic value	Ⓨ Ⓝ	Ⓨ Ⓝ	Ⓨ Ⓝ
Releases the air in the cuff slowly at about 2 to 3 mmHg per second (Note: when the first sound is heard and the last pulse is heard)	Ⓨ Ⓝ	Ⓨ Ⓝ	Ⓨ Ⓝ
Records and rechecks at regular intervals (5 to 10 mmHg difference may occur in opposite arms)	Ⓨ Ⓝ	Ⓨ Ⓝ	Ⓨ Ⓝ

The psychomotor skill was performed completely and in the appropriate order   0 1 2 3 4 5

The tester had control of the subject and the situation (showed confidence)   0 1 2 3 4 5

Method of performing the skill allowed the tester the ability to determine:
severity, proper progression, and the *fit* in the overall picture (Oral)   0 1 2 3 4 5

In order for a grade of *minimum standard* to be given, the total must be ≥11   TOTAL = _____

```
  1    2    3    4    5    6    7    8    9    10   11   12   13   14   15
  |    |    |    |    |    |    |    |    |    |    |    |    |    |    |
```

Not Acceptable   **Meets**   **Exceeds**
                                   Minimum Standards   **Minimum Standards**

TEST ENVIRONMENTS

L: Laboratory/Classroom Testing
C: Clinical/Field Testing
P: Practicum Testing
A: Assessment/Mock Exam Testing
S: Self-Reporting

SKILL TEST INFORMATION

Positive Finding:	High or Low blood pressure
Involved Structure:	Cardiovascular system
Special Consideration:	Ideally the athlete should be at rest for about 5 minutes prior to taking the BP
Reference(s):	Bickley et al; Starkey et al (2002)
Supplies Needed:	BP Cuff, stethoscope

GENERAL MEDICAL
(GMED-Test 4)

Peer Review _____ Peer Review _____

Skill Acquisition: _____   Practice Opportunities: _____

This problem allows you the opportunity to perform **cardiac auscultation** *to help identify abnormal heart sounds. You have 3 minutes to complete this task.*

Tester places athlete in appropriate position	Test 1	Test 2	Test 3
Supine	Ⓨ Ⓝ	Ⓨ Ⓝ	Ⓨ Ⓝ
Instructs the athlete to properly disrobe	Ⓨ Ⓝ	Ⓨ Ⓝ	Ⓨ Ⓝ
Tester placed in proper position	**Test 1**	**Test 2**	**Test 3**
Stands to the side of the athlete	Ⓨ Ⓝ	Ⓨ Ⓝ	Ⓨ Ⓝ
Places the stethoscope properly into his or her ears	Ⓨ Ⓝ	Ⓨ Ⓝ	Ⓨ Ⓝ
Tester performs test according to accepted guidelines	**Test 1**	**Test 2**	**Test 3**
Instructs the athlete to breathe normally	Ⓨ Ⓝ	Ⓨ Ⓝ	Ⓨ Ⓝ
Places the diaphragm of the stethoscope in the appropriate locations:			
Mitral valve (apex of the heart-fifth intercostal space/about 1 to 2 inches left of the inferior sternum)	Ⓨ Ⓝ	Ⓨ Ⓝ	Ⓨ Ⓝ
Tricuspid valve (inferior right sternal border at fifth intercostal space)	Ⓨ Ⓝ	Ⓨ Ⓝ	Ⓨ Ⓝ
Aortic valve (superior right sternal border at second intercostal space)	Ⓨ Ⓝ	Ⓨ Ⓝ	Ⓨ Ⓝ
Pulmonary valve (superior left sternal border at second intercostal space)	Ⓨ Ⓝ	Ⓨ Ⓝ	Ⓨ Ⓝ
Listens at each location during several contraction cycles	Ⓨ Ⓝ	Ⓨ Ⓝ	Ⓨ Ⓝ
Notes and records any findings	Ⓨ Ⓝ	Ⓨ Ⓝ	Ⓨ Ⓝ

The psychomotor skill was performed completely and in the appropriate order   0 1 2 3 4 5

The tester had control of the subject and the situation (showed confidence)   0 1 2 3 4 5

Method of performing the skill allowed the tester the ability to determine:
severity, proper progression, and the *fit* in the overall picture (Oral)   0 1 2 3 4 5

In order for a grade of *minimum standard* to be given, the total must be ≥11   TOTAL = _____

```
 1    2    3    4    5    6    7    8    9   10   11   12   13   14   15
 |    |    |    |    |    |    |    |    |    |    |    |    |    |    |
```
Not Acceptable   Meets   Exceeds
                          Minimum Standards   Minimum Standards

TEST ENVIRONMENTS

L: Laboratory/Classroom Testing
C: Clinical/Field Testing
P: Practicum Testing
A: Assessment/Mock Exam Testing
S: Self-Reporting

SKILL TEST INFORMATION

Positive Finding:	Abnormal sounds
Involved Structure:	Cardiovascular system
Special Considerations:	May repeat, sitting; squat to stand
Reference(s):	O'Connor
Supplies Needed:	Stethoscope, table, paper/pencil

GENERAL MEDICAL
(GMED-Test 5)

Skill Acquisition: _____   Practice Opportunities: _____

This problem allows you the opportunity to perform **pulmonary auscultation** *to help identify abnormal breath sounds. You have 3 minutes to complete this task.*

Tester places athlete in appropriate position	Test 1	Test 2	Test 3
Sitting	Ⓨ Ⓝ	Ⓨ Ⓝ	Ⓨ Ⓝ
Instructs the athlete to properly disrobe	Ⓨ Ⓝ	Ⓨ Ⓝ	Ⓨ Ⓝ
Tester placed in proper position	**Test 1**	**Test 2**	**Test 3**
Stands to the side of the athlete	Ⓨ Ⓝ	Ⓨ Ⓝ	Ⓨ Ⓝ
Places the stethoscope properly into his or her ears	Ⓨ Ⓝ	Ⓨ Ⓝ	Ⓨ Ⓝ
Tester performs test according to accepted guidelines	**Test 1**	**Test 2**	**Test 3**
Instructs the athlete to take a full, deep breath and let it out slowly (with each placement)	Ⓨ Ⓝ	Ⓨ Ⓝ	Ⓨ Ⓝ
Places the diaphragm of the stethoscope in the appropriate locations: Anterior thorax and posterior thorax	Ⓨ Ⓝ	Ⓨ Ⓝ	Ⓨ Ⓝ
Right Left			
1 1 Just below the clavicle—first intercostal space	Ⓨ Ⓝ	Ⓨ Ⓝ	Ⓨ Ⓝ
2 2 Medial—third intercostal space	Ⓨ Ⓝ	Ⓨ Ⓝ	Ⓨ Ⓝ
3 3 Lateral—third intercostal space	Ⓨ Ⓝ	Ⓨ Ⓝ	Ⓨ Ⓝ
4 4 Medial—fourth intercostal space	Ⓨ Ⓝ	Ⓨ Ⓝ	Ⓨ Ⓝ
5 5 Lateral—fourth intercostal space	Ⓨ Ⓝ	Ⓨ Ⓝ	Ⓨ Ⓝ
6 6 Mid-clavicular line of eference (eighth intercostal space)	Ⓨ Ⓝ	Ⓨ Ⓝ	Ⓨ Ⓝ
Assesses sounds at each location upon both inspiration and expiration	Ⓨ Ⓝ	Ⓨ Ⓝ	Ⓨ Ⓝ
Notes and records any findings	Ⓨ Ⓝ	Ⓨ Ⓝ	Ⓨ Ⓝ

The psychomotor skill was performed completely and in the appropriate order   0 1 2 3 4 5

The tester had control of the subject and the situation (showed confidence)   0 1 2 3 4 5

Method of performing the skill allowed the tester the ability to determine: severity, proper progression, and the *fit* in the overall picture (Oral)   0 1 2 3 4 5

In order for a grade of *minimum standard* to be given, the total must be ≥11   **TOTAL = _____**

```
  1    2    3    4    5    6    7    8    9    10   11   12   13   14   15
  |    |    |    |    |    |    |    |    |    |    |    |    |    |    |
```

Not Acceptable   **Meets**   **Exceeds**
                                        Minimum Standards   **Minimum Standards**

TEST ENVIRONMENTS

L: Laboratory/Classroom Testing
C: Clinical/Field Testing
P: Practicum Testing
A: Assessment/Mock Exam Testing
S: Self-Reporting

SKILL TEST INFORMATION

Positive Finding: Abnormal sounds
Involved Structure: Respiratory system
Special Considerations: May repeat having the athlete speak (whisper) "a"/"e" sounds
Reference(s): O'Connor
Supplies Needed: Stethoscope, pencil/paper

GENERAL MEDICAL
(GMED-Test 6)

Peer Review _____ Peer Review _____

Skill Acquisition: _____   Practice Opportunities: _____

*This problem allows you the opportunity to demonstrate the proper method for administering medicine through the use of an **asthma inhaler**. You have 2 minutes to complete this task.*

Tester places athlete limb in appropriate position	Test 1	Test 2	Test 3
Standing or seated	Ⓨ Ⓝ	Ⓨ Ⓝ	Ⓨ Ⓝ
Tester placed in proper position	**Test 1**	**Test 2**	**Test 3**
Stands in front of or to the side of the athlete	Ⓨ Ⓝ	Ⓨ Ⓝ	Ⓨ Ⓝ
Tester performs test according to accepted guidelines	**Test 1**	**Test 2**	**Test 3**
Shakes the inhaler (prior to the first puff)	Ⓨ Ⓝ	Ⓨ Ⓝ	Ⓨ Ⓝ
Attaches a 2- to 4-inch spacer to the inhaler (inhaler mouthpiece)	Ⓨ Ⓝ	Ⓨ Ⓝ	Ⓨ Ⓝ
Instructs the athlete to take a deep breath and exhale before placing the mouthpiece to the mouth	Ⓨ Ⓝ	Ⓨ Ⓝ	Ⓨ Ⓝ
Instructs the athlete to take slow, deep breaths (3 to 5 seconds) while administering the medication (sprays only one puff at a time)	Ⓨ Ⓝ	Ⓨ Ⓝ	Ⓨ Ⓝ
Instructs the athlete to hold the breath in for about 10 seconds	Ⓨ Ⓝ	Ⓨ Ⓝ	Ⓨ Ⓝ
Repeats (wait at least 30 seconds between puffs or longer depending on the medication)	Ⓨ Ⓝ	Ⓨ Ⓝ	Ⓨ Ⓝ

The psychomotor skill was performed completely and in the appropriate order   0 1 2 3 4 5

The tester had control of the subject and the situation (showed confidence)   0 1 2 3 4 5

Method of performing the skill allowed the tester the ability to determine: severity, proper progression, and the *fit* in the overall picture (Oral)   0 1 2 3 4 5

In order for a grade of *minimum standard* to be given, the total must be ≥11   **TOTAL = _____**

```
 1    2    3    4    5    6    7    8    9   10   11   12   13   14   15
 |    |    |    |    |    |    |    |    |    |    |    |    |    |    |
```

Not Acceptable   **Meets Minimum Standards**   **Exceeds Minimum Standards**

TEST ENVIRONMENTS

L: Laboratory/Classroom Testing
C: Clinical/Field Testing
P: Practicum Testing
A: Assessment/Mock Exam Testing
S: Self-Reporting

SKILL TEST INFORMATION

Positive Finding: N/A
Involved Structure: Respiratory system
Special Considerations: N/A
Reference(s): Goldman et al; *Physician's Desk Reference*
Supplies Needed: Empty inhaler, spacer

GENERAL MEDICAL
(GMED-Test 7)

Peer Review _____ Peer Review _____

Skill Acquisition: _____   Practice Opportunities: _____

In determining whether or not the vital signs of an athlete are normal, this problem allows you the opportunity to perform **respiration assessment**. *You have 2 minutes to complete this task.*

Tester places athlete in appropriate position	Test 1	Test 2	Test 3
Supine	Ⓨ Ⓝ	Ⓨ Ⓝ	Ⓨ Ⓝ
Tester placed in proper position	**Test 1**	**Test 2**	**Test 3**
Stands or kneels to the side of the athlete	Ⓨ Ⓝ	Ⓨ Ⓝ	Ⓨ Ⓝ
Positions to observe the rising and falling of the chest (look, listen, and/or feel)	Ⓨ Ⓝ	Ⓨ Ⓝ	Ⓨ Ⓝ
Tester performs test according to accepted guidelines	**Test 1**	**Test 2**	**Test 3**
Assesses rate of breath: Counts the number of breaths/minute (Note: 12 to 20)	Ⓨ Ⓝ	Ⓨ Ⓝ	Ⓨ Ⓝ
Assesses depth/character of breath (Note: Shallow, rapid, left/right side the same, etc)	Ⓨ Ⓝ	Ⓨ Ⓝ	Ⓨ Ⓝ
Assesses length of inspiration and expiration (Note: 1:1)	Ⓨ Ⓝ	Ⓨ Ⓝ	Ⓨ Ⓝ
Records and rechecks at regular intervals	Ⓨ Ⓝ	Ⓨ Ⓝ	Ⓨ Ⓝ

The psychomotor skill was performed completely and in the appropriate order   0   1   2   3   4   5

The tester had control of the subject and the situation (showed confidence)   0   1   2   3   4   5

Method of performing the skill allowed the tester the ability to determine:
severity, proper progression, and the *fit* in the overall picture (Oral)   0   1   2   3   4   5

In order for a grade of *minimum standard* to be given, the total must be ≥11   TOTAL = _____

```
  1    2    3    4    5    6    7    8    9    10   11   12   13   14   15
  |    |    |    |    |    |    |    |    |    |    |    |    |    |    |
```

Not Acceptable   **Meets**   **Exceeds**
                                         Minimum Standards   **Minimum Standards**

TEST ENVIRONMENTS

L: Laboratory/Classroom Testing
C: Clinical/Field Testing
P: Practicum Testing
A: Assessment/Mock Exam Testing
S: Self-Reporting

SKILL TEST INFORMATION

Positive Finding:	Improper rate and/or depth
Involved Structure:	Respiratory system
Special Considerations:	N/A
Reference(s):	O'Conner; Starkey et al (2002)
Supplies Needed:	Watch (with a second hand), paper/pencil

GENERAL MEDICAL
(GMED-Test 8)

Peer Review _____ Peer Review _____

Skill Acquisition: _____   Practice Opportunities: _____

This problem allows you the opportunity to demonstrate the proper method for administering a **peak flow meter** *on an athlete suspected of exercise-induced asthma. You have 2 minutes to complete this task.*

Tester places athlete in appropriate position	Test 1	Test 2	Test 3
Standing	Ⓨ Ⓝ	Ⓨ Ⓝ	Ⓨ Ⓝ
Tester placed in proper position	**Test 1**	**Test 2**	**Test 3**
Stands in front of the athlete	Ⓨ Ⓝ	Ⓨ Ⓝ	Ⓨ Ⓝ
Tester performs test according to accepted guidelines	**Test 1**	**Test 2**	**Test 3**
Instructs the athlete to take a deep breath	Ⓨ Ⓝ	Ⓨ Ⓝ	Ⓨ Ⓝ
Instructs the athlete to place the mouthpiece of the peak flow meter into his or her mouth	Ⓨ Ⓝ	Ⓨ Ⓝ	Ⓨ Ⓝ
Instructs the athlete to blow as hard and fast as possible into the peak flow meter	Ⓨ Ⓝ	Ⓨ Ⓝ	Ⓨ Ⓝ
Repeats steps	Ⓨ Ⓝ	Ⓨ Ⓝ	Ⓨ Ⓝ

The psychomotor skill was performed completely and in the appropriate order   **0 1 2 3 4 5**

The tester had control of the subject and the situation (showed confidence)   **0 1 2 3 4 5**

Method of performing the skill allowed the tester the ability to determine:
severity, proper progression, and the *fit* in the overall picture (Oral)   **0 1 2 3 4 5**

In order for a grade of *minimum standard* to be given, the total must be ≥11   **TOTAL = _____**

1	*2*	*3*	*4*	*5*	*6*	*7*	*8*	*9*	*10*	*11*	*12*	*13*	*14*	*15*

Not Acceptable   **Meets**   **Exceeds**
                          Minimum Standards   **Minimum Standards**

TEST ENVIRONMENTS

L: Laboratory/Classroom Testing
C: Clinical/Field Testing
P: Practicum Testing
A: Assessment/Mock Exam Testing
S: Self-Reporting

SKILL TEST INFORMATION

Positive Finding: Air not moving out of the lungs
Involved Structure: Respiratory system
Special Considerations: Do not allow the tongue to impede air flow
Reference(s): Starkey et al (2002)
Supplies Needed: Peak flow meter, mouthpiece

GENERAL MEDICAL
(GMED-Test 9)

Peer Review _____ Peer Review _____

Skill Acquisition: _____   Practice Opportunities: _____

This problem allows you the opportunity to inspect the ear canal and ear drum of an athlete by using an **otoscope**. *You have 2 minutes to complete this task.*

Tester places athlete in appropriate position	Test 1	Test 2	Test 3
Seated	Ⓨ Ⓝ	Ⓨ Ⓝ	Ⓨ Ⓝ
Position the athlete's head so that the tester can see comfortably through the otoscope	Ⓨ Ⓝ	Ⓨ Ⓝ	Ⓨ Ⓝ
Tester placed in proper position	**Test 1**	**Test 2**	**Test 3**
Stands or sits to the side of the athlete	Ⓨ Ⓝ	Ⓨ Ⓝ	Ⓨ Ⓝ
Grasps the auricle and pulls in an upward/backward direction	Ⓨ Ⓝ	Ⓨ Ⓝ	Ⓨ Ⓝ
Tester performs test according to accepted guidelines	**Test 1**	**Test 2**	**Test 3**
Turns on the light	Ⓨ Ⓝ	Ⓨ Ⓝ	Ⓨ Ⓝ
Holds the otoscope properly. (Note: Hand rests against the athlete's face)	Ⓨ Ⓝ	Ⓨ Ⓝ	Ⓨ Ⓝ
Inserts the otoscope (speculum) gently into the ear canal	Ⓨ Ⓝ	Ⓨ Ⓝ	Ⓨ Ⓝ
(Note: Uses the largest ear speculum that fits into the canal)			
Turns on the light	Ⓨ Ⓝ	Ⓨ Ⓝ	Ⓨ Ⓝ
Gently moves the speculum in multiple directions	Ⓨ Ⓝ	Ⓨ Ⓝ	Ⓨ Ⓝ

The psychomotor skill was performed completely and in the appropriate order   0 1 2 3 4 5

The tester had control of the subject and the situation (showed confidence)   0 1 2 3 4 5

Method of performing the skill allowed the tester the ability to determine:
severity, proper progression, and the *fit* in the overall picture (Oral)   0 1 2 3 4 5

In order for a grade of *minimum standard* to be given, the total must be ≥11   TOTAL = _____

```
   1    2    3    4    5    6    7    8    9   10   11   12   13   14   15
   |____|____|____|____|____|____|____|____|____|____|____|____|____|____|
```

Not Acceptable   Meets   Exceeds
                                            Minimum Standards   Minimum Standards

TEST ENVIRONMENTS

L: Laboratory/Classroom Testing
C: Clinical/Field Testing
P: Practicum Testing
A: Assessment/Mock Exam Testing
S: Self-Reporting

SKILL TEST INFORMATION

Positive Finding:	Abnormal structures and/or redness
Involved Structure:	Ear drum/canal
Special Considerations:	N/A
Reference(s):	Bickley et al
Supplies Needed:	Otoscope, chair

GENERAL MEDICAL
(GMED-Test 10)

Peer Review _____ Peer Review _____

Skill Acquisition: _____ Practice Opportunities: _____

*This problem allows you the opportunity to check the core temperature of an athlete using a **tympanic thermometer.** You have 2 minutes to complete this task.*

Tester places athlete in appropriate position	Test 1	Test 2	Test 3
Seated	Y N	Y N	Y N
Tester placed in proper position	**Test 1**	**Test 2**	**Test 3**
Stands to the side of the athlete	Y N	Y N	Y N
Tester performs test according to accepted guidelines	**Test 1**	**Test 2**	**Test 3**
Inserts the thermometer in the ear canal	Y N	Y N	Y N
Holds the thermometer in this position for about 3 seconds (until the digital reading appears)	Y N	Y N	Y N
Accurately reads and records the temperature	Y N	Y N	Y N

The psychomotor skill was performed completely and in the appropriate order   **0 1 2 3 4 5**

The tester had control of the subject and the situation (showed confidence)   **0 1 2 3 4 5**

Method of performing the skill allowed the tester the ability to determine:
severity, proper progression, and the *fit* in the overall picture (Oral)   **0 1 2 3 4 5**

In order for a grade of *minimum standard* to be given, the total must be ≥11   **TOTAL = _____**

1	2	3	4	5	6	7	8	9	10	11	12	13	14	15

Not Acceptable   **Meets**   **Exceeds**
                                    Minimum Standards   **Minimum Standards**

TEST ENVIRONMENTS

L: Laboratory/Classroom Testing
C: Clinical/Field Testing
P: Practicum Testing
A: Assessment/Mock Exam Testing
S: Self-Reporting

SKILL TEST INFORMATION

Positive Finding: Abnormal reading
Involved Structure: Body temperature
Special Considerations: Reading will be a little higher than using an oral thermometer (about 1.4° F higher)
Reference(s): Bickley et al
Supplies Needed: Tympanic thermometer, chair, pencil/paper

GENERAL MEDICAL
(GMED-Test 11)

Peer Review _____ Peer Review _____

Skill Acquisition: _____   Practice Opportunities: _____

*This problem allows you the opportunity to check the internal body temperature of an athlete using a **standard oral thermometer**. You have 2 minutes to complete this task.*

Tester places athlete in appropriate position	Test 1	Test 2	Test 3
Seated	Ⓨ Ⓝ	Ⓨ Ⓝ	Ⓨ Ⓝ
Tester placed in proper position	**Test 1**	**Test 2**	**Test 3**
Stands in front of the athlete	Ⓨ Ⓝ	Ⓨ Ⓝ	Ⓨ Ⓝ
Tester performs test according to accepted guidelines	**Test 1**	**Test 2**	**Test 3**
Sterilizes the thermometer	Ⓨ Ⓝ	Ⓨ Ⓝ	Ⓨ Ⓝ
Shakes the thermometer mercury down (Note: To about 96°F)	Ⓨ Ⓝ	Ⓨ Ⓝ	Ⓨ Ⓝ
Inserts the thermometer under the athlete's tongue	Ⓨ Ⓝ	Ⓨ Ⓝ	Ⓨ Ⓝ
Instructs the athlete to close both lips and hold the thermometer under the tongue	Ⓨ Ⓝ	Ⓨ Ⓝ	Ⓨ Ⓝ
Maintains this position for 3 minutes	Ⓨ Ⓝ	Ⓨ Ⓝ	Ⓨ Ⓝ
Removes the thermometer from the athlete's mouth	Ⓨ Ⓝ	Ⓨ Ⓝ	Ⓨ Ⓝ
Accurately reads and records the temperature	Ⓨ Ⓝ	Ⓨ Ⓝ	Ⓨ Ⓝ

The psychomotor skill was performed completely and in the appropriate order   **0 1 2 3 4 5**

The tester had control of the subject and the situation (showed confidence)   **0 1 2 3 4 5**

Method of performing the skill allowed the tester the ability to determine:
severity, proper progression, and the *fit* in the overall picture (Oral)   **0 1 2 3 4 5**

In order for a grade of *minimum standard* to be given, the total must be ≥11   **TOTAL = _____**

```
   1    2    3    4    5    6    7    8    9   10   11   12   13   14   15
   |____|____|____|____|____|____|____|____|____|____|____|____|____|____|
```

Not Acceptable   **Meets**   **Exceeds**
                                     Minimum Standards   **Minimum Standards**

TEST ENVIRONMENTS

L: Laboratory/Classroom Testing
C: Clinical/Field Testing
P: Practicum Testing
A: Assessment/Mock Exam Testing
S: Self-Reporting

SKILL TEST INFORMATION

Positive Finding:	Abnormal reading
Involved Structure:	Body temperature
Special Considerations:	N/A
Reference(s):	Bickley et al
Supplies Needed:	Glass oral thermometer, alcohol wipe, chair, paper/pencil

GENERAL MEDICAL
(GMED-Test 12)

Peer Review _____ Peer Review _____

Skill Acquisition: _____   Practice Opportunities: _____

This problem allows you the opportunity to inspect the posterior structures of the retinal surface of an athlete's eye by using an **ophthalmoscope**. *You have 3 minutes to complete this task.*

Tester places athlete in appropriate position	Test 1	Test 2	Test 3
Seated or standing	Ⓨ Ⓝ	Ⓨ Ⓝ	Ⓨ Ⓝ
Head placed in a neutral, upright position	Ⓨ Ⓝ	Ⓨ Ⓝ	Ⓨ Ⓝ

Tester placed in proper position	Test 1	Test 2	Test 3
Stands in front of the athlete	Ⓨ Ⓝ	Ⓨ Ⓝ	Ⓨ Ⓝ
Holds the ophthalmoscope in the right hand to evaluate the subject's right eye (switch left-to-left)	Ⓨ Ⓝ	Ⓨ Ⓝ	Ⓨ Ⓝ
Holds ophthalmoscope firmly under the medial aspect of the bony orbit (handle tilted laterally about 20 degrees)	Ⓨ Ⓝ	Ⓨ Ⓝ	Ⓨ Ⓝ

Tester performs test according to accepted guidelines	Test 1	Test 2	Test 3
Darkens the lights in the room	Ⓨ Ⓝ	Ⓨ Ⓝ	Ⓨ Ⓝ
Turns on the ophthalmoscope light (adjusts the light to a large, round beam of white light)	Ⓨ Ⓝ	Ⓨ Ⓝ	Ⓨ Ⓝ
Sets ophthalmoscope lens disk at 0 diopters (keeps index finger on lens disk in order to focus)	Ⓨ Ⓝ	Ⓨ Ⓝ	Ⓨ Ⓝ
Instructs the athlete to look over the tester's shoulder and gaze at a specific point on the wall	Ⓨ Ⓝ	Ⓨ Ⓝ	Ⓨ Ⓝ
Place hand on athlete's head/brow (stabilize head and provide the tester with a reference point)	Ⓨ Ⓝ	Ⓨ Ⓝ	Ⓨ Ⓝ
Positions the ophthalmoscope about 15 inches away from the athlete	Ⓨ Ⓝ	Ⓨ Ⓝ	Ⓨ Ⓝ
Shines the light on the pupil (focuses the light on the red reflex)	Ⓨ Ⓝ	Ⓨ Ⓝ	Ⓨ Ⓝ
Moves the ophthalmoscope slowly toward the eye (almost touching the lashes)	Ⓨ Ⓝ	Ⓨ Ⓝ	Ⓨ Ⓝ
Notes and records any findings	Ⓨ Ⓝ	Ⓨ Ⓝ	Ⓨ Ⓝ

The psychomotor skill was performed completely and in the appropriate order   **0 1 2 3 4 5**

The tester had control of the subject and the situation (showed confidence)   **0 1 2 3 4 5**

Method of performing the skill allowed the tester the ability to determine: severity, proper progression, and the *fit* in the overall picture (Oral)   **0 1 2 3 4 5**

In order for a grade of *minimum standard* to be given, the total must be ≥11   **TOTAL = _____**

1	2	3	4	5	6	7	8	9	10	11	12	13	14	15

Not Acceptable   **Meets**   **Exceeds**
                                     Minimum Standards   **Minimum Standards**

TEST ENVIRONMENTS

L: Laboratory/Classroom Testing
C: Clinical/Field Testing
P: Practicum Testing
A: Assessment/Mock Exam Testing
S: Self-Reporting

SKILL TEST INFORMATION

Positive Finding:	Abnormal structures/swelling
Involved Structure:	Eye
Special Considerations:	Do not dilate subject's pupils
Reference(s):	Bickley et al
Supplies Needed:	Ophthalmoscope, paper/pencil

GENERAL MEDICAL
(GMED-Test 13)

Peer Review _____   Peer Review _____

Skill Acquisition: _____   Practice Opportunities: _____

This problem allows you the opportunity to check the eyes for a normal reflex to light using the **Consensual Reaction Test (Pupillary Reflex Test)**. *You have 2 minutes to complete this task.*

Tester places athlete in appropriate position	Test 1	Test 2	Test 3
Standing or seated	Ⓨ Ⓝ	Ⓨ Ⓝ	Ⓨ Ⓝ

Tester placed in proper position	Test 1	Test 2	Test 3
Stands in front of the athlete	Ⓨ Ⓝ	Ⓨ Ⓝ	Ⓨ Ⓝ

Tester performs test according to accepted guidelines	Test 1	Test 2	Test 3
Instructs the athlete to keep both eyes open	Ⓨ Ⓝ	Ⓨ Ⓝ	Ⓨ Ⓝ
Shines the light into the pupil of one eye for about 1 second and observes for constriction of the opposite pupil	Ⓨ Ⓝ	Ⓨ Ⓝ	Ⓨ Ⓝ
Removes the light and observes for dilation of the opposite pupil	Ⓨ Ⓝ	Ⓨ Ⓝ	Ⓨ Ⓝ
Repeats above scenario using the other eye	Ⓨ Ⓝ	Ⓨ Ⓝ	Ⓨ Ⓝ

The psychomotor skill was performed completely and in the appropriate order   **0 1 2 3 4 5**

The tester had control of the subject and the situation (showed confidence)   **0 1 2 3 4 5**

Method of performing the skill allowed the tester the ability to determine: severity, proper progression, and the *fit* in the overall picture (Oral)   **0 1 2 3 4 5**

In order for a grade of *minimum standard* to be given, the total must be ≥11   **TOTAL = _____**

```
 1    2    3    4    5    6    7    8    9   10   11   12   13   14   15
 |----|----|----|----|----|----|----|----|----|----|----|----|----|----|
```

Not Acceptable   **Meets**   **Exceeds**
                                      Minimum Standards   **Minimum Standards**

TEST ENVIRONMENTS

L: Laboratory/Classroom Testing
C: Clinical/Field Testing
P: Practicum Testing
A: Assessment/Mock Exam Testing
S: Self-Reporting

SKILL TEST INFORMATION

Positive Finding: Inappropriate or no movement of the pupil
Involved Structure: Neurological
Special Considerations: Room should be darkened
Reference(s): Bickley et al
Supplies Needed: Penlight

GENERAL MEDICAL
(GMED-Test 14)

Peer Review _____   Peer Review _____

Skill Acquisition: _____   Practice Opportunities: _____

This problem allows you the opportunity to check the eyes for normal reaction to light (constriction/dilation) by using the **Pupillary Reaction Test**. *You have 2 minutes to complete this task.*

Tester places athlete in appropriate position	Test 1	Test 2	Test 3
Standing or seated	Ⓨ Ⓝ	Ⓨ Ⓝ	Ⓨ Ⓝ
Tester placed in proper position	**Test 1**	**Test 2**	**Test 3**
Stands in front of the athlete	Ⓨ Ⓝ	Ⓨ Ⓝ	Ⓨ Ⓝ
Tester performs test according to accepted guidelines	**Test 1**	**Test 2**	**Test 3**
Instructs athlete to cover one eye (may use hand or an eye patch/card)	Ⓨ Ⓝ	Ⓨ Ⓝ	Ⓨ Ⓝ
Instructs athlete to keep the uncovered eye open (Note: looking at a distant point)	Ⓨ Ⓝ	Ⓨ Ⓝ	Ⓨ Ⓝ
Shines the light from a penlight into the pupil of the open eye for about 1 second and observes for constriction of the eye	Ⓨ Ⓝ	Ⓨ Ⓝ	Ⓨ Ⓝ
Removes the light and checks for dilation of the pupil	Ⓨ Ⓝ	Ⓨ Ⓝ	Ⓨ Ⓝ

The psychomotor skill was performed completely and in the appropriate order   **0 1 2 3 4 5**

The tester had control of the subject and the situation (showed confidence)   **0 1 2 3 4 5**

Method of performing the skill allowed the tester the ability to determine:
severity, proper progression, and the *fit* in the overall picture (Oral)   **0 1 2 3 4 5**

In order for a grade of *minimum standard* to be given, the total must be ≥11   **TOTAL = _____**

```
 1    2    3    4    5    6    7    8    9   10   11   12   13   14   15
 |____|____|____|____|____|____|____|____|____|____|____|____|____|____|
```
Not Acceptable   **Meets**   **Exceeds**
                                              Minimum Standards   **Minimum Standards**

TEST ENVIRONMENTS

L: Laboratory/Classroom Testing
C: Clinical/Field Testing
P: Practicum Testing
A: Assessment/Mock Exam Testing
S: Self-Reporting

SKILL TEST INFORMATION

Positive Finding: Inappropriate or no movement of the pupil
Involved Structure: Iris
Special Considerations: Room should be darkened
Reference(s): Bickley et al; Starkey et al (2002);
Supplies Needed: Pen light, eye patch/card

GENERAL MEDICAL
(GMED-Test 15)

Peer Review _____   Peer Review _____

Skill Acquisition: _____   Practice Opportunities: _____

This problem allows you the opportunity to check the field of gaze for eye motility using the **Test for Eye Motility (Tracking)**. *You have 2 minutes to complete this task.*

Tester places athlete in appropriate position	Test 1	Test 2	Test 3
Standing or seated	Ⓨ Ⓝ	Ⓨ Ⓝ	Ⓨ Ⓝ
Tester placed in proper position	**Test 1**	**Test 2**	**Test 3**
Stands in front of the athlete	Ⓨ Ⓝ	Ⓨ Ⓝ	Ⓨ Ⓝ
Holds a pencil or index finger approximately 2 feet from the athlete's nose	Ⓨ Ⓝ	Ⓨ Ⓝ	Ⓨ Ⓝ
Tester performs test according to accepted guidelines	**Test 1**	**Test 2**	**Test 3**
Instructs the athlete to focus on the object (moving eyes only, not the head)	Ⓨ Ⓝ	Ⓨ Ⓝ	Ⓨ Ⓝ
Moves the object through the field of gaze—12-, 3-, 6-, 9-o'clock and 2-, 7-, 10-, 5-o'clock (Note: Smooth, symmetrical movement; equal distance traveled by both eyes)	Ⓨ Ⓝ	Ⓨ Ⓝ	Ⓨ Ⓝ

The psychomotor skill was performed completely and in the appropriate order   **0 1 2 3 4 5**

The tester had control of the subject and the situation (showed confidence)   **0 1 2 3 4 5**

Method of performing the skill allowed the tester the ability to determine: severity, proper progression, and the *fit* in the overall picture (Oral)   **0 1 2 3 4 5**

In order for a grade of *minimum standard* to be given, the total must be ≥11   **TOTAL = _____**

```
  1     2     3     4     5     6     7     8     9    10    11    12    13    14    15
  └─────┴─────┴─────┴─────┴─────┴─────┴─────┴─────┴─────┴─────┴─────┴─────┴─────┴─────┘
```

Not Acceptable   **Meets**   **Exceeds**
                                    Minimum Standards   **Minimum Standards**

TEST ENVIRONMENTS

L: Laboratory/Classroom Testing
C: Clinical/Field Testing
P: Practicum Testing
A: Assessment/Mock Exam Testing
S: Self-Reporting

SKILL TEST INFORMATION

Positive Finding: Asymmetrical movement
Involved Structure: Eye
Special Considerations: N/A
Reference(s): Starkey et al (2002)
Supplies Needed: Pencil/paper, pen light

GENERAL MEDICAL
(GMED-Test 16)

Peer Review _____ Peer Review _____

Skill Acquisition: _____   Practice Opportunities: _____

This problem allows you the opportunity to assess corrected visual acuity using a **Snellen eye chart**. *You have 2 minutes to complete this task.*

Tester places athlete in appropriate position	Test 1	Test 2	Test 3
Standing	Y N	Y N	Y N
Instructs the athlete to stand 20 feet away from the eye chart	Y N	Y N	Y N
Instructs the athlete to leave corrective eyewear (glasses/contacts) in place	Y N	Y N	Y N
Tester placed in proper position	**Test 1**	**Test 2**	**Test 3**
Stands in position to read the eye chart	Y N	Y N	Y N
Tester performs test according to accepted guidelines	**Test 1**	**Test 2**	**Test 3**
Instructs the athlete to cover one eye (may use hand or an eye patch/card)	Y N	Y N	Y N
Instructs the athlete to read each line (starting at the top)	Y N	Y N	Y N
Instructs the athlete to cover the other eye and read each line	Y N	Y N	Y N
Records the information	Y N	Y N	Y N

The psychomotor skill was performed completely and in the appropriate order   0 1 2 3 4 5

The tester had control of the subject and the situation (showed confidence)   0 1 2 3 4 5

Method of performing the skill allowed the tester the ability to determine:
severity, proper progression, and the *fit* in the overall picture (Oral)   0 1 2 3 4 5

In order for a grade of *minimum standard* to be given, the total must be ≥11   TOTAL = _____

```
  1    2    3    4    5    6    7    8    9   10   11   12   13   14   15
  |____|____|____|____|____|____|____|____|____|____|____|____|____|____|
```

Not Acceptable   **Meets**   **Exceeds**
                                    Minimum Standards   **Minimum Standards**

TEST ENVIRONMENTS

L: Laboratory/Classroom Testing
C: Clinical/Field Testing
P: Practicum Testing
A: Assessment/Mock Exam Testing
S: Self-Reporting

SKILL TEST INFORMATION

Positive Finding: Inability to read the appropriate letters
Involved Structure: Eye
Special Considerations: Area should be well-lit
Reference(s): Bickley et al; Hillman; Starkey et al (2002)
Supplies Needed: Snellen Eye Chart, 20-foot tape measure, pencil/paper

GENERAL MEDICAL
(GMED-Test 17)

Peer Review _____ Peer Review _____

Skill Acquisition: _____   Practice Opportunities: _____

This problem allows you the opportunity to administer a "clean catch" dipstick urinalysis in order to rule out hematuria. You have 2 minutes to complete this task.

Tester places athlete in appropriate position	Test 1	Test 2	Test 3
Gives instructions to the athlete	Ⓨ Ⓝ	Ⓨ Ⓝ	Ⓨ Ⓝ
Tester performs test according to accepted guidelines	**Test 1**	**Test 2**	**Test 3**
Instructs athlete to discard the initial flow of urine into the toilet bowl	Ⓨ Ⓝ	Ⓨ Ⓝ	Ⓨ Ⓝ
Delivers a "clean catch" specimen (mid-stream) into a specimen cup	Ⓨ Ⓝ	Ⓨ Ⓝ	Ⓨ Ⓝ
Collects about 2 oz of urine	Ⓨ Ⓝ	Ⓨ Ⓝ	Ⓨ Ⓝ
Immerses dipstick into the specimen cup for the recommended time (see manufacturer's recommendations)	Ⓨ Ⓝ	Ⓨ Ⓝ	Ⓨ Ⓝ
Records the results (matches the proper colors of the dipstick to the values provided by the manufacturer)	Ⓨ Ⓝ	Ⓨ Ⓝ	Ⓨ Ⓝ

The psychomotor skill was performed completely and in the appropriate order   0 1 2 3 4 5

The tester had control of the subject and the situation (showed confidence)   0 1 2 3 4 5

Method of performing the skill allowed the tester the ability to determine:
severity, proper progression, and the *fit* in the overall picture (Oral)   0 1 2 3 4 5

In order for a grade of *minimum standard* to be given, the total must be ≥11   TOTAL = _____

```
  1     2     3     4     5     6     7     8     9    10    11    12    13    14    15
  |_____|_____|_____|_____|_____|_____|_____|_____|_____|_____|_____|_____|_____|_____|
```

Not Acceptable   **Meets**   **Exceeds**
                                          Minimum Standards   **Minimum Standards**

TEST ENVIRONMENTS

L: Laboratory/Classroom Testing
C: Clinical/Field Testing
P: Practicum Testing
A: Assessment/Mock Exam Testing
S: Self-Reporting

SKILL TEST INFORMATION

Positive Finding: Results outside the norm
Involved Structure: N/A
Special Considerations: This test can be used to rule out protein, glucose, nitrite, ketones, and leucoytes in the urine.
Reference(s): Ferri; O'Conner; Starkey et al (2002); Tilkian et al
Supplies Needed: Clean specimen cup, dipstick, manufacturer's recommendations for time and interpretation

GENERAL MEDICAL
(GMED-Test 18)

Peer Review _____ Peer Review _____

Skill Acquisition: _____   Practice Opportunities: _____

*This problem allows you the opportunity to demonstrate the proper technique for administering a **"clean catch"** **dipstick urinalysis** in order to determine if the **specific gravity** and **pH** are within normal limits prior to the drug testing of an athlete. You have 2 minutes to complete this task.*

Tester places athlete in appropriate position	Test 1	Test 2	Test 3
Gives instructions to the athlete	Ⓨ Ⓝ	Ⓨ Ⓝ	Ⓨ Ⓝ
Tester performs test according to accepted guidelines	**Test 1**	**Test 2**	**Test 3**
Instructs athlete to discard the initial flow of urine into a toilet bowl	Ⓨ Ⓝ	Ⓨ Ⓝ	Ⓨ Ⓝ
Delivers a "clean catch" specimen (mid-stream) into a specimen cup	Ⓨ Ⓝ	Ⓨ Ⓝ	Ⓨ Ⓝ
Collects about 2 oz of urine	Ⓨ Ⓝ	Ⓨ Ⓝ	Ⓨ Ⓝ
Immerses dipstick into the specimen cup for the recommended time (see manufacturer's recommendations)	Ⓨ Ⓝ	Ⓨ Ⓝ	Ⓨ Ⓝ
Records the results (matches the proper colors of the dipstick to the values provided by the manufacturer)	Ⓨ Ⓝ	Ⓨ Ⓝ	Ⓨ Ⓝ

The psychomotor skill was performed completely and in the appropriate order   0 1 2 3 4 5

The tester had control of the subject and the situation (showed confidence)   0 1 2 3 4 5

Method of performing the skill allowed the tester the ability to determine: severity, proper progression, and the *fit* in the overall picture (Oral)   0 1 2 3 4 5

In order for a grade of *minimum standard* to be given, the total must be ≥11   **TOTAL =** _____

```
  1    2    3    4    5    6    7    8    9   10   11   12   13   14   15
  |____|____|____|____|____|____|____|____|____|____|____|____|____|____|
```

Not Acceptable   **Meets**   **Exceeds**
                                    Minimum Standards   **Minimum Standards**

TEST ENVIRONMENTS

L: Laboratory/Classroom Testing
C: Clinical/Field Testing
P: Practicum Testing
A: Assessment/Mock Exam Testing
S: Self-Reporting

SKILL TEST INFORMATION

Positive Finding: Results outside the norm
Involved Structure: N/A
Special Considerations: N/A
Reference(s): Ferri; O'Conner; Starkey et al (2002); Tilkian et al
Supplies Needed: Clean specimen cup, dipstick, manufacturer's recommendations for time and interpretation

GENERAL MEDICAL
(GMED-Test 19)

Peer Review _____ Peer Review _____

Skill Acquisition: _____   Practice Opportunities: _____

*This problem allows you the opportunity to demonstrate the proper technique for administering a **Fingerstick Blood Test (Fingerstick-Prick Test)** in order to determine if a 20-year old athlete's **hematocrit** level is within normal limits. You have 2 minutes to complete this task.*

Tester/Athlete Preparation	Test 1	Test 2	Test 3
Tester washes hands	Ⓨ Ⓝ	Ⓨ Ⓝ	Ⓨ Ⓝ
Tester uses surgical gloves	Ⓨ Ⓝ	Ⓨ Ⓝ	Ⓨ Ⓝ
Tester preps athlete by cleaning the area with an alcohol wipe	Ⓨ Ⓝ	Ⓨ Ⓝ	Ⓨ Ⓝ
Tester performs test according to accepted guidelines	**Test 1**	**Test 2**	**Test 3**
Performs a fingerstick using a lancet (wipe away the first drop of blood)	Ⓨ Ⓝ	Ⓨ Ⓝ	Ⓨ Ⓝ
Collects blood using small capillary tube	Ⓨ Ⓝ	Ⓨ Ⓝ	Ⓨ Ⓝ
Spins blood in a centrifuge	Ⓨ Ⓝ	Ⓨ Ⓝ	Ⓨ Ⓝ
Performs hematocrit reading (RBC falls to the bottom/WBC covers the RBC/liquid plasma rises to the top → the higher the RBC line the higher the hematocrit)	Ⓨ Ⓝ	Ⓨ Ⓝ	Ⓨ Ⓝ
Tester/Athlete Post Instructions	**Test 1**	**Test 2**	**Test 3**
Wipes off the involved areas (athlete/room)	Ⓨ Ⓝ	Ⓨ Ⓝ	Ⓨ Ⓝ
Assure adequate hemostasis at the fingerstick site	Ⓨ Ⓝ	Ⓨ Ⓝ	Ⓨ Ⓝ
Properly disposes of surgical gloves, lancet, gauze, and capillary tube	Ⓨ Ⓝ	Ⓨ Ⓝ	Ⓨ Ⓝ
Washes hands	Ⓨ Ⓝ	Ⓨ Ⓝ	Ⓨ Ⓝ
Records test results	Ⓨ Ⓝ	Ⓨ Ⓝ	Ⓨ Ⓝ

The psychomotor skill was performed completely and in the appropriate order   0 1 2 3 4 5

The tester had control of the subject and the situation (showed confidence)   0 1 2 3 4 5

Method of performing the skill allowed the tester the ability to determine:
severity, proper progression, and the *fit* in the overall picture (Oral)   0 1 2 3 4 5

In order for a grade of *minimum standard* to be given, the total must be ≥11   TOTAL = _____

1	2	3	4	5	6	7	8	9	10	11	12	13	14	15

Not Acceptable   **Meets**   **Exceeds**
                              Minimum Standards   **Minimum Standards**

SKILL TEST INFORMATION

Positive Finding:	Results outside the norm
Involved Structure:	Packed red blood cells
Special Considerations:	Male = 40% to 54%
	Female = 38% to 47%
Reference(s):	Manufacturer's guidelines; Tilkian et al
Supplies Needed:	Surgical gloves, alcohol pad, gauze, lancet, small capillary tube, centrifuge, biohazard waste container, bandage

TEST ENVIRONMENTS

L: Laboratory/Classroom Testing
C: Clinical/Field Testing
P: Practicum Testing
A: Assessment/Mock Exam Testing
S: Self-Reporting

GENERAL MEDICAL
(GMED-Test 20)

Peer Review _____ Peer Review _____

Skill Acquisition: _____   Practice Opportunities: _____

This problem allows you the opportunity to demonstrate the proper technique for administering a **Fingerstick Blood Test (Fingerstick-Prick Test)** *in order to determine the* **blood sugar level** *of an athlete with diabetes before practice. You have 2 minutes to complete this task.*

Tester/Athlete Preparation	Test 1	Test 2	Test 3
Tester washes hands	Ⓨ Ⓝ	Ⓨ Ⓝ	Ⓨ Ⓝ
Tester uses surgical gloves	Ⓨ Ⓝ	Ⓨ Ⓝ	Ⓨ Ⓝ
Tester preps the athlete by cleaning the area with an alcohol wipe	Ⓨ Ⓝ	Ⓨ Ⓝ	Ⓨ Ⓝ

Tester performs test according to accepted guidelines	Test 1	Test 2	Test 3
Performs a fingerstick using a lancet (wipes away the first drop of blood)	Ⓨ Ⓝ	Ⓨ Ⓝ	Ⓨ Ⓝ
Collects blood using a test stripInserts test strip into in glucose meter (see manufacturer's recommendations)	Ⓨ Ⓝ	Ⓨ Ⓝ	Ⓨ Ⓝ

Tester/Athlete Post Instructions	Test 1	Test 2	Test 3
Wipes off the involved areas (athlete/room)	Ⓨ Ⓝ	Ⓨ Ⓝ	Ⓨ Ⓝ
Assures adequate hemostasis at the fingerstick site	Ⓨ Ⓝ	Ⓨ Ⓝ	Ⓨ Ⓝ
Properly disposes of surgical gloves, lancet, gauze, and capillary tube	Ⓨ Ⓝ	Ⓨ Ⓝ	Ⓨ Ⓝ
Cleans glucose meter (as needed)	Ⓨ Ⓝ	Ⓨ Ⓝ	Ⓨ Ⓝ
Washes hands	Ⓨ Ⓝ	Ⓨ Ⓝ	Ⓨ Ⓝ
Records results	Ⓨ Ⓝ	Ⓨ Ⓝ	Ⓨ Ⓝ

The psychomotor skill was performed completely and in the appropriate order   **0 1 2 3 4 5**

The tester had control of the subject and the situation (showed confidence)   **0 1 2 3 4 5**

Method of performing the skill allowed the tester the ability to determine: severity, proper progression, and the *fit* in the overall picture (Oral)   **0 1 2 3 4 5**

In order for a grade of *minimum standard* to be given, the total must be ≥11   **TOTAL = _____**

1	2	3	4	5	6	7	8	9	10	11	12	13	14	15

Not Acceptable   **Meets Minimum Standards**   **Exceeds Minimum Standards**

TEST ENVIRONMENTS

L: Laboratory/Classroom Testing
C: Clinical/Field Testing
P: Practicum Testing
A: Assessment/Mock Exam Testing
S: Self-Reporting

SKILL TEST INFORMATION

Positive Finding: Results outside the norm
Purpose: Blood glucose (blood sugar)
Special Considerations Norm: 80 to 100 mg/dl
Mild Elevation: 120 to 130 mg/dl
Reference(s): Manufacturer's guidelines; Tilkian et al
Supplies Needed: Surgical gloves, alcohol pad, gauze, lancet, small capillary tube, centrifuge, biohazard waste container, bandage

GENERAL MEDICAL
(GMED-Test 21)

Peer Review _____ Peer Review _____

Skill Acquisition: _____   Practice Opportunities: _____

This task allows you the opportunity to demonstrate the assessment of **Romberg's Sign** *on an athlete. You have 2 minutes to complete this task.*

Tester places athlete in appropriate position	Test 1	Test 2	Test 3
Standing with feet together	Ⓨ Ⓝ	Ⓨ Ⓝ	Ⓨ Ⓝ
Tester performs test according to accepted guidelines	**Test 1**	**Test 2**	**Test 3**
Instructs athlete to close his or her eyes	Ⓨ Ⓝ	Ⓨ Ⓝ	Ⓨ Ⓝ
Stand ready to support/catch the athlete (if needed)	Ⓨ Ⓝ	Ⓨ Ⓝ	Ⓨ Ⓝ
Observes athlete's balance and behavior	Ⓨ Ⓝ	Ⓨ Ⓝ	Ⓨ Ⓝ

The psychomotor skill was performed completely and in the appropriate order   0 1 2 3 4 5

The tester had control of the subject and the situation (showed confidence)   0 1 2 3 4 5

Method of performing the skill allowed the tester the ability to determine:
severity, proper progression, and the *fit* in the overall picture (Oral)   0 1 2 3 4 5

In order for a grade of *minimum standard* to be given, the total must be ≥11   TOTAL = _____

```
 1    2    3    4    5    6    7    8    9   10   11   12   13   14   15
 |    |    |    |    |    |    |    |    |    |    |    |    |    |    |
```

Not Acceptable   **Meets**   **Exceeds**
                                     Minimum Standards   **Minimum Standards**

TEST ENVIRONMENTS

L: Laboratory/Classroom Testing
C: Clinical/Field Testing
P: Practicum Testing
A: Assessment/Mock Exam Testing
S: Self-Reporting

SKILL TEST INFORMATION

Positive Finding: Loss of balance, swaying, inability to keep eyes closed

Involved Structure: Head/brain

Special Considerations: May be repeated using single leg stance

Reference(s): Konin et al (2003); Prentice (2003)

Supplies Needed: N/A

GENERAL MEDICAL
(GMED-Test 22)

Peer Review _____ Peer Review _____

Skill Acquisition: _____   Practice Opportunities: _____

This problem allows you the opportunity to demonstrate wound care for a **forearm laceration** *of an athlete that is less then a ¼ inch deep. You have 3 minutes to complete this task.*

Tester places athlete and limb in appropriate position	Test 1	Test 2	Test 3
Uses latex gloves	Ⓨ Ⓝ	Ⓨ Ⓝ	Ⓨ Ⓝ
Avoids direct contact with blood and bodily fluids	Ⓨ Ⓝ	Ⓨ Ⓝ	Ⓨ Ⓝ
Tester evaluates injury and stops bleeding	**Test 1**	**Test 2**	**Test 3**
Checks laceration for foreign objects	Ⓨ Ⓝ	Ⓨ Ⓝ	Ⓨ Ⓝ
Applies direct pressure to control bleeding	Ⓨ Ⓝ	Ⓨ Ⓝ	Ⓨ Ⓝ
Elevates injured area above the heart until bleeding is controlled	Ⓨ Ⓝ	Ⓨ Ⓝ	Ⓨ Ⓝ
Checks sensation near and distal to injury site	Ⓨ Ⓝ	Ⓨ Ⓝ	Ⓨ Ⓝ
Tester treats wound according to accepted guidelines	**Test 1**	**Test 2**	**Test 3**
Cleans wound with antiseptic	Ⓨ Ⓝ	Ⓨ Ⓝ	Ⓨ Ⓝ
Applies antibiotic ointment	Ⓨ Ⓝ	Ⓨ Ⓝ	Ⓨ Ⓝ
Applies sterile dressing over the wound	Ⓨ Ⓝ	Ⓨ Ⓝ	Ⓨ Ⓝ
Secures dressing with bandage	Ⓨ Ⓝ	Ⓨ Ⓝ	Ⓨ Ⓝ
Disposes of biohazardous materials appropriately	Ⓨ Ⓝ	Ⓨ Ⓝ	Ⓨ Ⓝ
Cleans hands thoroughly (before and after)	Ⓨ Ⓝ	Ⓨ Ⓝ	Ⓨ Ⓝ

The psychomotor skill was performed completely and in the appropriate order   0 1 2 3 4 5

The tester had control of the subject and the situation (showed confidence)   0 1 2 3 4 5

Method of performing the skill allowed the tester the ability to determine:
severity, proper progression, and the *fit* in the overall picture (Oral)   0 1 2 3 4 5

In order for a grade of *minimum standard* to be given, the total must be ≥11   TOTAL = _____

```
   1    2    3    4    5    6    7    8    9    10   11   12   13   14   15
   |    |    |    |    |    |    |    |    |    |    |    |    |    |    |
```

Not Acceptable   **Meets**   **Exceeds**
                                   Minimum Standards   **Minimum Standards**

TEST ENVIRONMENTS

L: Laboratory/Classroom Testing
C: Clinical/Field Testing
P: Practicum Testing
A: Assessment/Mock Exam Testing
S: Self-Reporting

SKILL TEST INFORMATION

Positive Finding:	Wound care
Involved Structure:	Involved structure
Special Considerations:	N/A
Reference(s):	Prentice (2003)
Supplies Needed:	Latex gloves, sterile dressing, roller gauze, antibiotic ointment, antiseptic

GENERAL MEDICAL
(GMED-Test 23)

Peer Review _____ Peer Review _____

Skill Acquisition: _____   Practice Opportunities: _____

*This problem allows you the opportunity to demonstrate your **palpation skills**. You have to locate and mark each of the following eight anatomical landmarks (see table for dots). You have 15 seconds to find each landmark. Time begins immediately after the landmark is read to you.*

Tester locates the following landmarks	Test 1	Test 2	Test 3
Head of the fourth metatarsal	Y N	Y N	Y N
Lateral femoral condyle	Y N	Y N	Y N
Deltoid tuberosity of the humerus	Y N	Y N	Y N
Gerdy's tubercle	Y N	Y N	Y N
Thenar eminence	Y N	Y N	Y N
Anatomical snuffbox	Y N	Y N	Y N
Popliteal fossa	Y N	Y N	Y N
Head of the fibula	Y N	Y N	Y N

The psychomotor skill was performed completely and in the appropriate order   0 1 2 3 4 5

The tester had control of the subject and the situation (showed confidence)   0 1 2 3 4 5

Method of performing the skill allowed the tester the ability to determine:
severity, proper progression, and the *fit* in the overall picture (Oral)   0 1 2 3 4 5

In order for a grade of *minimum standard* to be given, the total must be ≥11   TOTAL = _____

```
 1     2     3     4     5     6     7     8     9    10    11    12    13    14    15
 |__|__|__|__|__|__|__|__|__|__|__|__|__|__|__|
```
Not Acceptable   Meets   Exceeds
                                          Minimum Standards   Minimum Standards

TEST ENVIRONMENTS

L: Laboratory/Classroom Testing
C: Clinical/Field Testing
P: Practicum Testing
A: Assessment/Mock Exam Testing
S: Self-Reporting

SKILL TEST INFORMATION

Findings: Correct marking
Reference(s): Any anatomy/evaluation book
Supplies Needed: Dots, table

GENERAL MEDICAL
(GMED-Test 24)

Peer Review _____ Peer Review _____

Skill Acquisition: _____   Practice Opportunities: _____

*This problem allows you the opportunity to demonstrate your **palpation skills**. You have to locate and mark each of the following eight anatomical landmarks (see table for dots). You have 15 seconds to find each landmark. Time begins immediately after the landmark is read to you.*

Tester locates the following landmarks	Test 1	Test 2	Test 3
Dorsal pedis artery (pulse)	Y N	Y N	Y N
Pes anserinus bursa	Y N	Y N	Y N
Acromion process	Y N	Y N	Y N
Greater trochanter	Y N	Y N	Y N
Head of the radius	Y N	Y N	Y N
Styloid process of the fifth metatarsal	Y N	Y N	Y N
Proximal attachment of pronator teres	Y N	Y N	Y N
Anterior talofibular ligament	Y N	Y N	Y N

The psychomotor skill was performed completely and in the appropriate order   **0 1 2 3 4 5**

The tester had control of the subject and the situation (showed confidence)   **0 1 2 3 4 5**

Method of performing the skill allowed the tester the ability to determine:
severity, proper progression, and the *fit* in the overall picture (Oral)   **0 1 2 3 4 5**

In order for a grade of *minimum standard* to be given, the total must be ≥11   **TOTAL = _____**

```
  1    2    3    4    5    6    7    8    9   10   11   12   13   14   15
  |    |    |    |    |    |    |    |    |    |    |    |    |    |    |
```

Not Acceptable   **Meets**   **Exceeds**
                              Minimum Standards   **Minimum Standards**

TEST ENVIRONMENTS

L: Laboratory/Classroom Testing
C: Clinical/Field Testing
P: Practicum Testing
A: Assessment/Mock Exam Testing
S: Self-Reporting

SKILL TEST INFORMATION

Findings: Correct marking
Reference(s): Any anatomy/evaluation book
Supplies Needed: Dots, table

General Medical
(GMED-Test 25)

Peer Review _____ Peer Review _____

Skill Acquisition: _____   Practice Opportunities: _____

This problem allows you the opportunity to demonstrate your **palpation skills.** *You have to locate and mark each of the following eight anatomical landmarks (see table for dots). You have 15 seconds to find each landmark. Time begins immediately after the landmark is read to you.*

Tester locates the following landmarks	Test 1	Test 2	Test 3
Bicipital groove	Ⓨ Ⓝ	Ⓨ Ⓝ	Ⓨ Ⓝ
Inferior angle of the scapula	Ⓨ Ⓝ	Ⓨ Ⓝ	Ⓨ Ⓝ
Olecranon process	Ⓨ Ⓝ	Ⓨ Ⓝ	Ⓨ Ⓝ
Mastoid process	Ⓨ Ⓝ	Ⓨ Ⓝ	Ⓨ Ⓝ
Anterior superior illiac spine	Ⓨ Ⓝ	Ⓨ Ⓝ	Ⓨ Ⓝ
Capitate	Ⓨ Ⓝ	Ⓨ Ⓝ	Ⓨ Ⓝ
Xiphoid process	Ⓨ Ⓝ	Ⓨ Ⓝ	Ⓨ Ⓝ
Coracoid process	Ⓨ Ⓝ	Ⓨ Ⓝ	Ⓨ Ⓝ

The psychomotor skill was performed completely and in the appropriate order   0 1 2 3 4 5

The tester had control of the subject and the situation (showed confidence)   0 1 2 3 4 5

Method of performing the skill allowed the tester the ability to determine:
severity, proper progression, and the *fit* in the overall picture (Oral)   0 1 2 3 4 5

In order for a grade of *minimum standard* to be given, the total must be ≥11   TOTAL = _____

```
  1    2    3    4    5    6    7    8    9    10   11   12   13   14   15
  |    |    |    |    |    |    |    |    |    |    |    |    |    |    |
```

Not Acceptable   **Meets**   **Exceeds**
                                        Minimum Standards   **Minimum Standards**

TEST ENVIRONMENTS

L: Laboratory/Classroom Testing
C: Clinical/Field Testing
P: Practicum Testing
A: Assessment/Mock Exam Testing
S: Self-Reporting

SKILL TEST INFORMATION

Findings:	Correct marking
Reference(s):	Any anatomy/evaluation book
Supplies Needed:	Dots, table

THERAPEUTIC EXERCISES/ RECONDITIONING

THERAPEUTIC EXERCISES/RECONDITIONING
(TE-U-Test 1)

Peer Review _____ Peer Review _____

Skill Acquisition: _____   Practice Opportunities: _____

This problem allows you the opportunity to demonstrate the proper technique for performing a **supraspinatus strengthening exercise** *in the* **"empty can" position.** *While performing this isotonic exercise, instruct the athlete to complete one set of five repetitions using a 5-pound cuff weight. You have 2 minutes to complete this task.*

Tester places athlete in appropriate position	Test 1	Test 2	Test 3
Standing	Y N	Y N	Y N
Elbow placed in 0 degrees of extension	Y N	Y N	Y N
Shoulder internally rotated (thumb pointed downward)	Y N	Y N	Y N
Shoulder horizontally adducted midway between the sagittal and frontal planes	Y N	Y N	Y N
Secure cuff weight to distal ulna/radius	Y N	Y N	Y N
Tester performs test according to accepted guidelines	**Test 1**	**Test 2**	**Test 3**
Athlete moves the limb through the plane of the Scapula (approximately 30 to 45 degrees horizontal adduction)	Y N	Y N	Y N
Athlete slowly raises the involved limb parallel to the floor (may go higher-if pain free)	Y N	Y N	Y N
Athlete slowly lowers the involved limb back to the starting position	Y N	Y N	Y N
Repeat (4 times)	Y N	Y N	Y N

The psychomotor skill was performed completely and in the appropriate order   0 1 2 3 4 5

The tester had control of the subject and the situation (showed confidence)   0 1 2 3 4 5

Method of performing the skill allowed the tester the ability to determine:
severity, proper progression, and the *fit* in the overall picture (Oral)   0 1 2 3 4 5

In order for a grade of *minimum standard* to be given, the total must be ≥11   TOTAL = _____

```
  1    2    3    4    5    6    7    8    9   10   11   12   13   14   15
  |----|----|----|----|----|----|----|----|----|----|----|----|----|----|
```

Not Acceptable   **Meets**   **Exceeds**
                                    Minimum Standards   **Minimum Standards**

TEST ENVIRONMENTS

L: Laboratory/Classroom Testing
C: Clinical/Field Testing
P: Practicum Testing
A: Assessment/Mock Exam Testing
S: Self-Reporting

SKILL TEST INFORMATION

Purpose: Strength development
Involved Structure: Supraspinatus
Special Considerations: N/A
Reference(s): Prentice (2004); Wilk et al
Supplies Needed: 5-lb cuff weight

THERAPEUTIC EXERCISES/RECONDITIONING
(TE-U-Test 2)

Peer Review _____ Peer Review _____

Skill Acquisition: _____   Practice Opportunities: _____

This problem allows you the opportunity to demonstrate the proper technique for performing **pendulum exercise (Codman's circumduction exercise)** *to create a slight distraction force to improve general motion of the glenohumeral joint. Instruct the athlete to perform the exercise in multiple directions. You have 2 minutes to complete this task.*

Tester places athlete in appropriate position	Test 1	Test 2	Test 3
Standing	Ⓨ Ⓝ	Ⓨ Ⓝ	Ⓨ Ⓝ
Lean over the table; supporting the upper body with the uninvolved armInvolved limb hangs straight down over the edge of the table	Ⓨ Ⓝ	Ⓨ Ⓝ	Ⓨ Ⓝ
Secure cuff weight to distal ulna/radius (do not hold the weight)	Ⓨ Ⓝ	Ⓨ Ⓝ	Ⓨ Ⓝ

Tester performs test according to accepted guidelines	Test 1	Test 2	Test 3
Maintains relaxation of the shoulder & scapula region throughout the exercise	Ⓨ Ⓝ	Ⓨ Ⓝ	Ⓨ Ⓝ
Gently swings the arm (movement starts at the hips, not the shoulder)			
Clockwise circles and counterclockwise circles	Ⓨ Ⓝ	Ⓨ Ⓝ	Ⓨ Ⓝ
Clockwise figure-8s and counterclockwise figure-8s	Ⓨ Ⓝ	Ⓨ Ⓝ	Ⓨ Ⓝ
Forward and backward (sagittal plane)	Ⓨ Ⓝ	Ⓨ Ⓝ	Ⓨ Ⓝ
Side-to-side (transverse plane)	Ⓨ Ⓝ	Ⓨ Ⓝ	Ⓨ Ⓝ

The psychomotor skill was performed completely and in the appropriate order   0 1 2 3 4 5

The tester had control of the subject and the situation (showed confidence)   0 1 2 3 4 5

Method of performing the skill allowed the tester the ability to determine: severity, proper progression, and the *fit* in the overall picture (Oral)   0 1 2 3 4 5

In order for a grade of *minimum standard* to be given, the total must be ≥11   **TOTAL =** _____

```
  1    2    3    4    5    6    7    8    9   10   11   12   13   14   15
  |    |    |    |    |    |    |    |    |    |    |    |    |    |    |
```
Not Acceptable   **Meets**   **Exceeds**
                                      Minimum Standards   **Minimum Standards**

TEST ENVIRONMENTS

L: Laboratory/Classroom Testing
C: Clinical/Field Testing
P: Practicum Testing
A: Assessment/Mock Exam Testing
S: Self-Reporting

SKILL TEST INFORMATION

Purpose: Increase motion to the glenohumeral joint; create a slight distraction force to the glenohumeral joint

Involved Structure: Glenohumeral joint

Special Considerations Greater distraction may be created by increasing the weight

Reference(s): Houglum; Prentice (2004); Wilk et al

Supplies Needed: Table; 5-lb cuff weight

THERAPEUTIC EXERCISES/RECONDITIONING
(TE-U-Test 3)

Peer Review _____   Peer Review _____

Skill Acquisition: _____   Practice Opportunities: _____

This problem allows you the opportunity to demonstrate the proper technique for performing a **reverse fly** **(prone fly/prone horizontal abduction)** *to help develop the muscle strength of the supraspinatus and the posterior deltoid. While performing this isotonic exercise, instruct the athlete to complete one set of five repetitions using a 5-pound dumbbell weight. You have 2 minutes to complete this task.*

Tester places athlete in appropriate position	Test 1	Test 2	Test 3
Prone	Ⓨ Ⓝ	Ⓨ Ⓝ	Ⓨ Ⓝ
Have athlete tightly grasp a 5-pound dumbbell	Ⓨ Ⓝ	Ⓨ Ⓝ	Ⓨ Ⓝ
Involved arm hanging off the table	Ⓨ Ⓝ	Ⓨ Ⓝ	Ⓨ Ⓝ
Shoulder placed in 100 degrees of abduction	Ⓨ Ⓝ	Ⓨ Ⓝ	Ⓨ Ⓝ
Shoulder externally rotated (thumb up)	Ⓨ Ⓝ	Ⓨ Ⓝ	Ⓨ Ⓝ

Tester performs test according to accepted guidelines	Test 1	Test 2	Test 3
Athlete horizontally abducts (horizontal extension)	Ⓨ Ⓝ	Ⓨ Ⓝ	Ⓨ Ⓝ
Athlete slowly raises the involved limb until parallel with the floor (may go higher if pain-free)	Ⓨ Ⓝ	Ⓨ Ⓝ	Ⓨ Ⓝ
Athlete slowly lowers the involved limb back to the starting position	Ⓨ Ⓝ	Ⓨ Ⓝ	Ⓨ Ⓝ
Repeat (4 times)	Ⓨ Ⓝ	Ⓨ Ⓝ	Ⓨ Ⓝ

The psychomotor skill was performed completely and in the appropriate order   **0 1 2 3 4 5**

The tester had control of the subject and the situation (showed confidence)   **0 1 2 3 4 5**

Method of performing the skill allowed the tester the ability to determine: severity, proper progression, and the *fit* in the overall picture (Oral)   **0 1 2 3 4 5**

In order for a grade of *minimum standard* to be given, the total must be ≥11   **TOTAL = _____**

1	*2*	*3*	*4*	*5*	*6*	*7*	*8*	*9*	*10*	*11*	*12*	*13*	*14*	*15*

Not Acceptable   **Meets**   **Exceeds**
                          Minimum Standards   **Minimum Standards**

TEST ENVIRONMENTS	**SKILL TEST INFORMATION**

TEST ENVIRONMENTS

L: Laboratory/Classroom Testing
C: Clinical/Field Testing
P: Practicum Testing
A: Assessment/Mock Exam Testing
S: Self-Reporting

SKILL TEST INFORMATION

Purpose: Strength development
Involved Structure: Supraspinatus posterior deltoid
Special Considerations: N/A
Reference(s): Prentice (2004), Wilk et al
Supplies Needed: Table, 5-lb dumbbell weight

THERAPEUTIC EXERCISES/RECONDITIONING
(TE-U-Test 4)

Peer Review _____ Peer Review _____

Skill Acquisition: _____   Practice Opportunities: _____

This problem allows you the opportunity to demonstrate the proper technique for performing a **concentric manual-resistance exercise** *to help develop the muscle strength of the* **rhomboid and inferior trapezius** *muscles. You have 2 minutes to complete this task.*

Tester places athlete in appropriate position	Test 1	Test 2	Test 3
Prone	Ⓨ Ⓝ	Ⓨ Ⓝ	Ⓨ Ⓝ
Involved limb placed behind the back	Ⓨ Ⓝ	Ⓨ Ⓝ	Ⓨ Ⓝ
Elbow of involved limb placed in approximately 90° of flexion (resting on the athletes back)	Ⓨ Ⓝ	Ⓨ Ⓝ	Ⓨ Ⓝ
Tester places one hand on the athlete's elbow	Ⓨ Ⓝ	Ⓨ Ⓝ	Ⓨ Ⓝ
Tester performs test according to accepted guidelines	**Test 1**	**Test 2**	**Test 3**
Athlete contracts the rhomboids against manual resistance at the elbow	Ⓨ Ⓝ	Ⓨ Ⓝ	Ⓨ Ⓝ
Applies manual resistance at the elbow through the full range of motion (bringing the arm upward away from the back)	Ⓨ Ⓝ	Ⓨ Ⓝ	Ⓨ Ⓝ
Athlete relaxes the involved limb, allowing it to move back into the starting position	Ⓨ Ⓝ	Ⓨ Ⓝ	Ⓨ Ⓝ

The psychomotor skill was performed completely and in the appropriate order   **0 1 2 3 4 5**

The tester had control of the subject and the situation (showed confidence)   **0 1 2 3 4 5**

Method of performing the skill allowed the tester the ability to determine: severity, proper progression, and the *fit* in the overall picture (Oral)   **0 1 2 3 4 5**

In order for a grade of *minimum standard* to be given, the total must be ≥11   **TOTAL = _____**

```
 1    2    3    4    5    6    7    8    9   10   11   12   13   14   15
 |    |    |    |    |    |    |    |    |    |    |    |    |    |    |
```

Not Acceptable   **Meets Minimum Standards**   **Exceeds Minimum Standards**

TEST ENVIRONMENTS

L: Laboratory/Classroom Testing
C: Clinical/Field Testing
P: Practicum Testing
A: Assessment/Mock Exam Testing
S: Self-Reporting

SKILL TEST INFORMATION

Purpose: Strength development
Involved Structure: Rhomboids; inferior trapezius
Special Considerations: N/A
Reference(s): Prentice (2004)
Supplies Needed: Table

THERAPEUTIC EXERCISES/RECONDITIONING
(TE-U-Test 5)

Peer Review _____ Peer Review _____

Skill Acquisition: _____   Practice Opportunities: _____

This problem allows you the opportunity to demonstrate the proper technique for performing a **tabletop push-up plus (with a punch)** *to help strengthen the serratus anterior muscle. While performing this isotonic exercise, instruct the athlete to complete one set of five repetitions. You have 2 minutes to complete this task.*

Tester places athlete in appropriate position	Test 1	Test 2	Test 3
Standing (feet flat on the floor; upper body leaning forward with both hands resting on the table)	Ⓨ Ⓝ	Ⓨ Ⓝ	Ⓨ Ⓝ
Elbow of the involved limb is flexed, allowing the athlete to be in an inclined push-up position	Ⓨ Ⓝ	Ⓨ Ⓝ	Ⓨ Ⓝ

Tester performs test according to accepted guidelines	Test 1	Test 2	Test 3
Athlete pushes the upper body upward, away from the hands	Ⓨ Ⓝ	Ⓨ Ⓝ	Ⓨ Ⓝ
Athlete continues to contract through the range of motion (typical push-up)	Ⓨ Ⓝ	Ⓨ Ⓝ	Ⓨ Ⓝ
Once the athlete has reached the normal end-feel, an additional push (punch) is performed, causing scapular protraction	Ⓨ Ⓝ	Ⓨ Ⓝ	Ⓨ Ⓝ
Athlete slowly lowers the upper body to the starting position	Ⓨ Ⓝ	Ⓨ Ⓝ	Ⓨ Ⓝ
Repeat (4 times)	Ⓨ Ⓝ	Ⓨ Ⓝ	Ⓨ Ⓝ

The psychomotor skill was performed completely and in the appropriate order   0 1 2 3 4 5

The tester had control of the subject and the situation (showed confidence)   0 1 2 3 4 5

Method of performing the skill allowed the tester the ability to determine:
severity, proper progression, and the *fit* in the overall picture (Oral)   0 1 2 3 4 5

In order for a grade of *minimum standard* to be given, the total must be ≥11   TOTAL = _____

```
 1    2    3    4    5    6    7    8    9   10   11   12   13   14   15
 |____|____|____|____|____|____|____|____|____|____|____|____|____|____|
```
Not Acceptable   **Meets**   **Exceeds**
                                         Minimum Standards   **Minimum Standards**

TEST ENVIRONMENTS

L: Laboratory/Classroom Testing
C: Clinical/Field Testing
P: Practicum Testing
A: Assessment/Mock Exam Testing
S: Self-Reporting

SKILL TEST INFORMATION

Purpose:	Strength development
Involved Structure:	Serratus anterior
Special Considerations	Exercise may be performed against a wall (decreases the amount of resistance on the working muscles)
Reference(s):	Adapted from Houglum; adapted from Prentice (2004)
Supplies Needed:	Table

THERAPEUTIC EXERCISES/RECONDITIONING
(TE-U-Test 6)

Peer Review _____ Peer Review _____

Skill Acquisition: _____   Practice Opportunities: _____

This problem allows you the opportunity to demonstrate the proper technique for performing a **pronation strengthening exercise.** *While performing this isotonic exercise, instruct the athlete to complete one set of five repetitions using light resistance surgical tubing. You have 2 minutes to complete this task.*

Tester places athlete in appropriate position	Test 1	Test 2	Test 3
Seated or standing	Y N	Y N	Y N
Elbow fully supinated	Y N	Y N	Y N
Elbow against athlete's side to stabilize the involved limb	Y N	Y N	Y N
Attach surgical tubing to a wall on the same side as the involved limb (parallel to the floor; inline with the elbow joint)	Y N	Y N	Y N
Have athlete tightly grasp the tubing (may want to use a tubing handle)	Y N	Y N	Y N
Position the body to allow for adequate tension on the tubing	Y N	Y N	Y N

Tester performs test according to accepted guidelines	Test 1	Test 2	Test 3
Athlete moves the limb through the transverse plane (full supination to full pronation)	Y N	Y N	Y N
Athlete slowly releases the tension of the surgical tubing, allowing the involved limb to move back into the starting position	Y N	Y N	Y N
Repeat (4 times)	Y N	Y N	Y N

The psychomotor skill was performed completely and in the appropriate order   **0 1 2 3 4 5**

The tester had control of the subject and the situation (showed confidence)   **0 1 2 3 4 5**

Method of performing the skill allowed the tester the ability to determine:
severity, proper progression, and the *fit* in the overall picture (Oral)   **0 1 2 3 4 5**

In order for a grade of *minimum standard* to be given, the total must be ≥11   **TOTAL = _____**

1   2   3   4   5   6   7   8   9   10   11   12   13   14   15

Not Acceptable   **Meets**   **Exceeds**
                              Minimum Standards   **Minimum Standards**

TEST ENVIRONMENTS

L: Laboratory/Classroom Testing
C: Clinical/Field Testing
P: Practicum Testing
A: Assessment/Mock Exam Testing
S: Self-Reporting

SKILL TEST INFORMATION

Purpose: Strength development
Involved Structure: Supraspinatus; posterior deltoid
Special Considerations: N/A
Reference(s): Prentice (2004); Wilk et al
Supplies Needed: Table, 5-lb dumbbell weight

THERAPEUTIC EXERCISES/RECONDITIONING
(TE-U-Test 7)

Peer Review _____ Peer Review _____

Skill Acquisition: _____   Practice Opportunities: _____

This problem allows you the opportunity to demonstrate the proper technique for performing a **supine elbow extension exercise** *to help strengthen the triceps muscle. While performing this isotonic exercise, instruct the athlete to complete one set of five repetitions using a 5-pound dumbbell. You have 2 minutes to complete this task.*

Tester places athlete in appropriate position	Test 1	Test 2	Test 3
Supine	Ⓨ Ⓝ	Ⓨ Ⓝ	Ⓨ Ⓝ
Have the athlete tightly grasp a 5-pound dumbbell	Ⓨ Ⓝ	Ⓨ Ⓝ	Ⓨ Ⓝ
Shoulder resting on the table; arm perpendicular to the floor (90 degrees of shoulder flexion)	Ⓨ Ⓝ	Ⓨ Ⓝ	Ⓨ Ⓝ
Elbow of the involved limb is fully flexed	Ⓨ Ⓝ	Ⓨ Ⓝ	Ⓨ Ⓝ
Tester performs test according to accepted guidelines	**Test 1**	**Test 2**	**Test 3**
Athlete extends the elbow	Ⓨ Ⓝ	Ⓨ Ⓝ	Ⓨ Ⓝ
Athlete slowly raises the involved limb until perpendicular to the floor	Ⓨ Ⓝ	Ⓨ Ⓝ	Ⓨ Ⓝ
Athlete slowly lowers the upper arm back to the starting position	Ⓨ Ⓝ	Ⓨ Ⓝ	Ⓨ Ⓝ
Repeat (4 times)	Ⓨ Ⓝ	Ⓨ Ⓝ	Ⓨ Ⓝ

The psychomotor skill was performed completely and in the appropriate order   **0 1 2 3 4 5**

The tester had control of the subject and the situation (showed confidence)   **0 1 2 3 4 5**

Method of performing the skill allowed the tester the ability to determine:
severity, proper progression, and the *fit* in the overall picture (Oral)   **0 1 2 3 4 5**

In order for a grade of *minimum standard* to be given, the total must be ≥11   **TOTAL = _____**

1	*2*	*3*	*4*	*5*	*6*	*7*	*8*	*9*	*10*	*11*	*12*	*13*	*14*	*15*

Not Acceptable   **Meets**   **Exceeds**
                                              Minimum Standards   **Minimum Standards**

TEST ENVIRONMENTS	**SKILL TEST INFORMATION**	
L: Laboratory/Classroom Testing	**Purpose:**	Strength development
C: Clinical/Field Testing	**Involved Structure:**	Triceps, anconeus
P: Practicum Testing	**Special Considerations:**	N/A
A: Assessment/Mock Exam Testing	**Reference(s):**	Houglum; Prentice (2004)
S: Self-Reporting	**Supplies Needed:**	Table, 5-lb dumbbell

THERAPEUTIC EXERCISES/RECONDITIONING
(TE-U-Test 8)

Peer Review _____ Peer Review _____

Skill Acquisition: _____   Practice Opportunities: _____

This problem allows you the opportunity to demonstrate the proper technique for performing a **radial deviation strengthening exercise** *with the wrist in neutral flexion and extension. While performing this isotonic exercise, instruct the athlete to complete one set of five repetitions using a 5-pound dumbbell. You have 2 minutes to complete this task.*

Tester places athlete in appropriate position	Test 1	Test 2	Test 3
Seated Have the athlete tightly grasp a 5-pound dumbbell	Ⓨ Ⓝ	Ⓨ Ⓝ	Ⓨ Ⓝ
Elbow/forearm supported by the table	Ⓨ Ⓝ	Ⓨ Ⓝ	Ⓨ Ⓝ
Elbow placed into a neutral position (thumb side pointing upward)	Ⓨ Ⓝ	Ⓨ Ⓝ	Ⓨ Ⓝ
Wrist placed in full ulnar deviation	Ⓨ Ⓝ	Ⓨ Ⓝ	Ⓨ Ⓝ
Tester performs test according to accepted guidelines	**Test 1**	**Test 2**	**Test 3**
Athlete moves the limb through the full range of motion (full ulnar deviation to full radial deviation)	Ⓨ Ⓝ	Ⓨ Ⓝ	Ⓨ Ⓝ
Athlete slowly lowers the hand/wrist to the starting position	Ⓨ Ⓝ	Ⓨ Ⓝ	Ⓨ Ⓝ
Repeat (4 times)	Ⓨ Ⓝ	Ⓨ Ⓝ	Ⓨ Ⓝ

The psychomotor skill was performed completely and in the appropriate order   0 1 2 3 4 5

The tester had control of the subject and the situation (showed confidence)   0 1 2 3 4 5

Method of performing the skill allowed the tester the ability to determine:
severity, proper progression, and the *fit* in the overall picture (Oral)   0 1 2 3 4 5

In order for a grade of *minimum standard* to be given, the total must be ≥11   TOTAL = _____

```
 1    2    3    4    5    6    7    8    9   10   11   12   13   14   15
 |    |    |    |    |    |    |    |    |    |    |    |    |    |    |
```
Not Acceptable   **Meets**   **Exceeds**
                                         Minimum Standards   **Minimum Standards**

TEST ENVIRONMENTS

L: Laboratory/Classroom Testing
C: Clinical/Field Testing
P: Practicum Testing
A: Assessment/Mock Exam Testing
S: Self-Reporting

SKILL TEST INFORMATION

Purpose:	Strength development
Involved Structure:	Flexor carpi radialis; extensor carpi radialis longus
Special Considerations:	N/A
Reference(s):	Prentice (2004)
Supplies Needed:	Chair, table, 5-lb dumbbell

THERAPEUTIC EXERCISES/RECONDITIONING
(TE-U-Test 9)

Peer Review _____ Peer Review _____

Skill Acquisition: _____   Practice Opportunities: _____

This problem allows you the opportunity to demonstrate the proper technique for performing an **eccentric manual-resistance** *exercise to help develop muscle strength for the* **wrist flexors**. *You have 2 minutes to complete this task.*

Tester places athlete in appropriate position	Test 1	Test 2	Test 3
Seated	Ⓨ Ⓝ	Ⓨ Ⓝ	Ⓨ Ⓝ
Wrist/lower arm hanging over the edge of the table	Ⓨ Ⓝ	Ⓨ Ⓝ	Ⓨ Ⓝ
Wrist placed in full flexion	Ⓨ Ⓝ	Ⓨ Ⓝ	Ⓨ Ⓝ
Tester places one hand on the palmer surface of the hand	Ⓨ Ⓝ	Ⓨ Ⓝ	Ⓨ Ⓝ
Tester places the other hand on the distal ulna/radius to stabilize the lower arm	Ⓨ Ⓝ	Ⓨ Ⓝ	Ⓨ Ⓝ

Tester performs test according to accepted guidelines	Test 1	Test 2	Test 3
Athlete holds an isometric contraction of the wrist flexors while the hand is in full flexion (resistance from tester is from anterior to posterior)	Ⓨ Ⓝ	Ⓨ Ⓝ	Ⓨ Ⓝ
Once the isometric contraction is maintained, the command of "Let Me Win" is given to the athlete	Ⓨ Ⓝ	Ⓨ Ⓝ	Ⓨ Ⓝ
Athlete continues to contract the wrist flexors; however, as resistance is applied by the tester, the wrist flexors gradually lengthen (moving from a flexed position to an extended position)	Ⓨ Ⓝ	Ⓨ Ⓝ	Ⓨ Ⓝ

The psychomotor skill was performed completely and in the appropriate order   **0 1 2 3 4 5**

The tester had control of the subject and the situation (showed confidence)   **0 1 2 3 4 5**

Method of performing the skill allowed the tester the ability to determine: severity, proper progression, and the *fit* in the overall picture (Oral)   **0 1 2 3 4 5**

In order for a grade of *minimum standard* to be given, the total must be ≥11   **TOTAL = _____**

1	2	3	4	5	6	7	8	9	10	11	12	13	14	15

Not Acceptable   **Meets Minimum Standards**   **Exceeds Minimum Standards**

TEST ENVIRONMENTS

L: Laboratory/Classroom Testing
C: Clinical/Field Testing
P: Practicum Testing
A: Assessment/Mock Exam Testing
S: Self-Reporting

SKILL TEST INFORMATION

Purpose: Strength development
Involved Structure: Flexor carpi radialis; flexor carpi ulnaris; palmaris longus
Special Considerations: N/A
Reference(s): Adapted from Dales et al
Supplies Needed: Table

THERAPEUTIC EXERCISES/RECONDITIONING
(TE-U-Test 10)

Peer Review _____ Peer Review _____

Skill Acquisition: _____   Practice Opportunities: _____

This problem allows you the opportunity to demonstrate the proper technique for performing an **aquatic therapy resistance exercise** *to help improve muscle strength of the* **biceps brachii** *muscle. Instruct the athlete to complete 1 set of 5 repetitions concentrating only on the elbow flexors (biceps brachii is the prime mover). You have 2 minutes to complete this task.*

Tester places athlete in appropriate position	Test 1	Test 2	Test 3
Standing or seated	Ⓨ Ⓝ	Ⓨ Ⓝ	Ⓨ Ⓝ
Webbed glove placed on the involved hand	Ⓨ Ⓝ	Ⓨ Ⓝ	Ⓨ Ⓝ
Upper arm, elbow and hand must be fully immersed in the water	Ⓨ Ⓝ	Ⓨ Ⓝ	Ⓨ Ⓝ
Involved limb actively moved into full extension	Ⓨ Ⓝ	Ⓨ Ⓝ	Ⓨ Ⓝ
Tester performs test according to accepted guidelines	**Test 1**	**Test 2**	**Test 3**
Athlete moves the lower arm into a flexed position as quickly as possible	Ⓨ Ⓝ	Ⓨ Ⓝ	Ⓨ Ⓝ
Athlete actively moves the arm back into an extended position	Ⓨ Ⓝ	Ⓨ Ⓝ	Ⓨ Ⓝ
Repeat (4 times)	Ⓨ Ⓝ	Ⓨ Ⓝ	Ⓨ Ⓝ

The psychomotor skill was performed completely and in the appropriate order   **0 1 2 3 4 5**

The tester had control of the subject and the situation (showed confidence)   **0 1 2 3 4 5**

Method of performing the skill allowed the tester the ability to determine:
severity, proper progression, and the *fit* in the overall picture (Oral)   **0 1 2 3 4 5**

In order for a grade of *minimum standard* to be given, the total must be ≥11   **TOTAL = _____**

```
  1     2     3     4     5     6     7     8     9    10    11    12    13    14    15
  |_____|_____|_____|_____|_____|_____|_____|_____|_____|_____|_____|_____|_____|_____|
```

Not Acceptable   **Meets**   **Exceeds**
                                   Minimum Standards   **Minimum Standards**

TEST ENVIRONMENTS

L: Laboratory/Classroom Testing
C: Clinical/Field Testing
P: Practicum Testing
A: Assessment/Mock Exam Testing
S: Self-Reporting

SKILL TEST INFORMATION

Purpose:	Strength development
Involved Structure:	Biceps brachii
Special Considerations:	N/A
Reference(s):	Adapted from Prentice (2004); Adapted from Thein-Nissenbaum
Supplies Needed:	Webbed glove

THERAPEUTIC EXERCISES/RECONDITIONING
(TE-U-Test 11)

Peer Review _____ Peer Review _____

Skill Acquisition: _____   Practice Opportunities: _____

Please demonstrate the **plyometric** *technique known at the* **medicine ball push-up**. *You have 2 minutes to complete this task.*

Tester places athlete and limb in appropriate position	Test 1	Test 2	Test 3
Prone on the floor	Ⓨ Ⓝ	Ⓨ Ⓝ	Ⓨ Ⓝ
Push-up position	Ⓨ Ⓝ	Ⓨ Ⓝ	Ⓨ Ⓝ
Hands on top of the medicine ball (elbows extended)	Ⓨ Ⓝ	Ⓨ Ⓝ	Ⓨ Ⓝ
Tester placed in proper position	**Test 1**	**Test 2**	**Test 3**
Standing (observation only)	Ⓨ Ⓝ	Ⓨ Ⓝ	Ⓨ Ⓝ
Tester performs task according to accepted guidelines	Ⓨ Ⓝ	Ⓨ Ⓝ	Ⓨ Ⓝ
Athlete: Drops the medicine ball (eccentric phase)	Ⓨ Ⓝ	Ⓨ Ⓝ	Ⓨ Ⓝ
Athlete: Completes the amortization phase (time between eccentric phase and concentric phase)	Ⓨ Ⓝ	Ⓨ Ⓝ	Ⓨ Ⓝ
Moving away from the floor and back to on top of the ball (concentric phase)	Ⓨ Ⓝ	Ⓨ Ⓝ	Ⓨ Ⓝ
Landing and bouncing on the ball	Ⓨ Ⓝ	Ⓨ Ⓝ	Ⓨ Ⓝ

The psychomotor skill was performed completely and in the appropriate order   0 1 2 3 4 5

The tester had control of the subject and the situation (showed confidence)   0 1 2 3 4 5

Method of performing the skill allowed the tester the ability to determine:
severity, proper progression, and the *fit* in the overall picture (Oral)   0 1 2 3 4 5

In order for a grade of *minimum standard* to be given, the total must be ≥11   TOTAL = _____

```
   1    2    3    4    5    6    7    8    9    10   11   12   13   14   15
   |    |    |    |    |    |    |    |    |    |    |    |    |    |    |
```
Not Acceptable   Meets   Exceeds
                                       Minimum Standards   Minimum Standards

TEST ENVIRONMENTS

L: Laboratory/Classroom Testing
C: Clinical/Field Testing
P: Practicum Testing
A: Assessment/Mock Exam Testing
S: Self-Reporting

SKILL TEST INFORMATION

Positive Finding: Power
Involved Structure: Anterior shoulder/triceps
Special Considerations: N/A
Reference(s): Baechle et al
Supplies Needed: Medicine ball

THERAPEUTIC EXERCISES/RECONDITIONING
(TE-L-Test 1)

Peer Review _____ Peer Review _____

Skill Acquisition: _____   Practice Opportunities: _____

This problem allows you the opportunity to demonstrate the proper technique for administering a **supine straight leg raise**, *incorporating a 5-pound cuff weight as fixed resistance. You have 2 minutes to complete this task.*

Tester places athlete and limb in appropriate position	Test 1	Test 2	Test 3
Supine	Y N	Y N	Y N
Hip/knee in anatomical position (heels on the table)	Y N	Y N	Y N
Attaches cuff weight securely to the involved limb	Y N	Y N	Y N

Tester performs test according to accepted guidelines	Test 1	Test 2	Test 3
Tightens involved quadriceps (hold)	Y N	Y N	Y N
Lifts involved limb off the table (6 to 8 inches)	Y N	Y N	Y N
Retightens involved quadriceps (hold)	Y N	Y N	Y N
Lowers involved limb slowly	Y N	Y N	Y N

The psychomotor skill was performed completely and in the appropriate order   **0 1 2 3 4 5**

The tester had control of the subject and the situation (showed confidence)   **0 1 2 3 4 5**

Method of performing the skill allowed the tester the ability to determine:
severity, proper progression, and the *fit* in the overall picture (Oral)   **0 1 2 3 4 5**

In order for a grade of *minimum standard* to be given, the total must be ≥11   **TOTAL = _____**

```
 1   2   3   4   5   6   7   8   9   10   11   12   13   14   15
 |   |   |   |   |   |   |   |   |   |    |    |    |    |    |
```

Not Acceptable   **Meets**   **Exceeds**
                          Minimum Standards   **Minimum Standards**

TEST ENVIRONMENTS

L: Laboratory/Classroom Testing
C: Clinical/Field Testing
P: Practicum Testing
A: Assessment/Mock Exam Testing
S: Self-Reporting

SKILL TEST INFORMATION

Purpose:	Muscle re-education
Involved Structure:	Quadriceps/hip flexors (iliopsoas)
Special Considerations:	Must have a good quad set
Reference(s):	Houglum; Prentice (2004)
Supplies Needed:	5-lb cuff weight, table

THERAPEUTIC EXERCISES/RECONDITIONING
(TE-L-Test 2)

Peer Review _____ Peer Review _____

Skill Acquisition: _____   Practice Opportunities: _____

This problem allows you the opportunity to demonstrate the proper technique for administering a **hip flexion exercise** *in a* **seated position**, *incorporating a 5-pound cuff weight as fixed resistance. The athlete is to avoid distraction of the knee joint. You have 2 minutes to complete this task.*

Tester places athlete and limb in appropriate position	Test 1	Test 2	Test 3
Seated	Y N	Y N	Y N
Knees flexed to approximately 90 degrees (hanging off the table)	Y N	Y N	Y N
Pelvis in neutral position (avoid anterior/posterior tilt)	Y N	Y N	Y N
Attaches cuff weight securely to distal thigh (just above the patella)	Y N	Y N	Y N

Tester performs test according to accepted guidelines	Test 1	Test 2	Test 3
Beginning position			
Athlete tightens quadriceps and hip flexors	Y N	Y N	Y N
Athlete maintains → good posture	Y N	Y N	Y N
Upward movement (concentric contraction)			
Athlete lifts involved limb toward chest so the thigh is 4 to 8 inches off table	Y N	Y N	Y N
Hold downward movement (eccentric contraction)	Y N	Y N	Y N
Athlete slowly lowers limb back to starting position	Y N	Y N	Y N

The psychomotor skill was performed completely and in the appropriate order   0 1 2 3 4 5

The tester had control of the subject and the situation (showed confidence)   0 1 2 3 4 5

Method of performing the skill allowed the tester the ability to determine:
severity, proper progression, and the *fit* in the overall picture (Oral)   0 1 2 3 4 5

In order for a grade of *minimum standard* to be given, the total must be ≥11   TOTAL = _____

```
1   2   3   4   5   6   7   8   9   10  11  12  13  14  15
```
Not Acceptable   **Meets**   **Exceeds**
                              Minimum Standards   **Minimum Standards**

TEST ENVIRONMENTS
L: Laboratory/Classroom Testing
C: Clinical/Field Testing
P: Practicum Testing
A: Assessment/Mock Exam Testing
S: Self-Reporting

SKILL TEST INFORMATION
Purpose: Strength development
Involved Structure: Quadriceps/hip flexors
Special Considerations: N/A
Reference(s): Prentice (2004)
Supplies Needed: 5-lb cuff weight, table or chair

THERAPEUTIC EXERCISES/RECONDITIONING
(TE-L-Test 3)

Peer Review _____ Peer Review _____

Skill Acquisition: _____   Practice Opportunities: _____

This problem allows you the opportunity to demonstrate the proper technique for administering a **hip adduction exercise** *using a 5-pound cuff weight. The athlete has no problems with the ankle or knee joints of the involved limb. You have 2 minutes to complete this task.*

Tester places athlete in appropriate position	Test 1	Test 2	Test 3
Side lying—involved side on the table	Ⓨ Ⓝ	Ⓨ Ⓝ	Ⓨ Ⓝ
Upper leg flexed at hip and knee, placing foot in front of bottom knee flat on the floor or with the upper leg supported by resting on the top of the chair	Ⓨ Ⓝ	Ⓨ Ⓝ	Ⓨ Ⓝ
Attaches cuff weight securely to distal tibia of the involved limb	Ⓨ Ⓝ	Ⓨ Ⓝ	Ⓨ Ⓝ
Tester performs test according to accepted guidelines	**Test 1**	**Test 2**	**Test 3**
Beginning position Athlete tightens hip adductors	Ⓨ Ⓝ	Ⓨ Ⓝ	Ⓨ Ⓝ
Upward movement (concentric contraction) Athlete slowly adducts bottom (involved) leg 6 to 10 inches off the floor or until the foot hits the supporting chair	Ⓨ Ⓝ	Ⓨ Ⓝ	Ⓨ Ⓝ
Hold	Ⓨ Ⓝ	Ⓨ Ⓝ	Ⓨ Ⓝ
Downward movement (eccentric contraction) Athlete slowly lowers the involved leg back to the starting position	Ⓨ Ⓝ	Ⓨ Ⓝ	Ⓨ Ⓝ

The psychomotor skill was performed completely and in the appropriate order   0 1 2 3 4 5

The tester had control of the subject and the situation (showed confidence)   0 1 2 3 4 5

Method of performing the skill allowed the tester the ability to determine:
severity, proper progression, and the *fit* in the overall picture (Oral)   0 1 2 3 4 5

In order for a grade of *minimum standard* to be given, the total must be ≥11   TOTAL = _____

```
 1    2    3    4    5    6    7    8    9   10   11   12   13   14   15
 |----|----|----|----|----|----|----|----|----|----|----|----|----|----|
```
Not Acceptable   **Meets**   **Exceeds**
                                     Minimum Standards   **Minimum Standards**

TEST ENVIRONMENTS

L: Laboratory/Classroom Testing
C: Clinical/Field Testing
P: Practicum Testing
A: Assessment/Mock Exam Testing
S: Self-Reporting

SKILL TEST INFORMATION

Purpose:	Strength development
Involved Structure:	Hip adductors (adductor magnus, brevis, longus)
Special Considerations:	N/A
Reference(s):	Houglum; Prentice (2004)
Supplies Needed:	5-lb cuff weight, table, chair

Therapeutic Exercises/Reconditioning
(TE-L-Test 4)

Peer Review _____ Peer Review _____

Skill Acquisition: _____   Practice Opportunities: _____

This problem allows you the opportunity to demonstrate the proper technique for administering a **straight leg hip extension exercise** *using a 5-pound cuff weight. The athlete has doctor restrictions to "avoid full extension/ prevent hyperextension of the tibiofemoral joint." You have 2 minutes to complete this task.*

Tester places athlete in appropriate position	Test 1	Test 2	Test 3
Prone	Ⓨ Ⓝ	Ⓨ Ⓝ	Ⓨ Ⓝ
Attaches cuff weight securely to distal femur of the involved limb	Ⓨ Ⓝ	Ⓨ Ⓝ	Ⓨ Ⓝ
Tester performs test according to accepted guidelines	**Test 1**	**Test 2**	**Test 3**
Beginning position			
Athlete tightens gluteus maximus and hamstrings	Ⓨ Ⓝ	Ⓨ Ⓝ	Ⓨ Ⓝ
Upward movement (concentric contraction)			
Athlete slowly extend the involved leg 6 to 10 inches off the table	Ⓨ Ⓝ	Ⓨ Ⓝ	Ⓨ Ⓝ
Athlete avoids hip and trunk rotation (movement within sagittal plane)	Ⓨ Ⓝ	Ⓨ Ⓝ	Ⓨ Ⓝ
Hold	Ⓨ Ⓝ	Ⓨ Ⓝ	Ⓨ Ⓝ
Downward movement (eccentric contraction)			
Athlete slowly lowers the involved leg back to the starting position	Ⓨ Ⓝ	Ⓨ Ⓝ	Ⓨ Ⓝ

The psychomotor skill was performed completely and in the appropriate order   0 1 2 3 4 5

The tester had control of the subject and the situation (showed confidence)   0 1 2 3 4 5

Method of performing the skill allowed the tester the ability to determine:
severity, proper progression, and the *fit* in the overall picture (Oral)   0 1 2 3 4 5

In order for a grade of *minimum standard* to be given, the total must be ≥11   TOTAL = _____

```
  1    2    3    4    5    6    7    8    9    10   11   12   13   14   15
  |    |    |    |    |    |    |    |    |    |    |    |    |    |    |
```
Not Acceptable   **Meets**   **Exceeds**
                                   Minimum Standards   **Minimum Standards**

TEST ENVIRONMENTS

L: Laboratory/Classroom Testing
C: Clinical/Field Testing
P: Practicum Testing
A: Assessment/Mock Exam Testing
S: Self-Reporting

SKILL TEST INFORMATION

Purpose:	Strength development
Involved Structure:	Gluteals and Hamstrings
Special Considerations	To isolate the gluteals, flex the knee
Reference(s):	Houglum, Prentice (2004)
Supplies Needed:	Table, 5-lb cuff weight

THERAPEUTIC EXERCISES/RECONDITIONING
(TE-L-Test 5)

Peer Review _____ Peer Review _____

Skill Acquisition: _____   Practice Opportunities: _____

*This problem allows you the opportunity to demonstrate the proper technique for administering a **standing leg curl** targeting the biceps femoris muscle using a 5-pound cuff weight. You have 2 minutes to complete this task.*

Tester places athlete in appropriate position	Test 1	Test 2	Test 3
Standing	Ⓨ Ⓝ	Ⓨ Ⓝ	Ⓨ Ⓝ
Attaches cuff weight securely to distal tibia of the involved limb	Ⓨ Ⓝ	Ⓨ Ⓝ	Ⓨ Ⓝ
Tester performs test according to accepted guidelines	**Test 1**	**Test 2**	**Test 3**
Beginning position			
Athlete tightens hamstrings	Ⓨ Ⓝ	Ⓨ Ⓝ	Ⓨ Ⓝ
Athlete actively rotates the tibia externally	Ⓨ Ⓝ	Ⓨ Ⓝ	Ⓨ Ⓝ
Upward movement (concentric contraction)			
Athlete slowly flexes the involved leg through a full range of motion	Ⓨ Ⓝ	Ⓨ Ⓝ	Ⓨ Ⓝ
Athlete avoids hip and trunk rotation (movement within sagittal plane)	Ⓨ Ⓝ	Ⓨ Ⓝ	Ⓨ Ⓝ
Hold	Ⓨ Ⓝ	Ⓨ Ⓝ	Ⓨ Ⓝ
Downward movement (eccentric contraction)			
Athlete slowly lowers the involved leg back to the starting position	Ⓨ Ⓝ	Ⓨ Ⓝ	Ⓨ Ⓝ

The psychomotor skill was performed completely and in the appropriate order   0   1   2   3   4   5

The tester had control of the subject and the situation (showed confidence)   0   1   2   3   4   5

Method of performing the skill allowed the tester the ability to determine: severity, proper progression, and the *fit* in the overall picture (Oral)   0   1   2   3   4   5

In order for a grade of *minimum standard* to be given, the total must be ≥11   **TOTAL = _____**

1	2	3	4	5	6	7	8	9	10	11	12	13	14	15

Not Acceptable   **Meets Minimum Standards**   **Exceeds Minimum Standards**

TEST ENVIRONMENTS

L: Laboratory/Classroom Testing
C: Clinical/Field Testing
P: Practicum Testing
A: Assessment/Mock Exam Testing
S: Self-Reporting

SKILL TEST INFORMATION

Purpose: Strength development
Involved Structure: Hamstrings
Special Considerations: Slight internal rotation needed to target semimembranosus and semitendinosus
Reference(s): Houglum; Wiksten et al
Supplies Needed: 5-lb cuff weight

THERAPEUTIC EXERCISES/RECONDITIONING
(TE-L-Test 6)

Peer Review _____ Peer Review _____

Skill Acquisition: _____   Practice Opportunities: _____

Using an 8-inch step (nesting block), demonstrate the proper technique for administering a **lateral step-up***. You have 2 minutes to complete this task.*

Tester places athlete in appropriate position	Test 1	Test 2	Test 3
Stands sideways on the step	Ⓨ Ⓝ	Ⓨ Ⓝ	Ⓨ Ⓝ
Involved foot resting flat on the 8-inch step	Ⓨ Ⓝ	Ⓨ Ⓝ	Ⓨ Ⓝ
Uninvolved limb resting on the floor	Ⓨ Ⓝ	Ⓨ Ⓝ	Ⓨ Ⓝ
Tester performs test according to accepted guidelines	**Test 1**	**Test 2**	**Test 3**
Upward movement (concentric contraction)			
Athlete slowly raises the uninvolved foot off the ground by extending the knee and hip of the involved limb	Ⓨ Ⓝ	Ⓨ Ⓝ	Ⓨ Ⓝ
Athlete continues the upward movement of the uninvolved limb until it is even with the block or the involved limb	Ⓨ Ⓝ	Ⓨ Ⓝ	Ⓨ Ⓝ
Hold	Ⓨ Ⓝ	Ⓨ Ⓝ	Ⓨ Ⓝ
Downward movement (eccentric contraction)			
Athlete slowly flexes the involved limb (knee/hip), lowering the uninvolved limb back to the starting position	Ⓨ Ⓝ	Ⓨ Ⓝ	Ⓨ Ⓝ
Athlete keeps the ankle of the uninvolved limb in full dorsiflexion	Ⓨ Ⓝ	Ⓨ Ⓝ	Ⓨ Ⓝ
Athlete allows the heel of the uninvolved foot to strike the floor first	Ⓨ Ⓝ	Ⓨ Ⓝ	Ⓨ Ⓝ

The psychomotor skill was performed completely and in the appropriate order   **0 1 2 3 4 5**

The tester had control of the subject and the situation (showed confidence)   **0 1 2 3 4 5**

Method of performing the skill allowed the tester the ability to determine: severity, proper progression, and the *fit* in the overall picture (Oral)   **0 1 2 3 4 5**

In order for a grade of *minimum standard* to be given, the total must be ≥11   **TOTAL = _____**

1	2	3	4	5	6	7	8	9	10	11	12	13	14	15

Not Acceptable   **Meets Minimum Standards**   **Exceeds Minimum Standards**

TEST ENVIRONMENTS

L: Laboratory/Classroom Testing
C: Clinical/Field Testing
P: Practicum Testing
A: Assessment/Mock Exam Testing
S: Self-Reporting

SKILL TEST INFORMATION

Purpose:	Strength development
Involved Structure:	Quadriceps
Special Considerations:	Do not allow the hip to adduct or internally rotate
Reference(s):	Houglum, Weber et al
Supplies Needed:	8-inch step

THERAPEUTIC EXERCISES/RECONDITIONING
(TE-L-Test 7)

Peer Review _____ Peer Review _____

Skill Acquisition: _____   Practice Opportunities: _____

Using manual resistance, demonstrate the proper technique for administering a **closed-chain terminal extension exercise (standing dontigney)** *in a standing position. You have 2 minutes to complete this task.*

Tester places athlete in appropriate position	Test 1	Test 2	Test 3
Athlete stands facing the tester	Ⓨ Ⓝ	Ⓨ Ⓝ	Ⓨ Ⓝ
Involved limb is about 6 inches in front of the uninvolved limb (creating 30 to 45 degrees of knee flexion)	Ⓨ Ⓝ	Ⓨ Ⓝ	Ⓨ Ⓝ
Majority of the body weight is placed on the involved limb	Ⓨ Ⓝ	Ⓨ Ⓝ	Ⓨ Ⓝ
Tester cups hands around the posterior aspect of the athlete's involved knee	Ⓨ Ⓝ	Ⓨ Ⓝ	Ⓨ Ⓝ
Tester performs test according to accepted guidelines	**Test 1**	**Test 2**	**Test 3**
Athlete contracts quadriceps	Ⓨ Ⓝ	Ⓨ Ⓝ	Ⓨ Ⓝ
Manual resistance is applied by the tester through the full range of motion	Ⓨ Ⓝ	Ⓨ Ⓝ	Ⓨ Ⓝ
Athlete relaxes and the involved knee is passively moved back into starting position	Ⓨ Ⓝ	Ⓨ Ⓝ	Ⓨ Ⓝ

The psychomotor skill was performed completely and in the appropriate order   **0 1 2 3 4 5**

The tester had control of the subject and the situation (showed confidence)   **0 1 2 3 4 5**

Method of performing the skill allowed the tester the ability to determine:
severity, proper progression, and the *fit* in the overall picture (Oral)   **0 1 2 3 4 5**

In order for a grade of *minimum standard* to be given, the total must be ≥11   **TOTAL = _____**

```
 1    2    3    4    5    6    7    8    9    10   11   12   13   14   15
 |    |    |    |    |    |    |    |    |    |    |    |    |    |    |
```
Not Acceptable   **Meets**   **Exceeds**
                                        Minimum Standards   **Minimum Standards**

TEST ENVIRONMENTS

L: Laboratory/Classroom Testing
C: Clinical/Field Testing
P: Practicum Testing
A: Assessment/Mock Exam Testing
S: Self-Reporting

SKILL TEST INFORMATION

Purpose:	Strength development
Involved Structure:	Quadriceps (vastus medialis)
Special Considerations	Do not allow knee to go into hyperextension; may be done in prone position
Reference(s):	Houglum, Prentice (2004)
Supplies Needed:	N/A (Surgical tubing maybe used instead of manual resistance)

THERAPEUTIC EXERCISES/RECONDITIONING
(TE-L-Test 8)

Peer Review _____ Peer Review _____

Skill Acquisition: _____   Practice Opportunities: _____

This problem allows you the opportunity to demonstrate the proper technique for administering an **eccentric quad set** *to help the athlete regain full active range of motion. You have 2 minutes to complete this task.*

Tester places athlete in appropriate position	Test 1	Test 2	Test 3
Seated	Y N	Y N	Y N
Knees flexed, hanging over the edge of the table	Y N	Y N	Y N
Tester performs test according to accepted guidelines	**Test 1**	**Test 2**	**Test 3**
Tester passively moves the involved limb in full extension	Y N	Y N	Y N
Athlete maximally contracts the quadriceps while the tester is holding the limb	Y N	Y N	Y N
Tester gradually releases pressure from under the involved limb	Y N	Y N	Y N
Athlete gradually lowers the involved limb	Y N	Y N	Y N

The psychomotor skill was performed completely and in the appropriate order   **0 1 2 3 4 5**

The tester had control of the subject and the situation (showed confidence)   **0 1 2 3 4 5**

Method of performing the skill allowed the tester the ability to determine:
severity, proper progression, and the *fit* in the overall picture (Oral)   **0 1 2 3 4 5**

In order for a grade of *minimum standard* to be given, the total must be ≥11   **TOTAL = _____**

1	2	3	4	5	6	7	8	9	10	11	12	13	14	15

Not Acceptable   **Meets**   **Exceeds**
                                Minimum Standards   **Minimum Standards**

TEST ENVIRONMENTS

L: Laboratory/Classroom Testing
C: Clinical/Field Testing
P: Practicum Testing
A: Assessment/Mock Exam Testing
S: Self-Reporting

SKILL TEST INFORMATION

Purpose: Strength development
Involved Structure: Quadriceps
Special Considerations: N/A
Reference(s): Houglum
Supplies Needed: Table

THERAPEUTIC EXERCISES/RECONDITIONING
(TE-L-Test 9)

Peer Review _____ Peer Review _____

Skill Acquisition: _____ Practice Opportunities: _____

This problem allows you the opportunity to demonstrate the proper technique for administering an **eccentric manual-resistance exercise** *to help develop muscle strength for the* **gastrocnemius** *muscle. You have 2 minutes to complete this task.*

Tester places athlete in appropriate position	Test 1	Test 2	Test 3
Seated	Ⓨ Ⓝ	Ⓨ Ⓝ	Ⓨ Ⓝ
Knee in full extension	Ⓨ Ⓝ	Ⓨ Ⓝ	Ⓨ Ⓝ
Ankle/lower leg hanging over the edge of the table	Ⓨ Ⓝ	Ⓨ Ⓝ	Ⓨ Ⓝ
Talocrural joint placed in full plantar flexion	Ⓨ Ⓝ	Ⓨ Ⓝ	Ⓨ Ⓝ
Tester places one hand on the plantar surface of the foot	Ⓨ Ⓝ	Ⓨ Ⓝ	Ⓨ Ⓝ
Tester places the other hand on the distal tibia to stabilize the lower leg	Ⓨ Ⓝ	Ⓨ Ⓝ	Ⓨ Ⓝ

Tester performs test according to accepted guidelines	Test 1	Test 2	Test 3
Athlete holds an isometric contraction of the gastrocnemius muscle while the foot is in full plantar flexion (resistance from the tester is from posterior to anterior)	Ⓨ Ⓝ	Ⓨ Ⓝ	Ⓨ Ⓝ
Once the isometric contraction is maintained, the command of "Let Me Win" is given to the athlete	Ⓨ Ⓝ	Ⓨ Ⓝ	Ⓨ Ⓝ
Athlete continues to contract the gastrocnemius; however, as resistance is applied by the tester, the gastrocnemius muscle gradually lengthens (moving from a plantar flexed position to a dorsiflexed position)	Ⓨ Ⓝ	Ⓨ Ⓝ	Ⓨ Ⓝ

The psychomotor skill was performed completely and in the appropriate order   0 1 2 3 4 5

The tester had control of the subject and the situation (showed confidence)   0 1 2 3 4 5

Method of performing the skill allowed the tester the ability to determine: severity, proper progression, and the *fit* in the overall picture (Oral)   0 1 2 3 4 5

In order for a grade of *minimum standard* to be given, the total must be ≥11   TOTAL = _____

```
 1   2   3   4   5   6   7   8   9   10  11  12  13  14  15
 |   |   |   |   |   |   |   |   |   |   |   |   |   |   |
```
Not Acceptable   **Meets Minimum Standards**   **Exceeds Minimum Standards**

TEST ENVIRONMENTS
L: Laboratory/Classroom Testing
C: Clinical/Field Testing
P: Practicum Testing
A: Assessment/Mock Exam Testing
S: Self-Reporting

SKILL TEST INFORMATION
Purpose: Strength development
Involved Structure: Gastrocnemius
Special Considerations: N/A
Reference(s): Adapted from Dale et al
Supplies Needed: Table

THERAPEUTIC EXERCISES/RECONDITIONING
(TE-L-Test 10)

Peer Review _____   Peer Review _____

Skill Acquisition: _____   Practice Opportunities: _____

This problem allows you the opportunity to demonstrate the proper technique for administering an **aquatic therapy resistance exercise** *to help increase the speed of the limb contraction for the* **tibialis anterior** *muscle. Instruct the athlete to complete one set of five repetitions concentrating only on the dorsiflexors (tibialis anterior is the prime mover). You have 2 minutes to complete this task.*

Tester places athlete in appropriate position	Test 1	Test 2	Test 3
Seated	Ⓨ Ⓝ	Ⓨ Ⓝ	Ⓨ Ⓝ
Buoyancy shoe securely anchored to the involved foot	Ⓨ Ⓝ	Ⓨ Ⓝ	Ⓨ Ⓝ
Knees flexed hanging over the edge of the pool (feet and lower legs must be fully immersed in the water)	Ⓨ Ⓝ	Ⓨ Ⓝ	Ⓨ Ⓝ
Involved foot actively moves into full plantar flexion	Ⓨ Ⓝ	Ⓨ Ⓝ	Ⓨ Ⓝ
Tester performs test according to accepted guidelines	**Test 1**	**Test 2**	**Test 3**
Athlete moves the foot into a dorsiflexed position as quickly as possible	Ⓨ Ⓝ	Ⓨ Ⓝ	Ⓨ Ⓝ
Athlete actively moves the foot back into a plantar flexed position	Ⓨ Ⓝ	Ⓨ Ⓝ	Ⓨ Ⓝ
Repeat (4 times)	Ⓨ Ⓝ	Ⓨ Ⓝ	Ⓨ Ⓝ

The psychomotor skill was performed completely and in the appropriate order   0 1 2 3 4 5

The tester had control of the subject and the situation (showed confidence)   0 1 2 3 4 5

Method of performing the skill allowed the tester the ability to determine: severity, proper progression, and the *fit* in the overall picture (Oral)   0 1 2 3 4 5

In order for a grade of *minimum standard* to be given, the total must be ≥11   TOTAL = _____

```
 1    2    3    4    5    6    7    8    9   10   11   12   13   14   15
 |    |    |    |    |    |    |    |    |    |    |    |    |    |    |
```

Not Acceptable   **Meets**   **Exceeds**
                            Minimum Standards   **Minimum Standards**

TEST ENVIRONMENTS

L: Laboratory/Classroom Testing
C: Clinical/Field Testing
P: Practicum Testing
A: Assessment/Mock Exam Testing
S: Self-Reporting

SKILL TEST INFORMATION

Purpose:	Strength development; improve speed of limb contraction
Involved Structure:	Tibialis anterior
Special Considerations:	Buoyancy shoe decreases the specific gravity of the foot which in turn increases the speed of the limb contraction
Reference(s):	Adapted from Thein-Nissenbaum
Supplies Needed:	Water (pool/large whirlpool); buoyancy shoe

THERAPEUTIC EXERCISES/RECONDITIONING
(TE-L-Test 11)

Peer Review _____ Peer Review _____

Skill Acquisition: _____   Practice Opportunities: _____

Using a broom handle, demonstrate the **proper technique for performing a back squat exercise to parallel depth**. *You have 3 minutes to complete this task.*

Tester places athlete and limb in appropriate position	Test 1	Test 2	Test 3
Standing	Ⓨ Ⓝ	Ⓨ Ⓝ	Ⓨ Ⓝ
Instructs the athlete to look toward the ceiling (head slightly extended)	Ⓨ Ⓝ	Ⓨ Ⓝ	Ⓨ Ⓝ

Tester performs test according to accepted guidelines	Test 1	Test 2	Test 3
Beginning position:			
Grasps the bar with a closed, pronated grip (slightly wider than shoulder width)	Ⓨ Ⓝ	Ⓨ Ⓝ	Ⓨ Ⓝ
Feet parallel to each other (shoulder width apart)	Ⓨ Ⓝ	Ⓨ Ⓝ	Ⓨ Ⓝ
Places the bar across posterior deltoids/middle trapezius (balanced position)	Ⓨ Ⓝ	Ⓨ Ⓝ	Ⓨ Ⓝ
Downward movement (descent):			
Allows the hips and knees to slowly flex (minimal trunk flexion is acceptable)	Ⓨ Ⓝ	Ⓨ Ⓝ	Ⓨ Ⓝ
Maintains flat back, elbows high, chest up and out	Ⓨ Ⓝ	Ⓨ Ⓝ	Ⓨ Ⓝ
Keeps heels on the floor	Ⓨ Ⓝ	Ⓨ Ⓝ	Ⓨ Ⓝ
Keeps knees over the feet	Ⓨ Ⓝ	Ⓨ Ⓝ	Ⓨ Ⓝ
Continues downward movement until thighs are parallel to the floor	Ⓨ Ⓝ	Ⓨ Ⓝ	Ⓨ Ⓝ
Upward movement (ascent):			
Extends the hips and knees	Ⓨ Ⓝ	Ⓨ Ⓝ	Ⓨ Ⓝ
Maintains flat back, elbows high, chest up and out	Ⓨ Ⓝ	Ⓨ Ⓝ	Ⓨ Ⓝ
Keeps heels on the floor	Ⓨ Ⓝ	Ⓨ Ⓝ	Ⓨ Ⓝ
Keeps knees over the feet	Ⓨ Ⓝ	Ⓨ Ⓝ	Ⓨ Ⓝ
Continues upward movement (does not fully "lock out")	Ⓨ Ⓝ	Ⓨ Ⓝ	Ⓨ Ⓝ

The psychomotor skill was performed completely and in the appropriate order   0   1   2   3   4   5

The tester had control of the subject and the situation (showed confidence)   0   1   2   3   4   5

Method of performing the skill allowed the tester the ability to determine: severity, proper progression, and the *fit* in the overall picture (Oral)   0   1   2   3   4   5

In order for a grade of *minimum standard* to be given, the total must be ≥11   **TOTAL = _____**

1	2	3	4	5	6	7	8	9	10	11	12	13	14	15

Not Acceptable   **Meets Minimum Standards**   **Exceeds Minimum Standards**

TEST ENVIRONMENTS

L: Laboratory/Classroom Testing
C: Clinical/Field Testing
P: Practicum Testing
A: Assessment/Mock Exam Testing
S: Self-Reporting

SKILL TEST INFORMATION

Positive Finding: Strength development
Involved Structure: Quadriceps
Special Considerations: N/A
Reference(s): Baechle et al
Supplies Needed: Broom handle

THERAPEUTIC EXERCISES/RECONDITIONING
(TE-L-Test 12)

Peer Review _____ Peer Review _____

Skill Acquisition: _____   Practice Opportunities: _____

*This problem allows you the opportunity to demonstrate the **proper spotting technique** for an athlete who is performing a **forward lunge**. You have 3 minutes to complete this task.*

Tester places athlete and limb in appropriate position	Test 1	Test 2	Test 3
Standing behind the athlete	Ⓨ Ⓝ	Ⓨ Ⓝ	Ⓨ Ⓝ
Tester performs test according to accepted guidelines	**Test 1**	**Test 2**	**Test 3**
Beginning position (spotter):			
Positions hands near the athlete's hips/wrist	Ⓨ Ⓝ	Ⓨ Ⓝ	Ⓨ Ⓝ
Feet side-by-side (shoulder width apart)	Ⓨ Ⓝ	Ⓨ Ⓝ	Ⓨ Ⓝ
Forward movement phase (spotter):			
Steps forward with the athlete (same foot as the athlete)	Ⓨ Ⓝ	Ⓨ Ⓝ	Ⓨ Ⓝ
Keeps the lead knee about 15 inches behind the athlete's foot	Ⓨ Ⓝ	Ⓨ Ⓝ	Ⓨ Ⓝ
Keeps hands near the athlete's torso	Ⓨ Ⓝ	Ⓨ Ⓝ	Ⓨ Ⓝ
Backward movement phase (spotter):			
Pushes backward with the lead leg at the same time the athlete moves (returns to legs in side-by-side)	Ⓨ Ⓝ	Ⓨ Ⓝ	Ⓨ Ⓝ
Keeps hands near the athlete's torso	Ⓨ Ⓝ	Ⓨ Ⓝ	Ⓨ Ⓝ
Repeat alternating lead leg	Ⓨ Ⓝ	Ⓨ Ⓝ	Ⓨ Ⓝ

The psychomotor skill was performed completely and in the appropriate order   0 1 2 3 4 5

The tester had control of the subject and the situation (showed confidence)   0 1 2 3 4 5

Method of performing the skill allowed the tester the ability to determine:
severity, proper progression, and the *fit* in the overall picture (Oral)   0 1 2 3 4 5

In order for a grade of *minimum standard* to be given, the total must be ≥11   TOTAL = _____

```
 1     2     3     4     5     6     7     8     9    10    11    12    13    14    15
 |     |     |     |     |     |     |     |     |     |     |     |     |     |     |
```
Not Acceptable   **Meets**   **Exceeds**
                                              Minimum Standards   **Minimum Standards**

TEST ENVIRONMENTS	**SKILL TEST INFORMATION**	
L: Laboratory/Classroom Testing	**Positive Finding:**	Safety
C: Clinical/Field Testing	**Involved Structure:**	N/A
P: Practicum Testing	**Special Considerations:**	N/A
A: Assessment/Mock Exam Testing	**Reference(s):**	Baechle et al
S: Self-Reporting	**Supplies Needed:**	Broom handle or dumbbells

THERAPEUTIC EXERCISES/RECONDITIONING
(TE-L-Test 13)

Peer Review _____ Peer Review _____

Skill Acquisition: _____   Practice Opportunities: _____

Using the athlete as your partner, demonstrate how you would perform a type of **plyometrics** *known as a* **medicine ball sit-up**. *You have 3 minutes to complete this task.*

Tester places athlete and limb in appropriate position	Test 1	Test 2	Test 3
Seated on the floor	Ⓨ Ⓝ	Ⓨ Ⓝ	Ⓨ Ⓝ
Sit-up position (knees bent, trunk flexed to 45 degrees)	Ⓨ Ⓝ	Ⓨ Ⓝ	Ⓨ Ⓝ
Hands/arms in an outstretched position (waiting to receive the ball)	Ⓨ Ⓝ	Ⓨ Ⓝ	Ⓨ Ⓝ
Tester placed in proper position	Ⓨ Ⓝ	Ⓨ Ⓝ	Ⓨ Ⓝ
Standing in front of the athlete (holding the medicine ball)	Ⓨ Ⓝ	Ⓨ Ⓝ	Ⓨ Ⓝ
Tester performs task according to accepted guidelines	**Test 1**	**Test 2**	**Test 3**
Tester throws the ball to the athlete	Ⓨ Ⓝ	Ⓨ Ⓝ	Ⓨ Ⓝ
Athlete: Catches the ball using both arms (eccentric phrase)	Ⓨ Ⓝ	Ⓨ Ⓝ	Ⓨ Ⓝ
Athlete: Completes the amortization phase (time between moving down toward the floor and coming back up)	Ⓨ Ⓝ	Ⓨ Ⓝ	Ⓨ Ⓝ
Athlete: Moves away from the floor and throws/pushes the ball back (concentric phase)	Ⓨ Ⓝ	Ⓨ Ⓝ	Ⓨ Ⓝ
Tester: Receives the ball from the athlete and repeats	Ⓨ Ⓝ	Ⓨ Ⓝ	Ⓨ Ⓝ

The psychomotor skill was performed completely and in the appropriate order   **0 1 2 3 4 5**

The tester had control of the subject and the situation (showed confidence)   **0 1 2 3 4 5**

Method of performing the skill allowed the tester the ability to determine:
severity, proper progression, and the *fit* in the overall picture (Oral)   **0 1 2 3 4 5**

In order for a grade of *minimum standard* to be given, the total must be ≥11   **TOTAL = _____**

```
 1    2    3    4    5    6    7    8    9    10   11   12   13   14   15
 |____|____|____|____|____|____|____|____|____|____|____|____|____|____|
```

Not Acceptable   **Meets**   **Exceeds**
                                     Minimum Standards   **Minimum Standards**

TEST ENVIRONMENTS

L: Laboratory/Classroom Testing
C: Clinical/Field Testing
P: Practicum Testing
A: Assessment/Mock Exam Testing
S: Self-Reporting

SKILL TEST INFORMATION

Positive Finding: Develop power
Involved Structure: Rectus abdominis (abdominal muscles)
Special Considerations: N/A
Reference(s): Bache et al
Supplies Needed: Medicine ball

THERAPEUTIC EXERCISES/RECONDITIONING
(TE-L-Test 14)

Peer Review _____ Peer Review _____

Skill Acquisition: _____   Practice Opportunities: _____

Please demonstrate the **plyometric** *technique known as the* **triple double-leg vertical jump (triple vertical jump-double leg)**. *You have 3 minutes to complete this task.*

Tester places athlete and limb in appropriate position	Test 1	Test 2	Test 3
Standing	Y N	Y N	Y N
Feet shoulder width apart	Y N	Y N	Y N
Arms flexed to 90 degrees	Y N	Y N	Y N
Tester placed in proper position	Y N	Y N	Y N
Observation only	Y N	Y N	Y N
Tester performs task according to accepted guidelines	**Test 1**	**Test 2**	**Test 3**
Instructs the athlete:			
To drop arms into hyperextension	Y N	Y N	Y N
To flex knees, hip, and trunk	Y N	Y N	Y N
To explosively jump up (vertical)	Y N	Y N	Y N
To land on two feet (in the starting place and position)	Y N	Y N	Y N
Repeats (double)	Y N	Y N	Y N
Repeats (triple)	Y N	Y N	Y N

The psychomotor skill was performed completely and in the appropriate order   0 1 2 3 4 5

The tester had control of the subject and the situation (showed confidence)   0 1 2 3 4 5

Method of performing the skill allowed the tester the ability to determine:
severity, proper progression, and the *fit* in the overall picture (Oral)   0 1 2 3 4 5

In order for a grade of *minimum standard* to be given, the total must be ≥11   **TOTAL = _____**

| 1 | 2 | 3 | 4 | 5 | 6 | 7 | 8 | 9 | 10 | 11 | 12 | 13 | 14 | 15 |

Not Acceptable   **Meets Minimum Standards**   **Exceeds Minimum Standards**

TEST ENVIRONMENTS	**SKILL TEST INFORMATION**	
L: Laboratory/Classroom Testing	**Positive Finding:**	Develop power
C: Clinical/Field Testing	**Involved Structure:**	Muscles of the lower body
P: Practicum Testing	**Special Considerations:**	N/A
A: Assessment/Mock Exam Testing	**Reference(s):**	Baechle et al
S: Self-Reporting	**Supplies Needed:**	N/A

Chapter **13**

THERAPEUTIC MEASUREMENTS

THERAPEUTIC MEASUREMENTS
(TM-U-Test 1)

Peer Review _____ Peer Review _____

Skill Acquisition: _____   Practice Opportunities: _____

Please demonstrate the proper use of a **goniometer** *for measuring an athlete's shoulder active range of motion for* **flexion at the glenohumeral joint**. *You have 3 minutes to complete this task.*

Tester places athlete and limb in appropriate position	Test 1	Test 2	Test 3
Supine	Ⓨ Ⓝ	Ⓨ Ⓝ	Ⓨ Ⓝ
Knee flexed to 90 degrees	Ⓨ Ⓝ	Ⓨ Ⓝ	Ⓨ Ⓝ
Shoulder adducted to 0 degrees	Ⓨ Ⓝ	Ⓨ Ⓝ	Ⓨ Ⓝ
Palm against the body	Ⓨ Ⓝ	Ⓨ Ⓝ	Ⓨ Ⓝ
Tester provides appropriate stabilization	**Test 1**	**Test 2**	**Test 3**
Scapula	Ⓨ Ⓝ	Ⓨ Ⓝ	Ⓨ Ⓝ
Tester places goniometer in appropriate position	**Test 1**	**Test 2**	**Test 3**
Fulcrum: Acromial process	Ⓨ Ⓝ	Ⓨ Ⓝ	Ⓨ Ⓝ
Stationary arm: Midaxillary line of the thorax	Ⓨ Ⓝ	Ⓨ Ⓝ	Ⓨ Ⓝ
Moving arm: Lateral midline of the humerus (lateral epicondyle)	Ⓨ Ⓝ	Ⓨ Ⓝ	Ⓨ Ⓝ
Tester performs test according to accepted guidelines	**Test 1**	**Test 2**	**Test 3**
Correct reading: Flexion	Ⓨ Ⓝ	Ⓨ Ⓝ	Ⓨ Ⓝ
Performs assessment bilaterally	Ⓨ Ⓝ	Ⓨ Ⓝ	Ⓨ Ⓝ

The psychomotor skill was performed completely and in the appropriate order   **0 1 2 3 4 5**

The tester had control of the subject and the situation (showed confidence)   **0 1 2 3 4 5**

Method of performing the skill allowed the tester the ability to determine: severity, proper progression, and the *fit* in the overall picture (Oral)   **0 1 2 3 4 5**

In order for a grade of *minimum standard* to be given, the total must be ≥11   **TOTAL = _____**

```
  1    2    3    4    5    6    7    8    9   10   11   12   13   14   15
  |    |    |    |    |    |    |    |    |    |    |    |    |    |    |
```
Not Acceptable   **Meets**   **Exceeds**
                                         Minimum Standards   **Minimum Standards**

TEST ENVIRONMENTS

L: Laboratory/Classroom Testing
C: Clinical/Field Testing
P: Practicum Testing
A: Assessment/Mock Exam Testing
S: Self-Reporting

SKILL TEST INFORMATION

Positive Finding: Range of motion (ROM)
Involved Structure: Glenohumeral joint
Special Considerations: N/A
Reference(s): Norkin et al
Supplies Needed: Goniometer, dots/markers

THERAPEUTIC MEASUREMENTS
(TM-U-Test 2)

Peer Review _____ Peer Review _____

Skill Acquisition: _____   Practice Opportunities: _____

Please demonstrate the proper use of a **goniometer** *for measuring an athlete's shoulder active range of motion for* **extension at the glenohumeral joint**. *You have 3 minutes to complete this task.*

Tester places athlete and limb in appropriate position	Test 1	Test 2	Test 3
Prone	Y N	Y N	Y N
Turns the head away from involved shoulder	Y N	Y N	Y N
Shoulder adducted to 0 degrees	Y N	Y N	Y N
Places elbow in slight flexion	Y N	Y N	Y N
Tester provides appropriate stabilization	**Test 1**	**Test 2**	**Test 3**
Scapula	Y N	Y N	Y N
Tester places goniometer in appropriate position	**Test 1**	**Test 2**	**Test 3**
Fulcrum: Greater tubercle of the shoulder	Y N	Y N	Y N
Stationary arm: Mid axillary line of the thorax	Y N	Y N	Y N
Moving arm: Lateral midline of the humerus (lateral epicondyle)	Y N	Y N	Y N
Tester performs test according to accepted guidelines	**Test 1**	**Test 2**	**Test 3**
Correct reading: Extension	Y N	Y N	Y N
Performs assessment bilaterally	Y N	Y N	Y N

The psychomotor skill was performed completely and in the appropriate order   0 1 2 3 4 5

The tester had control of the subject and the situation (showed confidence)   0 1 2 3 4 5

Method of performing the skill allowed the tester the ability to determine:
severity, proper progression, and the *fit* in the overall picture (Oral)   0 1 2 3 4 5

In order for a grade of *minimum standard* to be given, the total must be ≥11   **TOTAL = _____**

```
   1   2   3   4   5   6   7   8   9  10  11  12  13  14  15
```

Not Acceptable   **Meets**   **Exceeds**
                          Minimum Standards   **Minimum Standards**

TEST ENVIRONMENTS

L: Laboratory/Classroom Testing
C: Clinical/Field Testing
P: Practicum Testing
A: Assessment/Mock Exam Testing
S: Self-Reporting

SKILL TEST INFORMATION

Finding: Range of motion (ROM)
Involved Structure: Glenohumeral joint
Special Considerations N/A
Reference(s): Norkin et al
Supplies Needed: Goniometer; dot/marker

THERAPEUTIC MEASUREMENTS
(TM-U-Test 3)

Peer Review _____ Peer Review _____

Skill Acquisition: _____   Practice Opportunities: _____

Please demonstrate the proper use of a **goniometer** *for measuring an athlete's shoulder active range of motion for* **internal/external rotation at the glenohumeral joint.** *You have 3 minutes to complete this task.*

Tester places athlete and limb in appropriate position	Test 1	Test 2	Test 3
Supine	Ⓨ Ⓝ	Ⓨ Ⓝ	Ⓨ Ⓝ
Shoulder abducted to 90 degrees	Ⓨ Ⓝ	Ⓨ Ⓝ	Ⓨ Ⓝ
Forearm maintained at 0 degrees	Ⓨ Ⓝ	Ⓨ Ⓝ	Ⓨ Ⓝ
Pad/towel under humerus	Ⓨ Ⓝ	Ⓨ Ⓝ	Ⓨ Ⓝ
Tester provides appropriate stabilization	Ⓨ Ⓝ	Ⓨ Ⓝ	Ⓨ Ⓝ
Distal end of humerus (beginning of motion)	Ⓨ Ⓝ	Ⓨ Ⓝ	Ⓨ Ⓝ
Tester provides appropriate stabilization	**Test 1**	**Test 2**	**Test 3**
Scapula (end of motion)	Ⓨ Ⓝ	Ⓨ Ⓝ	Ⓨ Ⓝ
Tester places goniometer in appropriate position	**Test 1**	**Test 2**	**Test 3**
Fulcrum: Olecranon process	Ⓨ Ⓝ	Ⓨ Ⓝ	Ⓨ Ⓝ
Stationary arm: Parallel or perpendicular to the floor	Ⓨ Ⓝ	Ⓨ Ⓝ	Ⓨ Ⓝ
Moving arm: Align with the ulna; ulnar styloid	Ⓨ Ⓝ	Ⓨ Ⓝ	Ⓨ Ⓝ
Tester performs test according to accepted guidelines	**Test 1**	**Test 2**	**Test 3**
Correct reading: Internal/external rotation	Ⓨ Ⓝ	Ⓨ Ⓝ	Ⓨ Ⓝ
Performs assessment bilaterally	Ⓨ Ⓝ	Ⓨ Ⓝ	Ⓨ Ⓝ

The psychomotor skill was performed completely and in the appropriate order   **0 1 2 3 4 5**

The tester had control of the subject and the situation (showed confidence)   **0 1 2 3 4 5**

Method of performing the skill allowed the tester the ability to determine:
severity, proper progression, and the *fit* in the overall picture (Oral)   **0 1 2 3 4 5**

In order for a grade of *minimum standard* to be given, the total must be ≥11   **TOTAL = _____**

```
    1    2    3    4    5    6    7    8    9    10   11   12   13   14   15
    |____|____|____|____|____|____|____|____|____|____|____|____|____|____|
```
Not Acceptable   **Meets**   **Exceeds**
                               Minimum Standards   **Minimum Standards**

TEST ENVIRONMENTS

L: Laboratory/Classroom Testing
C: Clinical/Field Testing
P: Practicum Testing
A: Assessment/Mock Exam Testing
S: Self-Reporting

SKILL TEST INFORMATION

Positive Finding:	Range of motion (ROM)
Involved Structure:	Glenohumeral joint
Special Considerations:	N/A
Reference(s):	Norkin et al
Supplies Needed:	Goniometer, dots/markers, towel/pad

THERAPEUTIC MEASUREMENTS
(TM-U-Test 4)

Peer Review _____ Peer Review _____

Skill Acquisition: _____   Practice Opportunities: _____

Please demonstrate the proper use of a **goniometer** *for measuring an athlete's shoulder active range of motion for* **abduction at the glenohumeral joint**. *You have 3 minutes to complete this task..*

Tester places athlete and limb in appropriate position	Test 1	Test 2	Test 3
Supine	Ⓨ Ⓝ	Ⓨ Ⓝ	Ⓨ Ⓝ
Tester provides appropriate stabilization	**Test 1**	**Test 2**	**Test 3**
Scapula	Ⓨ Ⓝ	Ⓨ Ⓝ	Ⓨ Ⓝ
Tester places goniometer in appropriate position	**Test 1**	**Test 2**	**Test 3**
Fulcrum: Acromial Process	Ⓨ Ⓝ	Ⓨ Ⓝ	Ⓨ Ⓝ
Stationary Arm: Parallel to the sternum	Ⓨ Ⓝ	Ⓨ Ⓝ	Ⓨ Ⓝ
Moving Arm: Midline of the humerus	Ⓨ Ⓝ	Ⓨ Ⓝ	Ⓨ Ⓝ
Tester performs test according to accepted guidelines	**Test 1**	**Test 2**	**Test 3**
Correct reading: Abduction	Ⓨ Ⓝ	Ⓨ Ⓝ	Ⓨ Ⓝ
Performs assessment bilaterally	Ⓨ Ⓝ	Ⓨ Ⓝ	Ⓨ Ⓝ

The psychomotor skill was performed completely and in the appropriate order   **0 1 2 3 4 5**

The tester had control of the subject and the situation (showed confidence)   **0 1 2 3 4 5**

Method of performing the skill allowed the tester the ability to determine:
severity, proper progression, and the *fit* in the overall picture (Oral)   **0 1 2 3 4 5**

In order for a grade of *minimum standard* to be given, the total must be ≥11   **TOTAL = _____**

```
 1    2    3    4    5    6    7    8    9   10   11   12   13   14   15
 |    |    |    |    |    |    |    |    |    |    |    |    |    |    |
```
Not Acceptable   **Meets**   **Exceeds**
                                    Minimum Standards   **Minimum Standards**

TEST ENVIRONMENTS

L: Laboratory/Classroom Testing
C: Clinical/Field Testing
P: Practicum Testing
A: Assessment/Mock Exam Testing
S: Self-Reporting

SKILL TEST INFORMATION

Finding: Range of motion (ROM)
Involved Structure: Glenohumeral joint
Special Considerations: N/A
Reference(s): Norkin et al
Supplies Needed: Goniometer; dot/marker

THERAPEUTIC MEASUREMENTS
(TM-U-Test 5)

Peer Review _____ Peer Review _____

Skill Acquisition: _____   Practice Opportunities: _____

Please demonstrate the proper use of a **goniometer** *for measuring an athlete's elbow active range of motion for* **flexion/extension at the humeroulnar joint**. *You have 3 minutes to complete this task.*

Tester places athlete and limb in appropriate position	Test 1	Test 2	Test 3
Supine	Ⓨ Ⓝ	Ⓨ Ⓝ	Ⓨ Ⓝ
Anatomical position	Ⓨ Ⓝ	Ⓨ Ⓝ	Ⓨ Ⓝ
Pad/towel under the distal end of the humerus	Ⓨ Ⓝ	Ⓨ Ⓝ	Ⓨ Ⓝ
Tester provides appropriate stabilization	**Test 1**	**Test 2**	**Test 3**
Distal end of the humerus	Ⓨ Ⓝ	Ⓨ Ⓝ	Ⓨ Ⓝ
Tester places goniometer in appropriate position	**Test 1**	**Test 2**	**Test 3**
Fulcrum: Lateral epicondyle of humerus	Ⓨ Ⓝ	Ⓨ Ⓝ	Ⓨ Ⓝ
Stationary arm: Lateral midline of the humerus	Ⓨ Ⓝ	Ⓨ Ⓝ	Ⓨ Ⓝ
Moving arm: Lateral midline of the radius (radial head)	Ⓨ Ⓝ	Ⓨ Ⓝ	Ⓨ Ⓝ
Tester performs test according to accepted guidelines	**Test 1**	**Test 2**	**Test 3**
Correct reading: Flexion/extension	Ⓨ Ⓝ	Ⓨ Ⓝ	Ⓨ Ⓝ
Performs assessment bilaterally	Ⓨ Ⓝ	Ⓨ Ⓝ	Ⓨ Ⓝ

The psychomotor skill was performed completely and in the appropriate order   **0 1 2 3 4 5**

The tester had control of the subject and the situation (showed confidence)   **0 1 2 3 4 5**

Method of performing the skill allowed the tester the ability to determine:
severity, proper progression, and the *fit* in the overall picture (Oral)   **0 1 2 3 4 5**

In order for a grade of *minimum standard* to be given, the total must be ≥11   **TOTAL = _____**

1	2	3	4	5	6	7	8	9	10	11	12	13	14	15

Not Acceptable   **Meets**   **Exceeds**
                              Minimum Standards   **Minimum Standards**

TEST ENVIRONMENTS

L: Laboratory/Classroom Testing
C: Clinical/Field Testing
P: Practicum Testing
A: Assessment/Mock Exam Testing
S: Self-Reporting

SKILL TEST INFORMATION

Positive Finding: Range of motion (ROM)
Involved Structure: Humeroradial joint, humeroulnar joint
Special Considerations: N/A
Reference(s): Norkin et al
Supplies Needed: Goniometer, dots/markers, towel, table

THERAPEUTIC MEASUREMENTS
(TM-U-Test 6)

Peer Review _____ Peer Review _____

Skill Acquisition: _____   Practice Opportunities: _____

Please demonstrate the proper use of a **goniometer** *for measuring an athlete's elbow (forearm) active range of motion for* **pronation at the radioulnar joint**. *You have 3 minutes to complete this task.*

Tester places athlete and limb in appropriate position	Test 1	Test 2	Test 3
Sitting	Ⓨ Ⓝ	Ⓨ Ⓝ	Ⓨ Ⓝ
Shoulder adducted to 0 degrees	Ⓨ Ⓝ	Ⓨ Ⓝ	Ⓨ Ⓝ
Elbow flexed to 90 degrees	Ⓨ Ⓝ	Ⓨ Ⓝ	Ⓨ Ⓝ
Forearm supinated to 0 degrees (thumb pointing up)	Ⓨ Ⓝ	Ⓨ Ⓝ	Ⓨ Ⓝ
Tester provides appropriate stabilization	**Test 1**	**Test 2**	**Test 3**
Distal end of the humerus	Ⓨ Ⓝ	Ⓨ Ⓝ	Ⓨ Ⓝ
Tester places goniometer in appropriate position	**Test 1**	**Test 2**	**Test 3**
Fulcrum: Lateral to the ulnar styloid process	Ⓨ Ⓝ	Ⓨ Ⓝ	Ⓨ Ⓝ
Stationary arm: Parallel to the anterior midline of the humerus	Ⓨ Ⓝ	Ⓨ Ⓝ	Ⓨ Ⓝ
Moving arm: Across the dorsal aspect of the forearm	Ⓨ Ⓝ	Ⓨ Ⓝ	Ⓨ Ⓝ
Tester performs test according to accepted guidelines	**Test 1**	**Test 2**	**Test 3**
Correct reading: Pronation	Ⓨ Ⓝ	Ⓨ Ⓝ	Ⓨ Ⓝ
Performs assessment bilaterally	Ⓨ Ⓝ	Ⓨ Ⓝ	Ⓨ Ⓝ

The psychomotor skill was performed completely and in the appropriate order   0 1 2 3 4 5

The tester had control of the subject and the situation (showed confidence)   0 1 2 3 4 5

Method of performing the skill allowed the tester the ability to determine:
severity, proper progression, and the *fit* in the overall picture (Oral)   0 1 2 3 4 5

In order for a grade of *minimum standard* to be given, the total must be ≥11   TOTAL = _____

```
 1    2    3    4    5    6    7    8    9   10   11   12   13   14   15
 |    |    |    |    |    |    |    |    |    |    |    |    |    |    |
```

Not Acceptable   **Meets**   **Exceeds**
                              Minimum Standards   **Minimum Standards**

TEST ENVIRONMENTS

L: Laboratory/Classroom Testing
C: Clinical/Field Testing
P: Practicum Testing
A: Assessment/Mock Exam Testing
S: Self-Reporting

SKILL TEST INFORMATION

Positive Finding: Range of motion (ROM)
Involved Structure: Superior radioulnar joint, inferior radioulnar joint
Special Considerations: N/A
Reference(s): Norkin et al
Supplies Needed: Goniometer, dots/markers

THERAPEUTIC MEASUREMENTS
(TM-U-Test 7)

Skill Acquisition: _____   Practice Opportunities: _____

*Please demonstrate the proper use of a **goniometer** for measuring an athlete's wrist active range of motion for* **flexion/extension at the midcarpal joints**. *You have 3 minutes to complete this task.*

Tester places athlete and limb in appropriate position	Test 1	Test 2	Test 3
Sitting next to a supporting surface	Ⓨ Ⓝ	Ⓨ Ⓝ	Ⓨ Ⓝ
Shoulder abducted to 90 degrees/elbow flexed to 90 degrees	Ⓨ Ⓝ	Ⓨ Ⓝ	Ⓨ Ⓝ
Forearm supinated to 0 degrees (palm facing down, hanging off the table)	Ⓨ Ⓝ	Ⓨ Ⓝ	Ⓨ Ⓝ
Tester provides appropriate stabilization	**Test 1**	**Test 2**	**Test 3**
Radius and ulna	Ⓨ Ⓝ	Ⓨ Ⓝ	Ⓨ Ⓝ
Tester places goniometer in appropriate position	**Test 1**	**Test 2**	**Test 3**
Fulcrum: Lateral aspect of the wrist (triquetrum)	Ⓨ Ⓝ	Ⓨ Ⓝ	Ⓨ Ⓝ
Stationary arm: Lateral midline of the ulna	Ⓨ Ⓝ	Ⓨ Ⓝ	Ⓨ Ⓝ
Moving arm: Lateral midline of the fifth metacarpal	Ⓨ Ⓝ	Ⓨ Ⓝ	Ⓨ Ⓝ
Tester performs test according to accepted guidelines	**Test 1**	**Test 2**	**Test 3**
Correct reading: Flexion/extension	Ⓨ Ⓝ	Ⓨ Ⓝ	Ⓨ Ⓝ
Performs assessment bilaterally	Ⓨ Ⓝ	Ⓨ Ⓝ	Ⓨ Ⓝ

The psychomotor skill was performed completely and in the appropriate order   **0 1 2 3 4 5**

The tester had control of the subject and the situation (showed confidence)   **0 1 2 3 4 5**

Method of performing the skill allowed the tester the ability to determine: severity, proper progression, and the *fit* in the overall picture (Oral)   **0 1 2 3 4 5**

In order for a grade of *minimum standard* to be given, the total must be ≥11   **TOTAL = _____**

```
  1    2    3    4    5    6    7    8    9    10   11   12   13   14   15
  |    |    |    |    |    |    |    |    |    |    |    |    |    |    |
```

Not Acceptable   **Meets**   **Exceeds**
                                     Minimum Standards   **Minimum Standards**

TEST ENVIRONMENTS

L: Laboratory/Classroom Testing
C: Clinical/Field Testing
P: Practicum Testing
A: Assessment/Mock Exam Testing
S: Self-Reporting

SKILL TEST INFORMATION

Positive Finding: Range of motion (ROM)
Involved Structure: Wrist
Special Considerations: N/A
Reference(s): Norkin et al
Supplies Needed: Goniometer, dots/markers, chair, table

THERAPEUTIC MEASUREMENTS
(TM-U-Test 8)

Peer Review _____ Peer Review _____

Skill Acquisition: _____   Practice Opportunities: _____

Please demonstrate the proper use of a **goniometer** *for measuring an athlete's wrist active range of motion for* **radial deviation at the radiocarpal joint.** *You have 3 minutes to complete this task.*

Tester places athlete and limb in appropriate position	Test 1	Test 2	Test 3
Sitting next to a supporting surface	Y N	Y N	Y N
Shoulder abducted to 90 degrees/elbow flexed to 90 degrees	Y N	Y N	Y N
Forearm supinated to 0 degrees (palm facing down, supported by the table)	Y N	Y N	Y N
Tester provides appropriate stabilization	Test 1	Test 2	Test 3
Distal end of the radius and ulna	Y N	Y N	Y N
Tester places goniometer in appropriate position	Test 1	Test 2	Test 3
Fulcrum: Dorsal aspect of the wrist (capitate)	Y N	Y N	Y N
Stationary arm: Dorsal midline of the forearm	Y N	Y N	Y N
Moving arm: Dorsal midline of the third metacarpal	Y N	Y N	Y N
Tester performs test according to accepted guidelines	Test 1	Test 2	Test 3
Correct reading: Radial deviation	Y N	Y N	Y N
Performs assessment bilaterally	Y N	Y N	Y N

The psychomotor skill was performed completely and in the appropriate order   0 1 2 3 4 5

The tester had control of the subject and the situation (showed confidence)   0 1 2 3 4 5

Method of performing the skill allowed the tester the ability to determine:
severity, proper progression, and the *fit* in the overall picture (Oral)   0 1 2 3 4 5

In order for a grade of *minimum standard* to be given, the total must be ≥11   TOTAL = _____

```
1    2    3    4    5    6    7    8    9   10   11   12   13   14   15
```
Not Acceptable   **Meets**   **Exceeds**
                                    Minimum Standards   **Minimum Standards**

TEST ENVIRONMENTS
L: Laboratory/Classroom Testing
C: Clinical/Field Testing
P: Practicum Testing
A: Assessment/Mock Exam Testing
S: Self-Reporting

SKILL TEST INFORMATION
Positive Finding: Range of motion (ROM)
Involved Structure: Radiocarpal joint
Special Considerations: N/A
Reference(s): Norkin et al
Supplies Needed: Goniometer, dots/markers, chair, tables

THERAPEUTIC MEASUREMENTS
(TM-U-Test 9)

Peer Review _____ Peer Review _____

Skill Acquisition: _____   Practice Opportunities: _____

Please demonstrate the proper use of a **goniometer** *for measuring an athlete's second finger active range of motion for* **abduction at the metacarpophalangeal joint**. *You have 3 minutes to complete this task.*

Tester places athlete and limb in appropriate position	Test 1	Test 2	Test 3
Seated	Ⓨ Ⓝ	Ⓨ Ⓝ	Ⓨ Ⓝ
Rests forearm and hand on table (palm against on table)	Ⓨ Ⓝ	Ⓨ Ⓝ	Ⓨ Ⓝ
Places wrist, and fingers in a neutral position	Ⓨ Ⓝ	Ⓨ Ⓝ	Ⓨ Ⓝ
Tester provides appropriate stabilization	**Test 1**	**Test 2**	**Test 3**
Metacarpal	Ⓨ Ⓝ	Ⓨ Ⓝ	Ⓨ Ⓝ
Tester places goniometer in appropriate position	**Test 1**	**Test 2**	**Test 3**
Fulcrum: Dorsal Aspect of the MCP Joint	Ⓨ Ⓝ	Ⓨ Ⓝ	Ⓨ Ⓝ
Stationary arm: Dorsal midline of the second metacarpal	Ⓨ Ⓝ	Ⓨ Ⓝ	Ⓨ Ⓝ
Moving arm: Dorsal midline of the second proximal phalanx	Ⓨ Ⓝ	Ⓨ Ⓝ	Ⓨ Ⓝ
Tester performs test according to accepted guidelines	**Test 1**	**Test 2**	**Test 3**
Correct reading: Abduction (moves finger away from midline)	Ⓨ Ⓝ	Ⓨ Ⓝ	Ⓨ Ⓝ
Performs assessment bilaterally	Ⓨ Ⓝ	Ⓨ Ⓝ	Ⓨ Ⓝ

The psychomotor skill was performed completely and in the appropriate order   **0 1 2 3 4 5**

The tester had control of the subject and the situation (showed confidence)   **0 1 2 3 4 5**

Method of performing the skill allowed the tester the ability to determine:
severity, proper progression, and the *fit* in the overall picture (Oral)   **0 1 2 3 4 5**

In order for a grade of *minimum standard* to be given, the total must be ≥11   **TOTAL = _____**

```
  1    2    3    4    5    6    7    8    9   10   11   12   13   14   15
  |    |    |    |    |    |    |    |    |    |    |    |    |    |    |
```

Not Acceptable   **Meets**   **Exceeds**
                          Minimum Standards   **Minimum Standards**

TEST ENVIRONMENTS

L: Laboratory/Classroom Testing
C: Clinical/Field Testing
P: Practicum Testing
A: Assessment/Mock Exam Testing
S: Self-Reporting

SKILL TEST INFORMATION

Finding:	Range of motion (ROM)
Involved Structure:	Metacarpophalangeal joint
Special Considerations:	N/A
Reference(s):	Norkin et al
Supplies Needed:	Small goniometer, dot/marker, table, chair

THERAPEUTIC MEASUREMENTS
(TM-U-Test 10)

Peer Review _____ Peer Review _____

Skill Acquisition: _____   Practice Opportunities: _____

Using a fully inflated basketball and a flat surface (eg, floor), develop a **Balance Test** *that helps assess* **upper extremity proprioception**. *You have 3 minutes to develop and complete this task.*

Tester places athlete and limb in appropriate position	Test 1	Test 2	Test 3
Prone (push-up position)	Ⓨ Ⓝ	Ⓨ Ⓝ	Ⓨ Ⓝ
Tester performs test according to accepted guidelines	**Test 1**	**Test 2**	**Test 3**
Places the basketball under the athlete's uninvolved limb	Ⓨ Ⓝ	Ⓨ Ⓝ	Ⓨ Ⓝ
Moves the opposite limb away from the floor	Ⓨ Ⓝ	Ⓨ Ⓝ	Ⓨ Ⓝ
Instructs the athlete to balance on the uninvolved limb (as long possible or for a maximum of 1 minute)	Ⓨ Ⓝ	Ⓨ Ⓝ	Ⓨ Ⓝ
Repeats the above three steps with the involved limb	Ⓨ Ⓝ	Ⓨ Ⓝ	Ⓨ Ⓝ
Compares time in a balanced position (to determine deficit)	Ⓨ Ⓝ	Ⓨ Ⓝ	Ⓨ Ⓝ

The psychomotor skill was performed completely and in the appropriate order   **0 1 2 3 4 5**

The tester had control of the subject and the situation (showed confidence)   **0 1 2 3 4 5**

Method of performing the skill allowed the tester the ability to determine:
severity, proper progression, and the *fit* in the overall picture (Oral)   **0 1 2 3 4 5**

In order for a grade of *minimum standard* to be given, the total must be ≥11   **TOTAL = _____**

| 1 | 2 | 3 | 4 | 5 | 6 | 7 | 8 | 9 | 10 | 11 | 12 | 13 | 14 | 15 |

Not Acceptable   **Meets**   **Exceeds**
                              Minimum Standards   **Minimum Standards**

TEST ENVIRONMENTS	**SKILL TEST INFORMATION**	
L: Laboratory/Classroom Testing	**Positive Finding:**	Proprioception development
C: Clinical/Field Testing	**Involved Structure:**	Muscle spindles, etc
P: Practicum Testing	**Special Considerations:**	N/A
A: Assessment/Mock Exam Testing	**Reference(s):**	Prentice (2004)
S: Self-Reporting	**Supplies Needed:**	Stop watch, fully inflated ball

THERAPEUTIC MEASUREMENTS
(TM-U-Test 11)

Peer Review _____ Peer Review _____

Skill Acquisition: _____   Practice Opportunities: _____

Using a 10-pound dumbbell, develop an **Endurance-Based Strength Test** *in order to determine the percent fatigue of the* **middle deltoid muscle**. *This type of testing is also known as a "*% **Fatigue Test**.*" You have 3 minutes to develop and administer this test.*

Tester places athlete and limb in appropriate position	Test 1	Test 2	Test 3
Standing or seated	Ⓨ Ⓝ	Ⓨ Ⓝ	Ⓨ Ⓝ
Arms hanging to the side	Ⓨ Ⓝ	Ⓨ Ⓝ	Ⓨ Ⓝ
Tester performs test according to accepted guidelines	**Test 1**	**Test 2**	**Test 3**
Instructs the athlete to hold a 10-lb dumbbell with the uninvolved limb	Ⓨ Ⓝ	Ⓨ Ⓝ	Ⓨ Ⓝ
Instructs the athlete to fully abduct the shoulder (slow, controlled pace)	Ⓨ Ⓝ	Ⓨ Ⓝ	Ⓨ Ⓝ
Continues until the athlete cannot complete the next repetition or for 1 minute continuously (count the number of repetitions completed)	Ⓨ Ⓝ	Ⓨ Ⓝ	Ⓨ Ⓝ
Repeats the above three steps with the involved limb	Ⓨ Ⓝ	Ⓨ Ⓝ	Ⓨ Ⓝ
Compares the number of repetitions completed (determines deficit)	Ⓨ Ⓝ	Ⓨ Ⓝ	Ⓨ Ⓝ

The psychomotor skill was performed completely and in the appropriate order   **0 1 2 3 4 5**

The tester had control of the subject and the situation (showed confidence)   **0 1 2 3 4 5**

Method of performing the skill allowed the tester the ability to determine:
severity, proper progression, and the *fit* in the overall picture (Oral)   **0 1 2 3 4 5**

In order for a grade of *minimum standard* to be given, the total must be ≥11   **TOTAL = _____**

```
 1    2    3    4    5    6    7    8    9   10   11   12   13   14   15
 |----|----|----|----|----|----|----|----|----|----|----|----|----|----|
Not Acceptable                          Meets              Exceeds
                                  Minimum Standards    Minimum Standards
```

TEST ENVIRONMENTS

L: Laboratory/Classroom Testing
C: Clinical/Field Testing
P: Practicum Testing
A: Assessment/Mock Exam Testing
S: Self-Reporting

SKILL TEST INFORMATION

Positive Finding: Determine strength deficit
Involved Structure: Middle deltoid
Special Considerations: N/A
Reference(s): Adapted from Baechle et al
Supplies Needed: 10-lb dumbbell, stop watch

THERAPEUTIC MEASUREMENTS
(TM-U-Test 12)

Peer Review _____ Peer Review _____

Skill Acquisition: _____   Practice Opportunities: _____

*Using an imaginary wall pulley ("lateral pulldown" machine), develop a **Strength Test** in order to determine a 10 RM for an athlete's **shoulder extensors**. This type of testing is also known as "% **1 x 10 Test.**" You have 3 minutes to develop and administer this test.*

Tester places athlete and limb in appropriate position	Test 1	Test 2	Test 3
Seated or kneeling	Ⓨ Ⓝ	Ⓨ Ⓝ	Ⓨ Ⓝ
Tester performs test according to accepted guidelines	**Test 1**	**Test 2**	**Test 3**
Instructs the athlete to grip the wall pulley/lateral pulldown machine with the uninvolved limb	Ⓨ Ⓝ	Ⓨ Ⓝ	Ⓨ Ⓝ
Instructs the athlete to fully adduct the shoulder and flex the elbow (slow, controlled pace)	Ⓨ Ⓝ	Ⓨ Ⓝ	Ⓨ Ⓝ
Continues until the athlete cannot complete the 11th repetition (during this simulation, the amount of weight is only a guess; choose a weight that the uninvolved limb can only do 10 times)	Ⓨ Ⓝ	Ⓨ Ⓝ	Ⓨ Ⓝ
Repeats the above three steps with the involved limb (using the same weight)	Ⓨ Ⓝ	Ⓨ Ⓝ	Ⓨ Ⓝ
Compares the number repetitions completed (to determine deficit)	Ⓨ Ⓝ	Ⓨ Ⓝ	Ⓨ Ⓝ

The psychomotor skill was performed completely and in the appropriate order   **0 1 2 3 4 5**

The tester had control of the subject and the situation (showed confidence)   **0 1 2 3 4 5**

Method of performing the skill allowed the tester the ability to determine:
severity, proper progression, and the *fit* in the overall picture (Oral)   **0 1 2 3 4 5**

In order for a grade of *minimum standard* to be given, the total must be ≥11   **TOTAL = _____**

```
 1    2    3    4    5    6    7    8    9   10   11   12   13   14   15
 |    |    |    |    |    |    |    |    |    |    |    |    |    |    |
```
Not Acceptable   **Meets**   **Exceeds**
                                            Minimum Standards   **Minimum Standards**

TEST ENVIRONMENTS

L: Laboratory/Classroom Testing
C: Clinical/Field Testing
P: Practicum Testing
A: Assessment/Mock Exam Testing
S: Self-Reporting

SKILL TEST INFORMATION

Positive Finding: Determine strength deficit
Involved Structure: Latissimus dorsi, teres major
Special Considerations: N/A
Reference(s): Adapted from Baechle et al
Supplies Needed: Lateral pulldown machine (ideally)

THERAPEUTIC MEASUREMENTS
(TM-U-Test 13)

Peer Review _____ Peer Review _____

Skill Acquisition: _____   Practice Opportunities: _____

Using a dumbbell, develop a **Strength Test** *in order to determine a 5 RM for an athlete's* **wrist flexors.** *This type of testing is also known as a "% 1 x 5 Test." You have 3 minutes to develop and administer this test.*

Tester places athlete and limb in appropriate position	Test 1	Test 2	Test 3
Seated	Ⓨ Ⓝ	Ⓨ Ⓝ	Ⓨ Ⓝ
Wrist support hanging off the edge of the table	Ⓨ Ⓝ	Ⓨ Ⓝ	Ⓨ Ⓝ
Forearm supinated to 90 degrees	Ⓨ Ⓝ	Ⓨ Ⓝ	Ⓨ Ⓝ
Tester performs test according to accepted guidelines	**Test 1**	**Test 2**	**Test 3**
Instructs the athlete to hold the dumbbell with the uninvolved limb	Ⓨ Ⓝ	Ⓨ Ⓝ	Ⓨ Ⓝ
Instructs the athlete to fully flex the wrist (slow, controlled pace)	Ⓨ Ⓝ	Ⓨ Ⓝ	Ⓨ Ⓝ
Continues until the athlete cannot complete the sixth repetition (during this simulation the amount of weight is only a guess; choose a weight that the uninvolved limb can only do five times)	Ⓨ Ⓝ	Ⓨ Ⓝ	Ⓨ Ⓝ
Repeats the above three steps with the involved limb (using the same weight)	Ⓨ Ⓝ	Ⓨ Ⓝ	Ⓨ Ⓝ
Compares the number repetitions completed (determines deficit)	Ⓨ Ⓝ	Ⓨ Ⓝ	Ⓨ Ⓝ

The psychomotor skill was performed completely and in the appropriate order   **0 1 2 3 4 5**

The tester had control of the subject and the situation (showed confidence)   **0 1 2 3 4 5**

Method of performing the skill allowed the tester the ability to determine: severity, proper progression, and the *fit* in the overall picture (Oral)   **0 1 2 3 4 5**

In order for a grade of *minimum standard* to be given, the total must be ≥11   **TOTAL = _____**

1	2	3	4	5	6	7	8	9	10	11	12	13	14	15

Not Acceptable   **Meets**   **Exceeds**
                              Minimum Standards   **Minimum Standards**

TEST ENVIRONMENTS

L: Laboratory/Classroom Testing
C: Clinical/Field Testing
P: Practicum Testing
A: Assessment/Mock Exam Testing
S: Self-Reporting

SKILL TEST INFORMATION

Positive Finding: Determine strength deficit
Involved Structure: Wrist flexors
Special Considerations: N/A
Reference(s): Adapted from Baechle et al
Supplies Needed: Dumbbells

THERAPEUTIC MEASUREMENTS
(TM-U-Test 14)

Peer Review _____ Peer Review _____

Skill Acquisition: _____   Practice Opportunities: _____

Using a 10-pound dumbbell, develop a **Strength Test** *that will assess power bilaterally for the* **triceps**. *This type of testing is also known as a "% **Power Test**." You have 3 minutes to develop and administer this test.*

Tester places athlete and limb in appropriate position	Test 1	Test 2	Test 3
Supine or seated	Ⓨ Ⓝ	Ⓨ Ⓝ	Ⓨ Ⓝ

Tester performs test according to accepted guidelines	Test 1	Test 2	Test 3
Instructs the athlete to hold the 10-lb dumbbell with the uninvolved limb	Ⓨ Ⓝ	Ⓨ Ⓝ	Ⓨ Ⓝ
Instructs the athlete to fully extend the elbow (as quickly as possible)	Ⓨ Ⓝ	Ⓨ Ⓝ	Ⓨ Ⓝ
Continues contraction as quickly as possible for 20 seconds (during this simulation, the amount of time can vary; it is up to the tester to determine whether the time chosen is appropriate)	Ⓨ Ⓝ	Ⓨ Ⓝ	Ⓨ Ⓝ
Repeats the above three steps with the involved limb (using the same weight and amount of time)	Ⓨ Ⓝ	Ⓨ Ⓝ	Ⓨ Ⓝ
Compares the number repetitions completed (determines deficit)	Ⓨ Ⓝ	Ⓨ Ⓝ	Ⓨ Ⓝ

The psychomotor skill was performed completely and in the appropriate order   0 1 2 3 4 5

The tester had control of the subject and the situation (showed confidence)   0 1 2 3 4 5

Method of performing the skill allowed the tester the ability to determine:
severity, proper progression, and the *fit* in the overall picture (Oral)   0 1 2 3 4 5

In order for a grade of *minimum standard* to be given, the total must be ≥11   **TOTAL = _____**

```
 1    2    3    4    5    6    7    8    9   10   11   12   13   14   15
 |____|____|____|____|____|____|____|____|____|____|____|____|____|____|
```

Not Acceptable   **Meets**   **Exceeds**
                                    Minimum Standards   **Minimum Standards**

TEST ENVIRONMENTS

L: Laboratory/Classroom Testing
C: Clinical/Field Testing
P: Practicum Testing
A: Assessment/Mock Exam Testing
S: Self-Reporting

SKILL TEST INFORMATION

Positive Finding: Determine strength deficit
Involved Structure: Triceps
Special Considerations: N/A
Reference(s): Adapted from Baechle et al
Supplies Needed: Dumbbell, stop watch

THERAPEUTIC MEASUREMENTS
(TM-U-Test 15)

Peer Review _____ Peer Review _____

Skill Acquisition: _____   Practice Opportunities: _____

This problem allows you the opportunity to set up and assess an athlete using an **Isokinetic Device Test**. *This specific scenario requires you to set up the shoulder for abduction/adduction at 90, 180, and 270 degrees per second. You have 5 minutes to complete this task.*

Tester places athlete and limb in appropriate position	Test 1	Test 2	Test 3
Seated	Y N	Y N	Y N

Tester performs proper set-up of the Isokinetic Device	Test 1	Test 2	Test 3
All components of the isokinetic device are in proper working order	Y N	Y N	Y N
Proper attachments are collected and secured to the isokinetic device	Y N	Y N	Y N
Shoulder joint is in line with the axis of the isokinetic dynamometer	Y N	Y N	Y N
Lever arm is adjusted to match the length of the involved limb	Y N	Y N	Y N
All straps are properly placed and secured (if appropriate)	Y N	Y N	Y N

Tester performs test according to accepted guidelines	Test 1	Test 2	Test 3
Proper warm-up is provided	Y N	Y N	Y N
Proper instructions are given:			
Moves limb through full range of motion	Y N	Y N	Y N
Generates maximal contraction for each repetition	Y N	Y N	Y N
Moves limb as hard and as fast a possible	Y N	Y N	Y N
Velocities are preset at 90/180/270 degrees per second prior to the start of each set	Y N	Y N	Y N
Number of repetitions are given and explained to the athlete	Y N	Y N	Y N
Isokinetic test is administered and recorded/printed	Y N	Y N	Y N

The psychomotor skill was performed completely and in the appropriate order   0 1 2 3 4 5

The tester had control of the subject and the situation (showed confidence)   0 1 2 3 4 5

Method of performing the skill allowed the tester the ability to determine:
severity, proper progression, and the *fit* in the overall picture (Oral)   0 1 2 3 4 5

In order for a grade of *minimum standard* to be given, the total must be ≥11   TOTAL = _____

1	2	3	4	5	6	7	8	9	10	11	12	13	14	15

Not Acceptable   **Meets**   **Exceeds**
                              Minimum Standards   **Minimum Standards**

TEST ENVIRONMENTS

L: Laboratory/Classroom Testing
C: Clinical/Field Testing
P: Practicum Testing
A: Assessment/Mock Exam Testing
S: Self-Reporting

SKILL TEST INFORMATION

Positive Finding: Isokinetic testing
Involved Structure: Abduction/adduction
Special Considerations: Print reports available from testing device
Reference(s): Adapted from Prentice (2004)
Supplies Needed: Isokinetic device

THERAPEUTIC MEASUREMENTS
(TM-U-Test 16)

Peer Review _____ Peer Review _____

Skill Acquisition: _____   Practice Opportunities: _____

*Using a tennis ball, develop a **Functional Test** using only a "short toss," to help assure a safe return to participation for the **upper extremity**. You have 3 minutes to develop and complete this task.*

Tester places athlete and limb in appropriate position	Test 1	Test 2	Test 3
Standing	Ⓨ Ⓝ	Ⓨ Ⓝ	Ⓨ Ⓝ
Tester performs test according to accepted guidelines	**Test 1**	**Test 2**	**Test 3**
Instructs the athlete to go through the motion of throwing and letting go of the tennis ball	Ⓨ Ⓝ	Ⓨ Ⓝ	Ⓨ Ⓝ
Instructs the athlete to throw the ball so it hits a wall about 15 feet away			
Progression: Hits the wall and rolls back to the athlete	Ⓨ Ⓝ	Ⓨ Ⓝ	Ⓨ Ⓝ
Progression: Hits the wall, bounces once, then back to the athlete	Ⓨ Ⓝ	Ⓨ Ⓝ	Ⓨ Ⓝ
Progression: Hits the wall and comes back to the athlete in the air	Ⓨ Ⓝ	Ⓨ Ⓝ	Ⓨ Ⓝ
Instructs the athlete to throw the ball to a partner 20 feet away			
Progression: 1 to 60 throws	Ⓨ Ⓝ	Ⓨ Ⓝ	Ⓨ Ⓝ
Progression: Increases velocity of the throws	Ⓨ Ⓝ	Ⓨ Ⓝ	Ⓨ Ⓝ
Progression: Uses a glove to catch the ball	Ⓨ Ⓝ	Ⓨ Ⓝ	Ⓨ Ⓝ
Instructs the athlete to throw the ball to a partner 30 feet away			
Progression: 1 to 60 throws	Ⓨ Ⓝ	Ⓨ Ⓝ	Ⓨ Ⓝ

The psychomotor skill was performed completely and in the appropriate order   **0 1 2 3 4 5**

The tester had control of the subject and the situation (showed confidence)   **0 1 2 3 4 5**

Method of performing the skill allowed the tester the ability to determine:
severity, proper progression, and the *fit* in the overall picture (Oral)   **0 1 2 3 4 5**

In order for a grade of *minimum standard* to be given, the total must be ≥11   **TOTAL = _____**

```
 1    2    3    4    5    6    7    8    9   10   11   12   13   14   15
 |    |    |    |    |    |    |    |    |    |    |    |    |    |    |
```

Not Acceptable   **Meets**   **Exceeds**
                                Minimum Standards   **Minimum Standards**

TEST ENVIRONMENTS

L: Laboratory/Classroom Testing
C: Clinical/Field Testing
P: Practicum Testing
A: Assessment/Mock Exam Testing
S: Self-Reporting

SKILL TEST INFORMATION

Positive Finding: Throwing progression
Involved Structure: Throwing muscles
Special Considerations: N/A
Reference(s): Adapted from Prentice (2004)
Supplies Needed: Tennis ball, baseball, glove

THERAPEUTIC MEASUREMENTS
(TM-U-Test 17)

Skill Acquisition: _____　　　Practice Opportunities: _____

This problem allows you the opportunity to demonstrate proper technique for objectively measuring **hand and wrist swelling** *using a* **volumometer.** *You have 2 minutes to complete this task.*

Tester places athlete and limb in appropriate position	Test 1	Test 2	Test 3
Standing	Y N	Y N	Y N
Volumometer is placed on a table (the height of the table must allow the hand and wrist to move straight down into the volumometer)	Y N	Y N	Y N
Tank of the volumometer is filled with water to the appropriate markings	Y N	Y N	Y N
Overflow container is placed in the appropriate location on the table	Y N	Y N	Y N
Hand, wrist, and lower forearm are gently immersed into the water	Y N	Y N	Y N
Tester performs test according to accepted guidelines	**Test 1**	**Test 2**	**Test 3**
Collects and measures overflow water	Y N	Y N	Y N
Performs measurement bilaterally	Y N	Y N	Y N
Compares findings	Y N	Y N	Y N

The psychomotor skill was performed completely and in the appropriate order　　0　1　2　3　4　5

The tester had control of the subject and the situation (showed confidence)　　0　1　2　3　4　5

Method of performing the skill allowed the tester the ability to determine:
severity, proper progression, and the *fit* in the overall picture (Oral)　　0　1　2　3　4　5

In order for a grade of *minimum standard* to be given, the total must be ≥11　　TOTAL = _____

```
  1   2   3   4   5   6   7   8   9   10   11   12   13   14   15
  |   |   |   |   |   |   |   |   |   |    |    |    |    |    |
```

Not Acceptable　　　　　　　　　　**Meets**　　　　　　　　**Exceeds**
　　　　　　　　　　　　　　Minimum Standards　　　**Minimum Standards**

TEST ENVIRONMENTS

L: Laboratory/Classroom Testing
C: Clinical/Field Testing
P: Practicum Testing
A: Assessment/Mock Exam Testing
S: Self-Reporting

SKILL TEST INFORMATION

Positive Finding:	Increase/decrease in water displacement
Purpose:	Determine swelling or atrophy at the hand/wrist
Special Considerations:	Difference may be due to limb dominance
Reference(s):	Starkey et al (2002)
Supplies Needed:	Table, volumometer, overflow container, calibrated beaker, water

THERAPEUTIC MEASUREMENTS
(TM-U-Test 18)

Peer Review _____ Peer Review _____

Skill Acquisition: _____   Practice Opportunities: _____

This problem allows you the opportunity to demonstrate the proper technique for objectively measuring hand strength using a **hand grip dynamometer**. *You have 2 minutes to complete this task.*

Tester places athlete and limb in appropriate position	Test 1	Test 2	Test 3
Standing	Ⓨ Ⓝ	Ⓨ Ⓝ	Ⓨ Ⓝ
Arm to the side with the elbow flexed to 90 degrees	Ⓨ Ⓝ	Ⓨ Ⓝ	Ⓨ Ⓝ
Radioulnar joint position at 0 degrees (thumb toward the ceiling)	Ⓨ Ⓝ	Ⓨ Ⓝ	Ⓨ Ⓝ
Tester performs test according to accepted guidelines	**Test 1**	**Test 2**	**Test 3**
Based on hand size, the appropriate setting is selected (1, 1.5, 2, 2.5, 3)	Ⓨ Ⓝ	Ⓨ Ⓝ	Ⓨ Ⓝ
Grasps dynamometer and squeezes the handle with maximum force	Ⓨ Ⓝ	Ⓨ Ⓝ	Ⓨ Ⓝ
Performs measurement bilaterally	Ⓨ Ⓝ	Ⓨ Ⓝ	Ⓨ Ⓝ
Compare findings	Ⓨ Ⓝ	Ⓨ Ⓝ	Ⓨ Ⓝ

The psychomotor skill was performed completely and in the appropriate order   0 1 2 3 4 5

The tester had control of the subject and the situation (showed confidence)   0 1 2 3 4 5

Method of performing the skill allowed the tester the ability to determine:
severity, proper progression, and the *fit* in the overall picture (Oral)   0 1 2 3 4 5

In order for a grade of *minimum standard* to be given, the total must be ≥11   **TOTAL =** _____

```
 1    2    3    4    5    6    7    8    9   10   11   12   13   14   15
 |----|----|----|----|----|----|----|----|----|----|----|----|----|----|
```
Not Acceptable   **Meets**   **Exceeds**
                                          Minimum Standards   **Minimum Standards**

TEST ENVIRONMENTS

L: Laboratory/Classroom Testing
C: Clinical/Field Testing
P: Practicum Testing
A: Assessment/Mock Exam Testing
S: Self-Reporting

SKILL TEST INFORMATION

Positive Finding: Muscle strength not within normal limits

Purpose: Determine muscle strength of the hand

Special Considerations: Do not allow the athlete to use the total body when squeezing the dynamometer

Reference(s): Starkey et al (2002)

Supplies Needed: Hand grip dynamometer

THERAPEUTIC MEASUREMENTS
(TM-U-19)

Skill Acquisition: _____   Practice Opportunities: _____

*This task allows you the opportunity to determine the **body composition** of an athlete using a **skinfold caliper**. You have 3 minutes to complete this task.*

Tester places athlete and limb in appropriate position	Test 1	Test 2	Test 3
Standing	Ⓨ Ⓝ	Ⓨ Ⓝ	Ⓨ Ⓝ
Disrobe to shorts (male) or shorts and a sports bra (female)	Ⓨ Ⓝ	Ⓨ Ⓝ	Ⓨ Ⓝ
Tester placed in proper position (possible landmarks)	**Test 1**	**Test 2**	**Test 3**
Triceps-vertical pinch at midline of posterior upper arm	Ⓨ Ⓝ	Ⓨ Ⓝ	Ⓨ Ⓝ
Subscapular-oblique pinch below bottom tip of the scapula	Ⓨ Ⓝ	Ⓨ Ⓝ	Ⓨ Ⓝ
Suprailiac-oblique pinch just above hip bone	Ⓨ Ⓝ	Ⓨ Ⓝ	Ⓨ Ⓝ
Abdominal-vertical pinch 1 inch to the right of umbilicus	Ⓨ Ⓝ	Ⓨ Ⓝ	Ⓨ Ⓝ
Quadriceps-vertical pinch at midthigh	Ⓨ Ⓝ	Ⓨ Ⓝ	Ⓨ Ⓝ
Tester performs task according to accepted guidelines	**Test 1**	**Test 2**	**Test 3**
All measures should be taken on the right side of the body	Ⓨ Ⓝ	Ⓨ Ⓝ	Ⓨ Ⓝ
Grasps area with thumb and forefinger	Ⓨ Ⓝ	Ⓨ Ⓝ	Ⓨ Ⓝ
Pulls skin and fat away from underlying muscular tissue	Ⓨ Ⓝ	Ⓨ Ⓝ	Ⓨ Ⓝ
Pinches area with caliper	Ⓨ Ⓝ	Ⓨ Ⓝ	Ⓨ Ⓝ
Reads caliper dial within 2 seconds of pinching area	Ⓨ Ⓝ	Ⓨ Ⓝ	Ⓨ Ⓝ
Repeats measurement two to three times for each body site	Ⓨ Ⓝ	Ⓨ Ⓝ	Ⓨ Ⓝ
Takes average of two to three measurements and records results	Ⓨ Ⓝ	Ⓨ Ⓝ	Ⓨ Ⓝ

The psychomotor skill was performed completely and in the appropriate order   0 1 2 3 4 5

The tester had control of the subject and the situation (showed confidence)   0 1 2 3 4 5

Method of performing the skill allowed the tester the ability to determine:
severity, proper progression, and the *fit* in the overall picture (Oral)   0 1 2 3 4 5

In order for a grade of *minimum standard* to be given, the total must be ≥11   TOTAL = _____

```
  1    2    3    4    5    6    7    8    9   10   11   12   13   14   15
  |    |    |    |    |    |    |    |    |    |    |    |    |    |    |
```

Not Acceptable   **Meets**   **Exceeds**
                                    Minimum Standards   **Minimum Standards**

TEST ENVIRONMENTS

L: Laboratory/Classroom Testing
C: Clinical/Field Testing
P: Practicum Testing
A: Assessment/Mock Exam Testing
S: Self-Reporting

SKILL TEST INFORMATION

Positive Finding:	Body composition
Involved Structure:	Muscle/fat
Special Considerations:	N/A
Reference(s):	Manufacturer's recommendations
Supplies Needed:	Caliper, pencil/paper

THERAPEUTIC MEASUREMENTS
(TM-L-Test 1)

Peer Review _____ Peer Review _____

Skill Acquisition: _____   Practice Opportunities: _____

Please demonstrate the proper use of a **goniometer** *for measuring an athlete's ankle active range of motion for inversion/eversion at the* **subtalar joint**. *You have 3 minutes to complete this task.*

Tester places athlete and limb in appropriate position	Test 1	Test 2	Test 3
Prone	Ⓨ Ⓝ	Ⓨ Ⓝ	Ⓨ Ⓝ
Foot place over the edge of the table	Ⓨ Ⓝ	Ⓨ Ⓝ	Ⓨ Ⓝ
Tester provides appropriate stabilization	**Test 1**	**Test 2**	**Test 3**
Tibia and fibula	Ⓨ Ⓝ	Ⓨ Ⓝ	Ⓨ Ⓝ
Tester places goniometer in appropriate position	**Test 1**	**Test 2**	**Test 3**
Fulcrum: Posterior aspect, midway between the malleoli	Ⓨ Ⓝ	Ⓨ Ⓝ	Ⓨ Ⓝ
Stationary arm: Midline of the lower leg	Ⓨ Ⓝ	Ⓨ Ⓝ	Ⓨ Ⓝ
Moving arm: Posterior midline of the calcaneus	Ⓨ Ⓝ	Ⓨ Ⓝ	Ⓨ Ⓝ
Tester performs test according to accepted guidelines	**Test 1**	**Test 2**	**Test 3**
Correct reading: Inversion/eversion	Ⓨ Ⓝ	Ⓨ Ⓝ	Ⓨ Ⓝ
Performs assessment bilaterally	Ⓨ Ⓝ	Ⓨ Ⓝ	Ⓨ Ⓝ

The psychomotor skill was performed completely and in the appropriate order   0 1 2 3 4 5

The tester had control of the subject and the situation (showed confidence)   0 1 2 3 4 5

Method of performing the skill allowed the tester the ability to determine: severity, proper progression, and the *fit* in the overall picture (Oral)   0 1 2 3 4 5

In order for a grade of *minimum standard* to be given, the total must be ≥11   TOTAL = _____

```
 1    2    3    4    5    6    7    8    9   10   11   12   13   14   15
 |    |    |    |    |    |    |    |    |    |    |    |    |    |    |
```

Not Acceptable   **Meets Minimum Standards**   **Exceeds Minimum Standards**

TEST ENVIRONMENTS	**SKILL TEST INFORMATION**
L: Laboratory/Classroom Testing	**Positive Finding:** Range of motion (ROM)
C: Clinical/Field Testing	**Involved Structure:** Subtalar joint
P: Practicum Testing	**Special Considerations:** N/A
A: Assessment/Mock Exam Testing	**Reference(s):** Norkin et al
S: Self-Reporting	**Supplies Needed:** Goniometer, dots/markers

THERAPEUTIC MEASUREMENTS
(TM-L-Test 2)

Peer Review _____ Peer Review _____

Skill Acquisition: _____   Practice Opportunities: _____

Please demonstrate the proper use of a **goniometer** *for measuring an athlete's ankle active range of motion for dorsiflexion at the* **talocrural joint***. You have 2 minutes to complete this task.*

Tester places athlete and limb in appropriate position	Test 1	Test 2	Test 3
Supine or seated	Ⓨ Ⓝ	Ⓨ Ⓝ	Ⓨ Ⓝ
Knee flexed to 90 degrees	Ⓨ Ⓝ	Ⓨ Ⓝ	Ⓨ Ⓝ
Foot dorsiflexed to 0 degrees	Ⓨ Ⓝ	Ⓨ Ⓝ	Ⓨ Ⓝ
Tester provides appropriate stabilization	**Test 1**	**Test 2**	**Test 3**
Tibia and fibula	Ⓨ Ⓝ	Ⓨ Ⓝ	Ⓨ Ⓝ
Tester places goniometer in appropriate position	**Test 1**	**Test 2**	**Test 3**
Fulcrum: Lateral malleolus	Ⓨ Ⓝ	Ⓨ Ⓝ	Ⓨ Ⓝ
Stationary arm: Lateral midline of the fibula (reference head of the fibula)	Ⓨ Ⓝ	Ⓨ Ⓝ	Ⓨ Ⓝ
Moving arm: Parallel to the lateral aspect of the fifth metatarsal	Ⓨ Ⓝ	Ⓨ Ⓝ	Ⓨ Ⓝ
Tester performs test according to accepted guidelines	**Test 1**	**Test 2**	**Test 3**
Correct reading: Dorsiflexion	Ⓨ Ⓝ	Ⓨ Ⓝ	Ⓨ Ⓝ
Performs assessment bilaterally	Ⓨ Ⓝ	Ⓨ Ⓝ	Ⓨ Ⓝ

The psychomotor skill was performed completely and in the appropriate order   0 1 2 3 4 5

The tester had control of the subject and the situation (showed confidence)   0 1 2 3 4 5

Method of performing the skill allowed the tester the ability to determine:
severity, proper progression, and the *fit* in the overall picture (Oral)   0 1 2 3 4 5

In order for a grade of *minimum standard* to be given, the total must be ≥11   TOTAL = _____

```
  1   2   3   4   5   6   7   8   9   10  11  12  13  14  15
  |   |   |   |   |   |   |   |   |   |   |   |   |   |   |
```

Not Acceptable   **Meets**   **Exceeds**
                              Minimum Standards   **Minimum Standards**

TEST ENVIRONMENTS

L: Laboratory/Classroom Testing
C: Clinical/Field Testing
P: Practicum Testing
A: Assessment/Mock Exam Testing
S: Self-Reporting

SKILL TEST INFORMATION

Positive Finding:	Range of motion (ROM)
Involved Structure:	Talocrural joint
Special Considerations:	N/A
Reference(s):	Norkin et al
Supplies Needed:	Goniometer, dots/markers, table

THERAPEUTIC MEASUREMENTS
(TM-L-Test 3)

Peer Review _____ Peer Review _____

Skill Acquisition: _____   Practice Opportunities: _____

*Please demonstrate the proper use of a **goniometer** for measuring an athlete's knee active range of motion for flexion at the **tibiofemoral joint**. You have 3 minutes to complete this task.*

Tester places athlete and limb in appropriate position	Test 1	Test 2	Test 3
Supine	Ⓨ Ⓝ	Ⓨ Ⓝ	Ⓨ Ⓝ
Hip/knee in anatomical position	Ⓨ Ⓝ	Ⓨ Ⓝ	Ⓨ Ⓝ
Tester provides appropriate stabilization	**Test 1**	**Test 2**	**Test 3**
Femur	Ⓨ Ⓝ	Ⓨ Ⓝ	Ⓨ Ⓝ
Tester places goniometer in appropriate position	**Test 1**	**Test 2**	**Test 3**
Fulcrum: Lateral epicondyle of the femur	Ⓨ Ⓝ	Ⓨ Ⓝ	Ⓨ Ⓝ
Stationary arm: Lateral midline of the femur (reference greater trochanter)	Ⓨ Ⓝ	Ⓨ Ⓝ	Ⓨ Ⓝ
Moving arm: Lateral midline of the fibula (reference lateral malleolus)	Ⓨ Ⓝ	Ⓨ Ⓝ	Ⓨ Ⓝ
Tester performs test according to accepted guidelines	**Test 1**	**Test 2**	**Test 3**
Correct reading: Flexion	Ⓨ Ⓝ	Ⓨ Ⓝ	Ⓨ Ⓝ
Performs assessment bilaterally	Ⓨ Ⓝ	Ⓨ Ⓝ	Ⓨ Ⓝ

The psychomotor skill was performed completely and in the appropriate order   0 1 2 3 4 5

The tester had control of the subject and the situation (showed confidence)   0 1 2 3 4 5

Method of performing the skill allowed the tester the ability to determine:
severity, proper progression, and the *fit* in the overall picture (Oral)   0 1 2 3 4 5

In order for a grade of *minimum standard* to be given, the total must be ≥11   TOTAL = _____

1   2   3   4   5   6   7   8   9   10   11   12   13   14   15

Not Acceptable   **Meets**   **Exceeds**
                              Minimum Standards **Minimum Standards**

TEST ENVIRONMENTS

L: Laboratory/Classroom Testing
C: Clinical/Field Testing
P: Practicum Testing
A: Assessment/Mock Exam Testing
S: Self-Reporting

SKILL TEST INFORMATION

Positive Finding: Range of motion
Involved Structure: Tibiofemoral joint (knee)
Special Considerations: Maybe done in a prone position
Reference(s): Norkin et al
Supplies Needed: Goniometer, dots/markers, table

THERAPEUTIC MEASUREMENTS
(TM-L-Test 4)

Peer Review _____ Peer Review _____

Skill Acquisition: _____   Practice Opportunities: _____

*Please demonstrate the proper use of a **goniometer** for measuring an athlete's hip active range of motion for abduction at the **iliofemoral joint**. You have 3 minutes to complete this task.*

Tester places athlete and limb in appropriate position	Test 1	Test 2	Test 3
Supine	Ⓨ Ⓝ	Ⓨ Ⓝ	Ⓨ Ⓝ
Hip/knee in anatomical position	Ⓨ Ⓝ	Ⓨ Ⓝ	Ⓨ Ⓝ
Tester provides appropriate stabilization	**Test 1**	**Test 2**	**Test 3**
Pelvis	Ⓨ Ⓝ	Ⓨ Ⓝ	Ⓨ Ⓝ
Tester places goniometer in appropriate position	**Test 1**	**Test 2**	**Test 3**
Fulcrum: ASIS of extremity being tested	Ⓨ Ⓝ	Ⓨ Ⓝ	Ⓨ Ⓝ
Stationary arm: ASIS of extremity not being tested	Ⓨ Ⓝ	Ⓨ Ⓝ	Ⓨ Ⓝ
Moving arm: Anterior midline of the femur (reference patella)	Ⓨ Ⓝ	Ⓨ Ⓝ	Ⓨ Ⓝ
Tester performs test according to accepted guidelines	**Test 1**	**Test 2**	**Test 3**
Correct reading: Abduction	Ⓨ Ⓝ	Ⓨ Ⓝ	Ⓨ Ⓝ
Performs assessment bilaterally	Ⓨ Ⓝ	Ⓨ Ⓝ	Ⓨ Ⓝ

The psychomotor skill was performed completely and in the appropriate order   0 1 2 3 4 5

The tester had control of the subject and the situation (showed confidence)   0 1 2 3 4 5

Method of performing the skill allowed the tester the ability to determine:
severity, proper progression, and the *fit* in the overall picture (Oral)   0 1 2 3 4 5

In order for a grade of *minimum standard* to be given, the total must be ≥11   TOTAL = _____

```
  1    2    3    4    5    6    7    8    9   10   11   12   13   14   15
  |    |    |    |    |    |    |    |    |    |    |    |    |    |    |
```
Not Acceptable   **Meets**   **Exceeds**
                                       Minimum Standards   **Minimum Standards**

TEST ENVIRONMENTS	SKILL TEST INFORMATION	
L: Laboratory/Classroom Testing	**Positive Finding:**	Range of motion (ROM)
C: Clinical/Field Testing	**Involved Structure:**	Iliofemoral joint (hip)
P: Practicum Testing	**Special Considerations:**	N/A
A: Assessment/Mock Exam Testing	**Reference(s):**	Norkin et al
S: Self-Reporting	**Supplies Needed:**	Goniometer, dots/markers, table

THERAPEUTIC MEASUREMENTS
(TM-L-Test 5)

Peer Review _____ Peer Review _____

Skill Acquisition: _____   Practice Opportunities: _____

Please demonstrate the proper use of a **goniometer** *for measuring an athlete's hip active range of motion for lateral (external) rotation at the* **iliofemoral joint.** *You have 3 minutes to complete this task.*

Tester places athlete and limb in appropriate position	Test 1	Test 2	Test 3
Seated (knee flexed to 90 degrees)	Ⓨ Ⓝ	Ⓨ Ⓝ	Ⓨ Ⓝ
Hip in anatomical position	Ⓨ Ⓝ	Ⓨ Ⓝ	Ⓨ Ⓝ
Towel roll under distal end of femur	Ⓨ Ⓝ	Ⓨ Ⓝ	Ⓨ Ⓝ
Tester provides appropriate stabilization	**Test 1**	**Test 2**	**Test 3**
Distal end of femur	Ⓨ Ⓝ	Ⓨ Ⓝ	Ⓨ Ⓝ
Tester places goniometer in appropriate position	**Test 1**	**Test 2**	**Test 3**
Fulcrum: Anterior aspect of the patella	Ⓨ Ⓝ	Ⓨ Ⓝ	Ⓨ Ⓝ
Stationary arm: Perpendicular to or parallel to the floor	Ⓨ Ⓝ	Ⓨ Ⓝ	Ⓨ Ⓝ
Moving arm: Anterior midline of lower leg	Ⓨ Ⓝ	Ⓨ Ⓝ	Ⓨ Ⓝ
Tester performs test according to accepted guidelines	**Test 1**	**Test 2**	**Test 3**
Correct reading: Lateral/external rotation	Ⓨ Ⓝ	Ⓨ Ⓝ	Ⓨ Ⓝ
Performs assessment bilaterally	Ⓨ Ⓝ	Ⓨ Ⓝ	Ⓨ Ⓝ

The psychomotor skill was performed completely and in the appropriate order   0 1 2 3 4 5

The tester had control of the subject and the situation (showed confidence)   0 1 2 3 4 5

Method of performing the skill allowed the tester the ability to determine:
severity, proper progression, and the *fit* in the overall picture (Oral)   0 1 2 3 4 5

In order for a grade of *minimum standard* to be given, the total must be ≥11   TOTAL = _____

```
  1    2    3    4    5    6    7    8    9   10   11   12   13   14   15
  |----|----|----|----|----|----|----|----|----|----|----|----|----|----|
```

Not Acceptable   **Meets**   **Exceeds**
                                  Minimum Standards   **Minimum Standards**

TEST ENVIRONMENTS

L: Laboratory/Classroom Testing
C: Clinical/Field Testing
P: Practicum Testing
A: Assessment/Mock Exam Testing
S: Self-Reporting

SKILL TEST INFORMATION

Positive Finding: Range of motion (ROM)
Involved Structure: Iliofemoral joint (Hip)
Special Considerations: N/A
Reference(s): Norkin et al
Supplies Needed: Goniometer, dot/marker, table

THERAPEUTIC MEASUREMENTS
(TM-L-Test 6)

Peer Review _____ Peer Review _____

Skill Acquisition: _____   Practice Opportunities: _____

Please demonstrate the proper use of a **goniometer** *for measuring an athlete's hip active range of motion for* **extension at the iliofemoral joint**. *You have 3 minutes to complete this task.*

Tester places athlete and limb in appropriate position	Test 1	Test 2	Test 3
Prone	Ⓨ Ⓝ	Ⓨ Ⓝ	Ⓨ Ⓝ
Hip/knee in anatomical position	Ⓨ Ⓝ	Ⓨ Ⓝ	Ⓨ Ⓝ
Tester provides appropriate stabilization	**Test 1**	**Test 2**	**Test 3**
Pelvis (prevents anterior tilt)	Ⓨ Ⓝ	Ⓨ Ⓝ	Ⓨ Ⓝ
Tester places goniometer in appropriate position	**Test 1**	**Test 2**	**Test 3**
Fulcrum: greater trochanter of the femur	Ⓨ Ⓝ	Ⓨ Ⓝ	Ⓨ Ⓝ
Stationary arm: Midline of the pelvis	Ⓨ Ⓝ	Ⓨ Ⓝ	Ⓨ Ⓝ
Moving arm: Lateral epicondyle of the femur	Ⓨ Ⓝ	Ⓨ Ⓝ	Ⓨ Ⓝ
Tester performs test according to accepted guidelines	**Test 1**	**Test 2**	**Test 3**
Correct reading: Extension	Ⓨ Ⓝ	Ⓨ Ⓝ	Ⓨ Ⓝ
Performs assessment bilaterally	Ⓨ Ⓝ	Ⓨ Ⓝ	Ⓨ Ⓝ

The psychomotor skill was performed completely and in the appropriate order   0 1 2 3 4 5

The tester had control of the subject and the situation (showed confidence)   0 1 2 3 4 5

Method of performing the skill allowed the tester the ability to determine:
severity, proper progression, and the *fit* in the overall picture (Oral)   0 1 2 3 4 5

In order for a grade of *minimum standard* to be given, the total must be ≥11   TOTAL = _____

| 1 | 2 | 3 | 4 | 5 | 6 | 7 | 8 | 9 | 10 | 11 | 12 | 13 | 14 | 15 |

Not Acceptable   **Meets**   **Exceeds**
                          Minimum Standards   **Minimum Standards**

TEST ENVIRONMENTS

L: Laboratory/Classroom Testing
C: Clinical/Field Testing
P: Practicum Testing
A: Assessment/Mock Exam Testing
S: Self-Reporting

SKILL TEST INFORMATION

Positive Finding: Range of motion (ROM)
Involved Structure: Iliofemoral joint (Hip)
Special Considerations: N/A
Reference(s): Norkin et al
Supplies Needed: Goniometer, dot/marker, table

THERAPEUTIC MEASUREMENTS
(TM-L-Test 7)

Peer Review _____ Peer Review _____

Skill Acquisition: _____   Practice Opportunities: _____

Please demonstrate the proper use of a **goniometer** *for measuring an athlete's hip active range of motion for* **flexion at the ilio-femoral joint.** *You have 3 minutes to complete this task.*

Tester places athlete and limb in appropriate position	Test 1	Test 2	Test 3
Supine	Ⓨ Ⓝ	Ⓨ Ⓝ	Ⓨ Ⓝ
Hip/knee in anatomical position	Ⓨ Ⓝ	Ⓨ Ⓝ	Ⓨ Ⓝ
Tester provides appropriate stabilization	**Test 1**	**Test 2**	**Test 3**
Pelvis (prevents posterior tilting and rotation)	Ⓨ Ⓝ	Ⓨ Ⓝ	Ⓨ Ⓝ
Tester places goniometer in appropriate position	**Test 1**	**Test 2**	**Test 3**
Fulcrum: Greater trochanter of the femur	Ⓨ Ⓝ	Ⓨ Ⓝ	Ⓨ Ⓝ
Stationary arm: Midline of the pelvis	Ⓨ Ⓝ	Ⓨ Ⓝ	Ⓨ Ⓝ
Moving arm: Lateral epicondyle of the femur	Ⓨ Ⓝ	Ⓨ Ⓝ	Ⓨ Ⓝ
Tester performs test according to accepted guidelines	**Test 1**	**Test 2**	**Test 3**
Correct reading: Flexion (allows knee to actively flex while hip moves into flexion)	Ⓨ Ⓝ	Ⓨ Ⓝ	Ⓨ Ⓝ
Performs assessment bilaterally	Ⓨ Ⓝ	Ⓨ Ⓝ	Ⓨ Ⓝ

The psychomotor skill was performed completely and in the appropriate order   0 1 2 3 4 5

The tester had control of the subject and the situation (showed confidence)   0 1 2 3 4 5

Method of performing the skill allowed the tester the ability to determine:
severity, proper progression, and the *fit* in the overall picture (Oral)   0 1 2 3 4 5

In order for a grade of *minimum standard* to be given, the total must be ≥11   TOTAL = _____

1 2 3 4 5 6 7 8 9 10 11 12 13 14 15

Not Acceptable   **Meets Minimum Standards**   **Exceeds Minimum Standards**

TEST ENVIRONMENTS
L: Laboratory/Classroom Testing
C: Clinical/Field Testing
P: Practicum Testing
A: Assessment/Mock Exam Testing
S: Self-Reporting

SKILL TEST INFORMATION
Positive Finding: Range of motion (ROM)
Involved Structure: Iliofemoral joint (Hip)
Special Considerations: N/A
Reference(s): Norkin et al
Supplies Needed: Goniometer, dot/marker, table

THERAPEUTIC MEASUREMENTS
(TM-L-Test 8)

Peer Review _____ Peer Review _____

Skill Acquisition: _____   Practice Opportunities: _____

Please demonstrate the proper use of a **goniometer** *for measuring an athlete's* **trunk** *active range of motion for* **lateral rotation to the left.** *You have 3 minutes to complete this task.*

Tester places athlete and limb in appropriate position	Test 1	Test 2	Test 3
Seated on a stool with feet on the ground	Ⓨ Ⓝ	Ⓨ Ⓝ	Ⓨ Ⓝ
Cervical/thoracic/lumbar spine in anatomical position	Ⓨ Ⓝ	Ⓨ Ⓝ	Ⓨ Ⓝ
Tester provides appropriate stabilization	**Test 1**	**Test 2**	**Test 3**
Pelvis	Ⓨ Ⓝ	Ⓨ Ⓝ	Ⓨ Ⓝ
Tester places goniometer in appropriate position	**Test 1**	**Test 2**	**Test 3**
Fulcrum: Over the center of the cranial aspect of the head	Ⓨ Ⓝ	Ⓨ Ⓝ	Ⓨ Ⓝ
Stationary arm: Parallel to the line between the two prominent tubercles on the iliac crest	Ⓨ Ⓝ	Ⓨ Ⓝ	Ⓨ Ⓝ
Moving arm: Distal with a line between the two acromial processes	Ⓨ Ⓝ	Ⓨ Ⓝ	Ⓨ Ⓝ
Tester performs test according to accepted guidelines	**Test 1**	**Test 2**	**Test 3**
Correct reading: Lateral rotation left	Ⓨ Ⓝ	Ⓨ Ⓝ	Ⓨ Ⓝ
Performs assessment bilaterally	Ⓨ Ⓝ	Ⓨ Ⓝ	Ⓨ Ⓝ

The psychomotor skill was performed completely and in the appropriate order   0 1 2 3 4 5

The tester had control of the subject and the situation (showed confidence)   0 1 2 3 4 5

Method of performing the skill allowed the tester the ability to determine:
severity, proper progression, and the *fit* in the overall picture (Oral)   0 1 2 3 4 5

In order for a grade of *minimum standard* to be given, the total must be ≥11   TOTAL = _____

```
  1    2    3    4    5    6    7    8    9   10   11   12   13   14   15
  |----|----|----|----|----|----|----|----|----|----|----|----|----|----|
```

Not Acceptable   **Meets**   **Exceeds**
                                          Minimum Standards   **Minimum Standards**

TEST ENVIRONMENTS

L: Laboratory/Classroom Testing
C: Clinical/Field Testing
P: Practicum Testing
A: Assessment/Mock Exam Testing
S: Self-Reporting

SKILL TEST INFORMATION

Positive Finding:	Range of motion (ROM)
Involved Structure:	Trunk
Special Considerations:	N/A
Reference(s):	Norkin et al
Supplies Needed:	Goniometer, dots/markers, stationary stool

THERAPEUTIC MEASUREMENTS
(TM-L-Test 9)

Peer Review _____ Peer Review _____

Skill Acquisition: _____　　　Practice Opportunities: _____

Using a partially deflated soccer ball, develop a **Balance Test** *that helps assess* **lower extremity proprioception.** *You have 3 minutes to develop and complete this task.*

Tester places athlete and limb in appropriate position	Test 1	Test 2	Test 3
Standing	Ⓨ Ⓝ	Ⓨ Ⓝ	Ⓨ Ⓝ
Tester performs test according to accepted guidelines	**Test 1**	**Test 2**	**Test 3**
Places a deflated soccer ball under the athlete's uninvolved limb	Ⓨ Ⓝ	Ⓨ Ⓝ	Ⓨ Ⓝ
Removes the opposite limb away from the floor	Ⓨ Ⓝ	Ⓨ Ⓝ	Ⓨ Ⓝ
Instructs the athlete to balance on the uninvolved limb (as long as possible or for a maximum of 1 minute)	Ⓨ Ⓝ	Ⓨ Ⓝ	Ⓨ Ⓝ
Repeats the above three steps with the involved limb	Ⓨ Ⓝ	Ⓨ Ⓝ	Ⓨ Ⓝ
Compares time in a balanced position (to determine deficit)	Ⓨ Ⓝ	Ⓨ Ⓝ	Ⓨ Ⓝ

The psychomotor skill was performed completely and in the appropriate order　　0　1　2　3　4　5

The tester had control of the subject and the situation (showed confidence)　　0　1　2　3　4　5

Method of performing the skill allowed the tester the ability to determine: severity, proper progression, and the *fit* in the overall picture (Oral)　　0　1　2　3　4　5

In order for a grade of *minimum standard* to be given, the total must be ≥11　　TOTAL = _____

```
 1    2    3    4    5    6    7    8    9    10   11   12   13   14   15
 |    |    |    |    |    |    |    |    |    |    |    |    |    |    |
```
Not Acceptable　　　　　　　　　　　　　　　　　**Meets**　　　　　　　**Exceeds**
　　　　　　　　　　　　　　　　　　　　　　Minimum Standards　**Minimum Standards**

TEST ENVIRONMENTS

L: Laboratory/Classroom Testing
C: Clinical/Field Testing
P: Practicum Testing
A: Assessment/Mock Exam Testing
S: Self-Reporting

SKILL TEST INFORMATION

Positive Finding: Proprioception development
Involved Structure: Muscle spindles, etc
Special Considerations: N/A
Reference(s): Adapted from Prentice (2004)
Supplies Needed: Stopwatch, deflated soccer ball

THERAPEUTIC MEASUREMENTS
(TM-L-Test 10)

Peer Review _____ Peer Review _____

Skill Acquisition: _____   Practice Opportunities: _____

Using a 10-pound cuff weight, develop an **Endurance-Based Strength Test** *in order to determine the percent fatigue of the* **tibialis anterior**. *This type of testing is also known as a "*% **Fatigue Test**.*" You have 3 minutes to develop and administer this test.*

Tester places athlete and limb in appropriate position	Test 1	Test 2	Test 3
Seated (leg off the table)	Y N	Y N	Y N
Knee flexed to 90 degrees	Y N	Y N	Y N

Tester performs test according to accepted guidelines	Test 1	Test 2	Test 3
Fastens the 10-lb cuff weight around the foot of the uninvolved limb	Y N	Y N	Y N
Instructs the athlete to fully dorsiflex the ankle (slow, controlled pace)	Y N	Y N	Y N
Continues until the athlete cannot complete the next repetition or for 1 minute continuously (count the number of repetitions completed)	Y N	Y N	Y N
Repeats the above three steps with the involved limb	Y N	Y N	Y N
Compares the number of repetitions completed (to determine deficit)	Y N	Y N	Y N

The psychomotor skill was performed completely and in the appropriate order   0 1 2 3 4 5

The tester had control of the subject and the situation (showed confidence)   0 1 2 3 4 5

Method of performing the skill allowed the tester the ability to determine:
severity, proper progression, and the *fit* in the overall picture (Oral)   0 1 2 3 4 5

In order for a grade of *minimum standard* to be given, the total must be ≥11   **TOTAL = _____**

```
1    2    3    4    5    6    7    8    9    10   11   12   13   14   15
|____|____|____|____|____|____|____|____|____|____|____|____|____|____|
```

Not Acceptable   **Meets**   **Exceeds**
                                    Minimum Standards   **Minimum Standards**

TEST ENVIRONMENTS
L: Laboratory/Classroom Testing
C: Clinical/Field Testing
P: Practicum Testing
A: Assessment/Mock Exam Testing
S: Self-Reporting

SKILL TEST INFORMATION
Positive Finding: Determine strength deficit
Involved Structure: Tibialis anterior
Special Considerations: N/A
Reference(s): Adapted from Baechle et al
Supplies Needed: Cuff weight, stopwatch

THERAPEUTIC MEASUREMENTS
(TM-L-Test 11)

Peer Review _____   Peer Review _____

Skill Acquisition: _____   Practice Opportunities: _____

Using an imaginary prone leg curl machine (knee curl), develop a **Strength Test** *in order to determine a 10 RM for an athlete's* **hamstrings**. *This type of testing is also known as "% **1 x 10 Test**." You have 3 minutes to develop and administer this test.'*

Tester places athlete and limb in appropriate position	Test 1	Test 2	Test 3
Prone	Ⓨ Ⓝ	Ⓨ Ⓝ	Ⓨ Ⓝ

Tester performs test according to accepted guidelines	Test 1	Test 2	Test 3
Selects the appropriate weight needed for the uninvolved limb	Ⓨ Ⓝ	Ⓨ Ⓝ	Ⓨ Ⓝ
Instructs the athlete to fully flex the knee (slow, controlled pace)	Ⓨ Ⓝ	Ⓨ Ⓝ	Ⓨ Ⓝ
Continues until the athlete cannot complete the 11th repetition (during this simulation, the amount of weight is only a guess; choose a weight that the uninvolved limb can only do 10 times)	Ⓨ Ⓝ	Ⓨ Ⓝ	Ⓨ Ⓝ
Repeats the above three steps with the involved limb (using the same weight)	Ⓨ Ⓝ	Ⓨ Ⓝ	Ⓨ Ⓝ
Compares the number of repetitions completed (to determine deficit)	Ⓨ Ⓝ	Ⓨ Ⓝ	Ⓨ Ⓝ

The psychomotor skill was performed completely and in the appropriate order   0 1 2 3 4 5

The tester had control of the subject and the situation (showed confidence)   0 1 2 3 4 5

Method of performing the skill allowed the tester the ability to determine: severity, proper progression, and the *fit* in the overall picture (Oral)   0 1 2 3 4 5

In order for a grade of *minimum standard* to be given, the total must be ≥11   **TOTAL = _____**

1	2	3	4	5	6	7	8	9	10	11	12	13	14	15

Not Acceptable   **Meets**   **Exceeds**
                              Minimum Standards   **Minimum Standards**

TEST ENVIRONMENTS

L: Laboratory/Classroom Testing
C: Clinical/Field Testing
P: Practicum Testing
A: Assessment/Mock Exam Testing
S: Self-Reporting

SKILL TEST INFORMATION

Positive Finding:	Determine strength deficit
Involved Structure:	Hamstrings
Special Considerations:	N/A
Reference(s):	Adapted from Baechle et al
Supplies Needed:	Cuff weight, table (leg curl machine ideally)

THERAPEUTIC MEASUREMENTS
(TM-L-Test 12)

Peer Review _____ Peer Review _____

Skill Acquisition: _____   Practice Opportunities: _____

Using an imaginary leg press machine, develop a **Strength Test** *in order to determine a 5 RM for an athlete's* **ankle plantar flexors**. *This type of testing is also known as a* "**% 1 x 5 Test**." *You have 3 minutes to develop and administer this test.*

Tester places athlete and limb in appropriate position	Test 1	Test 2	Test 3
Seated	Ⓨ Ⓝ	Ⓨ Ⓝ	Ⓨ Ⓝ
Knee extended to 0 degrees	Ⓨ Ⓝ	Ⓨ Ⓝ	Ⓨ Ⓝ
Tester performs test according to accepted guidelines	**Test 1**	**Test 2**	**Test 3**
Selects the appropriate weight needed for the uninvolved limb	Ⓨ Ⓝ	Ⓨ Ⓝ	Ⓨ Ⓝ
Instructs the athlete to fully plantar flex the ankle (slow, controlled pace)	Ⓨ Ⓝ	Ⓨ Ⓝ	Ⓨ Ⓝ
Continues until the athlete cannot complete the sixth repetition (during this simulation the amount of weight is only a guess; choose a weight that the uninvolved limb can only do five times)	Ⓨ Ⓝ	Ⓨ Ⓝ	Ⓨ Ⓝ
Repeats the above three steps with the involved limb (using the same weight)	Ⓨ Ⓝ	Ⓨ Ⓝ	Ⓨ Ⓝ
Compares the number of repetitions completed (to determine deficit)	Ⓨ Ⓝ	Ⓨ Ⓝ	Ⓨ Ⓝ

The psychomotor skill was performed completely and in the appropriate order   **0 1 2 3 4 5**

The tester had control of the subject and the situation (showed confidence)   **0 1 2 3 4 5**

Method of performing the skill allowed the tester the ability to determine:
severity, proper progression, and the *fit* in the overall picture (Oral)   **0 1 2 3 4 5**

In order for a grade of *minimum standard* to be given, the total must be ≥11   **TOTAL = _____**

```
  1    2    3    4    5    6    7    8    9    10   11   12   13   14   15
  |    |    |    |    |    |    |    |    |    |    |    |    |    |    |
```

Not Acceptable   **Meets**   **Exceeds**
                                          Minimum Standards   **Minimum Standards**

TEST ENVIRONMENTS

L: Laboratory/Classroom Testing
C: Clinical/Field Testing
P: Practicum Testing
A: Assessment/Mock Exam Testing
S: Self-Reporting

SKILL TEST INFORMATION

Positive Finding: Determine strength deficit
Involved Structure: Gastrocnemius, soleus
Special Considerations: N/A
Reference(s): Adapted from Baechle et al
Supplies Needed: Leg press machine, ideally

THERAPEUTIC MEASUREMENTS
(TM-L-Test 13)

Peer Review _____ Peer Review _____

Skill Acquisition: _____   Practice Opportunities: _____

Using a 10-pound cuff weight, develop a **Srength Test** *that will assess power bilaterally for the* **knee extensors.** *This type of testing is also known as a "%* **Power Test.**" *You have 3 minutes to develop and administer this test.*

Tester places athlete and limb in appropriate position	Test 1	Test 2	Test 3
Seated (knee flexed)	Ⓨ Ⓝ	Ⓨ Ⓝ	Ⓨ Ⓝ
Tester performs test according to accepted guidelines	**Test 1**	**Test 2**	**Test 3**
Fastens the 10-lb cuff weight to the distal tibia/fibula of the uninvolved limb	Ⓨ Ⓝ	Ⓨ Ⓝ	Ⓨ Ⓝ
Instructs the athlete to fully extend the knee (as quickly as possible)	Ⓨ Ⓝ	Ⓨ Ⓝ	Ⓨ Ⓝ
Continues contractions as quickly as possible for 20 seconds (during this simulation, the amount time can vary; it is up to the tester to determine if the time chosen is appropriate)	Ⓨ Ⓝ	Ⓨ Ⓝ	Ⓨ Ⓝ
Repeats the above three steps with the involved limb (using the same weight and amount of time)	Ⓨ Ⓝ	Ⓨ Ⓝ	Ⓨ Ⓝ
Compares the number of repetitions completed (to determine deficit)	Ⓨ Ⓝ	Ⓨ Ⓝ	Ⓨ Ⓝ

The psychomotor skill was performed completely and in the appropriate order   0 1 2 3 4 5

The tester had control of the subject and the situation (showed confidence)   0 1 2 3 4 5

Method of performing the skill allowed the tester the ability to determine:
severity, proper progression, and the *fit* in the overall picture (Oral)   0 1 2 3 4 5

In order for a grade of *minimum standard* to be given, the total must be ≥11   TOTAL = _____

| 1 | 2 | 3 | 4 | 5 | 6 | 7 | 8 | 9 | 10 | 11 | 12 | 13 | 14 | 15 |

Not Acceptable   **Meets**   **Exceeds**
                              Minimum Standards   **Minimum Standards**

TEST ENVIRONMENTS
L: Laboratory/Classroom Testing
C: Clinical/Field Testing
P: Practicum Testing
A: Assessment/Mock Exam Testing
S: Self-Reporting

SKILL TEST INFORMATION
Positive Finding: Determine strength deficit
Involved Structure: Quadriceps
Special Considerations: N/A
Reference(s): Adapted from Baechle et al
Supplies Needed: Cuff weight, table, stopwatch

THERAPEUTIC MEASUREMENTS
(TM-L-Test 14)

Peer Review _____ Peer Review _____

Skill Acquisition: _____   Practice Opportunities: _____

This problem allows you the opportunity to set up and assess an athlete using an **Isokinetic Device Test.** *This specific scenario requires you to set up the* **knee** *for flexion/extension at 60, 120, and 210 degrees per second. You have 5 minutes to complete this task.*

Tester places athlete and limb in appropriate position	Test 1	Test 2	Test 3
Seated	Ⓨ Ⓝ	Ⓨ Ⓝ	Ⓨ Ⓝ

Tester performs proper set-up of the isokinetic device	Test 1	Test 2	Test 3
All components of the isokinetic device are in proper working order	Ⓨ Ⓝ	Ⓨ Ⓝ	Ⓨ Ⓝ
Proper attachments are collected and secured to the isokinetic device	Ⓨ Ⓝ	Ⓨ Ⓝ	Ⓨ Ⓝ
Knee joint is in line with the axis of the isokinetic dynamometer	Ⓨ Ⓝ	Ⓨ Ⓝ	Ⓨ Ⓝ
Lever arm is adjusted to match the length of the involved limb	Ⓨ Ⓝ	Ⓨ Ⓝ	Ⓨ Ⓝ
All straps are properly placed and secured (if appropriate)	Ⓨ Ⓝ	Ⓨ Ⓝ	Ⓨ Ⓝ

Tester performs test according to accepted guidelines	Test 1	Test 2	Test 3
Proper warm-up is provided	Ⓨ Ⓝ	Ⓨ Ⓝ	Ⓨ Ⓝ
Proper instructions are given:			
Moves limb through full range of motion	Ⓨ Ⓝ	Ⓨ Ⓝ	Ⓨ Ⓝ
Generates maximal contraction for each repetition	Ⓨ Ⓝ	Ⓨ Ⓝ	Ⓨ Ⓝ
Moves limb as hard and as fast a possible	Ⓨ Ⓝ	Ⓨ Ⓝ	Ⓨ Ⓝ
Velocities are preset at 60/120/210 degrees per second prior to the start of each set	Ⓨ Ⓝ	Ⓨ Ⓝ	Ⓨ Ⓝ
Number of repetitions are given and explained to the athlete	Ⓨ Ⓝ	Ⓨ Ⓝ	Ⓨ Ⓝ
Isokinetic test is administered and recorded/printed	Ⓨ Ⓝ	Ⓨ Ⓝ	Ⓨ Ⓝ

The psychomotor skill was performed completely and in the appropriate order   0 1 2 3 4 5

The tester had control of the subject and the situation (showed confidence)   0 1 2 3 4 5

Method of performing the skill allowed the tester the ability to determine:
severity, proper progression, and the *fit* in the overall picture (Oral)   0 1 2 3 4 5

In order for a grade of *minimum standard* to be given, the total must be ≥11   TOTAL = _____

1 2 3 4 5 6 7 8 9 10 11 12 13 14 15

Not Acceptable   **Meets Minimum Standards**   **Exceeds Minimum Standards**

TEST ENVIRONMENTS
L: Laboratory/Classroom Testing
C: Clinical/Field Testing
P: Practicum Testing
A: Assessment/Mock Exam Testing
S: Self-Reporting

SKILL TEST INFORMATION
Positive Finding: Isokinetic testing
Involved Structure: Knee: flexion/extension
Special Considerations: Print reports available from testing device
Reference(s): Adapted from Prentice (2004)
Supplies Needed: Isokinetic device

THERAPEUTIC MEASUREMENTS
(TM-L-Test 15)

Peer Review _____   Peer Review _____

Skill Acquisition: _____   Practice Opportunities: _____

This task gives you the opportunity to develop a **Functional Test** *using only "forward cutting," to help assure a safe return to participation for the* **lower extremity**. *You have 3 minutes to develop and complete this task.*

Tester places athlete and limb in appropriate position	Test 1	Test 2	Test 3
Standing	Ⓨ Ⓝ	Ⓨ Ⓝ	Ⓨ Ⓝ
Tester performs test according to accepted guidelines	**Test 1**	**Test 2**	**Test 3**
Instructs the athlete to warm up	Ⓨ Ⓝ	Ⓨ Ⓝ	Ⓨ Ⓝ
Cutting activities progress from easy to difficult	Ⓨ Ⓝ	Ⓨ Ⓝ	Ⓨ Ⓝ
Progression consists of speed:			
Progression: Half speed	Ⓨ Ⓝ	Ⓨ Ⓝ	Ⓨ Ⓝ
Progression: Three-quarter speed	Ⓨ Ⓝ	Ⓨ Ⓝ	Ⓨ Ⓝ
Progression: Full speed	Ⓨ Ⓝ	Ⓨ Ⓝ	Ⓨ Ⓝ
Progression consists of direction:			
Progression: Activities to the left	Ⓨ Ⓝ	Ⓨ Ⓝ	Ⓨ Ⓝ
Progression: Activities to the right	Ⓨ Ⓝ	Ⓨ Ⓝ	Ⓨ Ⓝ
Progression consists of angles/degrees:			
Progression: Running forward cutting at 15 degree angle	Ⓨ Ⓝ	Ⓨ Ⓝ	Ⓨ Ⓝ
Progression: Running forward cutting at 45 degree angle	Ⓨ Ⓝ	Ⓨ Ⓝ	Ⓨ Ⓝ
Progression: Running forward cutting at 90 degree angle	Ⓨ Ⓝ	Ⓨ Ⓝ	Ⓨ Ⓝ
Progression consist of commands:			
Progression: Instructs the athlete to cut left or right at the cone (instructions given prior to the activity	Ⓨ Ⓝ	Ⓨ Ⓝ	Ⓨ Ⓝ
Progression: Instructs the athlete to cut left or right on the whistle (instructions given during the activity)	Ⓨ Ⓝ	Ⓨ Ⓝ	Ⓨ Ⓝ
Progression consists of sport-specific activities:			
Progression (eg, catching, dribbling)	Ⓨ Ⓝ	Ⓨ Ⓝ	Ⓨ Ⓝ

The psychomotor skill was performed completely and in the appropriate order   0 1 2 3 4 5

The tester had control of the subject and the situation (showed confidence)   0 1 2 3 4 5

Method of performing the skill allowed the tester the ability to determine:
severity, proper progression, and the *fit* in the overall picture (Oral)   0 1 2 3 4 5

In order for a grade of *minimum standard* to be given, the total must be ≥11   **TOTAL =** _____

1	2	3	4	5	6	7	8	9	10	11	12	13	14	15

Not Acceptable   **Meets Minimum Standards**   **Exceeds Minimum Standards**

TEST ENVIRONMENTS

L: Laboratory/Classroom Testing
C: Clinical/Field Testing
P: Practicum Testing
A: Assessment/Mock Exam Testing
S: Self-Reporting

SKILL TEST INFORMATION

Positive Finding: Cutting progress
Involved Structure: Structures involved with running
Special Considerations: N/A
Reference(s): Adapted from Prentice (2004)
Supplies Needed: Cones, whistle, sport equipment

THERAPEUTIC MEASUREMENTS
(TM-L-Test 16)

Peer Review _____ Peer Review _____

Skill Acquisition: _____   Practice Opportunities: _____

*This problem allows you the opportunity to demonstrate the measurement of **thigh girth** for an athlete. You have 3 minutes to complete this task.*

	Test 1	Test 2	Test 3
Tester places athlete and limb in appropriate position	Test 1	Test 2	Test 3
Supine with feet completely on the table	Ⓨ Ⓝ	Ⓨ Ⓝ	Ⓨ Ⓝ
Tester prepares limb for measurement	Test 1	Test 2	Test 3
Marks superior pole of the patella with dot	Ⓨ Ⓝ	Ⓨ Ⓝ	Ⓨ Ⓝ
Marks thigh at 2, 6, and 10 inches above patella with dot (may vary depending on the length of the leg)	Ⓨ Ⓝ	Ⓨ Ⓝ	Ⓨ Ⓝ
Tester measures girth of thigh in appropriate manner	Test 1	Test 2	Test 3
Encircles thigh with cloth tape measure at each mark on thigh	Ⓨ Ⓝ	Ⓨ Ⓝ	Ⓨ Ⓝ
Instructs athlete to flex muscle (quadriceps set)	Ⓨ Ⓝ	Ⓨ Ⓝ	Ⓨ Ⓝ
Records girth of thigh at each mark	Ⓨ Ⓝ	Ⓨ Ⓝ	Ⓨ Ⓝ
Performs measurement bilaterally	Ⓨ Ⓝ	Ⓨ Ⓝ	Ⓨ Ⓝ

The psychomotor skill was performed completely and in the appropriate order   0 1 2 3 4 5

The tester had control of the subject and the situation (showed confidence)   0 1 2 3 4 5

Method of performing the skill allowed the tester the ability to determine:
severity, proper progression, and the *fit* in the overall picture (Oral)   0 1 2 3 4 5

In order for a grade of *minimum standard* to be given, the total must be ≥11   TOTAL = _____

```
 1    2    3    4    5    6    7    8    9    10   11   12   13   14   15
 |    |    |    |    |    |    |    |    |    |    |    |    |    |    |
```
Not Acceptable   **Meets   Exceeds**
                                       Minimum Standards   Minimum Standards

TEST ENVIRONMENTS
L: Laboratory/Classroom Testing
C: Clinical/Field Testing
P: Practicum Testing
A: Assessment/Mock Exam Testing
S: Self-Reporting

SKILL TEST INFORMATION
Positive Finding: Objective measurement
Involved Structure: Thigh (quadriceps)
Special Considerations: N/A
Reference(s): Starkey et al (2002)
Supplies Needed: Tape measure, dot, pencil/paper

THERAPEUTIC MEASUREMENTS
(TM-L-Test 17)

Peer Review _____ Peer Review _____

Skill Acquisition: _____   Practice Opportunities: _____

This task allows you the opportunity to demonstrate the measurement of **leg length (true/apparent)** *for an athlete. You have 3 minutes to complete this task.*

Tester places athlete and limb in appropriate position	Test 1	Test 2	Test 3
Supine with feet completely on the table	Ⓨ Ⓝ	Ⓨ Ⓝ	Ⓨ Ⓝ
Tester obtains measurements of true leg length	**Test 1**	**Test 2**	**Test 3**
Measures from ASIS to medial malleolus (tape measure)	Ⓨ Ⓝ	Ⓨ Ⓝ	Ⓨ Ⓝ
Measures both extremities	Ⓨ Ⓝ	Ⓨ Ⓝ	Ⓨ Ⓝ
Compares and records measurements	Ⓨ Ⓝ	Ⓨ Ⓝ	Ⓨ Ⓝ
Tester obtains measurements of apparent leg length	**Test 1**	**Test 2**	**Test 3**
Measures from navel to medial malleolus (tape measure)	Ⓨ Ⓝ	Ⓨ Ⓝ	Ⓨ Ⓝ
Measures both extremities	Ⓨ Ⓝ	Ⓨ Ⓝ	Ⓨ Ⓝ
Compares and records measurements	Ⓨ Ⓝ	Ⓨ Ⓝ	Ⓨ Ⓝ

The psychomotor skill was performed completely and in the appropriate order   0 1 2 3 4 5

The tester had control of the subject and the situation (showed confidence)   0 1 2 3 4 5

Method of performing the skill allowed the tester the ability to determine:
severity, proper progression, and the *fit* in the overall picture (Oral)   0 1 2 3 4 5

In order for a grade of *minimum standard* to be given, the total must be ≥11   TOTAL = _____

1   2   3   4   5   6   7   8   9   10   11   12   13   14   15

Not Acceptable   **Meets**   **Exceeds**
                              Minimum Standards   **Minimum Standards**

TEST ENVIRONMENTS

L: Laboratory/Classroom Testing
C: Clinical/Field Testing
P: Practicum Testing
A: Assessment/Mock Exam Testing
S: Self-Reporting

SKILL TEST INFORMATION

Positive Finding:	Leg length
Involved Structure:	Pelvis, legs
Special Considerations:	May measure to the lateral malleolus
Reference(s):	Magee
Supplies Needed:	Table, tape measure, pencil/paper

THERAPEUTIC MEASUREMENTS
(TM-L-Test 18)

Peer Review _____   Peer Review _____

Skill Acquisition: _____   Practice Opportunities: _____

*This task allows you the opportunity to demonstrate the measurement of the **Q-angle** of an athlete. You have 3 minutes to complete this task.*

Tester places athlete and limb in appropriate position	Test 1	Test 2	Test 3
Supine with foot on the table	Ⓨ Ⓝ	Ⓨ Ⓝ	Ⓨ Ⓝ
Tester obtains measurement in appropriate manner	**Test 1**	**Test 2**	**Test 3**
Marks the ASIS	Ⓨ Ⓝ	Ⓨ Ⓝ	Ⓨ Ⓝ
Draws an imaginary line from the ASIS to the midline of the patella (center point)	Ⓨ Ⓝ	Ⓨ Ⓝ	Ⓨ Ⓝ
Draws a line between the tibial tubercle and midpoint of the patella	Ⓨ Ⓝ	Ⓨ Ⓝ	Ⓨ Ⓝ
Uses the goniometer to measure the angle between lines that cross the patella	Ⓨ Ⓝ	Ⓨ Ⓝ	Ⓨ Ⓝ

The psychomotor skill was performed completely and in the appropriate order   0 1 2 3 4 5

The tester had control of the subject and the situation (showed confidence)   0 1 2 3 4 5

Method of performing the skill allowed the tester the ability to determine:
severity, proper progression, and the *fit* in the overall picture (Oral)   0 1 2 3 4 5

In order for a grade of *minimum standard* to be given, the total must be ≥11   TOTAL = _____

```
 1    2    3    4    5    6    7    8    9   10   11   12   13   14   15
 |----|----|----|----|----|----|----|----|----|----|----|----|----|----|
```

Not Acceptable   Meets   Exceeds
                                       Minimum Standards   Minimum Standards

TEST ENVIRONMENTS

L: Laboratory/Classroom Testing
C: Clinical/Field Testing
P: Practicum Testing
A: Assessment/Mock Exam Testing
S: Self-Reporting

SKILL TEST INFORMATION

Positive Finding: Angle >13 for male; Angle >18 for female
Involved Structure: Lower limb
Special Considerations: May be done with the knee flexed
Reference(s): Starkey et al (2002); Magee
Supplies Needed: Goniometer, pencil/paper, dots

THERAPEUTIC MEASUREMENTS
(TM-L-Test 19)

Peer Review _____ Peer Review _____

Skill Acquisition: _____   Practice Opportunities: _____

This problem allows you the opportunity to demonstrate the proper technique for **measuring swelling in and around the ankle joint** *using a* **figure-8** *girth measurement. You have 2 minutes to complete this task.*

Tester places athlete and limb in appropriate position	Test 1	Test 2	Test 3
Seated	Ⓨ Ⓝ	Ⓨ Ⓝ	Ⓨ Ⓝ
Foot hanging off the edge of the table	Ⓨ Ⓝ	Ⓨ Ⓝ	Ⓨ Ⓝ

Tester placed in proper position	Test 1	Test 2	Test 3
Facing the involved limb	Ⓨ Ⓝ	Ⓨ Ⓝ	Ⓨ Ⓝ

Tester performs test according to accepted guidelines	Test 1	Test 2	Test 3
Using a figure-8 technique, wraps the tape measure around the foot:			
Places one end of the tape measure on the lateral malleolus	Ⓨ Ⓝ	Ⓨ Ⓝ	Ⓨ Ⓝ
Moves the tape measure over the top of the foot down under the arch crossing the navicular	Ⓨ Ⓝ	Ⓨ Ⓝ	Ⓨ Ⓝ
Moves the tape measure under the arch, crossing the head of the fifth metatarsal	Ⓨ Ⓝ	Ⓨ Ⓝ	Ⓨ Ⓝ
Continues wrapping the tape measure over foot crossing the medial malleolus back behind the ankle	Ⓨ Ⓝ	Ⓨ Ⓝ	Ⓨ Ⓝ
Ends at the starting point (lateral malleolus)	Ⓨ Ⓝ	Ⓨ Ⓝ	Ⓨ Ⓝ
Performs measurement bilaterally	Ⓨ Ⓝ	Ⓨ Ⓝ	Ⓨ Ⓝ
Compares findings	Ⓨ Ⓝ	Ⓨ Ⓝ	Ⓨ Ⓝ

The psychomotor skill was performed completely and in the appropriate order   0 1 2 3 4 5

The tester had control of the subject and the situation (showed confidence)   0 1 2 3 4 5

Method of performing the skill allowed the tester the ability to determine:
severity, proper progression, and the *fit* in the overall picture (Oral)   0 1 2 3 4 5

In order for a grade of *minimum standard* to be given, the total must be ≥11   TOTAL = _____

```
   1     2     3     4     5     6     7     8     9    10    11    12    13    14    15
   |     |     |     |     |     |     |     |     |     |     |     |     |     |     |
```
Not Acceptable   **Meets**   **Exceeds**
                                          Minimum Standards   **Minimum Standards**

SKILL TEST INFORMATION

Positive Finding:	Increase or decrease circumference measurement
Purpose:	Determine swelling or atrophy at the hand/wrist
Special Considerations:	Difference may be due to dominant limb
Reference(s):	Starkey et al (2002)
Supplies Needed:	Tape measure

TEST ENVIRONMENTS
L: Laboratory/Classroom Testing
C: Clinical/Field Testing
P: Practicum Testing
A: Assessment/Mock Exam Testing
S: Self-Reporting

Chapter 14

PROPRIOCEPTIVE
NEUROMUSCULAR FACILITATION

PNF
(PNF-U-Test 1)

Peer Review _____   Peer Review _____

Skill Acquisition: _____   Practice Opportunities: _____

Please demonstrate how you would stretch the **wrist flexors** *using* **PNF Contract/Relax (Agonist/Antagonist)**. *You have 2 minutes to complete this task.*

Tester places athlete and limb in appropriate position	Test 1	Test 2	Test 3
Seated	Ⓨ Ⓝ	Ⓨ Ⓝ	Ⓨ Ⓝ
Wrist in full extension	Ⓨ Ⓝ	Ⓨ Ⓝ	Ⓨ Ⓝ
Tester performs test according to accepted guidelines	**Test 1**	**Test 2**	**Test 3**
Instructs the athlete on proper commands and sequence	Ⓨ Ⓝ	Ⓨ Ⓝ	Ⓨ Ⓝ
Stabilizes the ulna/radius with one hand	Ⓨ Ⓝ	Ⓨ Ⓝ	Ⓨ Ⓝ
Passively stretches the wrist flexors ("relax" command)	Ⓨ Ⓝ	Ⓨ Ⓝ	Ⓨ Ⓝ
Holds stretch for 4 to 10 seconds (wrist passively stretched in as much extension as possible)	Ⓨ Ⓝ	Ⓨ Ⓝ	Ⓨ Ⓝ
Passively moves the wrist from extension to flexion ("relax" command)	Ⓨ Ⓝ	Ⓨ Ⓝ	Ⓨ Ⓝ
Resists wrist extension using the "push" command through the full ROM with the other hand (moves isotonically against maximal resistance)	Ⓨ Ⓝ	Ⓨ Ⓝ	Ⓨ Ⓝ
Uses proper hand position for applying isotonic resistance	Ⓨ Ⓝ	Ⓨ Ⓝ	Ⓨ Ⓝ
Repeats above steps	Ⓨ Ⓝ	Ⓨ Ⓝ	Ⓨ Ⓝ

The psychomotor skill was performed completely and in the appropriate order   0 1 2 3 4 5

The tester had control of the subject and the situation (showed confidence)   0 1 2 3 4 5

Method of performing the skill allowed the tester the ability to determine:
severity, proper progression, and the *fit* in the overall picture (Oral)   0 1 2 3 4 5

In order for a grade of *minimum standard* to be given, the total must be ≥11   TOTAL = _____

1   2   3   4   5   6   7   8   9   10   11   12   13   14   15

Not Acceptable   **Meets**   **Exceeds**
                              Minimum Standards   **Minimum Standards**

TEST ENVIRONMENTS	**SKILL TEST INFORMATION**	
L: Laboratory/Classroom Testing	**Positive Finding:**	Increase flexibility
C: Clinical/Field Testing	**Involved Structure:**	Wrist flexors
P: Practicum Testing	**Special Considerations:**	N/A
A: Assessment/Mock Exam Testing	**Reference(s):**	Prentice (2004)
S: Self-Reporting	**Supplies Needed:**	N/A

PNF
(PNF-U-Test 2)

Peer Review _____ Peer Review _____

Skill Acquisition: _____   Practice Opportunities: _____

Please demonstrate how you would stretch the **elbow flexors** *using* **PNF Contract/Relax (Agonist/Agonist)***. You have 2 minutes to complete this task.*

Tester places athlete and limb in appropriate position	Test 1	Test 2	Test 3
Standing or seated	Ⓨ Ⓝ	Ⓨ Ⓝ	Ⓨ Ⓝ
Elbow in extension	Ⓨ Ⓝ	Ⓨ Ⓝ	Ⓨ Ⓝ
Tester performs test according to accepted guidelines	**Test 1**	**Test 2**	**Test 3**
Instructs the athlete with proper commands and sequence	Ⓨ Ⓝ	Ⓨ Ⓝ	Ⓨ Ⓝ
Stabilizes the humerus with one hand	Ⓨ Ⓝ	Ⓨ Ⓝ	Ⓨ Ⓝ
Passively stretches the elbow flexors (using the "relax" command, moves the forearm into full extension) with the other hand	Ⓨ Ⓝ	Ⓨ Ⓝ	Ⓨ Ⓝ
Holds stretch for 4 to 10 seconds using "relax" command	Ⓨ Ⓝ	Ⓨ Ⓝ	Ⓨ Ⓝ
Resists the elbow flexors using a "pull" command through the full ROM (extension ➔ flexion) with the hand previously applying the stretch	Ⓨ Ⓝ	Ⓨ Ⓝ	Ⓨ Ⓝ
Uses proper hand placement for applying maximal isotonic resistance	Ⓨ Ⓝ	Ⓨ Ⓝ	Ⓨ Ⓝ

The psychomotor skill was performed completely and in the appropriate order   **0 1 2 3 4 5**

The tester had control of the subject and the situation (showed confidence)   **0 1 2 3 4 5**

Method of performing the skill allowed the tester the ability to determine: severity, proper progression, and the fit in the overall picture (Oral)   **0 1 2 3 4 5**

In order for a grade of minimum standard to be given, the total must be ≥11   **TOTAL = _____**

```
   1     2     3     4     5     6     7     8     9    10    11    12    13    14    15
   |     |     |     |     |     |     |     |     |     |     |     |     |     |     |
```

Not Acceptable   **Meets**   **Exceeds**
                                              Minimum Standards   **Minimum Standards**

TEST ENVIRONMENTS

L: Laboratory/Classroom Testing
C: Clinical/Field Testing
P: Practicum Testing
A: Assessment/Mock Exam Testing
S: Self-Reporting

SKILL TEST INFORMATION

Purpose: Increase flexibility
Involved Structure: Biceps
Special Considerations: N/A
Reference(s): Prentice (2004)
Supplies Needed: Chair

PNF
(PNF-U-Test 3)

Peer Review _____   Peer Review _____

Skill Acquisition: _____   Practice Opportunities: _____

Please demonstrate how you would stretch the **shoulder horizontal flexors** *using* **PNF Hold/Relax (Agonist/ Antagonist)**. *You have 2 minutes to complete this task.*

Tester places athlete and limb in appropriate position	Test 1	Test 2	Test 3
Supine or seated	Ⓨ Ⓝ	Ⓨ Ⓝ	Ⓨ Ⓝ
Upper body supported by the table or back of a chair	Ⓨ Ⓝ	Ⓨ Ⓝ	Ⓨ Ⓝ
Shoulder in 90° of abduction	Ⓨ Ⓝ	Ⓨ Ⓝ	Ⓨ Ⓝ

Tester performs test according to accepted guidelines	Test 1	Test 2	Test 3
Instructs the athlete with proper commands and sequence	Ⓨ Ⓝ	Ⓨ Ⓝ	Ⓨ Ⓝ
Stabilizes the upper body with one hand	Ⓨ Ⓝ	Ⓨ Ⓝ	Ⓨ Ⓝ
Passively stretches the shoulder horizontal flexors (using the "relax" command, moves the shoulder into full horizontal extension) with the other hand	Ⓨ Ⓝ	Ⓨ Ⓝ	Ⓨ Ⓝ
Holds stretch for 4 to 10 seconds using the "relax" command	Ⓨ Ⓝ	Ⓨ Ⓝ	Ⓨ Ⓝ
Passively moves the shoulder from full horizontal extension to about 45 degrees of horizontal flexion ("relax" command)	Ⓨ Ⓝ	Ⓨ Ⓝ	Ⓨ Ⓝ
Resists the shoulder horizontal extensors using a "hold" command (isometric contraction) with the hand previously applying the stretch	Ⓨ Ⓝ	Ⓨ Ⓝ	Ⓨ Ⓝ
Uses proper hand placement for applying maximal isometric resistance	Ⓨ Ⓝ	Ⓨ Ⓝ	Ⓨ Ⓝ

The psychomotor skill was performed completely and in the appropriate order   0 1 2 3 4 5

The tester had control of the subject and the situation (showed confidence)   0 1 2 3 4 5

Method of performing the skill allowed the tester the ability to determine: severity, proper progression, and the *fit* in the overall picture (Oral)   0 1 2 3 4 5

In order for a grade of *minimum standard* to be given, the total must be ≥11   TOTAL = _____

```
 1    2    3    4    5    6    7    8    9    10   11   12   13   14   15
 |    |    |    |    |    |    |    |    |    |    |    |    |    |    |
```

Not Acceptable   **Meets**   **Exceeds**
                               Minimum Standards   **Minimum Standards**

TEST ENVIRONMENTS

L: Laboratory/Classroom Testing
C: Clinical/Field Testing
P: Practicum Testing
A: Assessment/Mock Exam Testing
S: Self-Reporting

SKILL TEST INFORMATION

Purpose: Increase flexibility
Involved Structure: Pectoralis major
Special Considerations: N/A
Reference(s): Prentice (2004)
Supplies Needed: Table

PNF
(PNF-U-Test 4)

Peer Review _____ Peer Review _____

Skill Acquisition: _____   Practice Opportunities: _____

Please demonstrate how you would stretch the **shoulder external rotators** *using* **PNF Hold/Relax (Agonist/Agonist)**. *You have 2 minutes to complete this task.*

Tester places athlete and limb in appropriate position	Test 1	Test 2	Test 3
Seated or supine	Ⓨ Ⓝ	Ⓨ Ⓝ	Ⓨ Ⓝ
Upper arm supported (90/90 position)	Ⓨ Ⓝ	Ⓨ Ⓝ	Ⓨ Ⓝ
Shoulder placed in full internal rotation	Ⓨ Ⓝ	Ⓨ Ⓝ	Ⓨ Ⓝ
Tester performs test according to accepted guidelines	**Test 1**	**Test 2**	**Test 3**
Instructs the athlete on proper commands and sequence	Ⓨ Ⓝ	Ⓨ Ⓝ	Ⓨ Ⓝ
Stabilizes the humerus with one hand	Ⓨ Ⓝ	Ⓨ Ⓝ	Ⓨ Ⓝ
Passively stretches the shoulder external rotators ("relax" command)	Ⓨ Ⓝ	Ⓨ Ⓝ	Ⓨ Ⓝ
Holds stretch for 4 to 10 seconds (shoulder passively stretched in as much internal rotation as possible)	Ⓨ Ⓝ	Ⓨ Ⓝ	Ⓨ Ⓝ
Passively moves the shoulder from full internal rotation about 20 degrees in the transverse plane toward external rotation ("relax" command)	Ⓨ Ⓝ	Ⓨ Ⓝ	Ⓨ Ⓝ
Resists shoulder external rotation using the "hold" command with the other hand (isometric contraction against maximal resistance)	Ⓨ Ⓝ	Ⓨ Ⓝ	Ⓨ Ⓝ
Holds isometric contraction for 4 to 10 seconds	Ⓨ Ⓝ	Ⓨ Ⓝ	Ⓨ Ⓝ
Uses proper hand position for applying isometric resistance	Ⓨ Ⓝ	Ⓨ Ⓝ	Ⓨ Ⓝ
Repeats above steps	Ⓨ Ⓝ	Ⓨ Ⓝ	Ⓨ Ⓝ

The psychomotor skill was performed completely and in the appropriate order   **0 1 2 3 4 5**

The tester had control of the subject and the situation (showed confidence)   **0 1 2 3 4 5**

Method of performing the skill allowed the tester the ability to determine:
severity, proper progression, and the *fit* in the overall picture (Oral)   **0 1 2 3 4 5**

In order for a grade of *minimum standard* to be given, the total must be ≥11   **TOTAL = _____**

1	2	3	4	5	6	7	8	9	10	11	12	13	14	15

Not Acceptable   **Meets**   **Exceeds**
                              Minimum Standards   **Minimum Standards**

TEST ENVIRONMENTS

L: Laboratory/Classroom Testing
C: Clinical/Field Testing
P: Practicum Testing
A: Assessment/Mock Exam Testing
S: Self-Reporting

SKILL TEST INFORMATION

Positive Finding: Increase flexibility
Involved Structure: External rotators
Special Considerations: N/A
Reference(s): Prentice (2004)
Supplies Needed: N/A

PNF
(PNF-U-Test 5)

Peer Review _____ Peer Review _____

Skill Acquisition: _____   Practice Opportunities: _____

Please demonstrate how you would strengthen the **shoulder internal rotators** *using* **PNF Slow Reversal**. *You have 2 minutes to complete this task.*

Tester places athlete and limb in appropriate position	Test 1	Test 2	Test 3
Supine	Ⓨ Ⓝ	Ⓨ Ⓝ	Ⓨ Ⓝ
Shoulder in 90 degree abduction; 90 degree external rotation	Ⓨ Ⓝ	Ⓨ Ⓝ	Ⓨ Ⓝ
Elbow in 90 degree flexion	Ⓨ Ⓝ	Ⓨ Ⓝ	Ⓨ Ⓝ
Tester performs test according to accepted guidelines	**Test 1**	**Test 2**	**Test 3**
Instructs the athlete with proper commands and sequence	Ⓨ Ⓝ	Ⓨ Ⓝ	Ⓨ Ⓝ
Stabilizes humerus with one hand	Ⓨ Ⓝ	Ⓨ Ⓝ	Ⓨ Ⓝ
Applies resistance at distal ulna/radius by the other hand	Ⓨ Ⓝ	Ⓨ Ⓝ	Ⓨ Ⓝ
Instructs the athlete to isotonically contract the internal rotators of the shoulder— moving from external rotation to full internal rotation ("pull" command)	Ⓨ Ⓝ	Ⓨ Ⓝ	Ⓨ Ⓝ
Instructs the athlete to immediately reverse the direction, contracting the external rotators moving from internal rotation to full external rotation ("push" command)	Ⓨ Ⓝ	Ⓨ Ⓝ	Ⓨ Ⓝ
Uses proper hand placement for applying isotonic and isometric resistance	Ⓨ Ⓝ	Ⓨ Ⓝ	Ⓨ Ⓝ

The psychomotor skill was performed completely and in the appropriate order   0 1 2 3 4 5

The tester had control of the subject and the situation (showed confidence)   0 1 2 3 4 5

Method of performing the skill allowed the tester the ability to determine:
severity, proper progression, and the *fit* in the overall picture (Oral)   0 1 2 3 4 5

In order for a grade of *minimum standard* to be given, the total must be ≥11   TOTAL = _____

```
  1    2    3    4    5    6    7    8    9   10   11   12   13   14   15
  |____|____|____|____|____|____|____|____|____|____|____|____|____|____|
```
Not Acceptable   **Meets**   **Exceeds**
                          Minimum Standards   **Minimum Standards**

TEST ENVIRONMENTS

L: Laboratory/Classroom Testing
C: Clinical/Field Testing
P: Practicum Testing
A: Assessment/Mock Exam Testing
S: Self-Reporting

SKILL TEST INFORMATION

Purpose:	Muscle education/strengthening
Involved Structure:	Pectoralis major; Latissimus Dorsi; Subscapularis
Special Considerations:	N/A
Reference(s):	Prentice (2004)
Supplies Needed:	Table

PNF
(PNF-U-Test 6)

Peer Review _____ Peer Review _____

Skill Acquisition: _____   Practice Opportunities: _____

Please demonstrate how you would strengthen **elbow extension** *using* **PNF Slow Reversal Hold.** *You have 2 minutes to complete this task.*

Tester places athlete and limb in appropriate position	Test 1	Test 2	Test 3
Seated	Ⓨ Ⓝ	Ⓨ Ⓝ	Ⓨ Ⓝ
Elbow in full flexion	Ⓨ Ⓝ	Ⓨ Ⓝ	Ⓨ Ⓝ
Tester performs test according to accepted guidelines	**Test 1**	**Test 2**	**Test 3**
Instructs the athlete on proper commands and sequence	Ⓨ Ⓝ	Ⓨ Ⓝ	Ⓨ Ⓝ
Stabilizes humerus with one hand	Ⓨ Ⓝ	Ⓨ Ⓝ	Ⓨ Ⓝ
Applies resistance at distal ulna/radius with the other hand	Ⓨ Ⓝ	Ⓨ Ⓝ	Ⓨ Ⓝ
Instructs the athlete to isotonically contract the extensors—moving from flexion to full extension ("push" command)	Ⓨ Ⓝ	Ⓨ Ⓝ	Ⓨ Ⓝ
Instructs the athlete to isometrically contract the extensors at the end of the range ("hold" command)	Ⓨ Ⓝ	Ⓨ Ⓝ	Ⓨ Ⓝ
Holds isometric contraction for 4 to 10 seconds	Ⓨ Ⓝ	Ⓨ Ⓝ	Ⓨ Ⓝ
Instructs the athlete to reverse the direction-isotonically contract the flexors, moving from extension to flexion ("pull" command)	Ⓨ Ⓝ	Ⓨ Ⓝ	Ⓨ Ⓝ
Instructs the athlete to isometrically contract the flexors at the end of the range ("hold" command)	Ⓨ Ⓝ	Ⓨ Ⓝ	Ⓨ Ⓝ
Hold isometric contraction for 4 to 10 seconds	Ⓨ Ⓝ	Ⓨ Ⓝ	Ⓨ Ⓝ
Uses proper hand placement for applying isotonic and isometric resistance	Ⓨ Ⓝ	Ⓨ Ⓝ	Ⓨ Ⓝ

The psychomotor skill was performed completely and in the appropriate order   **0 1 2 3 4 5**

The tester had control of the subject and the situation (showed confidence)   **0 1 2 3 4 5**

Method of performing the skill allowed the tester the ability to determine: severity, proper progression, and the *fit* in the overall picture (Oral)   **0 1 2 3 4 5**

In order for a grade of *minimum standard* to be given, the total must be ≥11   **TOTAL = _____**

1	2	3	4	5	6	7	8	9	10	11	12	13	14	15

Not Acceptable   **Meets**   **Exceeds**
                              Minimum Standards   **Minimum Standards**

TEST ENVIRONMENTS	**SKILL TEST INFORMATION**
L: Laboratory/Classroom Testing	**Purpose:** Muscle education/strengthening
C: Clinical/Field Testing	**Involved Structure:** Triceps
P: Practicum Testing	**Special Considerations:** N/A
A: Assessment/Mock Exam Testing	**Reference(s):** Prentice (2004)
S: Self-Reporting	**Supplies Needed:** Chair

PNF
(PNF-U-Test 7)

Peer Review _____ Peer Review _____

Skill Acquisition: _____   Practice Opportunities: _____

Please demonstrate how you would perform **PNF Repeated Contraction** *for the* **wrist extensors**. *You have 2 minutes to complete this task.*

Tester places athlete and limb in appropriate position	Test 1	Test 2	Test 3
Seated	Ⓨ Ⓝ	Ⓨ Ⓝ	Ⓨ Ⓝ
Wrist in full flexion	Ⓨ Ⓝ	Ⓨ Ⓝ	Ⓨ Ⓝ
Tester performs test according to accepted guidelines	**Test 1**	**Test 2**	**Test 3**
Instructs the athlete on proper commands and sequence	Ⓨ Ⓝ	Ⓨ Ⓝ	Ⓨ Ⓝ
Stabilizes radius/ulna with one hand	Ⓨ Ⓝ	Ⓨ Ⓝ	Ⓨ Ⓝ
Resist extension using the "push" command through the full ROM with the other hand (moves isotonically against maximal resistance)	Ⓨ Ⓝ	Ⓨ Ⓝ	Ⓨ Ⓝ
Repeats the above step until fatigue is evident	Ⓨ Ⓝ	Ⓨ Ⓝ	Ⓨ Ⓝ
Performs "quick stretch" (increases the amount of resistance quickly) at the weakest point of the motion or at the end of extension	Ⓨ Ⓝ	Ⓨ Ⓝ	Ⓨ Ⓝ
Uses proper hand placement for applying isotonic resistance	Ⓨ Ⓝ	Ⓨ Ⓝ	Ⓨ Ⓝ

The psychomotor skill was performed completely and in the appropriate order   0 1 2 3 4 5

The tester had control of the subject and the situation (showed confidence)   0 1 2 3 4 5

Method of performing the skill allowed the tester the ability to determine:
severity, proper progression, and the *fit* in the overall picture (Oral)   0 1 2 3 4 5

In order for a grade of *minimum standard* to be given, the total must be ≥11   TOTAL = _____

```
 1    2    3    4    5    6    7    8    9   10   11   12   13   14   15
 |    |    |    |    |    |    |    |    |    |    |    |    |    |    |
```

Not Acceptable   **Meets**   **Exceeds**
                                   Minimum Standards   **Minimum Standards**

TEST ENVIRONMENTS

L: Laboratory/Classroom Testing
C: Clinical/Field Testing
P: Practicum Testing
A: Assessment/Mock Exam Testing
S: Self-Reporting

SKILL TEST INFORMATION

Purpose:	Increase strengthening
Involved Structure:	Extensor Carpi Radialis; Longus/Brevis
Special Considerations:	N/A
Reference(s):	Prentice (2004)
Supplies Needed:	Chair

PNF
(PNF-U-Test 8)

Skill Acquisition: _____ Practice Opportunities: _____

*Please demonstrate how you would strengthen the **shoulder horizontal flexors** using **PNF Rhythmic Stabilization**.
You have 2 minutes to complete this task.*

Tester places athlete and limb in appropriate position	Test 1	Test 2	Test 3
Supine	Ⓨ Ⓝ	Ⓨ Ⓝ	Ⓨ Ⓝ
Shoulder horizontally flexed to 90 degrees	Ⓨ Ⓝ	Ⓨ Ⓝ	Ⓨ Ⓝ
Tester performs test according to accepted guidelines	**Test 1**	**Test 2**	**Test 3**
Instructs the athlete on proper commands and sequence	Ⓨ Ⓝ	Ⓨ Ⓝ	Ⓨ Ⓝ
Instructs the athlete to contract the muscles around the scapula	Ⓨ Ⓝ	Ⓨ Ⓝ	Ⓨ Ⓝ
Instructs the athlete to isometrically contract the horizontal flexors ("hold" command)	Ⓨ Ⓝ	Ⓨ Ⓝ	Ⓨ Ⓝ
Instructs the athlete to immediately reverse the direction, isometrically contracting the horizontal extensors ("hold" command)	Ⓨ Ⓝ	Ⓨ Ⓝ	Ⓨ Ⓝ
Uses proper hand position for applying isometric resistance	Ⓨ Ⓝ	Ⓨ Ⓝ	Ⓨ Ⓝ
Repeats above steps	Ⓨ Ⓝ	Ⓨ Ⓝ	Ⓨ Ⓝ

The psychomotor skill was performed completely and in the appropriate order   0 1 2 3 4 5

The tester had control of the subject and the situation (showed confidence)   0 1 2 3 4 5

Method of performing the skill allowed the tester the ability to determine:
severity, proper progression, and the *fit* in the overall picture (Oral)   0 1 2 3 4 5

In order for a grade of *minimum standard* to be given, the total must be ≥11   TOTAL = _____

```
 1    2    3    4    5    6    7    8    9   10   11   12   13   14   15
 |    |    |    |    |    |    |    |    |    |    |    |    |    |    |
```

Not Acceptable   **Meets**   **Exceeds**
                                    Minimum Standards   **Minimum Standards**

TEST ENVIRONMENTS

L: Laboratory/Classroom Testing
C: Clinical/Field Testing
P: Practicum Testing
A: Assessment/Mock Exam Testing
S: Self-Reporting

SKILL TEST INFORMATION

Positive Finding:	Muscle education/strengthening
Involved Structure:	Posterior deltoid; Pectoralis major
Special Considerations:	N/A
Reference(s):	Prentice (2004)
Supplies Needed:	N/A

PNF
(PNF-L-Test 1)

Peer Review _____ Peer Review _____

Skill Acquisition: _____ Practice Opportunities: _____

Please demonstrate how you would stretch the **ankle plantar flexors** *using* **PNF Contract/Relax (Agonist/ Antagonist)**. *You have 2 minutes to complete this task.*

Tester places athlete and limb in appropriate position	Test 1	Test 2	Test 3
Seated	Ⓨ Ⓝ	Ⓨ Ⓝ	Ⓨ Ⓝ
Foot/ankle hanging over the edge of the table	Ⓨ Ⓝ	Ⓨ Ⓝ	Ⓨ Ⓝ
Knee in full extension	Ⓨ Ⓝ	Ⓨ Ⓝ	Ⓨ Ⓝ
Tester performs test according to accepted guidelines	**Test 1**	**Test 2**	**Test 3**
Instructs the athlete on proper commands and sequence	Ⓨ Ⓝ	Ⓨ Ⓝ	Ⓨ Ⓝ
Stabilizes the lower leg with one hand	Ⓨ Ⓝ	Ⓨ Ⓝ	Ⓨ Ⓝ
Passively stretches the ankle planter flexors (using the "relax" command move the ankle into full dorsiflexion) with the other hand	Ⓨ Ⓝ	Ⓨ Ⓝ	Ⓨ Ⓝ
Holds stretch for 4 to 10 seconds using "relax" command	Ⓨ Ⓝ	Ⓨ Ⓝ	Ⓨ Ⓝ
Passively moves the ankle from dorsiflexion to plantar flexion ("relax" command)	Ⓨ Ⓝ	Ⓨ Ⓝ	Ⓨ Ⓝ
Resists the ankle dorsal flexors using a "pull" command through the full ROM (ankle plantar flexion ➜ ankle dorsiflexion) with the hand previously applying the stretch	Ⓨ Ⓝ	Ⓨ Ⓝ	Ⓨ Ⓝ
Uses proper hand placement for applying maximal isotonic resistance	Ⓨ Ⓝ	Ⓨ Ⓝ	Ⓨ Ⓝ

The psychomotor skill was performed completely and in the appropriate order　　0　1　2　3　4　5

The tester had control of the subject and the situation (showed confidence)　　0　1　2　3　4　5

Method of performing the skill allowed the tester the ability to determine:
severity, proper progression, and the *fit* in the overall picture (Oral)　　0　1　2　3　4　5

In order for a grade of *minimum standard* to be given, the total must be ≥11　　**TOTAL =** _____

```
 1    2    3    4    5    6    7    8    9   10   11   12   13   14   15
 |    |    |    |    |    |    |    |    |    |    |    |    |    |    |
```

Not Acceptable　　　　　　　　　　　**Meets**　　　　　　　　　**Exceeds**
　　　　　　　　　　　　　　　　　Minimum Standards　　　**Minimum Standards**

TEST ENVIRONMENTS	**SKILL TEST INFORMATION**	
L: Laboratory/Classroom Testing	**Purpose:**	Increase flexibility
C: Clinical/Field Testing	**Involved Structure:**	Gastrocnemius Soleus
P: Practicum Testing	**Special Considerations:**	N/A
A: Assessment/Mock Exam Testing	**Reference(s):**	Prentice (2004)
S: Self-Reporting	**Supplies Needed:**	Table

PNF
(PNF-L-Test 2)

Peer Review _____ Peer Review _____

Skill Acquisition: _____ Practice Opportunities: _____

Please demonstrate how you would stretch the **knee flexors** *using* **PNF Contract/Relax (Agonist/Agonist)**. *You have 2 minutes to complete this task.*

Tester places athlete and limb in appropriate position	Test 1	Test 2	Test 3
Supine	Ⓨ Ⓝ	Ⓨ Ⓝ	Ⓨ Ⓝ
Knee in full extension	Ⓨ Ⓝ	Ⓨ Ⓝ	Ⓨ Ⓝ
Hip in flexion	Ⓨ Ⓝ	Ⓨ Ⓝ	Ⓨ Ⓝ
Tester performs test according to accepted guidelines	**Test 1**	**Test 2**	**Test 3**
Instructs the athlete on proper commands and sequence	Ⓨ Ⓝ	Ⓨ Ⓝ	Ⓨ Ⓝ
Stabilizes the anterior femur with one hand	Ⓨ Ⓝ	Ⓨ Ⓝ	Ⓨ Ⓝ
Passively stretches the knee flexors (using the "relax" command, moves the hip into full flexion while maintaining knee extension) with the other hand	Ⓨ Ⓝ	Ⓨ Ⓝ	Ⓨ Ⓝ
Holds stretch for 4 to 10 seconds ("relax" command)	Ⓨ Ⓝ	Ⓨ Ⓝ	Ⓨ Ⓝ
Resists the knee flexors using a "pull" command through the full ROM (hip flexion → hip extension) with hand previously applying the stretch	Ⓨ Ⓝ	Ⓨ Ⓝ	Ⓨ Ⓝ
Uses proper hand placement for applying maximal isotonic resistance	Ⓨ Ⓝ	Ⓨ Ⓝ	Ⓨ Ⓝ

The psychomotor skill was performed completely and in the appropriate order   **0 1 2 3 4 5**

The tester had control of the subject and the situation (showed confidence)   **0 1 2 3 4 5**

Method of performing the skill allowed the tester the ability to determine:
severity, proper progression, and the *fit* in the overall picture (Oral)   **0 1 2 3 4 5**

In order for a grade of *minimum standard* to be given, the total must be ≥11   **TOTAL = _____**

| 1 | 2 | 3 | 4 | 5 | 6 | 7 | 8 | 9 | 10 | 11 | 12 | 13 | 14 | 15 |

Not Acceptable   **Meets Minimum Standards**   **Exceeds Minimum Standards**

TEST ENVIRONMENTS

L: Laboratory/Classroom Testing
C: Clinical/Field Testing
P: Practicum Testing
A: Assessment/Mock Exam Testing
S: Self-Reporting

SKILL TEST INFORMATION

Purpose: Increase flexibility
Involved Structure: Hamstring muscles
Special Considerations N/A
Reference(s): Prentice (2004)
Supplies Needed: Table

PNF
(PNF-L-Test 3)

Peer Review _____ Peer Review _____

Skill Acquisition: _____ Practice Opportunities: _____

*Please demonstrate how you would stretch the **ankle invertors** using **PNF Hold/Relax (Agonist/Antagonist)**. You have 2 minutes to complete this task.*

Tester places athlete and limb in appropriate position	Test 1	Test 2	Test 3
Seated	Ⓨ Ⓝ	Ⓨ Ⓝ	Ⓨ Ⓝ
Foot/ankle hanging off the edge of the table	Ⓨ Ⓝ	Ⓨ Ⓝ	Ⓨ Ⓝ
Tester performs test according to accepted guidelines	**Test 1**	**Test 2**	**Test 3**
Instructs the athlete on proper commands and sequence	Ⓨ Ⓝ	Ⓨ Ⓝ	Ⓨ Ⓝ
Stabilizes the lower leg with one hand	Ⓨ Ⓝ	Ⓨ Ⓝ	Ⓨ Ⓝ
Passively stretches the ankle invertors (using the "relax" command, moves the ankle into full eversion) with the other hand	Ⓨ Ⓝ	Ⓨ Ⓝ	Ⓨ Ⓝ
Holds stretch for 4 to 10 seconds using "relax" command	Ⓨ Ⓝ	Ⓨ Ⓝ	Ⓨ Ⓝ
Passively moves the ankle from full eversion to about 5 degrees of inversion ("relax" command)	Ⓨ Ⓝ	Ⓨ Ⓝ	Ⓨ Ⓝ
Resists the ankle evertors using a "hold" command (isometric contraction) with the hand previously applying the stretch (resistance is applied in an inward direction against the outward force of the foot)	Ⓨ Ⓝ	Ⓨ Ⓝ	Ⓨ Ⓝ
Holds isometric contraction for 6 to 10 seconds	Ⓨ Ⓝ	Ⓨ Ⓝ	Ⓨ Ⓝ
Uses proper hand placement for applying maximal isometric resistance	Ⓨ Ⓝ	Ⓨ Ⓝ	Ⓨ Ⓝ

The psychomotor skill was performed completely and in the appropriate order   **0 1 2 3 4 5**

The tester had control of the subject and the situation (showed confidence)   **0 1 2 3 4 5**

Method of performing the skill allowed the tester the ability to determine: severity, proper progression, and the *fit* in the overall picture (Oral)   **0 1 2 3 4 5**

In order for a grade of *minimum standard* to be given, the total must be ≥11   **TOTAL = _____**

```
   1    2    3    4    5    6    7    8    9   10   11   12   13   14   15
   |    |    |    |    |    |    |    |    |    |    |    |    |    |    |
```
Not Acceptable   **Meets**   **Exceeds**

                                               Minimum Standards   **Minimum Standards**

SKILL TEST INFORMATION

TEST ENVIRONMENTS

L: Laboratory/Classroom Testing
C: Clinical/Field Testing
P: Practicum Testing
A: Assessment/Mock Exam Testing
S: Self-Reporting

Purpose:	Increase flexibility
Involved Structure:	Tibialis Anterior; Tibialis Posterior
Special Considerations:	May be done with the knee extended
Reference(s):	Prentice (2004)
Supplies Needed:	Table

PNF
(PNF-L-Test 4)

Peer Review _____ Peer Review _____

Skill Acquisition: _____   Practice Opportunities: _____

Please demonstrate how you would stretch the **hip flexors** *using* **PNF Hold/Relax (Agonist/Agonist)**. *You have 2 minutes to complete this task.*

Tester places athlete and limb in appropriate position	Test 1	Test 2	Test 3
Prone	Ⓨ Ⓝ	Ⓨ Ⓝ	Ⓨ Ⓝ
Knee in full flexion	Ⓨ Ⓝ	Ⓨ Ⓝ	Ⓨ Ⓝ
Tester performs test according to accepted guidelines	**Test 1**	**Test 2**	**Test 3**
Instructs the athlete on proper commands and sequence	Ⓨ Ⓝ	Ⓨ Ⓝ	Ⓨ Ⓝ
Stabilizes the trunk with one hand	Ⓨ Ⓝ	Ⓨ Ⓝ	Ⓨ Ⓝ
Passively stretches the hip flexors (using the "relax" command, moves the hip into hyperextension) with the other hand	Ⓨ Ⓝ	Ⓨ Ⓝ	Ⓨ Ⓝ
Holds stretch for 4 to 10 seconds using "relax" command	Ⓨ Ⓝ	Ⓨ Ⓝ	Ⓨ Ⓝ
Resists the hip flexors using a "hold" command (isometric contraction) with the hand previously applying the stretch (resistance is applied in an upward direction against the downward force of the femur)	Ⓨ Ⓝ	Ⓨ Ⓝ	Ⓨ Ⓝ
Uses proper hand placement for applying maximal isometric resistance	Ⓨ Ⓝ	Ⓨ Ⓝ	Ⓨ Ⓝ

The psychomotor skill was performed completely and in the appropriate order   0 1 2 3 4 5

The tester had control of the subject and the situation (showed confidence)   0 1 2 3 4 5

Method of performing the skill allowed the tester the ability to determine:
severity, proper progression, and the *fit* in the overall picture (Oral)   0 1 2 3 4 5

In order for a grade of *minimum standard* to be given, the total must be ≥11   **TOTAL = _____**

```
 1    2    3    4    5    6    7    8    9   10   11   12   13   14   15
 |    |    |    |    |    |    |    |    |    |    |    |    |    |    |
```

Not Acceptable   **Meets**   **Exceeds**
                                            Minimum Standards   **Minimum Standards**

TEST ENVIRONMENTS

L: Laboratory/Classroom Testing
C: Clinical/Field Testing
P: Practicum Testing
A: Assessment/Mock Exam Testing
S: Self-Reporting

SKILL TEST INFORMATION

Purpose: Increase flexibility
Involved Structure: Iliopsoas; Rectus Femoris
Special Considerations: N/A
Reference(s): Prentice (2004)
Supplies Needed: Table

PNF
(PNF-L-Test 5)

Peer Review _____ Peer Review _____

Skill Acquisition: _____   Practice Opportunities: _____

Please demonstrate how you would strengthen the **knee flexors** *using* **PNF Slow Reversal.** *You have 2 minutes to complete this task.*

Tester places athlete and limb in appropriate position	Test 1	Test 2	Test 3
Seated or prone	Ⓨ Ⓝ	Ⓨ Ⓝ	Ⓨ Ⓝ
Knee in full extension	Ⓨ Ⓝ	Ⓨ Ⓝ	Ⓨ Ⓝ

Tester performs test according to accepted guidelines	Test 1	Test 2	Test 3
Instructs the athlete on proper commands and sequence	Ⓨ Ⓝ	Ⓨ Ⓝ	Ⓨ Ⓝ
Stabilizes femur	Ⓨ Ⓝ	Ⓨ Ⓝ	Ⓨ Ⓝ
Instructs the athlete to isotonically contract the hamstring—moving from extension to flexion ("pull" command)	Ⓨ Ⓝ	Ⓨ Ⓝ	Ⓨ Ⓝ
Instructs the athlete to immediately reverse the direction, contracting the quadriceps moving from flexion to extension ("push" command)	Ⓨ Ⓝ	Ⓨ Ⓝ	Ⓨ Ⓝ
Uses proper hand position for applying isotonic resistance	Ⓨ Ⓝ	Ⓨ Ⓝ	Ⓨ Ⓝ
Repeats above steps	Ⓨ Ⓝ	Ⓨ Ⓝ	Ⓨ Ⓝ

The psychomotor skill was performed completely and in the appropriate order   **0 1 2 3 4 5**

The tester had control of the subject and the situation (showed confidence)   **0 1 2 3 4 5**

Method of performing the skill allowed the tester the ability to determine:
severity, proper progression, and the *fit* in the overall picture (Oral)   **0 1 2 3 4 5**

In order for a grade of *minimum standard* to be given, the total must be ≥11   **TOTAL = _____**

```
  1     2     3     4     5     6     7     8     9    10    11    12    13    14    15
  |     |     |     |     |     |     |     |     |     |     |     |     |     |     |
```

Not Acceptable   **Meets**   **Exceeds**
                                    Minimum Standards   **Minimum Standards**

TEST ENVIRONMENTS	**SKILL TEST INFORMATION**

TEST ENVIRONMENTS

L: Laboratory/Classroom Testing
C: Clinical/Field Testing
P: Practicum Testing
A: Assessment/Mock Exam Testing
S: Self-Reporting

SKILL TEST INFORMATION

Positive Finding: Muscle education/strengthening
Involved Structure: Hamstrings
Special Considerations: N/A
Reference(s): Prentice (2004)
Supplies Needed: N/A

PNF
(PNF-L-Test 6)

Peer Review _____ Peer Review _____

Skill Acquisition: _____   Practice Opportunities: _____

*Please demonstrate how you would strengthen the **ankle invertors** using **PNF Slow Reversal-Hold**. You have 2 minutes to complete this task.*

Tester places athlete and limb in appropriate position	Test 1	Test 2	Test 3
Seated or supine	Ⓨ Ⓝ	Ⓨ Ⓝ	Ⓨ Ⓝ
Ankle placed in full eversion	Ⓨ Ⓝ	Ⓨ Ⓝ	Ⓨ Ⓝ
Tester performs test according to accepted guidelines	**Test 1**	**Test 2**	**Test 3**
Instructs the athlete on proper commands and sequence	Ⓨ Ⓝ	Ⓨ Ⓝ	Ⓨ Ⓝ
Stabilizes tibia	Ⓨ Ⓝ	Ⓨ Ⓝ	Ⓨ Ⓝ
Instructs the athlete to isotonically contract the invertors—moving from eversion to inversion ("pull" command)	Ⓨ Ⓝ	Ⓨ Ⓝ	Ⓨ Ⓝ
Instructs the athlete to isometrically contract the invertors at the end of the range ("hold" command)	Ⓨ Ⓝ	Ⓨ Ⓝ	Ⓨ Ⓝ
Holds isometric contraction for 4 to 10 seconds	Ⓨ Ⓝ	Ⓨ Ⓝ	Ⓨ Ⓝ
Instructs the athlete to reverse direction—isotonically contract the evertors, moving from inversion to eversion ("push" command)	Ⓨ Ⓝ	Ⓨ Ⓝ	Ⓨ Ⓝ
Instructs the athlete to isometrically contract the evertors at the end of the range ("hold" command)	Ⓨ Ⓝ	Ⓨ Ⓝ	Ⓨ Ⓝ
Holds isometric contraction for 4 to 10 seconds	Ⓨ Ⓝ	Ⓨ Ⓝ	Ⓨ Ⓝ
Uses proper hand position for applying isotonic and isometric resistance	Ⓨ Ⓝ	Ⓨ Ⓝ	Ⓨ Ⓝ
Repeats above steps	Ⓨ Ⓝ	Ⓨ Ⓝ	Ⓨ Ⓝ

The psychomotor skill was performed completely and in the appropriate order   0 1 2 3 4 5

The tester had control of the subject and the situation (showed confidence)   0 1 2 3 4 5

Method of performing the skill allowed the tester the ability to determine: severity, proper progression, and the *fit* in the overall picture (Oral)   0 1 2 3 4 5

In order for a grade of *minimum standard* to be given, the total must be ≥11   TOTAL = _____

1	2	3	4	5	6	7	8	9	10	11	12	13	14	15

Not Acceptable   **Meets**   **Exceeds**
                          Minimum Standards   **Minimum Standards**

TEST ENVIRONMENTS

L: Laboratory/Classroom Testing
C: Clinical/Field Testing
P: Practicum Testing
A: Assessment/Mock Exam Testing
S: Self-Reporting

SKILL TEST INFORMATION

Positive Finding: Muscle education/strengthening
Involved Structure: Tibialis anterior
Special Considerations: N/A
Reference(s): Prentice (2004)
Supplies Needed: N/A

PNF
(PNF-L-Test 7)

Peer Review _____ Peer Review _____

Skill Acquisition: _____   Practice Opportunities: _____

Please demonstrate how you would perform **PNF Repeated Contraction** *for the* **ankle dorsiflexors.** *You have 2 minutes to complete this task.*

Tester places athlete and limb in appropriate position	Test 1	Test 2	Test 3
Supine or seated	Ⓨ Ⓝ	Ⓨ Ⓝ	Ⓨ Ⓝ
Ankle placed in full plantar flexion	Ⓨ Ⓝ	Ⓨ Ⓝ	Ⓨ Ⓝ
Tester performs test according to accepted guidelines	**Test 1**	**Test 2**	**Test 3**
Stabilizes tibia	Ⓨ Ⓝ	Ⓨ Ⓝ	Ⓨ Ⓝ
Resists dorsiflexion using the "pull command" through the full ROM with the other hand (moves isotonically against maximal resistance)	Ⓨ Ⓝ	Ⓨ Ⓝ	Ⓨ Ⓝ
Repeats above step until fatigue is evident	Ⓨ Ⓝ	Ⓨ Ⓝ	Ⓨ Ⓝ
Performs "quick stretch" at the weakest point of the motion (or at the end of dorsiflexion)	Ⓨ Ⓝ	Ⓨ Ⓝ	Ⓨ Ⓝ

The psychomotor skill was performed completely and in the appropriate order   **0 1 2 3 4 5**

The tester had control of the subject and the situation (showed confidence)   **0 1 2 3 4 5**

Method of performing the skill allowed the tester the ability to determine: severity, proper progression, and the *fit* in the overall picture (Oral)   **0 1 2 3 4 5**

In order for a grade of *minimum standard* to be given, the total must be ≥11   **TOTAL = _____**

1	2	3	4	5	6	7	8	9	10	11	12	13	14	15

Not Acceptable   **Meets**   **Exceeds**
                              Minimum Standards   **Minimum Standards**

TEST ENVIRONMENTS

L: Laboratory/Classroom Testing
C: Clinical/Field Testing
P: Practicum Testing
A: Assessment/Mock Exam Testing
S: Self-Reporting

SKILL TEST INFORMATION

Positive Finding: Strengthening
Involved Structure: Tibialis anterior
Special Considerations: N/A
Reference(s): Prentice (2004)
Supplies Needed: Table

PNF
(PNF-L-Test 8)

Peer Review _____ Peer Review _____

Skill Acquisition: _____   Practice Opportunities: _____

Please demonstrate how you would strengthen the **ankle dorsiflexors** *using* **PNF Rhythmic Stabilization.** *Instruct the patient to complete 1 set of 3 repetitions in 2 directions/2 positions. You have 2 minutes to complete this task.*

Tester places athlete and limb in appropriate position	Test 1	Test 2	Test 3
Seated	Ⓨ Ⓝ	Ⓨ Ⓝ	Ⓨ Ⓝ
Foot/ankle hanging off the edge of the table	Ⓨ Ⓝ	Ⓨ Ⓝ	Ⓨ Ⓝ
Tester performs test according to accepted guidelines	**Test 1**	**Test 2**	**Test 3**
Instructs the athlete on proper commands and sequence	Ⓨ Ⓝ	Ⓨ Ⓝ	Ⓨ Ⓝ
Stabilizes tibia/fibula with one hand	Ⓨ Ⓝ	Ⓨ Ⓝ	Ⓨ Ⓝ
Passively move the foot into Position 1 (approximately 5 degrees of dorsiflexion) using the "relax" command with the other hand	Ⓨ Ⓝ	Ⓨ Ⓝ	Ⓨ Ⓝ
Resists the dorsiflexors using a "hold" command (resistance is applied in a downward direction against the upward force of the foot)	Ⓨ Ⓝ	Ⓨ Ⓝ	Ⓨ Ⓝ
Holds isometric contraction for 6 to 10 seconds	Ⓨ Ⓝ	Ⓨ Ⓝ	Ⓨ Ⓝ
Immediately reverse the force resisting the plantar flexors using a "hold" command (resistance is applied in an upward direction against the downward force of the foot)	Ⓨ Ⓝ	Ⓨ Ⓝ	Ⓨ Ⓝ
Holds isometric contraction for 6 to 10 seconds	Ⓨ Ⓝ	Ⓨ Ⓝ	Ⓨ Ⓝ
Repeats (2 times)	Ⓨ Ⓝ	Ⓨ Ⓝ	Ⓨ Ⓝ
Passively moves the foot into Position 2 (approximately 20 degrees of plantar flexion) using the "relax" command with the other hand	Ⓨ Ⓝ	Ⓨ Ⓝ	Ⓨ Ⓝ
Resists the dorsiflexors using a "hold" command (resistance is applied in a downward direction against the upward force of the foot)	Ⓨ Ⓝ	Ⓨ Ⓝ	Ⓨ Ⓝ
Holds isometric contraction for 6 to 10 seconds	Ⓨ Ⓝ	Ⓨ Ⓝ	Ⓨ Ⓝ
Immediately reverses the force resisting the plantar flexors using a "hold" command (resistance is applied in an upward direction against the downward force of the foot)	Ⓨ Ⓝ	Ⓨ Ⓝ	Ⓨ Ⓝ
Holds isometric contraction for 6 to 10 seconds	Ⓨ Ⓝ	Ⓨ Ⓝ	Ⓨ Ⓝ
Repeats (2 times)	Ⓨ Ⓝ	Ⓨ Ⓝ	Ⓨ Ⓝ

The psychomotor skill was performed completely and in the appropriate order   0 1 2 3 4 5

The tester had control of the subject and the situation (showed confidence)   0 1 2 3 4 5

Method of performing the skill allowed the tester the ability to determine:
severity, proper progression, and the *fit* in the overall picture (Oral)   0 1 2 3 4 5

In order for a grade of *minimum standard* to be given, the total must be ≥11   **TOTAL =** _____

```
 1    2    3    4    5    6    7    8    9   10   11   12   13   14   15
 |    |    |    |    |    |    |    |    |    |    |    |    |    |    |
```

Not Acceptable   **Meets**   **Exceeds**
                                   Minimum Standards   **Minimum Standards**

TEST ENVIRONMENTS

L: Laboratory/Classroom Testing
C: Clinical/Field Testing
P: Practicum Testing
A: Assessment/Mock Exam Testing
S: Self-Reporting

SKILL TEST INFORMATION

Purpose: Strengthening
Involved Structure: Tibialis Anterior
Special Considerations: N/A
Reference(s): Prentice (2004)
Supplies Needed: Table

Chapter 15

JOINT MOBILIZATION

Joint Mobilization
(JM-U-Test 1)

Peer Review _____ Peer Review _____

Skill Acquisition: _____   Practice Opportunities: _____

This problem allows you the opportunity to demonstrate the proper technique for administering an **Anterior-Posterior Glide of the radial head.** *You have 2 minutes to complete this task.*

Tester places athlete and limb in appropriate position	Test 1	Test 2	Test 3
Seated	Y N	Y N	Y N
Elbow resting supinated on a table (table serves as support)	Y N	Y N	Y N
Elbow flexed between 30 to 70 degrees	Y N	Y N	Y N
Tester placed in proper position	**Test 1**	**Test 2**	**Test 3**
Thumbs and index fingers are placed to control the proximal radius (radial head)	Y N	Y N	Y N
Tester performs test according to accepted guidelines	**Test 1**	**Test 2**	**Test 3**
Thumb and index finger apply a mobilization force in a posterior direction	Y N	Y N	Y N
Assess grades of excursion/glide	Y N	Y N	Y N
Oscillation of the posterior glide is performed → 2 to 3 times	Y N	Y N	Y N
Maintains relaxation of the limb	Y N	Y N	Y N
Performs assessment bilaterally	Y N	Y N	Y N

The psychomotor skill was performed completely and in the appropriate order   **0 1 2 3 4 5**

The tester had control of the subject and the situation (showed confidence)   **0 1 2 3 4 5**

Method of performing the skill allowed the tester the ability to determine:
severity, proper progression, and the *fit* in the overall picture (Oral)   **0 1 2 3 4 5**

In order for a grade of *minimum standard* to be given, the total must be ≥11   **TOTAL = _____**

```
  1     2     3     4     5     6     7     8     9    10    11    12    13    14    15
  |_____|_____|_____|_____|_____|_____|_____|_____|_____|_____|_____|_____|_____|_____|
```

Not Acceptable   **Meets**   **Exceeds**
                                    Minimum Standards   **Minimum Standards**

TEST ENVIRONMENTS

L: Laboratory/Classroom Testing
C: Clinical/Field Testing
P: Practicum Testing
A: Assessment/Mock Exam Testing
S: Self-Reporting

SKILL TEST INFORMATION

Purpose:	Increase pronation; decrease pain
Involved Structure:	Joint capsule
Special Considerations:	Assess grades of excursion/glide (I-IV)
Reference(s):	Edmond; Houglum; Konin et al (2004); Prentice (2004)
Supplies Needed:	Table

JOINT MOBILIZATION
(JM-U-Test 2)

This problem allows you the opportunity to demonstrate the proper technique for administering a **Posterior-Anterior Glide of the radial head**. *You have 2 minutes to complete this task.*

Tester places athlete and limb in appropriate position	Test 1	Test 2	Test 3
Seated	Y N	Y N	Y N
Athlete's involved elbow resting supinated on a table	Y N	Y N	Y N
Elbow flexed to approximately 70 degrees	Y N	Y N	Y N
Elbow supinated to approximately 35 degrees	Y N	Y N	Y N
Tester placed in proper position	**Test 1**	**Test 2**	**Test 3**
Thumbs and index fingers are placed to control the proximal radius (radial head)	Y N	Y N	Y N
Tester performs test according to accepted guidelines	**Test 1**	**Test 2**	**Test 3**
Instructs the athlete to "relax"	Y N	Y N	Y N
Thumb and index finger apply a mobilization force in an anterior direction	Y N	Y N	Y N
Assesses grades of excursion/glide	Y N	Y N	Y N
Oscillation of the anterior glide is performed → 2 to 3 times	Y N	Y N	Y N
Maintains relaxation of the involved limb	Y N	Y N	Y N

The psychomotor skill was performed completely and in the appropriate order   0 1 2 3 4 5

The tester had control of the subject and the situation (showed confidence)   0 1 2 3 4 5

Method of performing the skill allowed the tester the ability to determine:
severity, proper progression, and the *fit* in the overall picture (Oral)   0 1 2 3 4 5

In order for a grade of *minimum standard* to be given, the total must be ≥11   TOTAL = _____

1 2 3 4 5 6 7 8 9 10 11 12 13 14 15

Not Acceptable   **Meets Minimum Standards**   **Exceeds Minimum Standards**

SKILL TEST INFORMATION

TEST ENVIRONMENTS

L: Laboratory/Classroom Testing
C: Clinical/Field Testing
P: Practicum Testing
A: Assessment/Mock Exam Testing
S: Self-Reporting

Purpose: Increase supination; decrease pain
Involved Structure: Joint capsule
Special Considerations: Assess grades of excursion/glide (I-IV)
Reference(s): Edmond, Konin et al (2004); Prentice (2004)
Supplies Needed: Table

JOINT MOBILIZATION
(JM-U-Test 3)

Peer Review _____ Peer Review _____

Skill Acquisition: _____   Practice Opportunities: _____

This problem allows you the opportunity to demonstrate the proper technique for administering an **Posterior-Anterior (Volar) Glide of the wrist (radiocarpal joint)**. *You have 2 minutes to complete this task.*

Tester places athlete and limb in appropriate position	Test 1	Test 2	Test 3
Seated	Ⓨ Ⓝ	Ⓨ Ⓝ	Ⓨ Ⓝ
Forearm resting supinated on a table (table serves as support)	Ⓨ Ⓝ	Ⓨ Ⓝ	Ⓨ Ⓝ
Tester placed in proper position	**Test 1**	**Test 2**	**Test 3**
Stabilizes the (distal) radius and ulna with one hand	Ⓨ Ⓝ	Ⓨ Ⓝ	Ⓨ Ⓝ
Places the other hand around the carpal bones (proximal row)	Ⓨ Ⓝ	Ⓨ Ⓝ	Ⓨ Ⓝ
Tester performs test according to accepted guidelines	**Test 1**	**Test 2**	**Test 3**
Instructs the subject to "relax"	Ⓨ Ⓝ	Ⓨ Ⓝ	Ⓨ Ⓝ
Hand on the carpal bones applies a mobilization force in an anterior or ventral direction	Ⓨ Ⓝ	Ⓨ Ⓝ	Ⓨ Ⓝ
Assesses stages of distraction	Ⓨ Ⓝ	Ⓨ Ⓝ	Ⓨ Ⓝ
Assesses grades of excursion/glide	Ⓨ Ⓝ	Ⓨ Ⓝ	Ⓨ Ⓝ
Oscillation of the anterior glide is performed → 2 to 3 times	Ⓨ Ⓝ	Ⓨ Ⓝ	Ⓨ Ⓝ
Maintains relaxation of the limb	Ⓨ Ⓝ	Ⓨ Ⓝ	Ⓨ Ⓝ
Performs assessment bilaterally	Ⓨ Ⓝ	Ⓨ Ⓝ	Ⓨ Ⓝ

The psychomotor skill was performed completely and in the appropriate order   0 1 2 3 4 5

The tester had control of the subject and the situation (showed confidence)   0 1 2 3 4 5

Method of performing the skill allowed the tester the ability to determine:
severity, proper progression, and the *fit* in the overall picture (Oral)   0 1 2 3 4 5

In order for a grade of *minimum standard* to be given, the total must be ≥11   TOTAL = _____

```
 1    2    3    4    5    6    7    8    9   10   11   12   13   14   15
 |____|____|____|____|____|____|____|____|____|____|____|____|____|____|
```
Not Acceptable   **Meets**   **Exceeds**
                                    Minimum Standards   **Minimum Standards**

TEST ENVIRONMENTS

L: Laboratory/Classroom Testing
C: Clinical/Field Testing
P: Practicum Testing
A: Assessment/Mock Exam Testing
S: Self-Reporting

SKILL TEST INFORMATION

Purpose: Increase wrist extension; decrease pain
Involved Structure: Joint capsule
Special Considerations: Assess grades of distraction and excursion/glide (I-IV)
Reference(s): Edmond; Konin et al (2004); Prentice (2004)
Supplies Needed: Table

JOINT MOBILIZATION
(JM-U-Test 4)

Peer Review _____ Peer Review _____

Skill Acquisition: _____   Practice Opportunities: _____

This problem allows you the opportunity to demonstrate the proper technique for administering an **Anterior-Posterior (Dorsal) Glide of the Wrist (radiocarpal joint)**. *You have 2 minutes to complete this task.*

Tester places athlete and limb in appropriate position	Test 1	Test 2	Test 3
Seated	Ⓨ Ⓝ	Ⓨ Ⓝ	Ⓨ Ⓝ
Subject's involved forearm placed in slight ulnar deviation	Ⓨ Ⓝ	Ⓨ Ⓝ	Ⓨ Ⓝ
Tester placed in proper position	**Test 1**	**Test 2**	**Test 3**
Stabilizes the (distal) radius and ulna with one hand	Ⓨ Ⓝ	Ⓨ Ⓝ	Ⓨ Ⓝ
Place the other hand around the carpal bones (proximal row)	Ⓨ Ⓝ	Ⓨ Ⓝ	Ⓨ Ⓝ
Tester performs test according to accepted guidelines	**Test 1**	**Test 2**	**Test 3**
Instructs the subject to "relax"	Ⓨ Ⓝ	Ⓨ Ⓝ	Ⓨ Ⓝ
Assesses stages of distraction	Ⓨ Ⓝ	Ⓨ Ⓝ	Ⓨ Ⓝ
Applies a mobilization force in a posterior or dorsal direction on the carpal bones	Ⓨ Ⓝ	Ⓨ Ⓝ	Ⓨ Ⓝ
Assesses grades of excursion/glide	Ⓨ Ⓝ	Ⓨ Ⓝ	Ⓨ Ⓝ
Oscillation of the posterior glide is performed ➔ 2 to 3 times	Ⓨ Ⓝ	Ⓨ Ⓝ	Ⓨ Ⓝ
Maintains relaxation of the involved limb	Ⓨ Ⓝ	Ⓨ Ⓝ	Ⓨ Ⓝ

The psychomotor skill was performed completely and in the appropriate order   **0   1   2   3   4   5**

The tester had control of the subject and the situation (showed confidence)   **0   1   2   3   4   5**

Method of performing the skill allowed the tester the ability to determine:
severity, proper progression, and the *fit* in the overall picture (Oral)   **0   1   2   3   4   5**

In order for a grade of *minimum standard* to be given, the total must be ≥11   **TOTAL = _____**

1	2	3	4	5	6	7	8	9	10	11	12	13	14	15

Not Acceptable   **Meets**   **Exceeds**
                                        Minimum Standards   **Minimum Standards**

TEST ENVIRONMENTS

L: Laboratory/Classroom Testing
C: Clinical/Field Testing
P: Practicum Testing
A: Assessment/Mock Exam Testing
S: Self-Reporting

SKILL TEST INFORMATION

Purpose:	Increase wrist flexion; decrease pain
Involved Structure:	Joint capsule
Special Considerations:	Assess grades of distraction & excursion/glide (I-IV)
Reference(s):	Edmond, Konin et al (2004); Prentice (2004)
Supplies Needed:	Table

JOINT MOBILIZATION
(JM-U-Test 5)

Skill Acquisition: _____   Practice Opportunities: _____

This problem allows you the opportunity to demonstrate the proper technique for administering a **Distraction Glide of the Third Metacarpal on the Phalangeal Joint.** *You have 2 minutes to complete this task.*

Tester places athlete and limb in appropriate position	Test 1	Test 2	Test 3
Seated	Ⓨ Ⓝ	Ⓨ Ⓝ	Ⓨ Ⓝ
Elbow resting on a table; palm down	Ⓨ Ⓝ	Ⓨ Ⓝ	Ⓨ Ⓝ
Places MCP in slight flexion	Ⓨ Ⓝ	Ⓨ Ⓝ	Ⓨ Ⓝ

Tester placed in proper position	Test 1	Test 2	Test 3
Tester facing the MCP joint	Ⓨ Ⓝ	Ⓨ Ⓝ	Ⓨ Ⓝ
One hand grips the third metacarpal (thumb/dorsal surface & index finger/volar surface)	Ⓨ Ⓝ	Ⓨ Ⓝ	Ⓨ Ⓝ
Second hand grips the base of the proximal phalange (thumb & index finger)	Ⓨ Ⓝ	Ⓨ Ⓝ	Ⓨ Ⓝ

Tester performs test according to accepted guidelines	Test 1	Test 2	Test 3
Instructs the athlete to "relax"	Ⓨ Ⓝ	Ⓨ Ⓝ	Ⓨ Ⓝ
Hand on the proximal phalange applies a distraction force opening the joint	Ⓨ Ⓝ	Ⓨ Ⓝ	Ⓨ Ⓝ
Assesses stages of distractions	Ⓨ Ⓝ	Ⓨ Ⓝ	Ⓨ Ⓝ
Maintains relaxation of the involved limb	Ⓨ Ⓝ	Ⓨ Ⓝ	Ⓨ Ⓝ

The psychomotor skill was performed completely and in the appropriate order   **0 1 2 3 4 5**

The tester had control of the subject and the situation (showed confidence)   **0 1 2 3 4 5**

Method of performing the skill allowed the tester the ability to determine:
severity, proper progression, and the *fit* in the overall picture (Oral)   **0 1 2 3 4 5**

In order for a grade of *minimum standard* to be given, the total must be ≥11   **TOTAL = _____**

```
 1    2    3    4    5    6    7    8    9   10   11   12   13   14   15
 |    |    |    |    |    |    |    |    |    |    |    |    |    |    |
```
Not Acceptable   **Meets**   **Exceeds**
                                              Minimum Standards   **Minimum Standards**

TEST ENVIRONMENTS

L: Laboratory/Classroom Testing
C: Clinical/Field Testing
P: Practicum Testing
A: Assessment/Mock Exam Testing
S: Self-Reporting

SKILL TEST INFORMATION

Purpose: Increased overall motion; decrease pain
Involved Structure: Joint capsule
Special Considerations: Movement is minimal; maintain MCP joint flexion; assess stages of distraction
Reference(s): Edmond; Konin (2001)
Supplies Needed: Chair, Table

JOINT MOBILIZATION
(JM-U-Test 6)

Skill Acquisition: _____   Practice Opportunities: _____

This problem allows you the opportunity to demonstrate the proper technique for administering a **Posterior (Dorsal) Glide of the Carpometacarpal joint**. *You have 2 minutes to complete this task.*

Tester places athlete and limb in appropriate position	Test 1	Test 2	Test 3
Seated	Ⓨ Ⓝ	Ⓨ Ⓝ	Ⓨ Ⓝ
Elbow resting on a table; palm down	Ⓨ Ⓝ	Ⓨ Ⓝ	Ⓨ Ⓝ
Places CMC and radial carpal joint in slight flexion with minimal ulnar deviation	Ⓨ Ⓝ	Ⓨ Ⓝ	Ⓨ Ⓝ

Tester placed in proper position	Test 1	Test 2	Test 3
Tester facing the carpometacarpal joint	Ⓨ Ⓝ	Ⓨ Ⓝ	Ⓨ Ⓝ
One hand grips the individual carpal (thumb/dorsal surface & index finger/volar surface)	Ⓨ Ⓝ	Ⓨ Ⓝ	Ⓨ Ⓝ
Second hand grips the base of the individual metacarpal (thumb & index finger)	Ⓨ Ⓝ	Ⓨ Ⓝ	Ⓨ Ⓝ

Tester performs test according to accepted guidelines	Test 1	Test 2	Test 3
Instructs the athlete to "relax"	Ⓨ Ⓝ	Ⓨ Ⓝ	Ⓨ Ⓝ
Assesses stages of distraction	Ⓨ Ⓝ	Ⓨ Ⓝ	Ⓨ Ⓝ
Hand on the metacarpal applies a glide in a dorsal/posterior direction	Ⓨ Ⓝ	Ⓨ Ⓝ	Ⓨ Ⓝ
Assesses grades of excursion/glide	Ⓨ Ⓝ	Ⓨ Ⓝ	Ⓨ Ⓝ
Oscillation of the dorsal/posterior glide is performed ➜ 2 to 3 times	Ⓨ Ⓝ	Ⓨ Ⓝ	Ⓨ Ⓝ
Maintains relaxation of the involved limb	Ⓨ Ⓝ	Ⓨ Ⓝ	Ⓨ Ⓝ

The psychomotor skill was performed completely and in the appropriate order   0 1 2 3 4 5

The tester had control of the subject and the situation (showed confidence)   0 1 2 3 4 5

Method of performing the skill allowed the tester the ability to determine:
severity, proper progression, and the *fit* in the overall picture (Oral)   0 1 2 3 4 5

In order for a grade of *minimum standard* to be given, the total must be ≥11   TOTAL = _____

```
  1     2     3     4     5     6     7     8     9     10    11    12    13    14    15
  |     |     |     |     |     |     |     |     |     |     |     |     |     |     |
```
Not Acceptable   **Meets**   **Exceeds**
                                              Minimum Standards   **Minimum Standards**

SKILL TEST INFORMATION

Purpose:	Increase CMC joint extension; decrease Joint
Involved Structure:	Joint capsule
Special Considerations:	Movement is minimal; maintain CMC joint flexion; assess stages of distraction and grades of excursion/glide (I-IV)
Reference(s)	Edmond; Konin (2001); Prentice (2004)
Supplies Needed:	Chair, table

TEST ENVIRONMENTS
L: Laboratory/Classroom Testing
C: Clinical/Field Testing
P: Practicum Testing
A: Assessment/Mock Exam Testing
S: Self-Reporting

Joint Mobilization
(JM-U-Test 7)

Peer Review _____ Peer Review _____

Skill Acquisition: _____   Practice Opportunities: _____

This problem allows you the opportunity to demonstrate the proper technique for administering an **Anterior (PA/Volar) Glide of the DIP Joint of Second Finger**. *You have 2 minutes to complete this task.*

Tester places athlete and limb in appropriate position	Test 1	Test 2	Test 3
Seated	Y N	Y N	Y N
Elbow fully pronated (palm down)	Y N	Y N	Y N
Places the PIP joint in slight flexion and DIP in approximately 30 degrees of flexion	Y N	Y N	Y N

Tester placed in proper position	Test 1	Test 2	Test 3
Tester facing the involved joint	Y N	Y N	Y N
One hand grips the head of the middle phalanx (2nd finger) (thumb/dorsal surface & index finger/volar surface)	Y N	Y N	Y N
Second hand grips the base of the distal phalanx (2nd finger) (thumb/dorsal surface & index finger/volar surface)	Y N	Y N	Y N

Tester performs test according to accepted guidelines	Test 1	Test 2	Test 3
Instructs the athlete to "relax"	Y N	Y N	Y N
One hand stabilizes the middle phalanx	Y N	Y N	Y N
Assesses stages of distraction	Y N	Y N	Y N
Hand on the distal phalanx applies a glide in an anterior/volar direction	Y N	Y N	Y N
Assesses grades of excursion/glide	Y N	Y N	Y N
Oscillation of the anterior/volar glide is performed → 2 to 3 times	Y N	Y N	Y N
Maintains relaxation of the involved limb	Y N	Y N	Y N

The psychomotor skill was performed completely and in the appropriate order   0 1 2 3 4 5

The tester had control of the subject and the situation (showed confidence)   0 1 2 3 4 5

Method of performing the skill allowed the tester the ability to determine:
severity, proper progression, and the *fit* in the overall picture (Oral)   0 1 2 3 4 5

In order for a grade of *minimum standard* to be given, the total must be ≥11   TOTAL = _____

```
 1    2    3    4    5    6    7    8    9   10   11   12   13   14   15
 |____|____|____|____|____|____|____|____|____|____|____|____|____|____|
```

Not Acceptable   **Meets**   **Exceeds**
                              Minimum Standards   **Minimum Standards**

TEST ENVIRONMENTS

L: Laboratory/Classroom Testing
C: Clinical/Field Testing
P: Practicum Testing
A: Assessment/Mock Exam Testing
S: Self-Reporting

SKILL TEST INFORMATION

Purpose:	Increase flexion; decrease pain
Involved Structure:	Joint capsule
Special Considerations:	Movement is minimal; assess stages of distraction and grades of excursion/glide (I-IV)
Reference(s):	Edmond; Konin et al (2004)
Supplies Needed:	Chair, table

JOINT MOBILIZATION
(JM-U-Test 8)

Peer Review _____ Peer Review _____

Skill Acquisition: _____   Practice Opportunities: _____

This problem allows you the opportunity to demonstrate the proper technique for administering an **Inferior (Caudal) Glide of the Glenohumeral Joint**. *You have 2 minutes to complete this task.*

Tester places athlete and limb in appropriate position	Test 1	Test 2	Test 3
Supine	Y N	Y N	Y N
Shoulder abduction to approximately 55 degrees	Y N	Y N	Y N

Tester placed in proper position	Test 1	Test 2	Test 3
Tester stands behind the involved side	Y N	Y N	Y N
One hand grasps the distal humerus	Y N	Y N	Y N
Other hand is placed on the superior aspect of the proximal humerus	Y N	Y N	Y N

Tester performs test according to accepted guidelines	Test 1	Test 2	Test 3
Instructs the athlete to "relax"	Y N	Y N	Y N
Hand grasping the distal humerus applies a distraction force	Y N	Y N	Y N
Hand on the superior aspect of the proximal humerus applies an inferior/caudal glide	Y N	Y N	Y N
Assesses stages of distraction	Y N	Y N	Y N
Assesses grades of excursion/glide	Y N	Y N	Y N
Oscillation of the anterior glide is performed ➔ 2 to 3 times	Y N	Y N	Y N
Maintains relaxation of the involved limb	Y N	Y N	Y N

The psychomotor skill was performed completely and in the appropriate order   0 1 2 3 4 5

The tester had control of the subject and the situation (showed confidence)   0 1 2 3 4 5

Method of performing the skill allowed the tester the ability to determine:
severity, proper progression, and the *fit* in the overall picture (Oral)   0 1 2 3 4 5

In order for a grade of *minimum standard* to be given, the total must be ≥11   TOTAL = _____

```
 1    2    3    4    5    6    7    8    9    10   11   12   13   14   15
 |____|____|____|____|____|____|____|____|____|____|____|____|____|____|

 Not Acceptable                      Meets                    Exceeds
                               Minimum Standards         Minimum Standards
```

SKILL TEST INFORMATION

TEST ENVIRONMENTS

L: Laboratory/Classroom Testing
C: Clinical/Field Testing
P: Practicum Testing
A: Assessment/Mock Exam Testing
S: Self-Reporting

Purpose:	Increase glenohumeral abduction and elevation; decrease pain
Involved Structure:	Joint capsule
Special Considerations:	Assess stages of distraction and grades of excursion/glide (I-IV)
Reference(s):	Edmond; Konin et al (2004); Prentice (2004)
Supplies Needed	Chair, table

JOINT MOBILIZATION
(JM-U-Test 9)

Peer Review _____ Peer Review _____

Skill Acquisition: _____   Practice Opportunities: _____

This problem allows you the opportunity to demonstrate the proper technique for administering an **Anterior-Posterior Glide of the Glenohumeral Joint**. *You have 2 minutes to complete this task.*

Tester places athlete and limb in appropriate position	Test 1	Test 2	Test 3
Supine	Ⓨ Ⓝ	Ⓨ Ⓝ	Ⓨ Ⓝ
Shoulder at the edge of the table	Ⓨ Ⓝ	Ⓨ Ⓝ	Ⓨ Ⓝ
Shoulder abduction to approximately 55 degrees	Ⓨ Ⓝ	Ⓨ Ⓝ	Ⓨ Ⓝ

Tester placed in proper position	Test 1	Test 2	Test 3
Tester stands to the side of the athlete	Ⓨ Ⓝ	Ⓨ Ⓝ	Ⓨ Ⓝ
Scapula is stabilized by the table	Ⓨ Ⓝ	Ⓨ Ⓝ	Ⓨ Ⓝ
One hand grasps the distal humerus	Ⓨ Ⓝ	Ⓨ Ⓝ	Ⓨ Ⓝ
Other hand is placed on the anterior aspect of the humeral head	Ⓨ Ⓝ	Ⓨ Ⓝ	Ⓨ Ⓝ

Tester performs test according to accepted guidelines	Test 1	Test 2	Test 3
Hand grasping distal humerus applies distraction	Ⓨ Ⓝ	Ⓨ Ⓝ	Ⓨ Ⓝ
Hand on the humeral head applies a posterior force	Ⓨ Ⓝ	Ⓨ Ⓝ	Ⓨ Ⓝ
Assesses stages of distraction	Ⓨ Ⓝ	Ⓨ Ⓝ	Ⓨ Ⓝ
Assesses grades of excursion/glide	Ⓨ Ⓝ	Ⓨ Ⓝ	Ⓨ Ⓝ
Oscillation of the posterior glide is performed → 2 to 3 times	Ⓨ Ⓝ	Ⓨ Ⓝ	Ⓨ Ⓝ
Maintains relaxation of the limb	Ⓨ Ⓝ	Ⓨ Ⓝ	Ⓨ Ⓝ

The psychomotor skill was performed completely and in the appropriate order   0 1 2 3 4 5

The tester had control of the subject and the situation (showed confidence)   0 1 2 3 4 5

Method of performing the skill allowed the tester the ability to determine:
severity, proper progression, and the *fit* in the overall picture (Oral)   0 1 2 3 4 5

In order for a grade of *minimum standard* to be given, the total must be ≥11   TOTAL = _____

```
   1    2    3    4    5    6    7    8    9    10   11   12   13   14   15
   |    |    |    |    |    |    |    |    |    |    |    |    |    |    |
```

Not Acceptable   **Meets**   **Exceeds**
                               Minimum Standards   **Minimum Standards**

TEST ENVIRONMENTS

L: Laboratory/Classroom Testing
C: Clinical/Field Testing
P: Practicum Testing
A: Assessment/Mock Exam Testing
S: Self-Reporting

SKILL TEST INFORMATION

Purpose: Increase Glenohumeral joint; internal rotation; decrease pain

Involved Structure: Joint capsule

Special Considerations: Assess stages of distraction and grades of excursion/glide (I-IV)

Reference(s): Edmond; Konin et al (2004); Prentice (2004)

Supplies Needed: Table

JOINT MOBILIZATION
(JM-U-Test 10)

Peer Review _____ Peer Review _____

Skill Acquisition: _____   Practice Opportunities: _____

This problem allows you the opportunity to demonstrate the proper technique for administering a **Posterior-Anterior Glide of the Glenohumeral Joint**. *You have 2 minutes to complete this task.*

Tester places athlete and limb in appropriate position	Test 1	Test 2	Test 3
Prone	Y N	Y N	Y N
Shoulder abduction to approximately 55 degrees	Y N	Y N	Y N
Tester placed in proper position	**Test 1**	**Test 2**	**Test 3**
Tester stands to the side of the athlete	Y N	Y N	Y N
Scapula is stabilized by the table	Y N	Y N	Y N
One hand grasps the distal humerus	Y N	Y N	Y N
Other hand is placed on the posterior aspect of the humeral head	Y N	Y N	Y N
Tester performs test according to accepted guidelines	**Test 1**	**Test 2**	**Test 3**
Instructs the athlete to "relax"	Y N	Y N	Y N
Assesses stages of distraction	Y N	Y N	Y N
Hand on the humerus applies a mobilization force in an anterior direction	Y N	Y N	Y N
Assesses grades of excursion/glide	Y N	Y N	Y N
Oscillation of the anterior glide is performed → 2 to 3 times	Y N	Y N	Y N
Maintains relaxation of the involved limb	Y N	Y N	Y N

The psychomotor skill was performed completely and in the appropriate order   0 1 2 3 4 5

The tester had control of the subject and the situation (showed confidence)   0 1 2 3 4 5

Method of performing the skill allowed the tester the ability to determine: severity, proper progression, and the *fit* in the overall picture (Oral)   0 1 2 3 4 5

In order for a grade of *minimum standard* to be given, the total must be ≥11   TOTAL = _____

```
1    2    3    4    5    6    7    8    9    10   11   12   13   14   15
|    |    |    |    |    |    |    |    |    |    |    |    |    |    |
```

Not Acceptable   **Meets**   **Exceeds**
                                    Minimum Standards   **Minimum Standards**

TEST ENVIRONMENTS

L: Laboratory/Classroom Testing
C: Clinical/Field Testing
P: Practicum Testing
A: Assessment/Mock Exam Testing
S: Self-Reporting

SKILL TEST INFORMATION

Purpose:	Increase Glenohumeral joint external rotation; decrease pain
Involved Structure:	Joint capsule
Special Considerations:	Assess stages of distraction and grades of excursion/glide (I-IV)
Reference(s):	Edmond; Konin et al (2004; Prentice (2004)
Supplies Needed:	Table

Joint Mobilization
(JM-U-Test 11)

Peer Review _____   Peer Review _____

Skill Acquisition: _____   Practice Opportunities: _____

This problem allows you the opportunity to demonstrate the proper technique for administering **Rotational Mobilization of Cervical Vertebrae between C6 and C7**. *You have 2 minutes to complete this task.*

Tester places athlete and limb in appropriate position	Test 1	Test 2	Test 3
Prone with slight cervical flexion	Ⓨ Ⓝ	Ⓨ Ⓝ	Ⓨ Ⓝ
Tester placed in proper position	Ⓨ Ⓝ	Ⓨ Ⓝ	Ⓨ Ⓝ
Tester standing facing the cervical spine	**Test 1**	**Test 2**	**Test 3**
Thumb on one hand (nearest to the tester) is placed on the transverse process of the C7	Ⓨ Ⓝ	Ⓨ Ⓝ	Ⓨ Ⓝ
Other thumb (farthest from the tester) is placed on the transverse process of C6	Ⓨ Ⓝ	Ⓨ Ⓝ	Ⓨ Ⓝ
Tester performs test according to accepted guidelines	**Test 1**	**Test 2**	**Test 3**
Instructs the subject to "relax"	Ⓨ Ⓝ	Ⓨ Ⓝ	Ⓨ Ⓝ
Thumb on the transverse process at C7 stabilizes the vertebrae	Ⓨ Ⓝ	Ⓨ Ⓝ	Ⓨ Ⓝ
Thumb on the transverse process at C6 provides an anterior (ventral) glide	Ⓨ Ⓝ	Ⓨ Ⓝ	Ⓨ Ⓝ
Assesses grades of excursion/glide	Ⓨ Ⓝ	Ⓨ Ⓝ	Ⓨ Ⓝ
Oscillation of the anterior (ventral) glide is performed → 2 to 3 times	Ⓨ Ⓝ	Ⓨ Ⓝ	Ⓨ Ⓝ
Maintains relaxation of the cervical region	Ⓨ Ⓝ	Ⓨ Ⓝ	Ⓨ Ⓝ

The psychomotor skill was performed completely and in the appropriate order   0 1 2 3 4 5

The tester had control of the subject and the situation (showed confidence)   0 1 2 3 4 5

Method of performing the skill allowed the tester the ability to determine:
severity, proper progression, and the *fit* in the overall picture (Oral)   0 1 2 3 4 5

In order for a grade of *minimum standard* to be given, the total must be ≥11   **TOTAL = _____**

```
  1     2     3     4     5     6     7     8     9    10    11    12    13    14    15
  |     |     |     |     |     |     |     |     |     |     |     |     |     |     |
```

Not Acceptable   **Meets**   **Exceeds**
                                    Minimum Standards   **Minimum Standards**

TEST ENVIRONMENTS

L: Laboratory/Classroom Testing
C: Clinical/Field Testing
P: Practicum Testing
A: Assessment/Mock Exam Testing
S: Self-Reporting

SKILL TEST INFORMATION

Purpose:	Increase Cervical Spine rotation of C6 to the left; decrease pain
Involved Structure:	Joint capsule
Special Considerations:	Assess grades of excursion/ glides (I – IV)
Reference(s):	Edmond; Konin (2001)
Supplies Needed:	Table

JOINT MOBILIZATION
(JM-L-Test 1)

Peer Review _____ Peer Review _____

Skill Acquisition: _____   Practice Opportunities: _____

Please demonstrate the proper technique for administering **Rotational Mobilization of the Lumbar Vertebrae between L2 and L3**. *You have 2 minutes to complete this task.*

Tester places athlete and limb in appropriate position	Test 1	Test 2	Test 3
Prone Places pillow to maintain comfortable lumbar flexion	Ⓨ Ⓝ	Ⓨ Ⓝ	Ⓨ Ⓝ

Tester placed in proper position	Test 1	Test 2	Test 3
Tester standing facing the lumbar spine	Ⓨ Ⓝ	Ⓨ Ⓝ	Ⓨ Ⓝ
Thumb on one hand is placed on the lateral aspect of the spinous process of L3 on the right side	Ⓨ Ⓝ	Ⓨ Ⓝ	Ⓨ Ⓝ
Other thumb is placed on the lateral aspect of the spinous process of L2 on the left side	Ⓨ Ⓝ	Ⓨ Ⓝ	Ⓨ Ⓝ

Tester performs test according to accepted guidelines	Test 1	Test 2	Test 3
Instructs the subject to "relax"	Ⓨ Ⓝ	Ⓨ Ⓝ	Ⓨ Ⓝ
Thumb on the lateral aspect of the spinous process of L3 stabilizes the vertebrae	Ⓨ Ⓝ	Ⓨ Ⓝ	Ⓨ Ⓝ
Other thumb placed on the lateral aspect of the spinous process of L2 provides a lateral glide away from the examiner	Ⓨ Ⓝ	Ⓨ Ⓝ	Ⓨ Ⓝ
Assesses grades of excursion/glide	Ⓨ Ⓝ	Ⓨ Ⓝ	Ⓨ Ⓝ
Oscillation of the lateral glide is performed → 2to 3 times	Ⓨ Ⓝ	Ⓨ Ⓝ	Ⓨ Ⓝ
Maintains relaxation of the lumbar region	Ⓨ Ⓝ	Ⓨ Ⓝ	Ⓨ Ⓝ

The psychomotor skill was performed completely and in the appropriate order   0 1 2 3 4 5

The tester had control of the subject and the situation (showed confidence)   0 1 2 3 4 5

Method of performing the skill allowed the tester the ability to determine:
severity, proper progression, and the *fit* in the overall picture (Oral)   0 1 2 3 4 5

In order for a grade of *minimum standard* to be given, the total must be ≥11   **TOTAL =** _____

1	2	3	4	5	6	7	8	9	10	11	12	13	14	15

Not Acceptable   **Meets
Minimum Standards**   **Exceeds
Minimum Standards**

TEST ENVIRONMENTS

L: Laboratory/Classroom Testing
C: Clinical/Field Testing
P: Practicum Testing
A: Assessment/Mock Exam Testing
S: Self-Reporting

SKILL TEST INFORMATION

Purpose: Increase rotation to the left in the lumbar spine of L2; pain reduction

Involved Structure: Joint capsule

Special Considerations: L2 rotates to the left on L3; assesses grades of excursion/ glide (I – IV)

Reference(s): Edmond; Konin (2001)

Supplies Needed: Table, pillow

JOINT MOBILIZATION
(JM-L-Test 2)

Peer Review _____ Peer Review _____

Skill Acquisition: _____   Practice Opportunities: _____

Please demonstrate the proper technique for administering **Counternutation Mobilization of the Sacroiliac Joint**. *You have 2 minutes to complete this task.*

Tester places athlete and limb in appropriate position	Test 1	Test 2	Test 3
Prone	Ⓨ Ⓝ	Ⓨ Ⓝ	Ⓨ Ⓝ
Place pillow to maintain comfortable lumbar flexion	Ⓨ Ⓝ	Ⓨ Ⓝ	Ⓨ Ⓝ

Tester placed in proper position	Test 1	Test 2	Test 3
Tester standing to the side facing the sacroiliac joint	Ⓨ Ⓝ	Ⓨ Ⓝ	Ⓨ Ⓝ
One hand placed over the lumbar spine area (perpendicular to the spine)	Ⓨ Ⓝ	Ⓨ Ⓝ	Ⓨ Ⓝ
Other hand is placed over the inferior (caudal) portion to the sacrum	Ⓨ Ⓝ	Ⓨ Ⓝ	Ⓨ Ⓝ

Tester performs test according to accepted guidelines	Test 1	Test 2	Test 3
Instructs the subject to "relax"	Ⓨ Ⓝ	Ⓨ Ⓝ	Ⓨ Ⓝ
Hand over the lumbar area acts as a stabilizer	Ⓨ Ⓝ	Ⓨ Ⓝ	Ⓨ Ⓝ
Other hand glides the inferior surface of sacrum ventrally (forcing counternutation)	Ⓨ Ⓝ	Ⓨ Ⓝ	Ⓨ Ⓝ
Assesses grades of excursion/glide	Ⓨ Ⓝ	Ⓨ Ⓝ	Ⓨ Ⓝ
Oscillation of the counternutation mobilization is performed ➔ 2 to 3 times	Ⓨ Ⓝ	Ⓨ Ⓝ	Ⓨ Ⓝ
Maintains relaxation of the lumbar region	Ⓨ Ⓝ	Ⓨ Ⓝ	Ⓨ Ⓝ

The psychomotor skill was performed completely and in the appropriate order   0 1 2 3 4 5

The tester had control of the subject and the situation (showed confidence)   0 1 2 3 4 5

Method of performing the skill allowed the tester the ability to determine:
severity, proper progression, and the *fit* in the overall picture (Oral)   0 1 2 3 4 5

In order for a grade of *minimum standard* to be given, the total must be ≥11   TOTAL = _____

```
  1    2    3    4    5    6    7    8    9   10   11   12   13   14   15
  |    |    |    |    |    |    |    |    |    |    |    |    |    |    |
```

Not Acceptable   **Meets**   **Exceeds**
                              Minimum Standards   **Minimum Standards**

TEST ENVIRONMENTS

L: Laboratory/Classroom Testing
C: Clinical/Field Testing
P: Practicum Testing
A: Assessment/Mock Exam Testing
S: Self-Reporting

SKILL TEST INFORMATION

Purpose:	Increase sacral counternutation; reduce sacral nutation; positional fault; pain reduction
Involved Structure:	Joint capsule
Special Considerations:	Assesses grade of excursion/glide (I-IV)
Reference(s):	Edmond; Konin (2001)
Supplies Needed:	Table, pillow

Joint Mobilization
(JM-L-Test 3)

Peer Review _____ Peer Review _____

Skill Acquisition: _____   Practice Opportunities: _____

Please demonstrate the proper technique for administering **Posterior-Anterior Glide of the Hip Joint.** *You have 2 minutes to complete this task.*

Tester places athlete and limb in appropriate position	Test 1	Test 2	Test 3
Prone	Ⓨ Ⓝ	Ⓨ Ⓝ	Ⓨ Ⓝ
Place hip into approximately 30 degrees of flexion and abduction with slight external rotation off the end of the table	Ⓨ Ⓝ	Ⓨ Ⓝ	Ⓨ Ⓝ

Tester placed in proper position	Test 1	Test 2	Test 3
Tester standing at the foot of the table facing the involved hip joint	Ⓨ Ⓝ	Ⓨ Ⓝ	Ⓨ Ⓝ
One hand is placed on the pelvis	Ⓨ Ⓝ	Ⓨ Ⓝ	Ⓨ Ⓝ
The other hand, with a forearm grasp included, stabilizes the proximal-mid femur with the hand on the posterior aspect	Ⓨ Ⓝ	Ⓨ Ⓝ	Ⓨ Ⓝ

Tester performs test according to accepted guidelines	Test 1	Test 2	Test 3
Instructs the subject to "relax"	Ⓨ Ⓝ	Ⓨ Ⓝ	Ⓨ Ⓝ
Hand on the pelvis stabilizes it on the table	Ⓨ Ⓝ	Ⓨ Ⓝ	Ⓨ Ⓝ
The hand and forearm grasping the proximal-mid femur provides a distraction force	Ⓨ Ⓝ	Ⓨ Ⓝ	Ⓨ Ⓝ
Assesses stages of distraction	Ⓨ Ⓝ	Ⓨ Ⓝ	Ⓨ Ⓝ
The hand stabilizing the proximal-mid femur then applies an anterior glide	Ⓨ Ⓝ	Ⓨ Ⓝ	Ⓨ Ⓝ
Assesses grades of excursion/glide	Ⓨ Ⓝ	Ⓨ Ⓝ	Ⓨ Ⓝ
Oscillation of the PA Glide is performed → 2 to 3 times	Ⓨ Ⓝ	Ⓨ Ⓝ	Ⓨ Ⓝ
Maintains relaxation of the hip region	Ⓨ Ⓝ	Ⓨ Ⓝ	Ⓨ Ⓝ

The psychomotor skill was performed completely and in the appropriate order   0 1 2 3 4 5

The tester had control of the subject and the situation (showed confidence)   0 1 2 3 4 5

Method of performing the skill allowed the tester the ability to determine: severity, proper progression, and the *fit* in the overall picture (Oral)   0 1 2 3 4 5

In order for a grade of *minimum standard* to be given, the total must be ≥11   **TOTAL = _____**

1 2 3 4 5 6 7 8 9 10 11 12 13 14 15

Not Acceptable   **Meets Minimum Standards**   **Exceeds Minimum Standards**

TEST ENVIRONMENTS

L: Laboratory/Classroom Testing
C: Clinical/Field Testing
P: Practicum Testing
A: Assessment/Mock Exam Testing
S: Self-Reporting

SKILL TEST INFORMATION

Purpose: Increase hip extension and external rotation; pain reduction
Involved Structure: Joint capsule
Special Considerations: Support the uninvolved limb in some manner; additional clinician(s) and/or the use of a stabilizing device; subject comfort should be noted; assesses stages of distraction and grades of excursion/glide I-IV
Reference(s): Edmond; Konin (2001)
Supplies Needed: Table; stabilizing strap

Joint Mobilization
(JM-L-Test 4)

Peer Review _____ Peer Review _____

Skill Acquisition: _____   Practice Opportunities: _____

Please demonstrate the proper technique for administering an **Anterior-Posterior Glide of the Tibiofemoral Joint.** *You have 2 minutes to complete this task.*

Tester places athlete and limb in appropriate position	Test 1	Test 2	Test 3
Seated	Y N	Y N	Y N
Legs hanging off the table (table supporting distal femur)	Y N	Y N	Y N
Knee in slight flexion (30 to 40 degrees)	Y N	Y N	Y N
Tester placed in proper position	**Test 1**	**Test 2**	**Test 3**
Stands/sits in front of the involved side	Y N	Y N	Y N
Tester grasps proximal tibia and femur with both hands	Y N	Y N	Y N
Tester performs test according to accepted guidelines	**Test 1**	**Test 2**	**Test 3**
Applies distraction force to the tibia and holds with both hands	Y N	Y N	Y N
Applies a mobilization force in a posterior direction	Y N	Y N	Y N
Assesses stages of distraction	Y N	Y N	Y N
Assesses grades of excursions/glide	Y N	Y N	Y N
Oscillation of the posterior glide is performed → 2 to 3 times	Y N	Y N	Y N
Maintains relaxation of the limb	Y N	Y N	Y N

The psychomotor skill was performed completely and in the appropriate order   0 1 2 3 4 5

The tester had control of the subject and the situation (showed confidence)   0 1 2 3 4 5

Method of performing the skill allowed the tester the ability to determine:
severity, proper progression, and the *fit* in the overall picture (Oral)   0 1 2 3 4 5

In order for a grade of *minimum standard* to be given, the total must be ≥11   TOTAL = _____

```
    1     2     3     4     5     6     7     8     9    10    11    12    13    14    15
    |     |     |     |     |     |     |     |     |     |     |     |     |     |     |
    |     |     |     |     |     |     |     |     |     |     |     |     |     |     |
```

Not Acceptable   **Meets**   **Exceeds**
                                   Minimum Standards   **Minimum Standards**

TEST ENVIRONMENTS

L: Laboratory/Classroom Testing
C: Clinical/Field Testing
P: Practicum Testing
A: Assessment/Mock Exam Testing
S: Self-Reporting

SKILL TEST INFORMATION

Purpose: Increased joint motion (knee flexion); decrease pain

Involved Structure: Joint capsule

Special Considerations: May be done supine with towel roll under the knee joint; assesses stages of distraction and grades of excursion/glide (I-IV)

Reference(s): Edmond; Konin et al (2004); Prentice (2004)

Supplies Needed: Table, towel roll

JOINT MOBILIZATION
(JM-L-Test 5)

Peer Review _____ Peer Review _____

Skill Acquisition: _____   Practice Opportunities: _____

Please demonstrate the proper technique for administering an **Anterior-Posterior (Plantar) Glide of the Talocrural Joint***. You have 2 minutes to complete this task.*

Tester places athlete and limb in appropriate position	Test 1	Test 2	Test 3
Supine or seated	Ⓨ Ⓝ	Ⓨ Ⓝ	Ⓨ Ⓝ
Place talocrural joint into approximately 10 degrees of plantar flexion	Ⓨ Ⓝ	Ⓨ Ⓝ	Ⓨ Ⓝ

Tester placed in proper position	Test 1	Test 2	Test 3
Tester standing at the foot of the table facing the involved joint	Ⓨ Ⓝ	Ⓨ Ⓝ	Ⓨ Ⓝ
One hand grips the posterior surface of the distal tibia and fibula	Ⓨ Ⓝ	Ⓨ Ⓝ	Ⓨ Ⓝ
Other hand is placed over the anterior surface of the talus	Ⓨ Ⓝ	Ⓨ Ⓝ	Ⓨ Ⓝ

Tester performs test according to accepted guidelines	Test 1	Test 2	Test 3
Instructs the subject to "relax"	Ⓨ Ⓝ	Ⓨ Ⓝ	Ⓨ Ⓝ
Hand grasping the distal tibia/fibula acts as a stabilizer	Ⓨ Ⓝ	Ⓨ Ⓝ	Ⓨ Ⓝ
Other hand provides a distraction force to the talus and then glides the talus into a posterior (plantar) direction	Ⓨ Ⓝ	Ⓨ Ⓝ	Ⓨ Ⓝ
Assesses stages of distraction	Ⓨ Ⓝ	Ⓨ Ⓝ	Ⓨ Ⓝ
Assesses grades of excursion/glide	Ⓨ Ⓝ	Ⓨ Ⓝ	Ⓨ Ⓝ
Oscillation of the AP (plantar) Glide is performed → 2 to 3 times	Ⓨ Ⓝ	Ⓨ Ⓝ	Ⓨ Ⓝ
Maintains relaxation of the ankle region	Ⓨ Ⓝ	Ⓨ Ⓝ	Ⓨ Ⓝ

The psychomotor skill was performed completely and in the appropriate order   0 1 2 3 4 5

The tester had control of the subject and the situation (showed confidence)   0 1 2 3 4 5

Method of performing the skill allowed the tester the ability to determine:
severity, proper progression, and the *fit* in the overall picture (Oral)   0 1 2 3 4 5

In order for a grade of *minimum standard* to be given, the total must be ≥11   TOTAL = _____

```
 1     2     3     4     5     6     7     8     9    10    11    12    13    14    15
 |     |     |     |     |     |     |     |     |     |     |     |     |     |     |
```
Not Acceptable   **Meets**   **Exceeds**
                                             Minimum Standards   **Minimum Standards**

SKILL TEST INFORMATION

Purpose	Increase ankle dorsi flexion; pain reduction
Involved Structure:	Joint capsule
Special Considerations:	Assesses stages of distraction and grades of excursion/glide (I-IV); avoid closed pack position of ankle dorsiflexion
Reference(s):	Edmond; Konin et al (2004)
Supplies Needed:	Table

TEST ENVIRONMENTS

L: Laboratory/Classroom Testing
C: Clinical/Field Testing
P: Practicum Testing
A: Assessment/Mock Exam Testing
S: Self-Reporting

JOINT MOBILIZATION
(JM-L-Test 6)

Peer Review _____ Peer Review _____

Skill Acquisition: _____   Practice Opportunities: _____

Please demonstrate the proper technique for administering an **Anterior (Dorsal/PA) Glide of the Talocrural Joint***. You have 2 minutes to complete this task.*

Tester places athlete and limb in appropriate position	Test 1	Test 2	Test 3
Supine or seated	Ⓨ Ⓝ	Ⓨ Ⓝ	Ⓨ Ⓝ
Place ankle into approximately 10 degrees of plantar flexion	Ⓨ Ⓝ	Ⓨ Ⓝ	Ⓨ Ⓝ
Tester placed in proper position	**Test 1**	**Test 2**	**Test 3**
Tester standing at the foot of the table facing the involved ankle joint	Ⓨ Ⓝ	Ⓨ Ⓝ	Ⓨ Ⓝ
One hand grasps the anterior surface of the distal tibia and fibula	Ⓨ Ⓝ	Ⓨ Ⓝ	Ⓨ Ⓝ
Other hand grasps the calcaneus	Ⓨ Ⓝ	Ⓨ Ⓝ	Ⓨ Ⓝ
Tester performs test according to accepted guidelines	**Test 1**	**Test 2**	**Test 3**
Instructs the subject to "relax"	Ⓨ Ⓝ	Ⓨ Ⓝ	Ⓨ Ⓝ
Hand grasping the tibia and fibula acts as a stabilizer	Ⓨ Ⓝ	Ⓨ Ⓝ	Ⓨ Ⓝ
Hand grasping the calcaneus applies a distraction force followed by an anterior (dorsal) glide	Ⓨ Ⓝ	Ⓨ Ⓝ	Ⓨ Ⓝ
Assesses stages of distraction	Ⓨ Ⓝ	Ⓨ Ⓝ	Ⓨ Ⓝ
Assesses grades of excursion/glide	Ⓨ Ⓝ	Ⓨ Ⓝ	Ⓨ Ⓝ
Oscillation of the PA (dorsal)	Ⓨ Ⓝ	Ⓨ Ⓝ	Ⓨ Ⓝ
Glide is performed ➔ 2 to 3 times	Ⓨ Ⓝ	Ⓨ Ⓝ	Ⓨ Ⓝ
Maintains relaxation of the ankle region	Ⓨ Ⓝ	Ⓨ Ⓝ	Ⓨ Ⓝ

The psychomotor skill was performed completely and in the appropriate order   0 1 2 3 4 5

The tester had control of the subject and the situation (showed confidence)   0 1 2 3 4 5

Method of performing the skill allowed the tester the ability to determine:
severity, proper progression, and the *fit* in the overall picture (Oral)   0 1 2 3 4 5

In order for a grade of *minimum standard* to be given, the total must be ≥11   TOTAL = _____

```
  1   2   3   4   5   6   7   8   9   10   11   12   13   14   15
  |   |   |   |   |   |   |   |   |   |    |    |    |    |    |
```

Not Acceptable   **Meets**   **Exceeds**
                          Minimum Standards   **Minimum Standards**

TEST ENVIRONMENTS

L: Laboratory/Classroom Testing
C: Clinical/Field Testing
P: Practicum Testing
A: Assessment/Mock Exam Testing
S: Self-Reporting

SKILL TEST INFORMATION

Purpose:	Increase ankle plantar flexion; pain reduction
Involved Structure:	Joint capsule
Special Considerations:	Assesses stages of distraction and grades of excursion/glide (I-IV); avoid closed pack position of ankle dorsiflexion
Reference(s):	Edmond; Konin et al (2004)
Supplies Needed:	Table

JOINT MOBILIZATION
(JM-L-Test 7)

Peer Review _____   Peer Review _____

Skill Acquisition: _____   Practice Opportunities: _____

Please demonstrate the proper technique for administering an **Anterior-Posterior (Plantar) Glide of the Interphalangeal Joint** *involving the great toe. You have 2 minutes to complete this task.*

Tester places athlete and limb in appropriate position	Test 1	Test 2	Test 3
Supine or seated	Ⓨ Ⓝ	Ⓨ Ⓝ	Ⓨ Ⓝ
Places the joint into slight flexion	Ⓨ Ⓝ	Ⓨ Ⓝ	Ⓨ Ⓝ

Tester placed in proper position	Test 1	Test 2	Test 3
Tester positioned at the foot of the table facing the involved joint	Ⓨ Ⓝ	Ⓨ Ⓝ	Ⓨ Ⓝ
One hand grasps the head of the proximal phalanx of the 1st toe (thumb/dorsal surface & index finger/plantar surface)	Ⓨ Ⓝ	Ⓨ Ⓝ	Ⓨ Ⓝ
Other hand grasps the base of the distal phalanx of the 1st toe (thumb/dorsal surface & index finger/plantar surface)	Ⓨ Ⓝ	Ⓨ Ⓝ	Ⓨ Ⓝ

Tester performs test according to accepted guidelines	Test 1	Test 2	Test 3
Instructs the subject to "relax"	Ⓨ Ⓝ	Ⓨ Ⓝ	Ⓨ Ⓝ
Hand gripping the proximal phalanx acts as a stabilizer	Ⓨ Ⓝ	Ⓨ Ⓝ	Ⓨ Ⓝ
Other hand provides a distraction force followed by a posterior (plantar) glide to the base of the distal phalanx	Ⓨ Ⓝ	Ⓨ Ⓝ	Ⓨ Ⓝ
Assesses stages of distraction	Ⓨ Ⓝ	Ⓨ Ⓝ	Ⓨ Ⓝ
Assesses grades of excursion/glide	Ⓨ Ⓝ	Ⓨ Ⓝ	Ⓨ Ⓝ
Oscillation of the Plantar Glide is performed ➜ 2 to 3 times	Ⓨ Ⓝ	Ⓨ Ⓝ	Ⓨ Ⓝ
Maintains relaxation of the ankle & foot	Ⓨ Ⓝ	Ⓨ Ⓝ	Ⓨ Ⓝ

The psychomotor skill was performed completely and in the appropriate order   **0 1 2 3 4 5**

The tester had control of the subject and the situation (showed confidence)   **0 1 2 3 4 5**

Method of performing the skill allowed the tester the ability to determine: severity, proper progression, and the *fit* in the overall picture (Oral)   **0 1 2 3 4 5**

In order for a grade of *minimum standard* to be given, the total must be ≥11   **TOTAL = _____**

```
   1    2    3    4    5    6    7    8    9    10   11   12   13   14   15
   |    |    |    |    |    |    |    |    |    |    |    |    |    |    |
```

Not Acceptable   **Meets**   **Exceeds**
                                  Minimum Standards   **Minimum Standards**

TEST ENVIRONMENTS

L: Laboratory/Classroom Testing
C: Clinical/Field Testing
P: Practicum Testing
A: Assessment/Mock Exam Testing
S: Self-Reporting

SKILL TEST INFORMATION

Purpose:	Increase great toe IP flexion; pain reduction
Involved Structure:	Joint capsule
Special Considerations:	Assesses stages of distraction and grades of excursion/glide (I-IV)
Reference(s):	Edmond; Konin (2001)
Supplies Needed:	Table

JOINT MOBILIZATION
(JM-L-Test 8)

Peer Review _____ Peer Review _____

Skill Acquisition: _____   Practice Opportunities: _____

Please demonstrate the proper technique for administering a **Superior Glide of the Patellofemoral Joint**. *You have 2 minutes to complete this task.*

Tester places athlete and limb in appropriate position	Test 1	Test 2	Test 3
Supine	Ⓨ Ⓝ	Ⓨ Ⓝ	Ⓨ Ⓝ
Place the tibiofemoral joint into slight flexion	Ⓨ Ⓝ	Ⓨ Ⓝ	Ⓨ Ⓝ
Tester placed in proper position	**Test 1**	**Test 2**	**Test 3**
Tester positioned at the side of the table facing the involved joint	Ⓨ Ⓝ	Ⓨ Ⓝ	Ⓨ Ⓝ
Tester uses one or both hands to gently grasp the borders of the Patella	Ⓨ Ⓝ	Ⓨ Ⓝ	Ⓨ Ⓝ
Tester performs test according to accepted guidelines	**Test 1**	**Test 2**	**Test 3**
Instructs the subject to "relax"	Ⓨ Ⓝ	Ⓨ Ⓝ	Ⓨ Ⓝ
Hand(s) applies a gentle glide of the patella in the superior direction	Ⓨ Ⓝ	Ⓨ Ⓝ	Ⓨ Ⓝ
Assesses grades of excursion/glide	Ⓨ Ⓝ	Ⓨ Ⓝ	Ⓨ Ⓝ
Oscillation of the Superior Glide is performed → 2 to 3 times	Ⓨ Ⓝ	Ⓨ Ⓝ	Ⓨ Ⓝ
Maintains relaxation of the tibiofemoral joint	Ⓨ Ⓝ	Ⓨ Ⓝ	Ⓨ Ⓝ

The psychomotor skill was performed completely and in the appropriate order   0 1 2 3 4 5

The tester had control of the subject and the situation (showed confidence)   0 1 2 3 4 5

Method of performing the skill allowed the tester the ability to determine:
severity, proper progression, and the *fit* in the overall picture (Oral)   0 1 2 3 4 5

In order for a grade of *minimum standard* to be given, the total must be ≥11   TOTAL = _____

```
 1    2    3    4    5    6    7    8    9   10   11   12   13   14   15
 |    |    |    |    |    |    |    |    |    |    |    |    |    |    |
```

Not Acceptable   **Meets**   **Exceeds**
                              Minimum Standards   **Minimum Standards**

TEST ENVIRONMENTS

L: Laboratory/Classroom Testing
C: Clinical/Field Testing
P: Practicum Testing
A: Assessment/Mock Exam Testing
S: Self-Reporting

SKILL TEST INFORMATION

Purpose:	Increase knee joint extension; pain reduction
Involved Structure:	Joint capsule
Special Considerations:	Assesses grades of excursion/glide (I-IV)
Reference(s):	Edmond; Konin et al (2004)
Supplies Needed:	Table

THERAPEUTIC MODALITIES

THERAPEUTIC MODALITIES
(TMOD-Test 1)

Peer Review _____ Peer Review _____

Skill Acquisition: _____   Practice Opportunities: _____

This problem allows you the opportunity to use an **ice bag** *as a therapeutic modality. Your scenario is a sport-related acute injury of the quadriceps muscle. The physician's standing written acute injury protocol states that you are to use cryotherapy to decrease the metabolism and the tissue's need for oxygen. You have 3 minutes to review all the precautions with the athlete, perform the initial set-up, and begin treatment.*

	Test 1	Test 2	Test 3
Athlete Education	**Test 1**	**Test 2**	**Test 3**
Explains to the athlete why this modality is appropriate (rationale)	Y N	Y N	Y N
Explains to the athlete what are the expected treatment goals & outcomes	Y N	Y N	Y N
Explains to the athlete what they should or should not feel	Y N	Y N	Y N
Athlete Safety	**Test 1**	**Test 2**	**Test 3**
Prior to set-up of modality, checks all aspects for safety.	Y N	Y N	Y N
Reviews precautions/contraindications with the athlete.	Y N	Y N	Y N
Tester places athlete in appropriate position	**Test 1**	**Test 2**	**Test 3**
Supine	Y N	Y N	Y N
Places knee in slight flexion (form roll/towel roll)	Y N	Y N	Y N
Tester administers the therapeutic modality according to accepted guidelines	**Test 1**	**Test 2**	**Test 3**
Places an appropriate amount of ice into a bag (removes excess air; tie off bag)	Y N	Y N	Y N
Places the ice bag directly on the skin	Y N	Y N	Y N
Secures the ice bag in place with a plastic or elastic wrap	Y N	Y N	Y N
Termination of Treatment	**Test 1**	**Test 2**	**Test 3**
Inspects treatment area	Y N	Y N	Y N
Provides the athlete with feedback	Y N	Y N	Y N
Documents treatment	Y N	Y N	Y N

The psychomotor skill was performed completely and in the appropriate order   0 1 2 3 4 5

The tester had control of the subject and the situation (showed confidence)   0 1 2 3 4 5

Method of performing the skill allowed the tester the ability to determine:
severity, proper progression, and the *fit* in the overall picture (Oral)   0 1 2 3 4 5

In order for a grade of *minimum standard* to be given, the total must be ≥11   TOTAL = _____

1	2	3	4	5	6	7	8	9	10	11	12	13	14	15

Not Acceptable   **Meets**   **Exceeds**
                                Minimum Standards   **Minimum Standards**

TEST ENVIRONMENTS

L: Laboratory/Classroom Testing
C: Clinical/Field Testing
P: Practicum Testing
A: Assessment/Mock Exam Testing
S: Self-Reporting

SKILL TEST INFORMATION

Purpose:	Decrease inflammation and swelling
Involved Structure:	Quadriceps muscle
Special Considerations:	N/A
Reference(s):	Starkey (2004)
Supplies Needed:	Ice, plastic bag, wrap, towel roll

THERAPEUTIC MODALITIES
(TMOD-Test 2)

Peer Review _____ Peer Review _____

Skill Acquisition: _____   Practice Opportunities: _____

*This problem allows you the opportunity to use **moist heat** as a therapeutic modality for the purpose of applying superficial heat to an isolated area. Your scenario is a sport-related injury to the cervical spine. The physician's written orders state that you are to use superficial heat to reduce muscle spasm and pain. You have 3 minutes to review all the precautions with the athlete, perform the initial set-up, and begin treatment.*

Athlete Education	Test 1	Test 2	Test 3
Explains to the athlete why this modality is appropriate (rationale)	Y N	Y N	Y N
Explains to the athlete what are the expected treatment goals & outcomes	Y N	Y N	Y N
Explains to the athlete what they should or should not feel	Y N	Y N	Y N
Athlete Safety	**Test 1**	**Test 2**	**Test 3**
Prior to the set-up of the modality, checks all aspects for safety (ie, temperature, condition of the moist heat pack)	Y N	Y N	Y N
Reviews precautions/contraindications with the athlete	Y N	Y N	Y N
Tester places athlete in appropriate position	**Test 1**	**Test 2**	**Test 3**
Prone or seated	Y N	Y N	Y N
The treatment area is appropriately exposed	Y N	Y N	Y N
Tester administers the therapeutic modality according to accepted guidelines	**Test 1**	**Test 2**	**Test 3**
Places moist heat pack into terrycloth cover (uses a minimum of five layers of a towel between the pack and the athlete's skin)	Y N	Y N	Y N
Places the moist heat pack in the appropriate place (avoids lying on the moist heat pack)	Y N	Y N	Y N
Checks the athlete after 5 minutes (rechecks regularly thereafter)	Y N	Y N	Y N
Termination of Treatment	**Test 1**	**Test 2**	**Test 3**
Inspects treatment area	Y N	Y N	Y N
Provides the athlete with feedback	Y N	Y N	Y N
Documents treatment	Y N	Y N	Y N

The psychomotor skill was performed completely and in the appropriate order   0 1 2 3 4 5

The tester had control of the subject and the situation (showed confidence)   0 1 2 3 4 5

Method of performing the skill allowed the tester the ability to determine: severity, proper progression, and the *fit* in the overall picture (Oral)   0 1 2 3 4 5

In order for a grade of *minimum standard* to be given, the total must be ≥11   TOTAL = _____

Continued on the following page

Not Acceptable   Meets   Exceeds
                                                          Minimum Standards   Minimum Standards

TEST ENVIRONMENTS

L: Laboratory/Classroom Testing
C: Clinical/Field Testing
P: Practicum Testing
A: Assessment/Mock Exam Testing
S: Self-Reporting

SKILL TEST INFORMATION

Purpose:	Relieve subacute or chronic muscle spasm and pain
Involved Structure:	Cervical area
Special Considerations:	N/A
Reference(s):	Starkey (2004)
Supplies Needed:	Table/chair, Moist hot pack, cover/towel

THERAPEUTIC MODALITIES
(TMOD-Test 3)

Peer Review _____ Peer Review _____

Skill Acquisition: _____   Practice Opportunities: _____

*This problem allows you the opportunity to use a **paraffin bath** as a therapeutic modality for the purpose of heating an isolated area. Your scenario is a sport-related injury that has resulted in chronic inflammation to the PIP joint of the left ring finger. The physician's written orders state that you are to use a paraffin bath to reduce edema and promote healing. You have 3 minutes to review all the precautions with the athlete, perform the initial set-up, and begin treatment.*

Athlete Education	Test 1	Test 2	Test 3
Explains to the athlete why this modality is appropriate (rationale)	Ⓨ Ⓝ	Ⓨ Ⓝ	Ⓨ Ⓝ
Explains to the athlete what are the expected treatment goals & outcomes	Ⓨ Ⓝ	Ⓨ Ⓝ	Ⓨ Ⓝ
Explains to the athlete what they should or should not feel	Ⓨ Ⓝ	Ⓨ Ⓝ	Ⓨ Ⓝ
Athlete Safety	**Test 1**	**Test 2**	**Test 3**
Prior to the set-up of the modality, checks all aspects for safety (ie, temperature, etc)	Ⓨ Ⓝ	Ⓨ Ⓝ	Ⓨ Ⓝ
Reviews precautions/contraindications with the athlete	Ⓨ Ⓝ	Ⓨ Ⓝ	Ⓨ Ⓝ
Removes all jewelry on and around the involved area	Ⓨ Ⓝ	Ⓨ Ⓝ	Ⓨ Ⓝ
Cleans and dries the involved limb	Ⓨ Ⓝ	Ⓨ Ⓝ	Ⓨ Ⓝ
Tester administers the therapeutic modality according to accepted guidelines	**Test 1**	**Test 2**	**Test 3**
Instructs the athlete to dip and spread the fingers into the paraffin	Ⓨ Ⓝ	Ⓨ Ⓝ	Ⓨ Ⓝ
Removes hand/fingers from the paraffin	Ⓨ Ⓝ	Ⓨ Ⓝ	Ⓨ Ⓝ
Allows the wax coat to dry before reimmersing the limb back into the paraffin (dips the extremity 6 to 12 more times, allowing each coat to dry)	Ⓨ Ⓝ	Ⓨ Ⓝ	Ⓨ Ⓝ
Places the extremity back into the paraffin bath for the duration of the treatment or	Ⓨ Ⓝ	Ⓨ Ⓝ	Ⓨ Ⓝ
Wraps the involved area with a plastic bag and then a towel (leaves the limb out for the duration of the treatment)	Ⓨ Ⓝ	Ⓨ Ⓝ	Ⓨ Ⓝ
Termination of Treatment	**Test 1**	**Test 2**	**Test 3**
Removes hardened paraffin and return it back into heating unit	Ⓨ Ⓝ	Ⓨ Ⓝ	Ⓨ Ⓝ
Inspects treatment area	Ⓨ Ⓝ	Ⓨ Ⓝ	Ⓨ Ⓝ
Provides the athlete with feedback	Ⓨ Ⓝ	Ⓨ Ⓝ	Ⓨ Ⓝ
Documents treatment	Ⓨ Ⓝ	Ⓨ Ⓝ	Ⓨ Ⓝ

The psychomotor skill was performed completely and in the appropriate order   0 1 2 3 4 5

The tester had control of the subject and the situation (showed confidence)   0 1 2 3 4 5

Method of performing the skill allowed the tester the ability to determine:
severity, proper progression, and the *fit* in the overall picture (Oral)   0 1 2 3 4 5

In order for a grade of *minimum standard* to be given, the total must be ≥11   **TOTAL =** _____

Continued on the following page

Not Acceptable   Meets   Exceeds
                                               Minimum Standards   Minimum Standards

TEST ENVIRONMENTS

L: Laboratory/Classroom Testing
C: Clinical/Field Testing
P: Practicum Testing
A: Assessment/Mock Exam Testing
S: Self-Reporting

SKILL TEST INFORMATION

Purpose:	Superficially heating small body parts
Involved Structure:	Hand
Special Considerations:	Paraffin baths can be used if ROM is not part of the treatment protocol
Reference(s):	Starkey (2004)
Supplies Needed:	Paraffin bath, plastic bags, towel

THERAPEUTIC MODALITIES
(TMOD-Test 4)

Peer Review _____ Peer Review _____

Skill Acquisition: _____   Practice Opportunities: _____

*This problem allows you the opportunity to use a **cold whirlpool** as a therapeutic modality for combining therapeutic cold with active range of motion. Your scenario is a sport-related acute injury of the elbow. The physician's written orders state that you are to use cold therapy and exercise to reduce swelling and facilitate a normal range of motion. You have 3 minutes to review all the precautions with the athlete, perform the initial set-up, and begin treatment.*

Athlete Education	Test 1	Test 2	Test 3
Explains to the athlete why this modality is appropriate (rationale)	Y N	Y N	Y N
Explains to the athlete what are the expected treatment goals & outcomes	Y N	Y N	Y N
Explains to the athlete what they should or should not feel	Y N	Y N	Y N
Athlete Safety	**Test 1**	**Test 2**	**Test 3**
Prior to set-up of modality, checks all aspects for safety (water temperature; GFCI; etc)	Y N	Y N	Y N
Reviews precautions/contraindications with the athlete	Y N	Y N	Y N
Tester places athlete in appropriate position	**Test 1**	**Test 2**	**Test 3**
Seated (high chair or whirlpool bench) with the involved limb immersed in whirlpool	Y N	Y N	Y N
Tester administers the therapeutic modality according to accepted guidelines	**Test 1**	**Test 2**	**Test 3**
Water depth is enough to cover the involved limb	Y N	Y N	Y N
Water temperature is appropriate for the nature of the injury	Y N	Y N	Y N
Turns the turbine on before the athlete gets into the whirlpool	Y N	Y N	Y N
Instructs the athlete to actively move the involved limb throughout the full range of motion	Y N	Y N	Y N
Tester turns the turbine off after the athlete gets out of the whirlpool	Y N	Y N	Y N
Termination of Treatment	**Test 1**	**Test 2**	**Test 3**
Inspects treatment area	Y N	Y N	Y N
Provides the athlete with feedback	Y N	Y N	Y N
Documents treatment	Y N	Y N	Y N

The psychomotor skill was performed completely and in the appropriate order	0 1 2 3 4 5
The tester had control of the subject and the situation (showed confidence)	0 1 2 3 4 5
Method of performing the skill allowed the tester the ability to determine: severity, proper progression, and the *fit* in the overall picture (Oral)	0 1 2 3 4 5
In order for a grade of *minimum standard* to be given, the total must be ≥11	TOTAL = _____

Continued on the following page

Not Acceptable   Meets   Exceeds
                                         Minimum Standards   Minimum Standards

TEST ENVIRONMENTS

L: Laboratory/Classroom Testing
C: Clinical/Field Testing
P: Practicum Testing
A: Assessment/Mock Exam Testing
S: Self-Reporting

SKILL TEST INFORMATION

Purpose:	Application of cold to irregularly shaped body parts, AROM while receiving therapeutic cold
Involved Structure:	Lower leg
Special Considerations:	N/A
Reference(s):	Starkey (2004)
Supplies Needed:	Whirlpool, chair, towels

THERAPEUTIC MODALITIES
(TMOD-Test 5)

Peer Review _____ Peer Review _____

Skill Acquisition: _____   Practice Opportunities: _____

This problem allows you the opportunity to use **vapo-coolant spray** *as a therapeutic modality. Your scenario is a sport-related trauma to the hamstrings, resulting in muscle spasms. The physician's standing written acute injury protocol states that you are to use cryotherapy to decrease the muscle spasm. You have 3 minutes to review all precautions with the athlete, perform the initial set-up, and begin treatment.*

Athlete Education	Test 1	Test 2	Test 3
Explains to the athlete why this modality is appropriate (rationale)	Y N	Y N	Y N
Explains to the athlete what are the expected treatment goals & outcomes	Y N	Y N	Y N
Explains to the athlete what they should or should not feel	Y N	Y N	Y N
Athlete Safety	**Test 1**	**Test 2**	**Test 3**
Prior to the set-up of the modality, checks all aspects for safety	Y N	Y N	Y N
Reviews precautions/contraindications with the athlete	Y N	Y N	Y N
Tester places athlete in appropriate position	**Test 1**	**Test 2**	**Test 3**
Prone or standing	Y N	Y N	Y N
Tester administers the therapeutic modality according to accepted guidelines	**Test 1**	**Test 2**	**Test 3**
Holds the container about one foot from the involved surface of the skin	Y N	Y N	Y N
Delivers a mist of spray to the skin in a sweeping motion at about 4 inches/second	Y N	Y N	Y N
Sprays in a single direction in a slightly overlapping pattern	Y N	Y N	Y N
Covers the treatment area	Y N	Y N	Y N
Repeats treatment	Y N	Y N	Y N
Termination of Treatment	**Test 1**	**Test 2**	**Test 3**
Inspects treatment area	Y N	Y N	Y N
Provides the athlete with feedback	Y N	Y N	Y N
Documents treatment	Y N	Y N	Y N

The psychomotor skill was performed completely and in the appropriate order   0 1 2 3 4 5

The tester had control of the subject and the situation (showed confidence)   0 1 2 3 4 5

Method of performing the skill allowed the tester the ability to determine:
severity, proper progression, and the *fit* in the overall picture (Oral)   0 1 2 3 4 5

In order for a grade of *minimum standard* to be given, the total must be ≥11   **TOTAL =** _____

Continued on the following page

1   2   3   4   5   6   7   8   9   10   11   12   13   14   15

Not Acceptable   **Meets**   **Exceeds**
                                              Minimum Standards   **Minimum Standards**

TEST ENVIRONMENTS

L: Laboratory/Classroom Testing
C: Clinical/Field Testing
P: Practicum Testing
A: Assessment/Mock Exam Testing
S: Self-Reporting

SKILL TEST INFORMATION

Purpose:	Decrease muscle spasms
Involved Structure:	Hamstrings
Special Considerations:	Superficial cooling only; avoid frosting the skin
Reference(s):	Knight
Supplies Needed:	Spray container of liquid ethyl chloride or floromethane

THERAPEUTIC MODALITIES
(TMOD-Test 6)

Peer Review _____ Peer Review _____

Skill Acquisition: _____   Practice Opportunities: _____

*This problem allows you the opportunity to use **ice massage** as a therapeutic modality for the purpose of applying therapeutic cold to an isolated area. Your scenario is an exertional injury of the anterior lower leg. The physician's written orders state that you are to use ice massage to reduce inflammation in and around the anterior portion of the shin. You have 3 minutes to review all the precautions with the athlete, perform the initial set-up, and begin treatment.*

Athlete Education	Test 1	Test 2	Test 3
Explains to the athlete why this modality is appropriate (rationale)	Y N	Y N	Y N
Explains to the athlete what are the expected treatment goals & outcomes	Y N	Y N	Y N
Explains to the athlete what they should or should not feel	Y N	Y N	Y N
Athlete Safety	Test 1	Test 2	Test 3
Prior to set-up of modality, checks all aspects for safety	Y N	Y N	Y N
Reviews precautions/contraindications with the athlete	Y N	Y N	Y N
Tester places athlete in appropriate position	Test 1	Test 2	Test 3
Supine	Y N	Y N	Y N
Surrounds the area to be treated with a towel	Y N	Y N	Y N
Tester administers the therapeutic modality according to accepted guidelines	Test 1	Test 2	Test 3
Slowly moves the ice over the treatment area	Y N	Y N	Y N
Uses overlapping strokes and/or circles	Y N	Y N	Y N
Gradually increases the pressure of the strokes	Y N	Y N	Y N
Removes the paper from the cup as the ice melts	Y N	Y N	Y N
Termination of Treatment	Test 1	Test 2	Test 3
Inspects treatment area	Y N	Y N	Y N
Provides the athlete with feedback	Y N	Y N	Y N
Documents treatment	Y N	Y N	Y N

The psychomotor skill was performed completely and in the appropriate order   **0 1 2 3 4 5**

The tester had control of the subject and the situation (showed confidence)   **0 1 2 3 4 5**

Method of performing the skill allowed the tester the ability to determine:
severity, proper progression, and the *fit* in the overall picture (Oral)   **0 1 2 3 4 5**

In order for a grade of *minimum standard* to be given, the total must be ≥11   **TOTAL = _____**

Continued on the following page

Not Acceptable   **Meets**   **Exceeds**
                                                  Minimum Standards   **Minimum Standards**

TEST ENVIRONMENTS

L: Laboratory/Classroom Testing
C: Clinical/Field Testing
P: Practicum Testing
A: Assessment/Mock Exam Testing
S: Self-Reporting

SKILL TEST INFORMATION

Purpose:	Decrease pain and inflammation
Involved Structure:	Anterior lower leg
Special Considerations:	Treatment area should be no greater than two times the size of thecup
Reference(s):	Knight; Starkey (2004)
Supplies Needed:	5- to 10-ounce ice cup; towel

THERAPEUTIC MODALITIES
(TMOD-Test 7)

Peer Review _____ Peer Review _____

Skill Acquisition: _____   Practice Opportunities: _____

This problem allows you the opportunity to use a **contrast bath (hot/cold)** *as a therapeutic modality for the purpose of edema reduction as part of the secondary healing process. Your scenario is a sports-related injury to the ankle that presented with significant ecchymosis. The physician's written orders state that you are to use contrast bath to reduce ecchymosis in a nonacute injury. You have 3 minutes to review all the precautions with the athlete, perform the initial set-up, and begin treatment.*

Athlete Education	Test 1	Test 2	Test 3
Explains to the athlete why this modality is appropriate (rationale)	Y N	Y N	Y N
Explains to the athlete what are the expected treatment goals & outcomes	Y N	Y N	Y N
Explains to the athlete what they should or should not feel	Y N	Y N	Y N
Athlete Safety	**Test 1**	**Test 2**	**Test 3**
Prior to set-up of modality, checks all aspects for safety	Y N	Y N	Y N
Reviews the precautions/contraindications with the athlete	Y N	Y N	Y N
Tester places athlete in appropriate position	**Test 1**	**Test 2**	**Test 3**
Seated	Y N	Y N	Y N
Contrast tubs are as close to each other as possible	Y N	Y N	Y N
Tester administers the therapeutic modality according to accepted guidelines	**Test 1**	**Test 2**	**Test 3**
Begins with immersing the involved limb into the hot whirlpool for 3 to 4 minutes	Y N	Y N	Y N
Immediately follows by placing the involved limb into cold the whirlpool for 1 minute	Y N	Y N	Y N
Repeats the cycle (hot/cold) 4 times	Y N	Y N	Y N
Termination of Treatment	**Test 1**	**Test 2**	**Test 3**
Inspects treatment area	Y N	Y N	Y N
Provides the athlete with feedback	Y N	Y N	Y N
Documents treatment	Y N	Y N	Y N

The psychomotor skill was performed completely and in the appropriate order   0 1 2 3 4 5

The tester had control of the subject and the situation (showed confidence)   0 1 2 3 4 5

Method of performing the skill allowed the tester the ability to determine:
severity, proper progression, and the *fit* in the overall picture (Oral)   0 1 2 3 4 5

In order for a grade of *minimum standard* to be given, the total must be ≥11   **TOTAL = _____**

Continued on the following page

1	2	3	4	5	6	7	8	9	10	11	12	13	14	15

Not Acceptable   Meets   Exceeds
                                               Minimum Standards   Minimum Standards

TEST ENVIRONMENTS

L: Laboratory/Classroom Testing
C: Clinical/Field Testing
P: Practicum Testing
A: Assessment/Mock Exam Testing
S: Self-Reporting

SKILL TEST INFORMATION

Purpose:	Decreases ecchymosis and pain
Involved Structure:	Ankle
Special Considerations:	May end with either hot or cold treatment
Reference(s):	Starkey (2004)
Supplies Needed:	2 tubs, towels, chair/stool

THERAPEUTIC MODALITIES
(TMOD-Test 8)

Peer Review _____ Peer Review _____

Skill Acquisition: _____   Practice Opportunities: _____

This problem allows you the opportunity to use a **hot whirlpool** *as a therapeutic modality for combining therapeutic heat with active range of motion. Your scenario is a sport-related injury to the ankle in the secondary phase of healing. The physician's written orders state that you are to use heat therapy and exercise to facilitate a normal range of motion. You have 3 minutes to review all the precautions with the athlete, perform the initial set-up, and begin treatment.*

Athlete Education	Test 1	Test 2	Test 3
Explains to the athlete why this modality is appropriate (rationale)	Y N	Y N	Y N
Explains to the athlete what are the expected treatment goals and outcomes	Y N	Y N	Y N
Explains to the athlete what they should or should not feel	Y N	Y N	Y N
Athlete Safety	**Test 1**	**Test 2**	**Test 3**
Prior to the set-up of the modality, checks all aspects for safety (water temperature; GFCI; etc)	Y N	Y N	Y N
Reviews precautions/contraindications with the athlete	Y N	Y N	Y N
Tester places athlete in appropriate position	**Test 1**	**Test 2**	**Test 3**
Seated (high chair or whirlpool bench) with the involved limb immersed in whirlpool	Y N	Y N	Y N
Tester administers the therapeutic modality according to accepted guidelines	**Test 1**	**Test 2**	**Test 3**
Water depth is enough to cover the involved limb	Y N	Y N	Y N
Water temperature is appropriate for the nature of the injury and the size of area treated	Y N	Y N	Y N
Turns the turbine on before the athlete gets into the whirlpool	Y N	Y N	Y N
Instructs the athlete to actively move the involved limb throughout the full range of motion	Y N	Y N	Y N
Turns the turbine off after the athlete gets out of the whirlpool	Y N	Y N	Y N
Termination of Treatment	**Test 1**	**Test 2**	**Test 3**
Inspects treatment area	Y N	Y N	Y N
Provides the athlete with feedback	Y N	Y N	Y N
Documents treatment	Y N	Y N	Y N

The psychomotor skill was performed completely and in the appropriate order   0 1 2 3 4 5

The tester had control of the subject and the situation (showed confidence)   0 1 2 3 4 5

Method of performing the skill allowed the tester the ability to determine:
severity, proper progression, and the *fit* in the overall picture (Oral)   0 1 2 3 4 5

In order for a grade of *minimum standard* to be given, the total must be ≥11   **TOTAL = _____**

Continued on the following page

Not Acceptable

**Meets
Minimum Standards**

**Exceeds
Minimum Standards**

TEST ENVIRONMENTS

L: Laboratory/Classroom Testing
C: Clinical/Field Testing
P: Practicum Testing
A: Assessment/Mock Exam Testing
S: Self-Reporting

SKILL TEST INFORMATION

Purpose:	Application of heat to irregularly shaped body parts; AROM while receiving therapeutic heat
Involved Structure:	Lower leg
Special Considerations:	N/A
Reference(s):	Starkey (2004)
Supplies Needed:	Whirlpool, whirlpool table, towels

THERAPEUTIC MODALITIES
(TMOD-Test 9)

Peer Review _____ Peer Review _____

Skill Acquisition: _____   Practice Opportunities: _____

*This problem allows you the opportunity to use **effleurage**. Your scenario is a sports-related injury to the lumbar spine that has resulted in spasms of the muscles of the back. The physician's written orders state that you are to use **massage** to resolve muscle spasm. You have 3 minutes to review all the precautions with the athlete, perform the initial set-up, and begin treatment.*

Athlete Education	Test 1	Test 2	Test 3
Explains to the athlete why this treatment is appropriate (rationale)	Y N	Y N	Y N
Explains to the athlete what are the expected treatment goals & outcomes	Y N	Y N	Y N
Explains the type of massage to be used and the expected sensations	Y N	Y N	Y N
Athlete Safety	**Test 1**	**Test 2**	**Test 3**
Reviews precautions/contraindications with the athlete.	Y N	Y N	Y N
Tester places athlete in appropriate position	**Test 1**	**Test 2**	**Test 3**
Prone (positioned so that the muscles are relaxed)	Y N	Y N	Y N
Bolsters the ankles and places a pillow under the abdomen	Y N	Y N	Y N
Drapes the athlete for modesty and exposes of the area to be massaged	Y N	Y N	Y N
Tester administers the massage technique according to accepted guidelines	**Test 1**	**Test 2**	**Test 3**
Pre-heats the area to promote muscle relaxation, if applicable	Y N	Y N	Y N
Applies massage lubricant/powder, if applicable	Y N	Y N	Y N
Stands to the side and slightly behind the athlete	Y N	Y N	Y N
Begins with light effleurage gradually building to deep effleurage	Y N	Y N	Y N
Using both hands (side-by-side), pushes tissue downward and away from the tester running parallel with the back	Y N	Y N	Y N
Drags (glides) both hands back to the starting point (with no added pressure)	Y N	Y N	Y N
Repeats	Y N	Y N	Y N
Maintains contact throughout the treatment	Y N	Y N	Y N
Termination of Treatment	**Test 1**	**Test 2**	**Test 3**
Removes lubricant/powder with a towel	Y N	Y N	Y N
Inspects treatment area	Y N	Y N	Y N
Provides the athlete with feedback	Y N	Y N	Y N
Documents treatment	Y N	Y N	Y N

The psychomotor skill was performed completely and in the appropriate order   0 1 2 3 4 5

The tester had control of the subject and the situation (showed confidence)   0 1 2 3 4 5

Method of performing the skill allowed the tester the ability to determine:
severity, proper progression, and the *fit* in the overall picture (Oral)   0 1 2 3 4 5

In order for a grade of *minimum standard* to be given, the total must be ≥11   TOTAL = _____

Continued on the following page

| 1 | 2 | 3 | 4 | 5 | 6 | 7 | 8 | 9 | 10 | 11 | 12 | 13 | 14 | 15 |

Not Acceptable

**Meets
Minimum Standards**

**Exceeds
Minimum Standards**

TEST ENVIRONMENTS

L: Laboratory/Classroom Testing
C: Clinical/Field Testing
P: Practicum Testing
A: Assessment/Mock Exam Testing
S: Self-Reporting

SKILL TEST INFORMATION

Purpose:	Interrupt the pain/spasm cycle
Involved Structure:	Lower back
Special Considerations:	May use palms, fingers, or knuckles
Reference(s):	Salvo; Starkey (2004)
Supplies Needed:	Massage lubricant/powder, towel, draping material, pillow

THERAPEUTIC MODALITIES
(TMOD-Test 10)

Peer Review _____ Peer Review _____

Skill Acquisition: _____   Practice Opportunities: _____

*This problem allows you the opportunity to use **pétrissage**. Your scenario is a sport-related trauma to the upper back that has resulted in the development of adhesions and scar tissue. The physician's written orders state that you are to use **massage** to help reduce adhesions and try to break up the scar tissue. You have 3 minutes to review all the precautions with the athlete, perform the initial set-up, and begin treatment.*

Athlete Education	Test 1	Test 2	Test 3
Explains to the athlete why this treatment is appropriate (rationale)	Ⓨ Ⓝ	Ⓨ Ⓝ	Ⓨ Ⓝ
Explains to the athlete what are the expected treatment goals & outcomes	Ⓨ Ⓝ	Ⓨ Ⓝ	Ⓨ Ⓝ
Explains the type of massage to be used and the expected sensations	Ⓨ Ⓝ	Ⓨ Ⓝ	Ⓨ Ⓝ
Athlete Safety	**Test 1**	**Test 2**	**Test 3**
Reviews precautions/contraindications with the athlete	Ⓨ Ⓝ	Ⓨ Ⓝ	Ⓨ Ⓝ
Tester places athlete in appropriate position	**Test 1**	**Test 2**	**Test 3**
Prone (positioned so that the muscles are relaxed)	Ⓨ Ⓝ	Ⓨ Ⓝ	Ⓨ Ⓝ
Bolsters the ankles and used a pillow under the abdomen	Ⓨ Ⓝ	Ⓨ Ⓝ	Ⓨ Ⓝ
Drapes the athlete for modesty and exposes of the area to be massaged	Ⓨ Ⓝ	Ⓨ Ⓝ	Ⓨ Ⓝ
Tester administers the massage technique according to accepted guidelines	**Test 1**	**Test 2**	**Test 3**
Preheats the area to promote muscle relaxation	Ⓨ Ⓝ	Ⓨ Ⓝ	Ⓨ Ⓝ
Stands to the side of the athlete	Ⓨ Ⓝ	Ⓨ Ⓝ	Ⓨ Ⓝ
Using a "C" shape, grasp a fold of skin	Ⓨ Ⓝ	Ⓨ Ⓝ	Ⓨ Ⓝ
Lifts the underlying muscle tissue and skin	Ⓨ Ⓝ	Ⓨ Ⓝ	Ⓨ Ⓝ
Compresses the lifted tissue back and forth (kneading)	Ⓨ Ⓝ	Ⓨ Ⓝ	Ⓨ Ⓝ
Uses both hands intermittently	Ⓨ Ⓝ	Ⓨ Ⓝ	Ⓨ Ⓝ
Repeats several times and moves to a new area (does not lose contact with the body while moving the hands)	Ⓨ Ⓝ	Ⓨ Ⓝ	Ⓨ Ⓝ
Termination of Treatment	**Test 1**	**Test 2**	**Test 3**
Inspects treatment area	Ⓨ Ⓝ	Ⓨ Ⓝ	Ⓨ Ⓝ
Provides the athlete with feedback	Ⓨ Ⓝ	Ⓨ Ⓝ	Ⓨ Ⓝ
Documents treatment	Ⓨ Ⓝ	Ⓨ Ⓝ	Ⓨ Ⓝ

The psychomotor skill was performed completely and in the appropriate order   0 1 2 3 4 5

The tester had control of the subject and the situation (showed confidence)   0 1 2 3 4 5

Method of performing the skill allowed the tester the ability to determine:
severity, proper progression, and the *fit* in the overall picture (Oral)   0 1 2 3 4 5

In order for a grade of *minimum standard* to be given, the total must be ≥11   TOTAL = _____

Continued on the following page

1   2   3   4   5   6   7   8   9   10   11   12   13   14   15

Not Acceptable   **Meets**   **Exceeds**
                                          Minimum Standards   **Minimum Standards**

TEST ENVIRONMENTS

L: Laboratory/Classroom Testing
C: Clinical/Field Testing
P: Practicum Testing
A: Assessment/Mock Exam Testing
S: Self-Reporting

SKILL TEST INFORMATION

Purpose:	Breaks up scar tissue
Involved Structure:	Upper back
Special Considerations:	May follow effleurage
Reference(s):	Salvo; Starkey (2004)
Supplies Needed:	Towel, draping material, pillow

THERAPEUTIC MODALITIES
(TMOD-Test 11)

Peer Review _____ Peer Review _____

Skill Acquisition: _____ Practice Opportunities: _____

This problem allows you the opportunity to use **tapotement (precussion) massage** *to increase blood flow to the area. Your scenario is a sport-related trauma to the anterior upper arm. The physician's written orders state that you are to use massage to elicit the release of histamines and acetylcholine vasodilators. You have 3 minutes to review all the precautions with the athlete, perform the initial set-up, and begin treatment.*

Athlete Education	Test 1	Test 2	Test 3
Explains to the athlete why this treatment is appropriate (rationale)	Ⓨ Ⓝ	Ⓨ Ⓝ	Ⓨ Ⓝ
Explains to the athlete what are the expected treatment goals & outcomes	Ⓨ Ⓝ	Ⓨ Ⓝ	Ⓨ Ⓝ
Explains the type of massage to be used and the expected sensations	Ⓨ Ⓝ	Ⓨ Ⓝ	Ⓨ Ⓝ
Athlete Safety	**Test 1**	**Test 2**	**Test 3**
Reviews precautions/contraindications with the athlete	Ⓨ Ⓝ	Ⓨ Ⓝ	Ⓨ Ⓝ
Tester places athlete in appropriate position	**Test 1**	**Test 2**	**Test 3**
Supine (positioned so that the muscles are relaxed)	Ⓨ Ⓝ	Ⓨ Ⓝ	Ⓨ Ⓝ
Bolsters the athlete's knees	Ⓨ Ⓝ	Ⓨ Ⓝ	Ⓨ Ⓝ
Drapes the athlete for modesty and exposes of the area to be massaged	Ⓨ Ⓝ	Ⓨ Ⓝ	Ⓨ Ⓝ
Tester administers the massage technique according to accepted guidelines	**Test 1**	**Test 2**	**Test 3**
Gently taps or pounds the skin using one of the following techniques:			
Hacking: Contact with the skin is made with the lateral aspect of the hand and finger	Ⓨ Ⓝ	Ⓨ Ⓝ	Ⓨ Ⓝ
Cupping: The hands are cupped striking the skin with the heel and fingertips	Ⓨ Ⓝ	Ⓨ Ⓝ	Ⓨ Ⓝ
Pincement: The skin is pinched using the fingertips	Ⓨ Ⓝ	Ⓨ Ⓝ	Ⓨ Ⓝ
Rapping: The hand is held in a loose fist striking the skin with the distal phalanges	Ⓨ Ⓝ	Ⓨ Ⓝ	Ⓨ Ⓝ
Tapping (punctuation): The fingertips lightly drum the skin	Ⓨ Ⓝ	Ⓨ Ⓝ	Ⓨ Ⓝ
Executes the skill softly and slowly, while gradually increasing the pace and force	Ⓨ Ⓝ	Ⓨ Ⓝ	Ⓨ Ⓝ
Termination of Treatment	**Test 1**	**Test 2**	**Test 3**
Inspect treatment area	Ⓨ Ⓝ	Ⓨ Ⓝ	Ⓨ Ⓝ
Provides the athlete with feedback	Ⓨ Ⓝ	Ⓨ Ⓝ	Ⓨ Ⓝ
Document treatment	Ⓨ Ⓝ	Ⓨ Ⓝ	Ⓨ Ⓝ

The psychomotor skill was performed completely and in the appropriate order   0 1 2 3 4 5

The tester had control of the subject and the situation (showed confidence)   0 1 2 3 4 5

Method of performing the skill allowed the tester the ability to determine:
severity, proper progression, and the *fit* in the overall picture (Oral)   0 1 2 3 4 5

In order for a grade of *minimum standard* to be given, the total must be ≥11   TOTAL = _____

Continued on the following page

1   2   3   4   5   6   7   8   9   10   11   12   13   14   15

Not Acceptable

**Meets
Minimum Standards**

**Exceeds
Minimum Standards**

TEST ENVIRONMENTS

L: Laboratory/Classroom Testing
C: Clinical/Field Testing
P: Practicum Testing
A: Assessment/Mock Exam Testing
S: Self-Reporting

SKILL TEST INFORMATION

Purpose:	Increase blood flow, stimulate nerve endings, decrease pain
Involved Structure:	Upper arm
Special Considerations:	Many variations
Reference(s):	Salvo; Starkey (2004)
Supplies Needed:	Table

THERAPEUTIC MODALITIES
(TMOD-Test 12)

Peer Review _____ Peer Review _____

Skill Acquisition: _____   Practice Opportunities: _____

*This problem allows you the opportunity to use **fine vibration massage** to treat minor pain. Your scenario is a sports-related trauma to the posterior thigh. The physician's written orders state that you are to use massage to help decrease pain by eliciting the gate theory. You have 3 minutes to review all the precautions with the athlete, perform the initial set-up, and begin treatment.*

Athlete Education	Test 1	Test 2	Test 3
Explains to the athlete why this treatment is appropriate (rationale)	Ⓨ Ⓝ	Ⓨ Ⓝ	Ⓨ Ⓝ
Explains to the athlete what are the expected treatment goals & outcomes	Ⓨ Ⓝ	Ⓨ Ⓝ	Ⓨ Ⓝ
Explains the type of massage to be used and the expected sensations	Ⓨ Ⓝ	Ⓨ Ⓝ	Ⓨ Ⓝ
Athlete Safety	**Test 1**	**Test 2**	**Test 3**
Reviews precautions/contraindications with the athlete	Ⓨ Ⓝ	Ⓨ Ⓝ	Ⓨ Ⓝ
Tester places athlete in appropriate position	**Test 1**	**Test 2**	**Test 3**
Prone (positioned so that the muscles are relaxed)	Ⓨ Ⓝ	Ⓨ Ⓝ	Ⓨ Ⓝ
Drapes the athlete for modesty and exposes of the area to be massaged	Ⓨ Ⓝ	Ⓨ Ⓝ	Ⓨ Ⓝ
Tester administers the massage technique according to accepted guidelines	**Test 1**	**Test 2**	**Test 3**
Stands to the side of the athlete	Ⓨ Ⓝ	Ⓨ Ⓝ	Ⓨ Ⓝ
Places fingers firmly against the skin (perpendicular to the involved limb)	Ⓨ Ⓝ	Ⓨ Ⓝ	Ⓨ Ⓝ
Keeping the wrist and forearm in a locked position, moves the fingers up and down rapidly (fine, tremulous movements)	Ⓨ Ⓝ	Ⓨ Ⓝ	Ⓨ Ⓝ
The fingers should remain in contact with the skin (movement should come from the forearm)	Ⓨ Ⓝ	Ⓨ Ⓝ	Ⓨ Ⓝ
Termination of Treatment	**Test 1**	**Test 2**	**Test 3**
Inspects treatment area	Ⓨ Ⓝ	Ⓨ Ⓝ	Ⓨ Ⓝ
Provides the athlete with feedback	Ⓨ Ⓝ	Ⓨ Ⓝ	Ⓨ Ⓝ
Documents treatment	Ⓨ Ⓝ	Ⓨ Ⓝ	Ⓨ Ⓝ\

The psychomotor skill was performed completely and in the appropriate order	0 1 2 3 4 5
The tester had control of the subject and the situation (showed confidence)	0 1 2 3 4 5
Method of performing the skill allowed the tester the ability to determine: severity, proper progression, and the *fit* in the overall picture (Oral)	0 1 2 3 4 5
In order for a grade of *minimum standard* to be given, the total must be ≥11	TOTAL = _____

Continued on the following page

1   2   3   4   5   6   7   8   9   10   11   12   13   14   15

Not Acceptable

Meets Minimum Standards

Exceeds Minimum Standards

TEST ENVIRONMENTS

L: Laboratory/Classroom Testing
C: Clinical/Field Testing
P: Practicum Testing
A: Assessment/Mock Exam Testing
S: Self-Reporting

SKILL TEST INFORMATION

Purpose/:	Soothe peripheral nerves, increase circulation, decrease pain, and promote muscular relaxation
Involved Structure:	Posterior thigh
Special Considerations:	May be done with a vibratory mechanical device; other types of vibration include coarse and rocking
Reference(s):	Salvo; Starkey (2004)
Supplies Needed:	Table

THERAPEUTIC MODALITIES
(TMOD-Test 13)

Peer Review _____ Peer Review _____

Skill Acquisition: _____   Practice Opportunities: _____

This problem allows you the opportunity to use **cross-fiber (transverse) friction massage** *to break apart adhered tissue. Your scenario is a sports-related trauma to the anterior upper arm in the secondary phase of healing. The physician's written orders state that you are to use massage to help restore range of motion that has been restricted by adhesions within the healing muscle. You have 3 minutes to review all the precautions with the athlete, perform the initial set-up, and begin treatment*

Athlete Education	Test 1	Test 2	Test 3
Explains to the athlete why this treatment is appropriate (rationale)	Ⓨ Ⓝ	Ⓨ Ⓝ	Ⓨ Ⓝ
Explains to the athlete what are the expected treatment goals & outcomes	Ⓨ Ⓝ	Ⓨ Ⓝ	Ⓨ Ⓝ
Explains the type of massage to be used and the expected sensations	Ⓨ Ⓝ	Ⓨ Ⓝ	Ⓨ Ⓝ
Athlete Safety	**Test 1**	**Test 2**	**Test 3**
Reviews precautions/contraindications with the athlete	Ⓨ Ⓝ	Ⓨ Ⓝ	Ⓨ Ⓝ
Tester places athlete in appropriate position	**Test 1**	**Test 2**	**Test 3**
Supine (positioned so that the muscles are relaxed)	Ⓨ Ⓝ	Ⓨ Ⓝ	Ⓨ Ⓝ
Bolsters the knees	Ⓨ Ⓝ	Ⓨ Ⓝ	Ⓨ Ⓝ
Drapes the athlete for modesty and exposes of the area to be massaged	Ⓨ Ⓝ	Ⓨ Ⓝ	Ⓨ Ⓝ
Tester administers the massage technique according to accepted guidelines	**Test 1**	**Test 2**	**Test 3**
Preheats the tissue prior to treatment (ultrasound, moist hot pack, etc)	Ⓨ Ⓝ	Ⓨ Ⓝ	Ⓨ Ⓝ
Thumbs or fingertip strokes are performed in opposite directions	Ⓨ Ⓝ	Ⓨ Ⓝ	Ⓨ Ⓝ
Performs strokes perpendicular to the muscle fibers with firm consistent pressure	Ⓨ Ⓝ	Ⓨ Ⓝ	Ⓨ Ⓝ
Begins with light strokes; progresses to heavy pressure (adequate force should be used reach target tissue)	Ⓨ Ⓝ	Ⓨ Ⓝ	Ⓨ Ⓝ
Termination of Treatment	**Test 1**	**Test 2**	**Test 3**
Inspects treatment area	Ⓨ Ⓝ	Ⓨ Ⓝ	Ⓨ Ⓝ
Provides the athlete with feedback	Ⓨ Ⓝ	Ⓨ Ⓝ	Ⓨ Ⓝ
Documents treatment	Ⓨ Ⓝ	Ⓨ Ⓝ	Ⓨ Ⓝ

The psychomotor skill was performed completely and in the appropriate order   **0   1   2   3   4   5**

The tester had control of the subject and the situation (showed confidence)   **0   1   2   3   4   5**

Method of performing the skill allowed the tester the ability to determine:
severity, proper progression, and the *fit* in the overall picture (Oral)   **0   1   2   3   4   5**

In order for a grade of *minimum standard* to be given, the total must be ≥11   **TOTAL = _____**

Continued on the following page

Not Acceptable   Meets   Exceeds
                                          Minimum Standards   Minimum Standards

TEST ENVIRONMENTS

L: Laboratory/Classroom Testing
C: Clinical/Field Testing
P: Practicum Testing
A: Assessment/Mock Exam Testing
S: Self-Reporting

SKILL TEST INFORMATION

Purpose:	Mobilizes muscle and breaks down adhesions and scar tissue
Involved Structure:	Anterior upper leg
Special Considerations:	There are additional types of friction massage: rolling, etc
Reference(s):	Salvo; Starkey (2004)
Supplies Needed:	Table

THERAPEUTIC MODALITIES
(TMOD-Test 14)

Peer Review _____ Peer Review _____

Skill Acquisition: _____   Practice Opportunities: _____

This problem allows you the opportunity to use **intermittent compression** *as a therapeutic modality for the purpose of encouraging lymphatic and venous return. Your scenario is a sports-related injury to the knee in the secondary phase of healing. The physician's written orders state that you are to use intermittent compression to reduce edema. You have 3 minutes to review all precautions with the athlete, perform the initial set-up, and begin treatment.*

Athlete Education	Test 1	Test 2	Test 3
Explains to the athlete why this modality is appropriate (rationale)	Y N	Y N	Y N
Explains to the athlete what are the expected treatment goals & outcomes	Y N	Y N	Y N
Explains to the athlete what they should or should not feel	Y N	Y N	Y N
Athlete Safety	**Test 1**	**Test 2**	**Test 3**
Prior to set-up of the modality, checks all aspects for safety	Y N	Y N	Y N
Reviews precautions/contraindications with the athlete	Y N	Y N	Y N
Removes any jewelry in the area being treated	Y N	Y N	Y N
Takes athlete's blood pressure	Y N	Y N	Y N
Tester places athlete in appropriate position	**Test 1**	**Test 2**	**Test 3**
Supine	Y N	Y N	Y N
Elevates the involved limb	Y N	Y N	Y N
Tester administers the therapeutic modality according to accepted guidelines	**Test 1**	**Test 2**	**Test 3**
Measures/records the girth measurements of the involved limb	Y N	Y N	Y N
Covers the involved area with stockinette	Y N	Y N	Y N
Selects the appropriate sized appliance	Y N	Y N	Y N
Places the involved limb into the appliance	Y N	Y N	Y N
Connects the appliance to the compression unit	Y N	Y N	Y N
Selects the proper settings:			
Temperature (if applicable)	Y N	Y N	Y N
Maximum pressure	Y N	Y N	Y N
On-off times	Y N	Y N	Y N
Treatment duration	Y N	Y N	Y N
Encourages the athlete to move toes/foot throughout the treatment	Y N	Y N	Y N
Termination of Treatment	**Test 1**	**Test 2**	**Test 3**
Removes the air/water from the appliance	Y N	Y N	Y N
Inspects treatment area (remeasures the girth)	Y N	Y N	Y N
Provides the athlete with feedback (applies compression wrap)	Y N	Y N	Y N
Documents treatment	Y N	Y N	Y N

The psychomotor skill was performed completely and in the appropriate order   0 1 2 3 4 5

The tester had control of the subject and the situation (showed confidence)   0 1 2 3 4 5

Method of performing the skill allowed the tester the ability to determine:
severity, proper progression, and the *fit* in the overall picture (Oral)   0 1 2 3 4 5

In order for a grade of *minimum standard* to be given, the total must be ≥11   **TOTAL = _____**

Continued on the following page

1   2   3   4   5   6   7   8   9   10   11   12   13   14   15

Not Acceptable   **Meets**   **Exceeds**
                                                       Minimum Standards   **Minimum Standards**

TEST ENVIRONMENTS

L: Laboratory/Classroom Testing
C: Clinical/Field Testing
P: Practicum Testing
A: Assessment/Mock Exam Testing
S: Self-Reporting

SKILL TEST INFORMATION

Purpose:	Encourage lymphatic/venous return
Involved Structure:	Knee
Special Considerations:	Pressure should not exceed diastolic; blood pressure
Reference(s):	Starkey (2004)
Supplies Needed:	Compression unit with appliances, stockinette, elevation pillow, BP Cuff, stethoscope

THERAPEUTIC MODALITIES
(TMOD-Test 15)

Peer Review _____ Peer Review _____

Skill Acquisition: _____   Practice Opportunities: _____

This problem allows you the opportunity to use the **immersion technique** *for administering ultrasound as a therapeutic modality to treat chronic inflammation of the distal forearm. Your scenario is a sports-related injury to the hand that has resulted in chronic inflammation in the ulnocarpal joint. The physician's written orders state that you are to use underwater ultrasound to reduce the inflammation and pain. You have 3 minutes to review all the precautions with the athlete, perform the initial set-up, and begin treatment.*

Athlete Education	Test 1	Test 2	Test 3
Explains to the athlete why this modality is appropriate (rationale)	Ⓨ Ⓝ	Ⓨ Ⓝ	Ⓨ Ⓝ
Explains to the athlete what are the expected treatment goals & outcomes	Ⓨ Ⓝ	Ⓨ Ⓝ	Ⓨ Ⓝ
Explains to the athlete what they should or should not feel	Ⓨ Ⓝ	Ⓨ Ⓝ	Ⓨ Ⓝ
Athlete Safety	**Test 1**	**Test 2**	**Test 3**
Prior to the set-up of modality, checks all aspects for safety	Ⓨ Ⓝ	Ⓨ Ⓝ	Ⓨ Ⓝ
Reviews precautions/contraindications with the athlete	Ⓨ Ⓝ	Ⓨ Ⓝ	Ⓨ Ⓝ
Tester places athlete in appropriate position	Ⓨ Ⓝ	Ⓨ Ⓝ	Ⓨ Ⓝ
Seated	Ⓨ Ⓝ	Ⓨ Ⓝ	Ⓨ Ⓝ
Places hand in a water tub (ceramic, plastic, rubber tub recommended)	Ⓨ Ⓝ	Ⓨ Ⓝ	Ⓨ Ⓝ
Tester administers the therapeutic modality according to accepted guidelines	**Test 1**	**Test 2**	**Test 3**
Places transducer in the water	Ⓨ Ⓝ	Ⓨ Ⓝ	Ⓨ Ⓝ
Places surface head about 1 inch away from the involved area	Ⓨ Ⓝ	Ⓨ Ⓝ	Ⓨ Ⓝ
Transducer should be parallel to the surface of the involved area	Ⓨ Ⓝ	Ⓨ Ⓝ	Ⓨ Ⓝ
Should not submerse hand in the water	Ⓨ Ⓝ	Ⓨ Ⓝ	Ⓨ Ⓝ
Treatment parameters are consistent with the intended goals:			
Intensity	Ⓨ Ⓝ	Ⓨ Ⓝ	Ⓨ Ⓝ
Frequency	Ⓨ Ⓝ	Ⓨ Ⓝ	Ⓨ Ⓝ
Treatment Time	Ⓨ Ⓝ	Ⓨ Ⓝ	Ⓨ Ⓝ
Termination of Treatment	**Test 1**	**Test 2**	**Test 3**
Inspects treatment area	Ⓨ Ⓝ	Ⓨ Ⓝ	Ⓨ Ⓝ
Provides the athlete with feedback	Ⓨ Ⓝ	Ⓨ Ⓝ	Ⓨ Ⓝ
Documents treatment	Ⓨ Ⓝ	Ⓨ Ⓝ	Ⓨ Ⓝ

The psychomotor skill was performed completely and in the appropriate order   0 1 2 3 4 5

The tester had control of the subject and the situation (showed confidence)   0 1 2 3 4 5

Method of performing the skill allowed the tester the ability to determine:
severity, proper progression, and the *fit* in the overall picture (Oral)   0 1 2 3 4 5

In order for a grade of *minimum standard* to be given, the total must be ≥11   **TOTAL = _____**

Continued on the following page

1   2   3   4   5   6   7   8   9   10   11   12   13   14   15

Not Acceptable   **Meets**   **Exceeds**
                                                              Minimum Standards   **Minimum Standards**

TEST ENVIRONMENTS

L: Laboratory/Classroom Testing
C: Clinical/Field Testing
P: Practicum Testing
A: Assessment/Mock Exam Testing
S: Self-Reporting

SKILL TEST INFORMATION

Purpose:	Treat chronic inflammation and pain
Involved Structure:	Wrist
Special Considerations:	N/A
Reference(s):	Starkey (2004)
Supplies Needed:	Ultrasound unit, tub of water, towel, chair

THERAPEUTIC MODALITIES
(TMOD-Test 16)

Peer Review _____ Peer Review _____

Skill Acquisition: _____   Practice Opportunities: _____

*This problem allows you the opportunity to use **ultrasound at 1 MHz** as a therapeutic modality to treat a deep thigh contusion. Your scenario is a sports-related injury to the thigh in the secondary phase of healing. The physician's written orders state that you are to use ultrasound to treat muscle injuries in the secondary phase of healing. You have 3 minutes to review all the precautions with the athlete, perform the initial set-up, and begin treatment.*

Athlete Education	Test 1	Test 2	Test 3
Explains to the athlete why this modality is appropriate (rationale)	Ⓨ Ⓝ	Ⓨ Ⓝ	Ⓨ Ⓝ
Explains to the athlete what are the expected treatment goals & outcomes	Ⓨ Ⓝ	Ⓨ Ⓝ	Ⓨ Ⓝ
Explains to the athlete what they should or should not feel	Ⓨ Ⓝ	Ⓨ Ⓝ	Ⓨ Ⓝ
Athlete Safety	**Test 1**	**Test 2**	**Test 3**
Prior to set-up of modality, checks all aspects for safety	Ⓨ Ⓝ	Ⓨ Ⓝ	Ⓨ Ⓝ
Reviews the precautions/contraindications with the athlete	Ⓨ Ⓝ	Ⓨ Ⓝ	Ⓨ Ⓝ
Identifies the BNR, ERA	Ⓨ Ⓝ	Ⓨ Ⓝ	Ⓨ Ⓝ
Tester places athlete in appropriate position	**Test 1**	**Test 2**	**Test 3**
Supine	Ⓨ Ⓝ	Ⓨ Ⓝ	Ⓨ Ⓝ
Properly drapes the athlete	Ⓨ Ⓝ	Ⓨ Ⓝ	Ⓨ Ⓝ
Tester administers the therapeutic modality according to accepted guidelines	**Test 1**	**Test 2**	**Test 3**
Applies the appropriate transmission medium (coupling agent) to the involved area	Ⓨ Ⓝ	Ⓨ Ⓝ	Ⓨ Ⓝ
Using the transducer, applies firm overlapping circular strokes with constant pressure to the involved area throughout the treatment	Ⓨ Ⓝ	Ⓨ Ⓝ	Ⓨ Ⓝ
Treatment parameters are consistent with the intended goals:			
Intensity	Ⓨ Ⓝ	Ⓨ Ⓝ	Ⓨ Ⓝ
Frequency	Ⓨ Ⓝ	Ⓨ Ⓝ	Ⓨ Ⓝ
Treatment duration	Ⓨ Ⓝ	Ⓨ Ⓝ	Ⓨ Ⓝ
Duty cycle	Ⓨ Ⓝ	Ⓨ Ⓝ	Ⓨ Ⓝ
Depresses the start button after the transducer is slowly moved in overlapping circles	Ⓨ Ⓝ	Ⓨ Ⓝ	Ⓨ Ⓝ
Termination of Treatment	**Test 1**	**Test 2**	**Test 3**
Inspects treatment area	Ⓨ Ⓝ	Ⓨ Ⓝ	Ⓨ Ⓝ
Provides the athlete with feedback	Ⓨ Ⓝ	Ⓨ Ⓝ	Ⓨ Ⓝ
Documents treatment	Ⓨ Ⓝ	Ⓨ Ⓝ	Ⓨ Ⓝ

The psychomotor skill was performed completely and in the appropriate order   **0 1 2 3 4 5**

The tester had control of the subject and the situation (showed confidence)   **0 1 2 3 4 5**

Method of performing the skill allowed the tester the ability to determine:
severity, proper progression, and the *fit* in the overall picture (Oral)   **0 1 2 3 4 5**

In order for a grade of *minimum standard* to be given, the total must be ≥11   **TOTAL = _____**

Continued on the following page

Not Acceptable   **Meets**   **Exceeds**
                                                           Minimum Standards   **Minimum Standards**

TEST ENVIRONMENTS

L: Laboratory/Classroom Testing
C: Clinical/Field Testing
P: Practicum Testing
A: Assessment/Mock Exam Testing
S: Self-Reporting

SKILL TEST INFORMATION

Purpose:	Increase the temperature of the tissue
Involved Structure:	Anterior upper leg
Special Considerations:	N/A
Reference(s):	Starkey (2004)
Supplies Needed:	Ultrasound unit, ultrasound gel, towel

THERAPEUTIC MODALITIES
(TMOD-Test 17)

Peer Review _____ Peer Review _____

Skill Acquisition: _____   Practice Opportunities: _____

This problem allows you the opportunity to use **ultrasound at 3 MHz** *as a therapeutic modality to reduce inflammation to the upper arm. Your scenario is a baseball pitcher who has developed bicipital tendonitis. The physician's written orders state that you are to use ultrasound to treat this type of overuse injury. You have 3 minutes to review all the precautions with the patient, perform the initial set-up, and begin treatment.*

Athlete Education	Test 1	Test 2	Test 3
Explains to the athlete why this modality is appropriate (rationale)	Y N	Y N	Y N
Explains to the athlete what are the expected treatment goals & outcomes	Y N	Y N	Y N
Explains to the athlete what they should or should not feel	Y N	Y N	Y N
Athlete Safety	**Test 1**	**Test 2**	**Test 3**
Prior to the set-up of modality, checks all aspects for safety	Y N	Y N	Y N
Reviews the precautions/contraindications with the athlete	Y N	Y N	Y N
Identifies the BNR, ERA	Y N	Y N	Y N
Tester places athlete in appropriate position	**Test 1**	**Test 2**	**Test 3**
Supine	Y N	Y N	Y N
Properly drapes the athlete	Y N	Y N	Y N
Tester administers the therapeutic modality according to accepted guidelines	**Test 1**	**Test 2**	**Test 3**
Applies the appropriate transmission medium (coupling agent) to the involved area	Y N	Y N	Y N
Using the transducer, applies firm overlapping circular strokes with constant pressure to the involved area throughout the treatment	Y N	Y N	Y N
Treatment parameters are consistent with the intended goals:			
Intensity	Y N	Y N	Y N
Frequency	Y N	Y N	Y N
Treatment duration	Y N	Y N	Y N
Duty cycle	Y N	Y N	Y N
Depresses the start button after the transducer is slowly moved in overlapping circles	Y N	Y N	Y N
Termination of Treatment	**Test 1**	**Test 2**	**Test 3**
Inspects treatment area	Y N	Y N	Y N
Provides athlete feedback	Y N	Y N	Y N
Documents treatment	Y N	Y N	Y N

The psychomotor skill was performed completely and in the appropriate order   0 1 2 3 4 5

The tester had control of the subject and the situation (showed confidence)   0 1 2 3 4 5

Method of performing the skill allowed the tester the ability to determine:
severity, proper progression, and the *fit* in the overall picture (Oral)   0 1 2 3 4 5

In order for a grade of *minimum standard* to be given, the total must be ≥11   **TOTAL = _____**

Continued on the following page

1 2 3 4 5 6 7 8 9 10 11 12 13 14 15

Not Acceptable   **Meets**   **Exceeds**
                              Minimum Standards   **Minimum Standards**

TEST ENVIRONMENTS

L: Laboratory/Classroom Testing
C: Clinical/Field Testing
P: Practicum Testing
A: Assessment/Mock Exam Testing
S: Self-Reporting

SKILL TEST INFORMATION

Purpose:	Increase temperature of the tissue
Involved Structure:	Bicips tendon
Special Considerations:	NA
Reference(s):	Starkey (2004)
Supplies Needed:	Ultrasound unit, ultrasound gel, towel

THERAPEUTIC MODALITIES
(TMOD-Test 18)

Peer Review _____ Peer Review _____

Skill Acquisition: _____   Practice Opportunities: _____

This problem allows you the opportunity to use **phonophoresis** *to assist in diffusing medication through the skin. Your scenario is a sport-related injury of a wrestler who has developed prepatellar bursitis. The physician's written orders state that you are to use phonophoresis to treat this type of injury. You have 3 minutes to review all the precautions with the athlete, perform the initial set-up, and begin treatment.*

Athlete Education	Test 1	Test 2	Test 3
Explains to the athlete why this modality is appropriate (rationale)	Y N	Y N	Y N
Explains to the athlete what are the expected treatment goals and outcomes	Y N	Y N	Y N
Explains to the athlete what they should or should not feel	Y N	Y N	Y N
Athlete Safety	**Test 1**	**Test 2**	**Test 3**
Prior to the set-up of the modality, checks all aspects for safety	Y N	Y N	Y N
Reviews the precautions/contraindications with the athlete	Y N	Y N	Y N
Identifies the BNR, ERA	Y N	Y N	Y N
Tester places athlete in appropriate position	**Test 1**	**Test 2**	**Test 3**
Supine	Y N	Y N	Y N
Tester administers the therapeutic modality according to accepted guidelines	**Test 1**	**Test 2**	**Test 3**
Preheats the area to increase local blood flow	Y N	Y N	Y N
Applies the appropriate prescription or nonprescription medication to the involved area (massaging the medication into the area)	Y N	Y N	Y N
Using the transducer, applies firm overlapping circular strokes with constant pressure to the involved area throughout the treatment	Y N	Y N	Y N
Treatment parameters are consistent with the intended goals:			
Intensity	Y N	Y N	Y N
Frequency	Y N	Y N	Y N
Treatment duration	Y N	Y N	Y N
Duty cycle	Y N	Y N	Y N
Depresses the start button after the transducer is slowly moved in overlapping circles	Y N	Y N	Y N
Termination of Treatment	**Test 1**	**Test 2**	**Test 3**
Leaves the remaining medication on the skin after treatment Inspects treatment area	Y N	Y N	Y N
Provides the athlete with feedback	Y N	Y N	Y N
Documents treatment	Y N	Y N	Y N

The psychomotor skill was performed completely and in the appropriate order   0 1 2 3 4 5

The tester had control of the subject and the situation (showed confidence)   0 1 2 3 4 5

Method of performing the skill allowed the tester the ability to determine:
severity, proper progression, and the *fit* in the overall picture (Oral)   0 1 2 3 4 5

In order for a grade of *minimum standard* to be given, the total must be ≥11   TOTAL = _____

Continued on the following page

1   2   3   4   5   6   7   8   9   10   11   12   13   14   15

Not Acceptable   **Meets**   **Exceeds**
                                               Minimum Standards   **Minimum Standards**

TEST ENVIRONMENTS

L: Laboratory/Classroom Testing
C: Clinical/Field Testing
P: Practicum Testing
A: Assessment/Mock Exam Testing
S: Self-Reporting

SKILL TEST INFORMATION

Purpose: Allow medication to absorb into the involved area
Involved Structure: Patella tendon
Special Considerations: Commonly used medications include: corticosteroids and salicylates
Reference(s): Starkey (2004)
Supplies Needed: Ultrasound unit, ultrasound gel, towel, preheating device

THERAPEUTIC MODALITIES
(TMOD-Test 19)

Peer Review _____ Peer Review _____

Skill Acquisition: _____   Practice Opportunities: _____

This problem allows you the opportunity to use **interferential electrical stimulation** *to treat shoulder pain. Your scenario is a sport-related injury of a tennis player with an acutely painful shoulder. The physician's written orders state that you are to use electrical stimulation to treat the anterior shoulder pain. You have 3 minutes to review all the precautions with the athlete, perform the initial set-up, and begin treatment.*

Athlete Education	Test 1	Test 2	Test 3
Explains to the athlete why this modality is appropriate (rationale)	Ⓨ Ⓝ	Ⓨ Ⓝ	Ⓨ Ⓝ
Explains to the athlete what are the expected treatment goals & outcomes	Ⓨ Ⓝ	Ⓨ Ⓝ	Ⓨ Ⓝ
Explains to the athlete what they should or should not feel	Ⓨ Ⓝ	Ⓨ Ⓝ	Ⓨ Ⓝ
Athlete Safety	**Test 1**	**Test 2**	**Test 3**
Prior to the set-up of the modality, checks all aspects for safety	Ⓨ Ⓝ	Ⓨ Ⓝ	Ⓨ Ⓝ
Reviews the precautions/contraindications with the athlete	Ⓨ Ⓝ	Ⓨ Ⓝ	Ⓨ Ⓝ
Tester places athlete in appropriate position	**Test 1**	**Test 2**	**Test 3**
Supine	Ⓨ Ⓝ	Ⓨ Ⓝ	Ⓨ Ⓝ
Drapes the athlete for modesty and exposes the area to be treated	Ⓨ Ⓝ	Ⓨ Ⓝ	Ⓨ Ⓝ
Tester administers the therapeutic modality according to accepted guidelines	**Test 1**	**Test 2**	**Test 3**
Places the electrodes appropriately around the painful area (clean area with alcohol swabs)	Ⓨ Ⓝ	Ⓨ Ⓝ	Ⓨ Ⓝ
Turns the power on and depresses the reset button	Ⓨ Ⓝ	Ⓨ Ⓝ	Ⓨ Ⓝ
Treatment parameters are consistent with the intended goals:			
Selects the proper application mode	Ⓨ Ⓝ	Ⓨ Ⓝ	Ⓨ Ⓝ
Adjusts the beat frequency	Ⓨ Ⓝ	Ⓨ Ⓝ	Ⓨ Ⓝ
Adjusts the sweep frequency	Ⓨ Ⓝ	Ⓨ Ⓝ	Ⓨ Ⓝ
Adjusts the duration by setting the timer	Ⓨ Ⓝ	Ⓨ Ⓝ	Ⓨ Ⓝ
Depresses the start switch after all parameters are set	Ⓨ Ⓝ	Ⓨ Ⓝ	Ⓨ Ⓝ
Adjusts the intensity to the appropriate current level	Ⓨ Ⓝ	Ⓨ Ⓝ	Ⓨ Ⓝ
Adjusts the balance to control comfort	Ⓨ Ⓝ	Ⓨ Ⓝ	Ⓨ Ⓝ
Termination of Treatment	**Test 1**	**Test 2**	**Test 3**
Inspects treatment area	Ⓨ Ⓝ	Ⓨ Ⓝ	Ⓨ Ⓝ
Provides the athlete with feedback	Ⓨ Ⓝ	Ⓨ Ⓝ	Ⓨ Ⓝ
Documents treatment	Ⓨ Ⓝ	Ⓨ Ⓝ	Ⓨ Ⓝ

The psychomotor skill was performed completely and in the appropriate order   0 1 2 3 4 5

The tester had control of the subject and the situation (showed confidence)   0 1 2 3 4 5

Method of performing the skill allowed the tester the ability to determine:
severity, proper progression, and the *fit* in the overall picture (Oral)   0 1 2 3 4 5

In order for a grade of *minimum standard* to be given, the total must be ≥11   TOTAL = _____

Continued on the following page

| 1 | 2 | 3 | 4 | 5 | 6 | 7 | 8 | 9 | 10 | 11 | 12 | 13 | 14 | 15 |

Not Acceptable   **Meets**   **Exceeds**
                                           Minimum Standards   **Minimum Standards**

TEST ENVIRONMENTS

L: Laboratory/Classroom Testing
C: Clinical/Field Testing
P: Practicum Testing
A: Assessment/Mock Exam Testing
S: Self-Reporting

SKILL TEST INFORMATION

Purpose:	Modulate pain
Involved Structure:	Anterior shoulder
Special Considerations:	N/A
Reference(s):	Starkey (2004); manufacturer's operating instructions
Supplies Needed:	Interferential stimulation generator, 4 electrodes, alcohol swabs

THERAPEUTIC MODALITIES
(TMOD-Test 20)

Peer Review _____ Peer Review _____

Skill Acquisition: _____   Practice Opportunities: _____

This problem allows you the opportunity to use **microcurrent electrical stimulation (low–intensity stimulation)** *to treat an acute inflammation of the SI joint. Your scenario is a sports-related injury during the primary phase of healing. The physician's written orders state that you are to use electrical stimulation to treat the inflamed sacroiliac joint. You have 3 minutes to review all the precautions with the athlete, perform the initial set-up, and begin treatment.*

Athlete Education	Test 1	Test 2	Test 3
Explains to the athlete why this modality is appropriate (rationale)	Ⓨ Ⓝ	Ⓨ Ⓝ	Ⓨ Ⓝ
Explains to the athlete what are the expected treatment goals & outcomes	Ⓨ Ⓝ	Ⓨ Ⓝ	Ⓨ Ⓝ
Explains to the athlete what they should or should not feel	Ⓨ Ⓝ	Ⓨ Ⓝ	Ⓨ Ⓝ
Athlete Safety	**Test 1**	**Test 2**	**Test 3**
Prior to the set-up of the modality, checks all aspects for safety	Ⓨ Ⓝ	Ⓨ Ⓝ	Ⓨ Ⓝ
Reviews the precautions/contraindications with the athlete	Ⓨ Ⓝ	Ⓨ Ⓝ	Ⓨ Ⓝ
Tester places athlete in appropriate position	**Test 1**	**Test 2**	**Test 3**
Prone	Ⓨ Ⓝ	Ⓨ Ⓝ	Ⓨ Ⓝ
Bolsters the athlete's ankles and places a pillow under the abdomen	Ⓨ Ⓝ	Ⓨ Ⓝ	Ⓨ Ⓝ
Tester administers the therapeutic modality according to accepted guidelines	**Test 1**	**Test 2**	**Test 3**
Selects and wets the appropriate electrodes with saline solution	Ⓨ Ⓝ	Ⓨ Ⓝ	Ⓨ Ⓝ
Places the electrodes appropriately in the painful area (clean area with alcohol swabs)	Ⓨ Ⓝ	Ⓨ Ⓝ	Ⓨ Ⓝ
Begins treatment by depressing the start switch	Ⓨ Ⓝ	Ⓨ Ⓝ	Ⓨ Ⓝ
Treatment parameters are consistent with the intended goals:			
Selects the appropriate output frequency	Ⓨ Ⓝ	Ⓨ Ⓝ	Ⓨ Ⓝ
Increases the output frequency	Ⓨ Ⓝ	Ⓨ Ⓝ	Ⓨ Ⓝ
Repositions the electrodes about every 10 minutes (removes, rewets, repositions)	Ⓨ Ⓝ	Ⓨ Ⓝ	Ⓨ Ⓝ
Adjusts the duration by setting the timer throughout the treatment	Ⓨ Ⓝ	Ⓨ Ⓝ	Ⓨ Ⓝ
Termination of Treatment	**Test 1**	**Test 2**	**Test 3**
Inspects treatment area	Ⓨ Ⓝ	Ⓨ Ⓝ	Ⓨ Ⓝ
Provides the athlete with feedback	Ⓨ Ⓝ	Ⓨ Ⓝ	Ⓨ Ⓝ
Documents treatment	Ⓨ Ⓝ	Ⓨ Ⓝ	Ⓨ Ⓝ

The psychomotor skill was performed completely and in the appropriate order   **0 1 2 3 4 5**

The tester had control of the subject and the situation (showed confidence)   **0 1 2 3 4 5**

Method of performing the skill allowed the tester the ability to determine:
severity, proper progression, and the *fit* in the overall picture (Oral)   **0 1 2 3 4 5**

In order for a grade of *minimum standard* to be given, the total must be ≥11   **TOTAL = _____**

Continued on the following page

1   2   3   4   5   6   7   8   9   10   11   12   13   14   15

Not Acceptable

**Meets
Minimum Standards**

**Exceeds
Minimum Standards**

SKILL TEST INFORMATION

Purpose:	Treat acute inflammation
Involved Structure:	Sacroiliac joint
Special Considerations:	May perform the treatment on the contralateral side
Reference(s):	Starkey (2004); manufacturer's operating instructions
Supplies Needed:	Microcurrent generator, 2 MET electrodes, saline solution, pillows, alcohol swabs

TEST ENVIRONMENTS

L: Laboratory/Classroom Testing
C: Clinical/Field Testing
P: Practicum Testing
A: Assessment/Mock Exam Testing
S: Self-Reporting

THERAPEUTIC MODALITIES
(TMOD-Test 21)

Peer Review _____ Peer Review _____

Skill Acquisition: _____   Practice Opportunities: _____

This problem allows you the opportunity to use **iontophoresis.** *Your scenario is an activity-related chronic inflammation of the shoulder. The physician's written orders state that you are to use iontophoresis to administer an anti-inflammatory medication to the shoulder. You have 3 minutes to review all the precautions with the athlete, perform the initial set-up, and begin treatment.*

Athlete Education	Test 1	Test 2	Test 3
Explains to the athlete why this modality is appropriate (rationale)	Y N	Y N	Y N
Explains to the athlete what are the expected treatment goals & outcomes	Y N	Y N	Y N
Explains to the athlete what they should or should not feel	Y N	Y N	Y N
Athlete Safety	**Test 1**	**Test 2**	**Test 3**
Prior to the set-up of the modality, checks all aspects for safety	Y N	Y N	Y N
Reviews the precautions/contraindications with the athlete	Y N	Y N	Y N
Tester places athlete in appropriate position	**Test 1**	**Test 2**	**Test 3**
Seated or supine	Y N	Y N	Y N
Tester administers the therapeutic modality according to accepted guidelines	Y N	Y N	Y N
Prepares the treatment area by cleaning with alcohol wipes (shave area if necessary)	Y N	Y N	Y N
Fills the active electrode with the appropriate medication	Y N	Y N	Y N
Wets (buffering solution) the return electrode	Y N	Y N	Y N
Places the active electrode (delivery electrode) over the target area	Y N	Y N	Y N
Places the return electrode 4 to 6 inches away from target site	Y N	Y N	Y N
Turns the power on	Y N	Y N	Y N
Treatment parameters are consistent with the intended goals:			
Sets the treatment duration (based on intensity and desired treatment dose)	Y N	Y N	Y N
Selects the electrode polarity	Y N	Y N	Y N
Sets the treatment dosage (recommended by physician)	Y N	Y N	Y N
Adjusts the intensity to the appropriate level (may increase throughout the treatment)	Y N	Y N	Y N
Shuts down power and discards electrodes	Y N	Y N	Y N
Termination of Treatment	**Test 1**	**Test 2**	**Test 3**
Inspects treatment area (may apply lotion to prevent skin irritation)	Y N	Y N	Y N
Provides the athlete with feedback	Y N	Y N	Y N
Documents treatment	Y N	Y N	Y N

The psychomotor skill was performed completely and in the appropriate order   **0 1 2 3 4 5**

The tester had control of the subject and the situation (showed confidence)   **0 1 2 3 4 5**

Method of performing the skill allowed the tester the ability to determine:
severity, proper progression, and the *fit* in the overall picture (Oral)   **0 1 2 3 4 5**

In order for a grade of *minimum standard* to be given, the total must be ≥11   **TOTAL = _____**

Continued on the following page

Not Acceptable   Meets   Exceeds
                                              Minimum Standards   Minimum Standards

TEST ENVIRONMENTS

L: Laboratory/Classroom Testing
C: Clinical/Field Testing
P: Practicum Testing
A: Assessment/Mock Exam Testing
S: Self-Reporting

SKILL TEST INFORMATION

Positive Finding:	Anterior displacement
Involved Structure:	ACL; posteriormedial capsule
Special Considerations:	Hamstring guarding
Reference(s):	Konin; Magee
Supplies Needed:	Tables

THERAPEUTIC MODALITIES
(TMOD-Test 22)

Peer Review _____ Peer Review _____

Skill Acquisition: _____   Practice Opportunities: _____

This problem allows you the opportunity to demonstrate the appropriate **cleaning of a therapeutic whirlpool.**
You have 3 minutes to complete this task.

Equipment Maintenance	Test 1	Test 2	Test 3
Uses appropriate personal protective attire	Ⓨ Ⓝ	Ⓨ Ⓝ	Ⓨ Ⓝ
Drains the whirlpool	Ⓨ Ⓝ	Ⓨ Ⓝ	Ⓨ Ⓝ
Refills the tub with hot water (120°)	Ⓨ Ⓝ	Ⓨ Ⓝ	Ⓨ Ⓝ
Adds a cleaning agent (antibacterial/chlorine bleach)	Ⓨ Ⓝ	Ⓨ Ⓝ	Ⓨ Ⓝ
Turns on the turbine for 1 minute (water level must be sufficient not to cause damage)	Ⓨ Ⓝ	Ⓨ Ⓝ	Ⓨ Ⓝ
Drains whirlpool	Ⓨ Ⓝ	Ⓨ Ⓝ	Ⓨ Ⓝ
Cleans the interior of the whirlpool (with a brush and the appropriate cleaner)	Ⓨ Ⓝ	Ⓨ Ⓝ	Ⓨ Ⓝ
Rinses the interior of the whirlpool	Ⓨ Ⓝ	Ⓨ Ⓝ	Ⓨ Ⓝ
Cleans the exterior of the whirlpool (use appropriate cleaner)	Ⓨ Ⓝ	Ⓨ Ⓝ	Ⓨ Ⓝ

The psychomotor skill was performed completely and in the appropriate order   0 1 2 3 4 5

The tester had control of the subject and the situation (showed confidence)   0 1 2 3 4 5

Method of performing the skill allowed the tester the ability to determine:
severity, proper progression, and the *fit* in the overall picture (Oral)   0 1 2 3 4 5

In order for a grade of *minimum standard* to be given, the total must be ≥11   TOTAL = _____

```
  1    2    3    4    5    6    7    8    9   10   11   12   13   14   15
  |----|----|----|----|----|----|----|----|----|----|----|----|----|----|
```
Not Acceptable   **Meets**   **Exceeds**
                                          Minimum Standards   **Minimum Standards**

TEST ENVIRONMENTS

L: Laboratory/Classroom Testing
C: Clinical/Field Testing
P: Practicum Testing
A: Assessment/Mock Exam Testing
S: Self-Reporting

SKILL TEST INFORMATION

Purpose: Demonstrate the appropriate cleaning of a whirlpool
Special Considerations: May want to use a culture kit to determine the amount of bacteria growing the whirlpool
Reference(s): Starkey (2004)
Supplies Needed: Whirlpool, cleaning and disinfecting supplies, brush protective attire, towel

B

BIBLIOGRAPHY

Anderson MK, Hall SJ. *Sports Injury Management*. Baltimore, Md: Williams & Wilkins; 1995.

Baechle TR, Earle RW. *Essentials of Strength Training and Conditioning*. Champaign, Ill: Human Kinetics; 2000.

Bickley LS, Szilagyi PG. *Bates' Guide to Physical Examination and History Taking*. Philadelphia, Pa: Lippincott; 2003.

Cecil, RL, Goldman L, Bennett JC. *Cecil Textbook of Medicine*. Philadelphia, Pa: WB Saunders; 2000.

Dale, BR, Harrelson GL, Leaver-Dunn D. Principles of rehabilitation. In: Andrews J, ed. *Physical Rehabilitation of the Injured Athlete*. Philadelphia, Pa: Saunders; 2004:173.

Edmond SL. *Manipulation Mobilization*. St. Louis, Mo: Mosby; 1993.

Ferri, FF. *Clinical Advisor: Instant Diagnosis and Treatment*. St. Louis, Mo: Mosby; 2000.

Hillman SK. *Introduction to Athletic Training*. Champaign, Ill: Human Kinetics; 2000.

Hoppenfeld S. *Physical Examination of the Spine and Extremities*. Norwalk, Conn: Appleton-Century-Crofts; 1976.

Houglum PA. *Therapeutic Exercise for Athletic Injuries*. Champaign, Ill: Human Kinetics; 2001.

Kendall FP, McCreary EK, Provance PG, Rodgers M, Romani, W. *Muscles: Testing and Function*. 5th ed. Baltimore, Md: Lippincott Williams & Wilkins; 2005.

Knight KL. *Cryotherapy in Sport Injury Management*. Champaignm Ill: Human Kinetics; 1995

Konin JG. *Joint Mobilization, Workshop Series Handbook*. Lewes, Del: Coastal Health Consultants; 2001.

Konin JG, Harrelson GL, Leaver-Dunn D. Range of motion and flexibility. In: Andrews J, ed. Physical Rehabilitation of the Injured Athlete. Philadelphia, Pa: Saunders; 2004:136-156.

Konin JG, Wiksten DL, Isear JA, Brader H. *Special Tests for Orthopedic Examination*. Thorofare, NJ: SLACK Incorporated; 2002.

Limmer D, O'Keefe, MF. *Emergency Care*. 10th ed. Upper Saddle River, NJ: Pearson Prentice Hall; 2005.

Magee DJ. Orthopedic *Physical Assessment*. 3rd ed. Philadelphia, Pa: Saunders; 2002.

NATA. *Athletic Training Educational Competencies*. 4th ed. Dallas, Tex: NATA; 2006.

Norkin CC, White DJ. *Measurement of Joint Motion: A Guide to Goniometry*. Philadelphia, Pa: FA Davis; 2003.

O'Connor DP. *Clinical Pathology for Athletic Trainers: Recognizing Systemic Disease*. Thorofare, NJ: SLACK Incorporated; 2001.

Perrin DH. *Athletic Taping and Bracing*. Champaign, Ill: Human Kinetics; 2005.

Physician's Desk Reference. 54th ed. Montvale, NJ: Medical Economics Co; 2000.

Prentice WE. *Arnheim's Principles of Athletic Training*. Boston, Mass: McGraw Hill; 2003.

Prentice WE. *Rehabilitation Techniques in Sports Medicine and Athletic Training*. Boston Mass: McGraw Hill; 2004.

Salvo, SG. *Massage Therapy: Principles and Practice*. Philadelphia, Pa: WB Saunders; 2003

Shultz SJ, Houglum PA, Perrin DH. *Assessment of Athletic Injuries*. Champaign, Ill: Human Kinetics; 2000.

Starkey C. *Therapeutic Modalities*. Philadelphia, Pa: FA Davis; 2004.

Starkey C, Ryan K. *Evaluation of Orthopedic and Athletic Injuries*. Philadelphia, Pa: FA Davis; 2002.

Street SA, Runkle D. *Athletic Protective Equipment: Care, Selection, and Fitting*. Boston, Mass: McGraw Hill; 2000.

Thein-Nissenbaum JM. Principles of rehabilitation. In Andrews J, ed. *Physical Rehabilitation of the Injured Athlete* Philadelphia, PA: Saunders; 2004:298-300.

Tilkian SM, Conover MB, Tilkian AG. *Clinical Implications of Laboratory Tests.* St. Louis, Mo; 1983.

Van Ost L, Manfre K. *Athletic Training: Student Guide to Success.* Thorofare, NJ: SLACK Incorporated; 2000.

Weber MD, Woodall WR. Knee rehabilitation. In: Andrews J, ed. *Physical Rehabilitation of the Injured Athlete.* Philadelphia, PA: Saunders; 2004:377-428.

Wiksten D, Peters C. *The Athletic Trainer's Guide to Strength and Endurance Training.* Thorofare, NJ: SLACK Incorporated; 2000.

Wilk, KE, Harrelson GL, Arrigo, C. Range of motion and flexibility. In: Andrews J, ed. *Shoulder Rehabilitation.* Philadelphia, PA: Saunders; 2004:513-589.

Wright KE, Whitehill WR. *The Comprehensive Manual of Taping and Wrapping Techniques.* Gardner, Kan: Cramer Products; 1996.

WAIT

...*There's More!*

SLACK Incorporated's Book Division offers a wide selection of products in the field of Athletic Training. We are dedicated to providing important works that educate, inform and improve the knowledge of our customers. Don't miss out on our other informative titles that will enhance your collection.

Athletic Training Exam Review: A Student Guide to Success, Third Edition
Lynn Van Ost, RN, PT, ATC, MEd; Karen Manfre, ATR, MA; and Karen Lew, MEd, ATC, LAT
272 pp., Soft Cover, 2006, ISBN 1-55642-764-6, Order# 47646, **$42.95**

Athletic Training Exam Review: A Student Guide to Success has been revised and updated into a new *Third Edition* that guides students throughout the entire testing process, from the day they fill out the application to the day they sit for the actual exam. With new written examination and written on-line simulation questions, this *Third Edition* prepares students better than ever before!

Quick Reference Dictionary for Athletic Training, Second Edition
Julie N. Bernier, EdD, ATC
416 pp., Soft Cover, 2005, ISBN 1-55642-666-6, Order# 46666, **$28.95**

The expanded and updated *Second Edition* of *Quick Reference Dictionary for Athletic Training* is a pocket sized, comprehensive, and user-friendly guide to athletic training. This *Second Edition* contains over 2,100 terms and 20 appendices on revised and new topics such as manual muscle testing and joint mobility positioning.

Special Tests for Orthopedic Examination, Third Edition
Jeff G. Konin, PhD, ATC, PT; Denise L. Wiksten, PhD, ATC; Jerome A. Isear Jr., MS, PT, ATC-L; and Holly Brader, MPH, RN, BSN, ATC
400 pp., Soft Cover, 2006, ISBN 1-55642-741-7, Order# 47417, **$38.95**

Special Tests for Orthopedic Examination has been used for 10 years by thousands of students, clinicians, and rehab professionals and is now available in a revised and updated *Third Edition.* Concise and pocket-sized, this handbook is an invaluable guide filled with the most current and practical clinical exam techniques used during an orthopedic examination. This *Third Edition* takes a user-friendly approach to visualizing and explaining more than 150 commonly used orthopedic special tests, including 11 new and modern tests.

Clinical Skills Documentation Guide for Athletic Training, Second Edition
Herb Amato, DA, ATC; Christy D. Hawkins, MS, ATC; and Steven L. Cole, MEd, ATC, CSCS
464 pp., Soft Cover, 2006, ISBN 1-55642-758-1, Order# 47581, **$34.95**

Clinical Pathology for Athletic Trainers: Recognizing Systemic Disease
Dan O'Connor, PhD, ATC
288 pp., Soft Cover, 2001, ISBN 1-55642-469-8, Order# 44698, **$38.95**

Principles of Pharmacology for Athletic Trainers
Joel Houglum, PhD; Gary Harrelson, EdD, ATC; and Deidre Leaver-Dunn, PhD, ATC
440 pp., Hard Cover, 2005, ISBN 1-55642-594-5, Order# 45945, **$44.95**

Assessment of Nonorthopedic Sports Injuries: A Sideline Reference Manual
Jeff Lewandowski, DPT, SCS, ATC
176 pp., Soft Cover, 2000, ISBN 1-55642-444-2, Order# 44442, **$34.95**

Athletic Training Student Primer: A Foundation for Success
Andrew P. Winterstein, PhD, ATC
256 pp., Soft Cover, 2003, ISBN 1-55642-570-8, Order# 45708, **$37.95**

Gait Analysis: Normal and Pathological Function
Jacquelin Perry, MD
556 pp., Hard Cover, 1992, ISBN 1-55642-192-3, Order# 11923, **$64.95**